A Companion to Specialist Surgical Practice
Third Edition

Series Editors
O. James Garden
Simon Paterson-Brown

Hepatobiliary and Pancreatic Surgery
Third Edition

Edited by
O. James Garden
Regius Professor of Clinical Surgery
Clinical and Surgical Sciences (Surgery)
University of Edinburgh
and
Honorary Consultant Surgeon
Royal Infirmary of Edinburgh

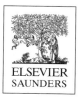

ELSEVIER
SAUNDERS

ELSEVIER
SAUNDERS

An imprint of Elsevier Limited

First edition 1997
Second edition 2001
Third edition 2005
Reprinted 2006, 2007

The right of O.J. Garden to be identified as editor of this work has been asserted by him in accordance with the Copyright, Designs and Patents Act 1988

ISBN 0 7020 2736 7

British Library Cataloguing in Publication Data
A catalogue record for this book is available from the British Library

Library of Congress Cataloging in Publication Data
A catalog record for this book is available from the Library of Congress

Notice
Medical knowledge is constantly changing. Standard safety precautions must be followed, but as new research and clinical experience broaden our knowledge, changes in treatment and drug therapy may become necessary or appropriate. Readers are advised to check the most current product information provided by the manufacturer of each drug to be administered to verify the recommended dose, the method and duration of administration, and contraindications. It is the responsibility of the practitioner, relying on experience and knowledge of the patient, to determine dosages and the best treatment for each individual patient. Neither the Publisher nor the editor assumes any liability for any injury and/or damage to persons or property arising from this publication.
The Publisher

Printed in The Netherlands
Last digit is the print number: 9 8 7 6 5 4 3

Commissioning Editor: Michael Houston
Project Development Manager: Sheila Black
Editorial Assistants: Kathryn Mason, Liz Brown
Project Manager: Cheryl Brant
Design Manager: Jayne Jones
Illustration Manager: Mick Ruddy
Illustrator: Martin Woodward
Marketing Managers: Gaynor Jones (UK), Ethel Cathers (USA)

Hepatobiliary and Pancreatic Surgery
Third Edition

Take a look at the other great titles in the Companion Series...

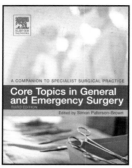

Paterson-Brown
Core Topics in
General and
Emergency Surgery
3rd Edition
0702027332

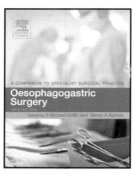

Griffin & Raimes
Oesophagogastric
Surgery
3rd Edition
0702027359

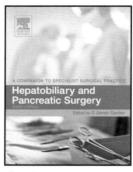

Garden
Hepatobiliary and
Pancreatic Surgery
3rd Edition
0702027367

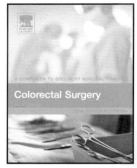

Phillips
Colorectal Surgery
3rd Edition
0702027324

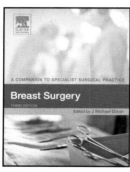

Dixon
Breast Surgery
3rd Edition
0702027383

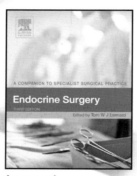

Lennard
Endocrine Surgery
3rd Edition
0702027391

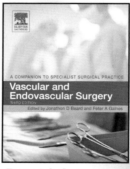

Beard & Gaines
Vascular and
Endovascular
Surgery
3rd Edition
0702027340

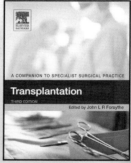

Forsythe
Transplantation
3rd Edition
0702027375

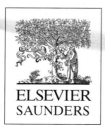

Contents

Colour plate section follows p. 20

Contributors

Jacques Belghiti MD
Professor of Surgery and Head of Department
Department of Hepato-Bilio-Pancreatic Surgery and Transplantation
Hôpital Beaujon
Paris, France

Willem A. Bemelman MD PhD
Gastrointestinal Surgeon
Department of Surgery
Academic Medical Center
Amsterdam, The Netherlands

Irving S. Benjamin BSc MB ChB MD FRCS(Glasg) FRCS
Emeritus Professor of Surgery
King's College London;
Honorary Consultant Surgeon
King's College Hospital
London, UK

Cynthia-Michelle Borg MD MRCS
Research Fellow/ Registrar
Department of Surgery
King's College Hospital
London, UK

Philippus C. Bornman MB ChB MMED(Surg) FRCS(Ed) FCS(SA) FRCS(Glasg)
Professor of Surgery
University of Cape Town and Grooteschuur Hospital
Cape Town, South Africa

John A.C. Buckels CBE MD FRCS
Consultant Hepatobiliary and Liver Transplant Surgeon
Liver Unit
Queen Elizabeth Hospital
Birmingham, UK

Olivier R.C. Busch MD PhD
Gastrointestinal Surgeon
Department of Surgery
Academic Medical Center
Amsterdam, The Netherlands

C. Ross Carter MD FRCS (Gen Surg)
Consultant Pancreaticobiliary Surgeon
Lister Department of Surgery
Glasgow Royal Infirmary
Glasgow, UK

John J. Casey MB ChB PhD FRCS
Consultant Surgeon/Honorary Senior Lecturer
Department of Surgical and Clinical Sciences
Royal Infirmary of Edinburgh
Edinburgh, UK

Kevin C. Conlon MCh MBA FRCSI FACS
Department of Surgery
Adelaide & Meath Hospital
Dublin, Ireland

Olivier Farges MD PhD
Professor of Surgery
Hôpital Beaujon
Université Paris VII
Paris, France

O. James Garden BSc MB ChB MD FRCS(Glasg) FRCS(Ed) FRCP(Ed)
Regius Professor of Clinical Surgery
Clinical and Surgical Sciences (Surgery)
University of Edinburgh;
Honorary Consultant Surgeon
Royal Infirmary of Edinburgh
Edinburgh, UK

Paula Ghaneh MB ChB MD FRCS
Senior Lecturer
Honorary Consultant Surgeon
Department of Surgery and Oncology
University of Liverpool
Liverpool, UK

Dirk J. Gouma MD PhD
Professor of Surgery
Chair of the Department of Surgery
Academic Medical Center
Amsterdam, The Netherlands

Geoffrey H. Haydon MB ChB MD FRCP(Ed)
Consultant Hepatologist
Liver Unit
Queen Elizabeth Hospital
Birmingham, UK

Thomas J. Hugh MD FRACS
Upper Gastrointestinal Surgical Unit
Department of Surgery
Royal North Shore Hospital
St Leonards, NSW, Australia

Clement W. Imrie BSc MB ChB FRCS
Professor and Consultant Surgeon
Lister Department of Surgery
Glasgow Royal Infirmary
Glasgow, UK

Colin J. McKay MD FRCS
Senior Lecturer in Surgery
West of Scotland
Pancreatic Unit
Royal Infirmary
Glasgow, UK

Leslie K. Nathanson MB ChB FRACS
Consultant Surgeon
Royal Brisbane and Women's Hospital
Brisbane, Australia

Simon P. Olliff MRCP FRCR
Consultant Radiologist
Department of Radiology
Queen Elizabeth Hospital
Birmingham, UK

Rowan W. Parks MD FRCSI FRCS(Ed)
Senior Lecturer in Surgery and
Honorary Consultant
Department of Clinical and Surgical
Sciences
Royal Infirmary of Edinburgh
Edinburgh, UK

Graeme J. Poston MB BS MS FRCS
Consultant Hepatobiliary Surgeon
Department of Surgery
University Hospital Aintree
Liverpool, UK

Paul F. Ridgway MD MMedSc(Anat) AFRCSI
Senior (Specialist) Registrar
Department of Surgery
Trinity College Dublin;
Adelaide and Meath Hospital
Dublin, Ireland;
Honorary Clinical Research Fellow
Imperial College
St Mary's Hospital
London, UK

Ian M. Shaw MB BS FRACS
Royal Brisbane Hospital
Herston
Brisbane, Australia

Steven M. Strasberg MD FACS FRCSC
Pruett Professor of Surgery and
Head Hepatobiliary–Pancreatic
Surgery
Washington University in Saint
Louis
St Louis, MO, USA

Benjamin N.J. Thomson MB BS FRACS
Consultant Hepatobiliary Surgeon
Department of Surgical Oncology
Peter MacCallum Cancer Centre;
Department of General Surgery
Royal Melbourne Hospital
Melbourne, VIC, Australia

Otto M. van Delden MD PhD
Interventional Radiologist
Department of Radiology
Academic Medical Center
Amsterdam, The Netherlands

Fenella K.S. Welsh MA MD FRCS
Consultant Surgeon at the
Hepatobiliary Unit
The North Hampshire Hospital
NHS Trust
Basingstoke, UK

Preface

The *Companion to Specialist Surgical Practice* series was designed to meet the needs of surgeons in higher training and the practising consultant who wish up-to-date and evidence-based information on the subspecialist areas relevant to their surgical practice. In trying to meet this aim, we have recognised that the series will never be as all-encompassing as many of the larger reference surgical textbooks. However, by their very size, it is rare that the latter are completely up to date at the time of publication. The first edition of this series was published in 1997, with the second following in 2001. In this third edition, we have been able to bring up to date the relevant specialist information that we and the individual volume editors consider important for the practising subspecialist surgeon. Where possible, all contributors have attempted to identify evidence-based references to support key recommendations within each chapter. These should all be interpreted with the help of the guidance summary 'Evidence-based practice in surgery', which follows this preface.

We are extremely grateful to all volume editors and to their contributors to this third edition. It is thanks to their enthusiasm and hard work that the relatively short time frame between each of the editions has been maintained, thereby providing to the reader the most accurate and up-to-date infor-mation possible. We were all immensely saddened by the sudden and tragic death of Professor John Farndon, who edited the first and second editions of the volumes *Breast Surgery* and *Endocrine Surgery*. While recognising that he was a unique and talented individual, we are pleased to welcome the additional editorial skills of Mike Dixon and Tom Lennard for this third edition.

We are also grateful for the support and encourage-ment of Elsevier Ltd and hope that our aim – of providing up-to-date and affordable surgical texts – has been met and that all readers, whether in training or in consultant practice, will find this third edition a valuable resource.

O. James Garden BSc, MB, ChB, MD, FRCS(Glasg), FRCS(Ed), FRCP(Ed)
Regius Professor of Clinical Surgery, Clinical and Surgical Sciences (Surgery), University of Edinburgh, and Honorary Consultant Surgeon, Royal Infirmary of Edinburgh

Simon Paterson-Brown MB, BS, MPhil, MS, FRCS(Ed), FRCS
Honorary Senior Lecturer, Clinical and Surgical Sciences (Surgery), University of Edinburgh, and Consultant General and Upper Gastrointestinal Surgeon, Royal Infirmary of Edinburgh

EVIDENCE-BASED PRACTICE IN SURGERY

The third edition of the *Companion to Specialist Surgical Practice* series has attempted to incorporate, where appropriate, **evidence-based practice in surgery**, which has been highlighted in the text and relevant references. A detailed chapter on evidence-based practice in surgery written by Kathryn Rigby and Jonathan Michaels has been included in the volume on *Core Topics in General and Emergency Surgery*, to which the reader is referred for further information on assessing levels of evidence. We are grateful to them for providing this summary for each volume.

Critical appraisal for developing evidence-based practice can be obtained from a number of sources, the most reliable being randomised controlled clinical trials, systematic literature reviews, meta-analyses and observational studies. For practical purposes three grades of evidence can be used, analogous to the levels of 'proof' required in a court of law:

1. **Beyond reasonable doubt** – such evidence is likely to have arisen from high-quality randomised controlled trials, systematic reviews, or high-quality synthesised evidence such as decision analysis, cost-effectiveness analysis or large observational data sets. The studies need to be directly applicable to the population of concern and have clear results. The grade is analogous to burden of proof within a crimimal court and may be thought of as corresponding to the usual standard of 'proof' within the medical literature (i.e. $P<0.05$).

2. **On the balance of probabilities** – in many cases a high-quality review of literature may fail to reach firm conclusions owing to conflicting or inconclusive results, trials of poor methodological quality or the lack of evidence in the population to which the guidelines apply. In such cases it may still be possible to make a statement as to the best treatment on the 'balance of probabilities'. This is analogous to the decision in a civil court where all the available evidence will be weighed up and the verdict will depend upon the balance of probabilities.

3. **Not proven** – insufficient evidence upon which to base a decision or contradictory evidence.

Depending on the information available three grades of recommendation can be used:

a. strong recommendation, which should be followed unless there are compelling reasons to act otherwise

b. a recommendaton based on evidence of effectiveness, but where there may be other factors to take into account in decision-making, for example the user of the guidelines may be expected to take into account patient preferences, local facilities, local audit results or available resources

c. a recommendation made where there is no adequate evidence as to the most effective practice, although there may be reasons for making a recommendation in order to minimise cost or reduce the chance of error through a locally agreed protocol.

The text and references that are considered to be associated with reasonable evidence are highlighted in this volume with a 'scalpel code', leaving the reader to reach his or her own conclusion.

Acknowledgements

This new edition has benefited greatly from the dedication of the contributing authors, many of whom have supported this book since 1997. We have introduced new material in this edition and sought to refresh some areas by recruiting authors who have given this edition a stronger international feel. I would like to recognise the support of our departmental secretaries and, in particular, Anne McKeller, who has served me well over a number of years but has just moved on to new challenges. As always, my family has been extremely tolerant and I trust that I will now be able to spend more time with my wife, Amanda, and my children, Stephen and Katie.

OJG

One

Hepatic, biliary and pancreatic anatomy

Steven M. Strasberg

This chapter is an introduction to surgical anatomy of the liver, biliary tract and the pancreas. It is intended to provide an anatomical foundation for performing surgical procedures in these three areas. Therefore, the reader will find description of a particular anatomical structure such as the bile duct in more than one part of the chapter. Surgically unimportant anatomic features are omitted. Anatomical distortions due to pathological processes, which may confuse anatomical orientation during surgery, are included. This chapter is only an introduction – entire books have been written about the component parts of the overall anatomy of these organs. A key point about hepatopancreaticobiliary (HPB) surgical anatomy is that there is a prevailing pattern of anatomy, i.e. a pattern that is most commonly found, but that variations from the prevailing pattern are frequent. Each surgical patient should be approached with the idea that the prevailing pattern of anatomy may not be present.

LIVER

Overview of hepatic anatomy and terminology

HEPATIC ARTERIES, BILE DUCTS AND THE DIVISIONS OF THE LIVER

The terminology used in this chapter is based on the new terminology of hepatic anatomy sanctioned

by the International Hepatobiliary Pancreatic Association.[1] The anatomical divisions of the liver are based on vascular and biliary anatomy rather than surface markings. This is of obvious importance because anatomical surgical resection is a process of isolation of liver volumes serviced by specific vascular and biliary structures. The anatomical ramifications of the hepatic artery and bile ducts are regular and virtually identical. Liver anatomy is best understood by first following these structures through a series of orderly divisions.

The first-order division of the proper hepatic artery and common hepatic duct into the right and left hepatic arteries (**Fig. 1.1**) and bile ducts, respectively, results in division of the liver into two parts, or volumes, referred to as **right** and **left hemilivers** or **livers** (**Fig. 1.2**). The right hepatic artery supplies the right hemiliver and the left hepatic artery supplies the left hemiliver. The right and left bile ducts drain the corresponding hemilivers. If the two arteries were injected with different dyes the dyes would fill the right and left hemilivers, respectively. The plane between these two zones of vascular supply is called a watershed. The border, or watershed, of the first-order division is a plane that intersects the gallbladder fossa and the fossa for the inferior vena cava (IVC) (**Fig. 1.2**). This plane is referred to as the **mid-plane of the liver**. It has previously had many other names, most of which are either linguistically or anatomically incorrect (e.g. Cantlie's line). The right liver usually

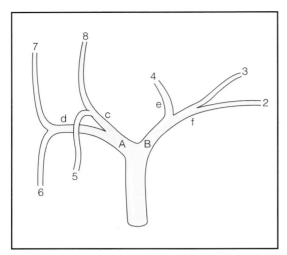

Figure 1.1 • Ramification of the hepatic artery in the liver. The prevailing pattern is shown. The proper hepatic divides into the right (A) and left (B) hepatic arteries, which supply right and left hemilivers (see **Fig. 1.2**) respectively. The right hepatic artery divides into anterior (c) and posterior (d) sectional arteries, which supply the right anterior and right posterior sections (see **Fig. 1.3**). The right anterior sectional artery divides into two segmental arteries, which supply Sg5 and Sg8 (see **Fig. 1.4**), and the right posterior sectional artery divides into arteries that supply Sg6 and Sg7. The left hepatic artery (B) also divides into two sectional arteries, the left medial (e) and left lateral (f). The former supplies the left medial section (see **Fig. 1.3**), also called Sg4, while the latter supplies the left lateral section. The left lateral sectional artery divides into segmental arteries to Sg2 and 3 (see **Fig. 1.4**). The caudate lobe (Sg1 and Sg9) is supplied by branches from A and B. Bile duct anatomy and nomenclature are similar to that of the hepatic artery.

has a larger volume than the left liver (60:40), although this is variable.

The second-order division (**Figs 1.1** and **1.3**) divides the right and left livers into two parts. Each of these parts is referred to as a **section**. On the right side there is a **right anterior section** and a **right posterior section**. These sections are supplied by the right anterior sectional hepatic artery and a right posterior sectional hepatic artery (**Fig. 1.1**). Also these sections are drained by a right anterior sectional hepatic duct and a right posterior sectional hepatic duct. The plane between these sections is the **right intersectional plane**. Unlike the mid-plane and the left intersectional plane, the right inter-sectional plane does not have markings on the

surface of the liver. The left liver is divided into a **left medial section** and a **left lateral section** (**Fig. 1.3**) and, as on the right side, is supplied by a left medial sectional hepatic artery and a left lateral sectional hepatic artery (**Fig. 1.1**) and drained by left medial sectional hepatic duct and a left lateral sectional hepatic duct. The plane between these sections is referred to as the **left intersectional plane** and corresponds to the umbilical fissure and the line of attachment of the falciform ligament to the anterior surface of the liver.

The third-order divisions are referred to as **segments** (Sg) and are numbered from 1 to 8 (or 9) (**Figs 1.1** and **1.4**). Each of the segments has its own segmental artery and bile duct. Sg1 and 9 make up the **caudate lobe**. The caudate lobe is a unique portion of the liver that is separate from the right and left hemilivers. It is a third and distinct part of the liver that lies behind the plane of the porta hepatis and anterior and lateral to the vena cava.[2,3] It is referred appropriately to as a lobe because it is demarcated by visible fissures. It receives vascular supply from both right and left hepatic arteries (and portal veins). Caudate bile ducts drain into both right and left hepatic ducts.

The left lateral section is divided into Sg2 and Sg3. The left medial section and Sg4 are synonymous. The pattern or ramification of vessels within the left medial section does not permit subdivision of this section into two segments each with its own blood supply and biliary drainage. Some do divide the left medial section into Sg4a and Sg4b. This division in not based on blood supply, but is an arbitrary division of the segment into superior (4a) and inferior (4b) halves. The right anterior section is divided into two segments, Sg5 and Sg8. The right posterior section is divided into Sg6 and Sg7. The planes between segments are referred to as **inter-segmental planes**.

PORTAL VEINS

On the right side of the liver the portal vein divisions correspond exactly to those of the hepatic artery and bile duct and they supply the same hepatic volumes. Hence, there is a right portal vein that supplies the entire right hemiliver (**Fig. 1.5**). It divides into two sectional and four segmental veins as do the arteries and bile ducts. On the left side of the liver, however, the left portal vein is unusual

Anatomical term	Couinaud segments referred to	Term for surgical resection	Diagram (pertinent area is shaded)
Right hemiliver or Right liver	Sg5–8 (+/–Sg1)	Right hepatectomy or Right hemihepatectomy (stipulate +/– segment 1)	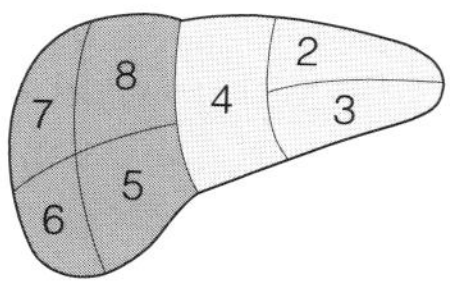
Left hemiliver or Left liver	Sg2–4 (+/–Sg1)	Left hepatectomy or Left hemihepatectomy (stipulate +/– segment 1)	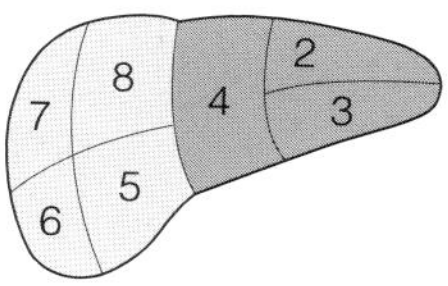

Border or watershed: The border or watershed of the first-order division which separates the two hemilivers is a plane which intersects the gallbladder fossa and the fossa for the IVC and is called the midplane of the liver.

Figure 1.2 • Nomenclature for first-order division anatomy (hemilivers) and resections. With permission from Washington University in Saint Louis School of Medicine.

because its structure was adapted to function in utero as a conduit between the umbilical vein and the ductus venosus. The left portal vein consists of two portions, a **horizontal** or **transverse portion**, which is located under Sg4, and a **vertical part** or **umbilical portion**, which is situated in the umbilical fissure (Fig. 1.5). The vein may be exposed in the umbilical fissure or hidden by a bridge of tissue passing between the left medial and lateral sections. This bridge may simply be a fibrous band, but more commonly is composed of liver tissue. The junction of the transverse and umbilical portions of the left portal vein is marked by the attachment of a stout cord – the ligamentum venosum. This structure, the remnant of the fetal ductus venosus, runs in the groove between the left lateral section and the caudate lobe and attaches to the left hepatic vein/IVC junction.

Ramification of the left portal vein

The transverse portion of the left portal vein sends only a few small branches to Sg4. Large branches from the portal vein to the left liver arise exclusively beyond the attachment of the ligamentum venosum, i.e. from the umbilical part of the vein.[4] These branches come off both sides of the vein – those arising from the right side pass into Sg4 and those

from the left supply Sg2 and Sg3. There is usually only one branch to Sg2 but commonly there is more than one branch to Sg3 and 4. The left portal vein terminates where it joins the ligamentum teres at the free edge of the left liver. Note that the umbilical portion of the portal vein has a unique pattern of ramification. The pattern is similar to an air-conditioning duct that sends branches at right angles from both of its sides to supply rooms (segments), tapering as it does so, finally to end blindly (in the ligamentum teres). Other vascular and biliary structures normally ramify by dividing into two other structures at their termination and not by sending out branches along their length.

HEPATIC VEINS (Fig. 1.6)

There are normally three large hepatic veins. Respectively these run in the mid-plane of the liver (middle hepatic vein), the right intersectional plane (right hepatic vein) and the left intersectional plane (left hepatic vein). The left hepatic vein actually begins in the plane between Sg2 and Sg3 and travels in that plane for most of its length. It becomes a fairly large vein even in that location. About 1 cm from its termination in the IVC it enters the left intersectional plane, where it receives the umbilical vein from Sg4 (Fig. 1.6). It is important not to

4

Figure 1.3 • Nomenclature for second-order division anatomy (sections) and resections including extended resections. With permission from Washington University in Saint Louis School of Medicine.

Anatomical term	Couinaud segments referred to	Term for surgical resection	Diagram (pertinent area is shaded)
Right anterior section	Sg5,8	Add (-ectomy) to any of the anatomical terms as in Right anterior sectionectomy	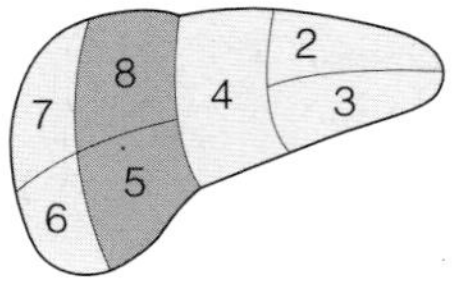
Right posterior section	Sg6,7	Right posterior sectionectomy	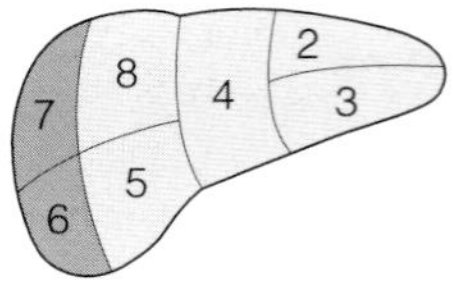
Left medial section	Sg4	Left medial sectionectomy or Resection segment 4 (also see third order) or Segmentectomy 4 (also see third order)	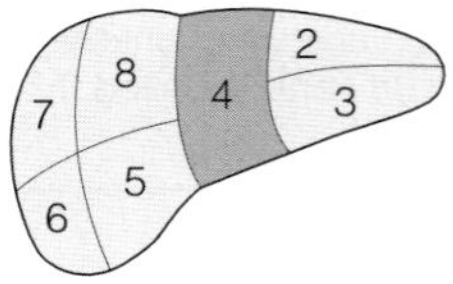
Left lateral section	Sg2,3	Left lateral sectionectomy or Bisegmentectomy 2,3 (also see third order)	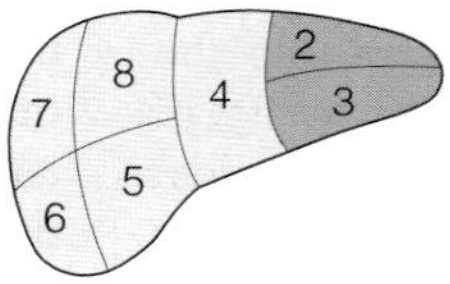

Other sectional liver resections

| | Sg4–8 (+/–Sg1) | Right trisectionectomy (preferred item) or Extended right hepatectomy or Extended right hemihepatectomy (stipulate +/– segment 1) | 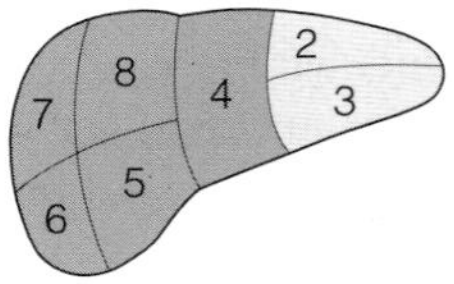 |
| | Sg2,3,4,5,8 (+/–Sg1) | Left trisectionectomy (preferred term) or Extended left hepatectomy or Extended left hemihepatectomy (stipulate +/– segment 1) | 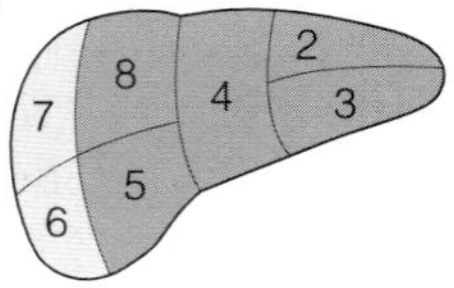 |

Border or watershed: The borders or watersheds of the sections are planes referred to as the right and left intersectional planes. The left intersectional plane passes through the umbilical fissure and the attachment of the falciform ligament. There is no surface marking of the right intersectional plane.

confuse the 'umbilical portion of the left portal vein' with the 'umbilical vein'. The latter is a tributary of the left hepatic vein that normally drains the most leftward part of Sg4.[5,6] The length of the left hepatic vein in the left intersectional plane is short. It lies between the point where it receives the **umbilical vein** from Sg4 and the IVC, a distance of only about 1 cm. The left and middle hepatic veins normally fuse at a distance of about 1 cm from the IVC, so that when viewed from within the IVC there are only two hepatic vein openings. Rarely, hepatic veins join the IVC above the diaphragm.

In about 10% of individuals there is more than one large right hepatic vein. In these persons in addition to the right superior hepatic vein (normally called the right hepatic vein), which enters the IVC just below the level of the diaphragm, there is a right inferior hepatic vein, which enters the IVC 5–6 cm below this level. In the presence of this vein resections of Sg7 and Sg8 may be performed including resection of the right superior vein without compromising the venous drainage of Sg5 and Sg6.

The caudate lobe is drained by its own veins – several short veins that enter the IVC directly from the caudate lobe. The number and size are variable. On occasion they are relatively short and wide and must be isolated and divided with great care.

SURFACE ANATOMY

Numerous terms for surface anatomy exist. They are of minimal surgical importance. Since the term 'lobe' has been used in different ways by various anatomists and surgeons it is best avoided except in reference to the caudate lobe. Fissure and scissure or scissura are similarly confusing terms since they apply only to clefts in casts of the liver. The ligaments of the liver are of surgical importance and are described below.

LIVER CAPSULE AND ATTACHMENTS

The liver is encased in a thin fibrous capsule that covers the entire organ except for a large bare area posteriorly where the organ is in contact with the IVC and with the diaphragm to the right of the IVC. The bare area stretches superiorly to include the termination of the three hepatic veins and ends in a point that is also where the attachment of the falciform ligament ends. The limit of the bare area, where the peritoneum passes between the body wall and the liver, is called the **coronary ligament**. It is one of three structures that connect the liver to the abdominal wall 'dorsally', the other two being the right and left triangular ligaments. The liver also has another bare area, best thought of as a bare crease where the hepatoduodenal ligament and the lesser omentum attach on the 'ventral' surface. It is through this crease that the portal structures enter the liver at the hilum (hilum = 'a crease on a seed'). The other ligamentous structures of interest to surgeons are the ligamentum teres, falciform ligament and the ligamentum venosum. The **ligamentum teres** (teres = 'round') is the obliterated left umbilical vein and runs in the free edge of the falciform ligament from the umbilicus to the termination of the umbilical portion of the left portal vein. The **falciform** (falciform = 'scythe shaped') is the filmy fold that runs between the anterior abdominal wall above the umbilicus and attaches to the anterior surface of the liver between the left medial and left lateral sections.

PORTAL SHEATHS AND 'LIVER PLATES'

As the portal structures approach the liver they become invested in fibrous **sheaths**, which are condensations of the liver capsule in the region of the hilum.[3] These sheaths are carried into the liver surrounding the portal structures, i.e. portal vein hepatic artery and bile duct. The gallbladder rests on a fibrous plate referred to as the cystic plate, which is part of this perihilar system of fibrous tissue. The combined structure consisting of a hepatic artery, bile duct and portal vein surrounded by its fibrous sheath is referred to as a '**portal pedicle**'. There is no **sheathed** main portal pedicle because the main portal vein, proper hepatic artery and common hepatic duct are not close enough to the liver to be enclosed in a sheath. However, when the right hepatic artery, bile duct and portal vein approach the liver they become encased in a tubular fibrous coating, and the combined entity is referred to as the **right portal pedicle** (pedicle = 'little foot'). As the right portal pedicle enters the liver it divides into a right anterior and right posterior portal pedicle supplying the respective sections, and then segmental pedicles supplying the four segments. On the left side the arrangement is somewhat less

Anatomical term	Couinaud segments referred to	Term for surgical resection	Diagram (pertinent area is shaded)
Segments 1–9	Any one of Sg1 to Sg9	Segmentectomy (e.g. seg-mentectomy 6)	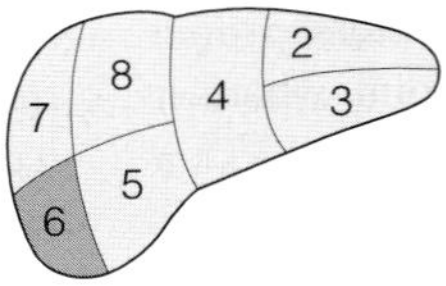
Two contiguous segments	Any two of Sg1 to Sg9 in continuity	Bisegmentectomy (e.g. bi-segmentectomy 5,6)	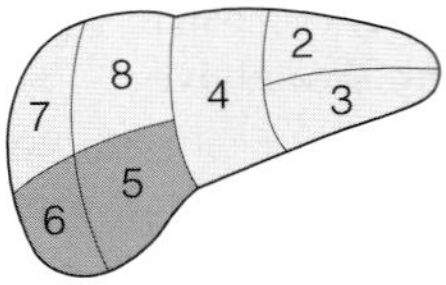

For clarity Sg1 and 9 are not shown. It is also acceptable to refer to any resection by its third-order segments, e.g. right hemihepatectomy can also be called resection Sg5–8.

Border or watershed: The borders or watersheds of the segments are planes referred to as intersegmental planes.

Figure 1.4 • Nomenclature for third-order division anatomy (segments) and resections. With permission from Washington University in Saint Louis School of Medicine.

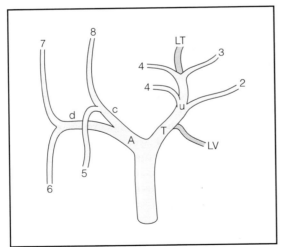

Figure 1.5 • Ramification of the portal vein in the liver. The portal vein divides into right (A) and left (T) branches. The branches in the right liver correspond to those of the hepatic artery and bile duct (see **Fig. 1.1**). The branching pattern on the left is unique. The left portal vein has transverse (T) and umbilical (U) portions. The transition point between the two parts is marked by the attachment of the ligamentum venosum (LV). All major branches come off the umbilical portion (see text). The vein ends blindly in the ligamentum teres (LT).

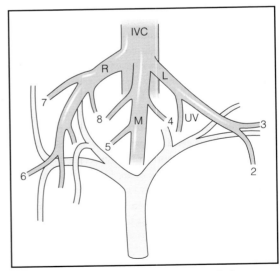

Figure 1.6 • Hepatic veins. There are normally three hepatic veins, right (R), middle (M) and left (L). Note the segments drained. UV is the umbilical vein, which normally drains part of Sg4 into the left hepatic vein. The latter is proof that the terminal portion of the left vein lies in the intersectional plane of the left liver.

complete in that the left bile duct and the transverse portion of the left portal vein become wrapped in a fibrous sheath on the underside of Sg4 but the hepatic arteries do not enter the sheaths on the underside of Sg4 but in the umbilical fissure.

The cystic plate attaches directly onto the anterior surface of the right portal pedicle. This is an anatomical point of importance because if the anterior surface of the right portal pedicle is to be visualised, the attachment of the cystic plate to the anterior surface of the right portal pedicle must be divided as described by Strasberg et al.[7] The cystic plate is the fibrous surface encountered during cholecystectomy, deep to which lies the hepatic parenchyma.

The terminology of hepatic resections is based upon the terminology of hepatic anatomy. Therefore resection of one side of the liver is called a **hepatectomy** or **hemihepatectomy** (**Fig. 1.2**). Resection of the right side of the liver is right hepatectomy or right hemihepatectomy and resection of the left side of the liver is left hepatectomy or left hemihepatectomy. Resection of a liver section is referred to as a **sectionectomy** (**Fig. 1.3**). Resection of the liver to the left side of the umbilical fissure would be referred to as a left lateral sectionectomy. The other sectionectomies are named accordingly, e.g. right anterior sectionectomy. Resection of the whole right liver plus Sg4 is referred to as a right trisectionectomy (**Fig. 1.3**). It can also be called a right hepatectomy extended to Sg4. The former is preferred since it implies that all of Sg4 is resected whereas the latter does not. Similarly, resection of the left hemiliver plus the right anterior section is referred to as a left trisectionectomy.

Resection of one of the numbered segments is referred to as a **segmentectomy** (**Fig. 1.4**). Resection of the caudate lobe can be referred to as a caudate lobectomy or resection of Sg1 (and Sg9). It is always appropriate to refer to a resection by the numbered segments. For instance, it would be appropriate to call a left lateral sectionectomy a resection of Sg 2 and 3.

Surgical anatomy for liver resections

The following is intended as an introduction to those interested in liver resection. Much more detailed descriptions are available in standard texts of hepatic surgery. In performing a right hepatectomy there are two methods of managing the right-sided portal vessels and bile ducts. The first is to isolate the hepatic artery, portal vein and bile duct individually and either control them or ligate them extrahepatically, whereas the second is to isolate the entire portal pedicle and staple the pedicle. Isolation of the right portal pedicle involves making hepatotomies in the liver above the right portal pedicle in Sg4 and in the gallbladder fossa after removing the gallbladder. A finger is passed through the hepatotomy to isolate the right portal pedicle. It is advisable to divide the caudate veins going into the inferior vena cava at least in the lower half of the distance over which the liver is attached to the IVC before performing pedicle isolation, since bleeding from these veins can be considerable if they are ruptured during the manoeuvre of isolation of the right portal pedicle.

HEPATIC ARTERIES AND LIVER RESECTIONS

The usual branching pattern of the hepatic artery is for the common hepatic artery to arise where the coeliac artery terminates by dividing into splenic artery and common hepatic artery. The latter runs for 2–3 cm to divide into gastroduodenal and proper hepatic artery branches. The proper hepatic artery normally runs for 2–3 cm along the left side of the common bile duct to terminate into the right and left hepatic arteries, the right hepatic artery immediately passing behind the common hepatic duct. The four sectional arteries arise from the right and left arteries 1–2 cm from the liver. Although this is the commonest pattern, variations from this pattern are also common. The surgeon is wise not to make assumptions regarding hepatic arteries based on size or position, but rely instead on complete dissection, trial occlusions and radiological support. When an artery that is to be ligated appears unusually large it is especially important to dissect until identification is unquestionable.

The most important arterial variation is 'replaced' arteries. The terminology here is confusing. 'Replaced' means that the artery supplying a particular volume is in an unusual location and also that it is the sole supply to that volume. 'Aberrant' means the replaced structure is in an unusual location. 'Accessory' refers to an artery that is additional; it is a structure that is not normally present and is **not** the sole supply to a volume, i.e. the normal structure is also present. It may be ligated without loss of supply. While the dictionary definition of 'aberrant' does not state whether the structure provides sole supply, it is used most often as being synonymous with replaced, i.e. that it is the sole supply to a volume.

In about 25% of patients part or all of the liver is supplied by a replaced (or aberrant) artery. The **replaced right hepatic artery** is a structure arising from the superior mesenteric artery that runs from left to right behind the lower end of the bile duct to emerge and course on its right posterior border. It may supply a segment, section or the whole right hemiliver. Rarely this artery supplies the entire liver and then it is called a **replaced hepatic artery**. The **replaced left hepatic artery** arises from the left gastric artery and courses in the lesser omentum in conjunction with vagal branches to the liver (hepatic nerve). Like the right artery it may supply a segment, section (usually the left lateral section), hemiliver or, very rarely, the whole liver. Sometimes left hepatic arteries arising from the left gastric artery are actually accessory arteries, which exist in conjunction with normally situated left hepatic arteries. This is less commonly true of right hepatic arteries arising from the superior mesenteric artery (SMA). Knowledge of these particular arterial variations is important not only in hepatobiliary surgery, including transplantation, but in gastric surgery and pancreatic surgery. Transection of the left gastric artery at its origin during gastrectomy has led to devascularisation of the left hemiliver in the presence of a replaced left artery, and the same has occurred on the right side as a result of injury to a replaced right artery. In some cases there is no proper hepatic artery because the entire liver is supplied by right or left replaced arteries or both. That this is so may be suspected when opening the peritoneum at the base of the hepatoduodenal ligament, because in these cases the portal vein is immediately seen. Rarely, the hepatic artery arises directly from the aorta. Replaced arteries occasionally confer an advantage during surgery. For instance, in the case of a replaced left artery supplying the left lateral section, it is possible to resect the entire proper hepatic artery when performing a right

trisectionectomy for hilar cholangiocarcinoma. The replaced right artery is sometimes invaded by pancreatic head tumours and is in danger of injury during pancreato-duodenectomy.

The variations described above are only a few of the possible variations. There is great variation in the distance from the liver at which the various divisions occur. For instance, the right and left hepatic arteries may arise from the proper hepatic artery just a few millimetres from the gastroduodenal artery, or the common hepatic artery may simply trifurcate into gastroduodenal artery, right hepatic and left hepatic artery. On rare occasions the common hepatic artery may divide into a right and left artery and the gastroduodenal artery arise as a branch of one of these structures. Also hepatic arteries, including the proper hepatic artery, may pass behind the bile duct to emerge on its right side before ramifying.

In performing hepatectomies by the standard technique, it is important to isolate the arteries going to the side of the liver to be resected. An anatomical point of importance is that an artery located to the right side of the bile duct always supplies the right side of the liver, but arteries found on the left side of the bile duct may also supply the right side of the liver. Therefore, when using the individual vessel ligation method it is important to be aware of the position of the common hepatic duct. A trial occlusion of an artery with an atraumatic clamp should always be performed in order to establish that there is a good pulse to the side of the liver to be retained.

HEPATIC DUCTS AND LIVER RESECTIONS

In approximately 25% of cases there is no true right hepatic duct. In these cases either the right anterior sectional hepatic duct or right posterior sectional hepatic duct joins the left hepatic duct.[2] It is not of consequence in a right hepatectomy if these ducts are divided separately during the transection of the liver. However, there is danger in left hepatectomy because when coming through the liver just to the left of the mid-plane it is possible to divide the aberrant right duct leaving one-half of the remnant right liver without biliary drainage into the intestine. For this reason, it is highly advisable to divide the biliary system close to the umbilical fissure when doing a left hepatectomy, i.e. not to resect the medial part of the left hepatic duct, which is the portion that receives the aberrant right duct. Also, because of the frequency of this anomaly, it is the author's practice to perform intraoperative cystic duct cholangiography or preoperative magnetic resonance cholangiopancreatography (MRCP), if a previous cholecystectomy has been done, whenever performing a left hepatectomy. For those doing more advanced resections on the right side, it is advisable to be aware of the fact that the right posterior sectional hepatic duct loops over the right anterior sectional portal vein before passing inferiorly to supply the right posterior section. This exposes this duct to injury when the right anterior sectional pedicle is divided. One should always divide this pedicle as least 1 cm away from the bifurcation of the main right portal pedicle into the anterior and posterior portal pedicles. This anatomical danger point was first pointed out by Hjortsjo[8] and is referred to as 'Hjortsjo's crook'.

There are also many variations of the union of ducts from Sg2 to 4. The prevailing pattern is for the Sg2 and Sg3 ducts to unite within the umbilical fissure behind the portal vein to form a left lateral sectional duct, which is then joined by the duct from Sg4 at the right side of the fissure to form the left hepatic duct. However, there are many variations of these unions, including the rare occurrence of an absent left hepatic duct, in which ducts from one or more segments (Sg2–4) join the right duct centrally in the porta hepatis. These variations are important in split liver transplantation and in repair of biliary injuries. The bile duct to Sg3 has been used to perform biliary bypass and can be isolated by following the superior surface of the ligamentum teres down to isolate the portal pedicle to Sg3. The technique is less commonly used now that internal endoscopic bypass has been developed.

PORTAL VEIN AND LIVER RESECTIONS

Although the divisions of the portal vein are unusual for the embryonic reasons described above, it is uncommon to have variations from this unusual pattern. Probably the most common variation is absence of the right portal vein, which is replaced by a pattern in which right posterior and right anterior sectional veins originate independently from the main portal vein. When this occurs the anterior sectional vein is usually quite high in the porta hepatis and may not be obvious. An unsuspecting surgeon may divide the posterior sectional vein thinking that it is the right portal vein and become confused when the anterior sectional vein is encountered during hepatic transection.

A rare but potentially devastating anomaly is the absent extrahepatic left portal vein. In this case the apparent right vein is really the main portal vein, a structure that enters the liver, gives off the right veins and then loops back within the liver substance to supply the left side. The vein looks like a right vein in terms of position but is larger. Transection results in total portal vein disconnection from the liver. This anomaly should always be searched for on computed tomography (CT) scans because right hepatectomy is not usually possible when it is present. The presence of the vertical portion of the left vein in the umbilical fissure on CT scan precludes this problem.

The portal vein branches to Sg4 may be isolated in the umbilical fissure on the right side of the umbilical portion of the left portal vein. The veins here are associated with the bile ducts and the arteries passing to Sg4. Isolation in this location may provide extra margin when resecting a tumour in Sg4 that impinges upon the umbilical fissure. Normally the branches to Sg4 are isolated after dividing the parenchyma of the liver of Sg4 close to the umbilical fissure, an approach used to avoid injury to the umbilical portion of the left portal vein. Injury to this vein would of course deprive Sg2 and Sg3 of portal vein supply, as well as Sg4. For instance, if this occurs when performing a right trisectionectomy, the only portion of the liver to be retained would be devascularised of portal vein flow. However, isolation of these structures does provide extra margin and can be done safely if care is taken to ascertain the position of the portal vein. Likewise, it is possible to isolate the portal vein branches going into Sg2 and Sg3 in the umbilical fissure and to extend a margin when resecting a tumour in the left lateral section. In order to access the portal vein in this location it is usually necessary to divide the bridge of liver tissue, between the left medial and lateral sections. This is done by passing a blunt instrument behind the bridge before dividing it, usually with cautery. Note that arteries and bile ducts passing to the left lateral section are in danger of being injured as one isolates the most posterior-superior portion of the bridge. To facilitate passage of an instrument behind the bridge the peritoneum at the base of the bridge may be opened in a preliminary step. The instrument being passed behind the bridge should never be forced.

HEPATIC VEINS AND LIVER RESECTION

When performing a right hepatectomy, caudate veins are usually divided in the preliminary portion of the dissection. These veins can be thin-walled, wide and short, and in those cases should be managed by suture ligation rather than simple ligation. As dissection moves up the anterior surface of the vena cava to isolate the right hepatic vein, one encounters a bridge of tissue lateral to the IVC that connects the posterior portion of the right liver to the caudate lobe behind the IVC. This bridge of tissue prevents exposure of the right side of the IVC at a point just below the right hepatic vein. The bridge of tissue is referred to as the **inferior vena caval ligament**. Its importance was first described by Makuuchi and in Japan is referred to eponymously.[9] This 'ligament' is a point of potential hazard in mobilisation of the liver, since it may contain a large vein. Therefore dissection under this ligament is done with great care and it is divided using a method that assumes it is vascular. Isolation of the right hepatic vein requires that a passage be created on the anterior surface of the vena cava on the left side of the right hepatic vein, a passage that emerges superiorly in the space between the right and middle hepatic veins. Formation of this passage is facilitated by first dividing fibrous tissue (from a vantage point above the liver) between the right and middle hepatic veins down to the surface of the vena cava.

The left and middle veins can also be isolated prior to division of the liver in performing hepatectomy. There are several ways to achieve this anatomically. One method is to divide all the caudate veins as well as the right hepatic vein. This exposes the entire anterior surface of the retrohepatic vena cava and leaves the liver attached to the vena cava only by the middle and left hepatic veins, which are then easily isolated. This is suitable when performing a right hepatectomy or extended right hepatectomy especially when the caudate lobe is also to be resected. The advantage of having control of these veins during operations on the right liver is that total vascular occlusion is possible without occlusion of the IVC, and haemodynamically the effect is no greater than occlusion of the main portal pedicle (Pringle manoeuvre). However, in performing a left hepatectomy the right hepatic vein is conserved and a different anatomical approach to isolation of the left and middle hepatic veins is required. They may be isolated from the left side by dividing the ligamentum venosum where it attaches to the left hepatic vein, dividing the peritoneum at the superior tip of the caudate lobe, and gently passing an instrument on the anterior surface of the vena cava to come out between the middle and right veins and/or between the left and middle veins. Again, great care is needed when performing this manoeuvre in order to avoid injury to the structures. Isolation of the vena cava above and below the hepatic veins is also a technique that should be in the armamentarium of every surgeon performing major hepatic resection. It is not always necessary but surgeons should be familiar with the anatomical technique of doing so. Isolation of the vena cava superior to the hepatic veins is done by dividing the left triangular ligament and the lesser omentum, being careful to first look for a replaced left hepatic artery. Next, the peritoneum on the superior border of the caudate lobe is divided and a finger is passed behind the vena cava to come out just inferior to the crus of the diaphragm. The crus of the diaphragm makes an easily identified column of the right side. This column passes across the vena cava and dissection of the space inferior to this column and behind the vena cava facilitates passage of the finger from the left side to the right side of the space behind the vena cava. Isolation of the vena cava below the liver is more straightforward but one should be aware of the position of the adrenal vein; in some cases it is necessary to isolate the adrenal vein if bleeding is persisting after occlusion of the vena cava above and below the liver.

Finally, the surgeon should be aware that, during transection of the liver, large veins will be encountered in certain planes of transection. For instance, the middle hepatic vein enters the left side of the vena cava superiorly and in its passage along the mid-plane of the liver it usually receives two large tributaries, one from Sg5 anteriorly and the other from Sg8 posteriorly. Both are encountered routinely in performing right hepatectomy. The venous drainage of the right side of the liver is highly variable and additional large veins, including one from Sg6, may also enter the middle hepatic vein.

Pathological conditions may distort normal hepatic structures. Tumours may invade and occlude or invade and fill vessels. They may cause structures such as bile ducts to dilate to a size many times normal. Tumours may push vessels so that they are stretched and curved over the surface of the tumour. These pathological effects can occur in all organs. However, in the liver there is another important process, called **atrophy**, that affects normal anatomical relationships. Atrophy of a liver volume will be induced by processes that occlude either the portal vein or bile duct. Since the liver will undergo hyperplasia to maintain a constant volume of liver cells, atrophy of one part of the liver is usually accompanied by growth of another. This has anatomical consequence of importance to the surgeon. For instance, if the right portal vein is occluded by a tumour, the right liver will atrophy and the left liver will grow. When seen from below this process will exert a counterclockwise rotational effect on the porta hepatis, rotating the bile duct posteriorly, the hepatic artery to the right, and the portal vein to the left and anteriorly.

GALLBLADDER AND EXTRAHEPATIC BILE DUCTS

Gallbladder

The gallbladder is a cystic structure that lies on the gallbladder plate. The gallbladder forms one side of the hepatocystic triangle. The other two sides are the right side of the common hepatic duct and the liver. The eponyms covering this anatomy (Calot, Moosman, etc.) are particularly confusing and should be abandoned. The hepatocystic triangle contains the cystic artery and cystic node and a portion of the right hepatic artery as well as fat and fibrous tissue. Clearance of this triangle along with isolation of the cystic duct and elevation of the base of the gallbladder off the lower portion of the cystic plate gives the critical view of safety that we have described for identification of the cystic structures during laparoscopic cholecystectomy.[10]

A large number of curiosities of the gallbladder, e.g. phrygian cap, have been described but are not anomalies of much importance to the biliary surgeon.

AGENESIS OF THE GALLBLADDER

The gallbladder may be absent, a condition seen in about 1 out of 8000 patients. This may be difficult to recognise since an ultrasonographer looking in the right upper quadrant may describe a 'shrunken' gallbladder. When agenesis of the gallbladder is suspected it may be confirmed by axial imaging and if any doubt remains, it can be confirmed by laparoscopy. Patients should always be made aware of the possibility that there is agenesis of the gallbladder prior to undertaking a procedure, in these circumstances.

DOUBLE GALLBLADDER

This is also a very rare anomaly but can be the cause of persistent symptoms after resection of one gallbladder. A gallbladder may also be bifid, which usually does not cause symptoms or have an hourglass constriction that may cause symptoms due to obstruction of the upper segment.

Cystic duct

This structure is normally 1–2 cm in length and 2–3 mm in diameter. It joins the common hepatic duct at an acute angle to form the common bile duct. The cystic duct normally joins the common hepatic duct approximately 4 cm above the duodenum. However, the cystic duct may enter at any level down to the ampulla. While it normally enters the right side of the common hepatic duct it may enter posteriorly or on the left side. More importantly, it may run alongside the common hepatic duct for part of its course and be adherent to it in such a way that two structures appear to be a single structure. This is of surgical importance, because when making a choledochotomy at this level the incision should be started slightly to the left side of the mid-plane of the duct in order to avoid entering a septum between the two fused structures. The cystic duct may also join the right hepatic duct in its normal or aberrant location. Because of the close association of the cystic duct with the common bile duct, it is possible to injure the latter if one is persistent in attempting to ligate the cystic duct close to the common bile duct during a cholecystectomy. Although it is important that the cystic duct be free of stones at the end of cholecystectomy, it is not important that it be ligated flush with the bile duct. There is no evidence that ligation of the cystic duct at the union with the gallbladder results in residual symptoms. For that reason, one should attempt to occlude the cystic duct so that there is a clear remnant of cystic duct in order to avoid injury to the common bile duct.

Although a gallbladder with two cystic ducts has been described, this must be an anomaly of extreme rarity. When it is suspected that there are two cystic ducts, it is much more likely that a surgeon is looking at a gallbladder with a short cystic duct and that the two structures thought to be dual cystic ducts are, in fact, the common bile duct and the common hepatic duct.

Other anomalies of the cystic duct are also of surgical importance. As suggested above, the cystic duct can be very short and as a result contribute to the misconception that the cystic duct is being dissected when, in fact, the surgeon is dissecting on the common bile duct. Anatomical distortions caused by pathological conditions are also important here. A large gallstone impacted in the bottom of the gallbladder, severe acute and chronic inflammation, and adhesions between the gallbladder and the common bile duct or common hepatic duct tend to **hide** the cystic and contribute to the possibility of biliary injury.

Cystic artery

The cystic artery, about 1 mm in diameter, normally arises from the right hepatic artery in the hepato-cystic triangle and runs for 1–2 cm to meet the gallbladder superior to the insertion of the cystic duct. It ramifies into an anterior and posterior branch at the point of contact with the gallbladder, and these branches continue to divide on their respective surfaces. The cystic artery may divide into branches before the gallbladder edge is reached. In that case the anterior branch may be mistaken as the cystic artery proper and the

posterior branch will not be discovered until later in the dissection when it may be divided inadvertently. The anterior and posterior branches may arise independently from the right hepatic artery, giving rise to two distinct cystic arteries. The artery may ramify into several branches before arriving at the gallbladder giving the impression that there is no cystic artery.

The cystic artery may arise from a right hepatic artery that runs anterior to the common hepatic duct. The cystic artery can also arise from the right hepatic artery on the left side of the common hepatic duct and run anterior to this duct, while the right hepatic artery runs behind it. Such cystic arteries tend to tether the gallbladder and make dissection of the hepatocystic triangle more difficult. The cystic artery can arise from an aberrant right hepatic artery coming off the SMA. In this case the cystic artery and not the cystic duct tends to be in the free edge of the fold leading from the hepatoduodenal ligament to the gallbladder. This should be suspected whenever the 'cystic duct' looks smaller than the 'cystic artery'.

The cystic veins are multiple and drain into the portal vein by passing into the liver around or through the cystic plate. Sometimes there are cystic veins in the hepatocystic triangle that run parallel to the cystic artery to enter the main portal vein.

The **cystic plate** has been described above. Small bile ducts may penetrate the cystic plate to enter the gallbladder. These ducts of Luschka are sub-millimetre accessory ducts, which when cut may lead to postoperative bilomas. Bilomas and haemorrhage may also be caused by penetration of the cystic plate during dissection. In about 10% of patients there is a large peripheral bile duct immediately deep to the plate, disruption of which will cause copious bile drainage. The origin of the middle hepatic vein is also in this location. There is areolar tissue between the muscularis of the gallbladder and the cystic plate. At the top of the gallbladder the layer is very thin. As one progresses downwards the areolar layer thickens. If dissection from the top of the gallbladder downward is carried on the gallbladder leaving the areolar tissue on the cystic plate, one will arrive onto the posterior surface of the cystic artery and bile duct. If it is carried downward on the cystic plate leaving the areolar tissue on the gallbladder, one will arrive onto the surface of the right portal pedicle. If this is not anticipated, structures in the right portal pedicle may be injured.

Extrahepatic bile ducts

The common hepatic duct (CHD) is a structure formed by the union of left and right ducts. The union normally occurs at the right extremity of the base of Sg4 anterior and superior to the bifurcation of the portal vein. The CHD travels in the right edge of the hepatoduodenal ligament for 2–3 cm where it joins with the cystic duct to form the common bile duct (CBD). The latter has a supra-duodenal course of 3–4 cm and then passes behind the duodenum to run in or occasionally behind the pancreas to enter the second portion of the duo-denum. Details of its lower section and relation to the pancreatic duct are described under 'Pancreas' below. The external diameter of the common bile duct varies from 5 to 13 mm when distended to physiological pressures. However, the duct diameter at surgery, i.e. in fasting patients with low duct pressures, may be as small as 3 mm. Radiologically the internal duct diameter is measured on fasting patients. Under these conditions the upper limit of normal is 8 mm. Size should never be used as a sole criterion for identifying a bile duct. Great caution is advised in situations in which a structure seems larger than the expected norm. Although the cystic duct may be enlarged due to passage of stones, the surgeon should take extra precautions before dividing a 'cystic duct' that is greater than 2 mm in diameter. As noted the common bile duct can be a very small structure and aberrant ducts can be extremely small.

ANOMALIES OF EXTRAHEPATIC BILE DUCTS

As already noted there are biliary anomalies of the right and left ductal systems that can affect the out-come of hepatic surgery. The same is true for biliary surgery. The most important clinical anomalies are low insertions of right hepatic ducts. In approxi-mately 2% of patients one of the right hepatic sectional ducts, usually the posterior, joins the common hepatic duct at a level close to the point where the cystic duct normally enters the common hepatic duct. Sometimes the aberrant duct is a segmental duct and rarely it is the main right hepatic duct itself. Because of its low location, it may be mistaken for the cystic duct and be injured. This is even more likely to occur when the cystic duct enters an aberrant duct as opposed to joining with the common hepatic duct. An extremely rare and even more hazardous anomaly occurs when an aberrant right hepatic duct joins the infundibulum of the gallbladder. This anomaly will in most instances not be recognised and lead to an injury of the duct. Left hepatic ducts can also join the common hepatic duct at a low level. They are less prone to be injured since the dissection during cholecystectomy is on the right side of the biliary tree.

Extrahepatic arteries

The course of these arteries has been described above. Anomalies of the hepatic artery are also important in gallbladder surgery. In 80% of cases the right hepatic artery passes posterior to the bile duct and gives off the cystic artery in the hepato-cystic triangle. However, in 20% of cases the right hepatic artery runs anterior to the bile duct. The right hepatic artery may lie very close to the gall-bladder, and in cases where there is inflammation, scarring can bring the right hepatic artery directly onto the gallbladder, where it forms an inverse U-loop. In this position it is very easily injured. In the classical injury in laparoscopic cholecystectomy, in which the common bile duct is mistaken for the cystic duct, an associated right hepatic artery injury is very common, since that right hepatic artery is considered to be the cystic artery.

Blood supply of bile ducts

Unlike the liver, which has dual supply from the portal vein and hepatic artery, the bile ducts are supplied only by the hepatic artery. An important advance in biliary surgery was the description of the blood supply of the bile duct by Northover and Terblanche in 1979.[11] These authors discovered that blood supply to the bile duct is axial. The bile duct receives blood supply inferiorly from retroduodenal arteries, which are branches of the gastroduodenal arcade. Superiorly, branches pass from the main hepatic artery or right and left hepatic arteries onto the bile duct at the level of the bifurcation of the bile duct. Between the level of the duodenum and the bifurcation there are very few arteries that pass directly into the bile duct. This portion of the bile duct is supplied by two longitudinal arteries, which pass down the bile duct at 3 and 9 o'clock positions. These are readily seen when the bile duct is transected, for instance, during a Whipple procedure. The important clinical significance of this is that there is a watershed of blood supply in the mid-bile duct. If the bile duct is transected at a high level, i.e. close to the bifurcation, one must consider the possibility that the inferior cut edge of the bile duct will be ischaemic. Similarly, when the bile duct is transected at the level of the duodenum, the upper cut edge of the bile duct may be ischaemic. For that reason whenever hepato-jejunostomy is performed the bile duct should be divided close to its upper end to ensure good blood supply. For the same reason, choledocho-choledochotomy is somewhat risky because of the potential for one or other of the cut ends to be ischaemic depending on the level of transection.

The fact that only the hepatic artery supplies the bile ducts has other surgical implications. For instance, occlusion of a hepatic artery can lead to necrosis of bile duct without necrosis of hepatic parenchyma, which will still be supplied by the portal vein. This scenario is seen with some frequency when hepatic artery thrombosis complicates liver transplantation, and it is seen occasionally in association with trauma, including iatrogenic injuries.

PANCREAS

The pancreas is a retroperitoneal organ that is disposed across the upper abdomen so that the tail is higher than the head. This is easily appreciated in CT scans. On average it is 22 cm in length. The **head** of the pancreas is discoid in shape and terminates inferiorly and medially in the hooklike **uncinate process**. The neck, body and tail are shaped like a flattened cylinder but often somewhat triangular in cross-section with a flat anterior and pointed posterior surface, which explains why it can be an unsatisfactory organ for stapling. These divisions of the organ are somewhat arbitrary; the neck of the pancreas is the portion behind which the superior

mesenteric artery and vein run. Normally the consistency of the gland is soft.

Pancreatic ducts

The pancreatic duct is composed of the union of the ducts of the embryonic ventral and dorsal pancreas. The prevailing pattern develops as a result of union of the ventral duct (Wirsung) with the dorsal duct (Santorini) along with partial regression of the dorsal duct in the head. The 'genu' of the duct (genu = 'knee') is the bend in the duct concave inferiorly where the ventral duct joins the dorsal. In the prevailing pattern both ducts communicate with the duodenum, the dorsal duct entering at the minor papilla about 2 cm above and 5 mm anterior to the major papilla. Various other patterns are possible, which involve various degrees of dominance or regression of the portions of the ducts in the head of the pancreas. For instance, the ducts may not unite resulting in separate drainage from the ventral and dorsal pancreas (pancreas divisum), the dorsal duct may lose its connection to the duodenum, or the dorsal duct in the head may lose its connection to the rest of the ductal system and drain only a small section of the head into the duodenum. Alternatively, the ventral duct may regress and the dorsal duct drain more or all of the pancreas through the minor pupilla.

The pancreatic duct (and pancreas) are often referred to as proximal (head) and distal (tail). These are extremely poor and confusing terms – as are the terms proximal and distal on the bile duct. Note that confusingly 'distal' on the bile duct is near the ampulla, which is the location for 'proximal' on the pancreatic duct. Instead, that part of the bile duct should be referred to as pancreatic portion or lower bile duct while that near the bifurcation should be called the upper extrahepatic or hilar bile duct. In the case of the pancreas, the duct should be referred to as the 'pancreatic head duct', 'pancreatic body duct', etc.

The ventral duct usually joins the common bile duct to form a common channel several millimetres from the ampulla of Vater, usually within the wall of the duodenum. The bile duct traverses the duodenal wall obliquely and the pancreatic duct at a right angle. Each duct and the common channel have their own sphincters. The sphincter of the common channel can be palpated from within the duodenum. The common channel may be longer or absent, with both ducts entering the duodenum separately, the pancreatic duct more inferiorly. In performing a sphincteroplasty it is advisable to open the common channel superiorly (10–12 o'clock position in the mobilised duodenum) to avoid the orifice of the pancreatic duct (4 o'clock). The ampulla is normally at the midpoint of the second part of the duodenum. It is rarely higher but can be as low as the midpoint of the third part of the duodenum.

Blood supply of the pancreas

The arterial supply of the pancreas consists of two systems of arteries, one supplying the head and uncinate and the other the body and tail. The neck is a watershed between these two areas of supply.[12] The head and uncinate process are supplied by the pancreatico-duodenal arcade, which consists of two to several loops of vessels that arise from the superior pancreatico-duodenal (branch of gastro-duodenal) and inferior pancreatico-duodenal (branch of the SMA), and which run on the anterior and posterior surface of the pancreas along the edge of the duodenum, the anterior arcade being somewhat closer to the duodenum. The second system arises from the splenic artery, which gives three arteries into the dorsal surface of the gland (**Fig. 1.7**). The dorsal pancreatic artery is the most medial of the three and the most important. It anastomoses with the pancreatico-duodenal arcade in the neck of the pancreas. It is the most aberrant

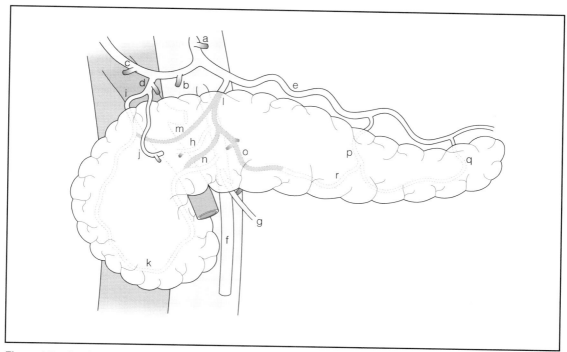

Figure 1.7 • Arterial blood supply to the pancreas. The dorsal pancreatic artery is shown shaded. Alternative origins of the artery are shown as black stumps. Key: a, coeliac artery; b, common hepatic artery; c, right hepatic artery; d, gastroduodenal artery; e, splenic artery; f, superior mesenteric artery; g, middle colic artery; h, right hepatic artery (aberrant); i, superior pancreatico-duodenal artery; j, right gastroepiploic artery; k, inferior pancreatico-duodenal artery; l, dorsal pancreatic artery (DPA); m, right anastomotic branch of DPA to superior part of pancreatico-duodenal arcade; n, right anastomotic branch of DPA to inferior part of pancreatico-duodenal arcade; o, left anastomotic branch of DPA becomes transverse pancreatic artery; p, pancreatica magna artery; q, caudal pancreatic artery; r, transverse pancreatic artery. From Strasberg SM, McNevin MS. Results of a technique of a pancreaticojejunostomy that optimizes blood supply to the pancreas. J Am Coll Surg 1998; 187:591–6, with permission from American College of Surgeons.

artery in the upper abdomen and may arise from vessels that are routinely occluded during pancreatico-duodenectomy, and this may account in part for fistula formation after this procedure.

Venous drainage generally follows arterial supply. The veins of the body and tail of the pancreas drain into the splenic vein where it lies embedded in the gland. These veins are short and fragile. The head and uncinate process veins drain into the SMV and portal vein on the right lateral side of these structures. Uncinate veins often drain into a large first jejunal tributary vein, which then empties into the superior mesenteric vein (SMV). A nearly constant posterior superior pancreatico-duodenal vein enters the right lateral side of the portal vein at the level of the duodenum.

Lymphatics of the pancreas

For surgical purposes the lymphatic drainage of the pancreas is best considered in relation to the two main surgical procedures, resection of the pancreatic head and resection of the pancreatic body and tail. The aim of lymphatic resection during these pro-

cedures is to resect the primary lymph nodes, i.e. those nodes that receive lymph directly from pancreatic tissue (N1 nodes) as opposed to nodes that receive drainage from N1 nodes (N2 nodes). There is a ring of nodes around the pancreas that drain the adjacent gland. These in turn drain into nodes along the SMA, coeliac artery and aorta (axial nodes). The nodes of the ring are N1 for the adjacent pancreas, but the situation is complicated in that the axial nodes are also N1 for adjacent central portions of the pancreatic head, body and uncinate process. The lymphatics of the body and tail are shown in **Fig. 1.8**. The lymphatics of the head and uncinate process drain into a nodal ring for this part of the gland, consisting of lymph nodes in the pancreatico-duodenal groove anteriorly and posteriorly, into subpyloric nodes inferiorly, into nodes adjacent to the common bile duct and hepatic artery superiorly, and into nodes along the SMA medially. These are N1, but as noted above so are some of the axial nodes. The standard node dissection for a Whipple procedure removes all of these nodal groups. This removes the N1 nodes unless there is direct lymphatic drainage to the left side of the SMA or to nodes around the coeliac

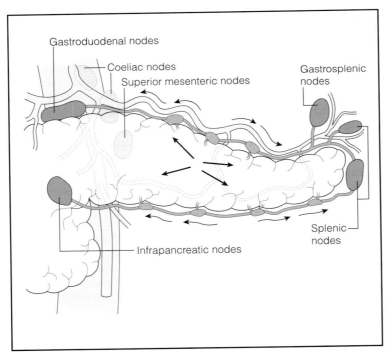

Figure 1.8 • Lymphatic drainage of the body and tail of the pancreas. The intraparenchymal lymphatics from the four quadrants empty into lymphatic vessels on the superior and inferior borders of the pancreas (arrows). Small nodes are found along these vessels. The lymph flows to the nodes of the 'ring'. These are N1 nodes although some of the lymph may have passed through the smaller nodes as described. The nodes of the ring empty into nodes along the superior mesenteric artery (SMA), coeliac artery and aorta. The latter are therefore N2 nodes, but they are also N1 nodes for the more central part of the pancreas. From Strasberg SM, Drebin JA, Linehan D. Radical antegrade modular pancreatosplendectomy. Surgery 2003; 133:521–7, with permission.

Gastroduodenal nodes

Coeliac nodes
Superior mesenteric nodes

Gastrosplenic nodes

Splenic nodes

Infrapancreatic nodes

artery, which does occur in a small proportion of patients.

Anatomical relations and ligaments of the pancreas

The pancreas is a deep-seated organ that, unlike the liver and most of the biliary tree, is not obvious when opening the abdomen. The anatomical relations of the pancreas are very important in pancreatic surgery, e.g. compared to the anatomical relations of the liver in liver surgery. The structures emphasised in the following section are those that are commonly invaded by tumours.

Posteriorly the pancreas is related, from right to left, to the right kidney and perinephric fat, to the IVC and right gonadal vein, aorta, the left renal vein (slightly inferior), **retropancreatic fat**, the **left adrenal gland** and the superior pole of the left kidney. The **SMV** and **portal vein** are posterior relations of the neck of the pancreas, and the **splenic vein** is related to the body and tail. The **SMA** is a posterior relation of the junction of the neck of the gland. The SMA and SMV are both related to the uncinate process and give branches into (SMA) and receive **tributaries from** (SMV) the uncinate process. These short arteries and veins are of importance surgically as they are divided when the head of the pancreas is resected; the veins tend to be thin and fragile. The **coeliac artery** arises vertically superior to the SMA close to the superior edge of the pancreas, where it gives off the common hepatic artery and the **splenic artery**. The former runs anteriorly and to the left in approximation to the superior border of the pancreas. At the point where the hepatic artery passes in front of the portal vein it divides into the **gastroduodenal artery**, which passes anterior to the neck of the pancreas, sometimes buried within it. It terminates in the right gastroepiploic artery, which arises in a fold of tissue toward the pylorus, a fold that also contains the right gastroepiploic vein and subpyloric nodes. The splenic artery snakes along the superior border of the pancreas to leave it 2–3 cm from the termination of the pancreas. The head of the pancreas is wrapped in the first three parts of the duodenum, and the tail ends in relation to the splenic hilum. There is variability in the proximity

of the tail of the pancreas to the spleen. In some cases the pancreas terminates 2 cm from the splenic substance and in others it abuts it. The anterior surface of the body and tail of the pancreas is covered by peritoneum, which is the posterior wall of the lesser sac, and then by the posterior wall of the stomach anterior to this. The transverse mesocolon is related to the inferior border of the pancreas, and the right and left extremities of the transverse colon are related to the head and tail of the gland. The inferior mesenteric vein is related to the inferior border of the neck of the pancreas and may pass behind it to enter the splenic vein or turn medially to enter the SMV.

The pancreas is normally accessed surgically by entering the lesser sac either by division of the greater omentum below the gastroepiploic arcade or by releasing the greater omentum from its attachment to the transverse colon. When the lesser sac is entered the anterior surface of the neck body and tail are often visible but may be obscured by congenital filmy adhesions to the posterior wall of the stomach. To expose the head of the pancreas it is necessary to mobilise the right side of the transverse colon and hepatic flexure inferiorly and to divide the right gastroepiploic vein. The latter crosses the inferior border of the pancreas to join with the middle colic vein to form the gastrocolic trunk, which then enters the SMV. For complete exposure, e.g. for a Frey procedure, the right gastroepiploic artery is also divided, and it and the subpyloric nodes are swept upwards off the pancreas. To access the SMV at the inferior border of the pancreas the peritoneum at the inferior border of the neck is divided and the dissection is carried inferiorly and laterally to open a groove between the uncinate process and the mesentery. Division of the right gastroepiploic vein at the inferior border of the pancreas greatly facilitates this manoeuvre. There are normally no veins entering the SMC or portal vein from the posterior surface of the neck of the pancreas. For this reason it is usually possible to free the neck of the pancreas from these veins in an avascular plane. The peritoneum at the inferior border of the neck, body and tail of the pancreas is avascular and may be divided to roll up the pancreas to access the posterior surface. However, the middle colic artery and inferior mesenteric vein lie in a slightly posterior plane and can be injured if the dissection is carried too deep. The splenic vein is embedded in the back of the pancreas from the point that it reaches the gland on the left to about 1 cm from its termination.

SUMMARY OF LIVER ANATOMY AND TERMINOLOGY

As noted above the term 'lobe' should be reserved for structures that are demarcated by clefts visible in the intact organ. It is a suitable descriptor for the caudate lobe. It can also be used to describe the two parts of the liver demarcated by the umbilical fissure and attachment of the falciform ligament, i.e. the 'right lobe' and the 'left lobe'. However, this usage should be discouraged because it divides the liver on a basis other than internal anatomy – i.e. it divides it according to surface appearance rather than vascular supply. It is also confused with the 'true lobes' of Cantlie – the hemilivers. Therefore, with regard to the liver, the term 'lobe' should be reserved for the caudate lobe. Similarly 'lobectomy' should be reserved for 'caudate lobectomy'. Some authors still use right lobectomy and left lobectomy in the sense of right trisectionectomy (Sg4–8) and left lateral sectionectomy (Sg2,3). The disadvantage of a surgical term dependent on surface anatomy rather than vascular supply, which is the basis of resection, is obvious.

'Sector' is a term used to describe a second-order division based on the portal vein rather than the hepatic artery and bile duct. Sectors and sections are anatomically identical in the right liver, where the three elements of the portal triad ramify similarly. But on the left side the left medial sector is composed of Sg3,4 and the left lateral sector of Sg2 alone. This division is based upon two contentions. The first is that the transverse portion of the portal vein terminally ramifies into the branch to Sg2 and the umbilical portion of the portal vein. One might draw this conclusion from corrosion casts in which the ligamentum venosum has been digested away. However, in the intact liver, in which the ligamentum venosum is available to demarcate the transition from transverse to umbilical portions of the vein, it becomes clear that there is a smooth transition from transverse to umbilical portions

without branching at this point. The branch to Sg2 does not originate for about 1 cm beyond this point and is therefore a branch of the umbilical portion, as are the branches to Sg3 and Sg4. The other contention is that the left hepatic vein does not run in the plane that separates Sg4 from Sg2 and Sg3, i.e. the plane of the umbilical fissure and the attachment of the falciform ligament. Although the left hepatic vein runs in the Sg2/Sg3 intersegmental plane for most of its course, its terminal portion, which begins where it receives the umbilical vein, must be in the plane between Sg4 and Sg2/Sg3. Therefore, the anatomical basis for 'sectorifying' the left liver is suspect. Also as a practical matter for the surgeon, sections relate much more meaningfully to common resections performed through the umbilical fissure.

REFERENCES

1. Terminology Committee of the IHPBA. The Brisbane 2000 Terminology of Liver Anatomy and Resections. HPB 2000; 2:333–9.
2. Healey JE, Schroy PC. Anatomy of the biliary ducts within the human liver; analysis of the prevailing pattern of branchings and the major variations of the biliary ducts. Arch Surg 1953; 66:599–616.
3. Couinaud C. Le Foie. Etudes Anatomiques et Chirugicales. Paris, Masson & Cie, 1957.
4. Botero AC, Strasberg SM. Division of the left hemiliver in man – segments, sectors, or sections. Liver Transplant Surg 1998; 4:226–31.
5. Masselot R, Leborgne J. Anatomical study of hepatic veins. Anat Clin 1978; 1:109–25.
6. Kawasaki S, Makuuchi M, Miyagawa S et al. Extended lateral segmentectomy using intraoperative ultrasound to obtain a partial liver graft. Am J Surg 1996; 171:286–8.
7. Strasberg SM, Picus DD, Drebin JA. Results of a new strategy for reconstruction of biliary injuries having an isolated right-sided component. J Gastrointest Surg 2001; 5:266–74.
8. Hjortsjo C-H. The topography of the intrahepatic duct systems. Acta Anat 1951; 11:599–615.
9. Makuuchi M, Yamamoto J, Takayama T et al. Extrahepatic division of the right hepatic vein in hepatectomy. Hepatogastroenterology 1991; 38:176–9.
10. Strasberg SM, Hertl M, Soper NJ. An analysis of the problem of biliary injury during laparoscopic cholecystectomy. J Am Coll Surg 1995; 180:101–25.

11. Northover JM, Terblanche J. A new look at the arterial supply of the bile duct in man and its surgical implications. Br J Surg 1979; 66:379–84.

12. Michels NA. Blood Supply and Anatomy of the Upper Abdominal Organs. Philadelphia and Montreal: JB Lippincott, 1955.

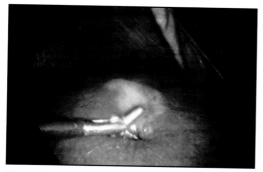

Plate 1 • Visual guided biopsy during laparoscopy.

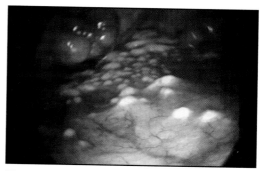

Plate 2 • Peritoneal metastases from pancreatic cancer.

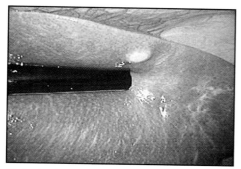

Plate 3 • Small liver metastases from pancreatic cancer during laparotomy.

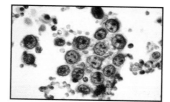

Plate 4 • Peritoneal washing with malignant cells from pancreatic cancer.

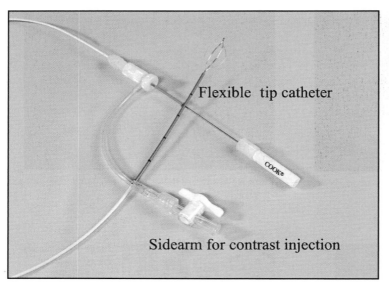

Flexible tip catheter

Sidearm for contrast injection

Plate 5 • Composite cholangiogram catheter and stone extraction basket used for laparoscopic transcystic exploration of the common bile duct. Reproduced with permission of Cook Australia.

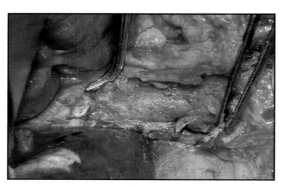

Plate 6 • Operative picture of an early repair of an E4 injury. A right-angle forceps is placed in the opening of the left hepatic duct whilst the open right hepatic duct is visible below. The portal vein is skeletonised with ligation and excision of both the extrahepatic biliary tree and right hepatic artery (held by forceps).

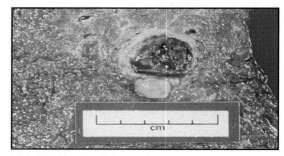

Plate 7 • Hepatocellular carcinoma as a consequence of biliary injury. This patient required a liver transplant for secondary biliary cirrhosis. At pathological examination a hepatocellular carcinoma was detected in the explanted liver.

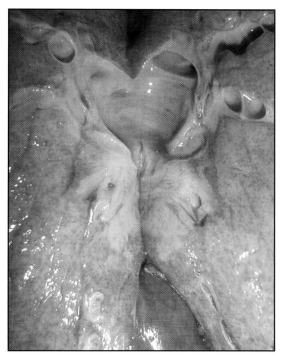

Plate 8 • Macroscopic appearance of hilar cholangiocarcinoma. The resected specimen is opened and shows stenosis of the hepatic duct at the hilus, and local invasion of the adjacent hepatic parenchyma.

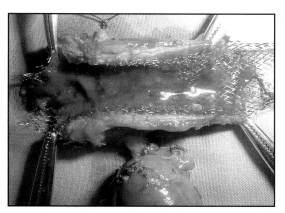

Plate 9 • Local excision of a short localised cholangiocarcinoma of the common hepatic duct. A metallic stent had been previously placed, and was excised in situ within the duct. The mesh has already become firmly embedded in the duct lining. The gallbladder is attached at the bottom of the picture.

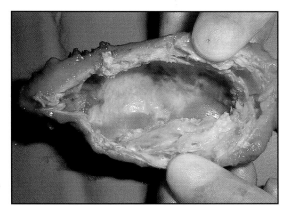

Plate 10 • CT scan showing heavy intramural calcification in a 'porcelain' gallbladder.

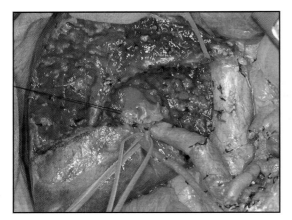

Plate 11 • Operative appearance after extended left hepatectomy (Sg1–5 + 8) for a hilar cholangiocarcinoma. On the right the vena cava is exposed. A blue sling is placed around the right hepatic vein. Red slings mark the residual right hepatic artery, and above this the opened ducts of Sg 6 and 7 are seen. The portal vein was involved by the tumour at the bifurcation, and has been resected and reconstructed end to end: the anastomosis is clearly shown. Resection margins were all clear.

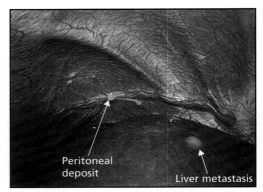

Plate 12 • Staging laparoscopy demonstrating small-volume hepatic and peritoneal deposits not seen on pancreas protocol CT.

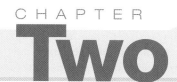

Two

Laparoscopy in staging and assessment of hepatobiliary diseases

Olivier R.C. Busch, Willem A. Bemelman,
Otto M. van Delden and Dirk J. Gouma

INTRODUCTION

Diagnostic laparoscopy for hepato-pancreato-biliary (HPB) tumours was introduced (or reintroduced) as an additional staging procedure in the late 1980s by Cuschieri and Warshaw.[1,2] During that time there was a need for more appropriate tumour staging to differentiate patients who can benefit from a resection from those who require palliative treatment. Accurate staging is only of importance in patients who can be treated non-surgically for palliation of advanced disease. If surgical palliation is preferred exploratory laparotomy is indicated regardless of tumour resectability, and palliation can be performed during the same operation.

In the early days of laparoscopic staging for HPB tumours, preoperative staging consisted of ultrasonography and conventional CT scanning. At that time, metastases were found in about 10–40% of the patients during exploratory laparotomy. Diagnostic laparoscopy enabled the detection of small metastases on the liver surface and peritoneum, which could easily be missed with standard radiological techniques. Additional laparoscopic ultrasonography was helpful to detect small intrahepatic metastases and local ingrowth in vascular structures surrounding the tumour.

Several studies on diagnostic laparoscopy and laparoscopic ultrasonography have shown beneficial results in HPB tumours but the benefit is highly influenced by various factors. Furthermore, the benefit depends on the determination of endpoints for success of the procedure. For example, success can be defined as additional findings such as liver cysts or a change in treatment strategy (bypass instead of resection) or the avoidance of unnecessary laparotomies (detection of metastases followed by non-surgical palliation). The success of laparoscopy also depends on the localisation of the tumour, since tumours with a high suspicion of metastases or advanced local tumour ingrowth tend to have a higher yield of diagnostic laparoscopy. The quality of the prelaparoscopy non-invasive imaging modalities, and the timing of the laparoscopy in the staging process are also important factors influencing the yield of diagnostic laparoscopy. Other factors are the skills of the surgeon and the effort taken in finding metastases, suspected lymph nodes and determination of local resectability. Lastly, success of diagnostic laparoscopy depends on the indication for which it is performed – either for the selection of patients to undergo a curative resection or for selection of the type of palliative treatment (radiotherapy for locally advanced disease or systemic chemotherapy for metastatic disease). These factors may be used to identify patients to increase the yield of diagnostic laparoscopy when it is used in a selective way.

During the past decade diagnostic laparoscopy and laparoscopic ultrasonography in patients with HPB malignancies have been evaluated in our institution. These studies focused on different aspects of diagnostic laparoscopy as a procedure to prevent unnecessary laparotomies, because we believe that this has to be the most important measurement of success of this procedure. A change in success rate was found over the years for several HPB tumours due to factors such as improvements in radiological staging techniques, especially the introduction of (multislice) spiral computed tomography (CT) scanning. In this chapter the findings of these studies and subsequent changes in the yield of laparoscopic staging of HPB patients in our department as well as results from the literature will be reviewed. Some issues will be discussed for HPB tumours in general, whereas other key management points will be dealt with for each specific tumour location (pancreatic, proximal bile duct and liver).

SPECIAL TECHNICAL DETAILS

Diagnostic laparoscopy and subsequent therapeutic laparotomy are performed in a separate session for logistical reasons at our institution. Others have performed laparoscopic staging directly before the laparotomy. In doing so, the time needed for operation is difficult to schedule, but the patient can be spared a second procedure under general anaesthesia. Usually, the procedure is performed under general anaesthesia with the patient in a supine position and the surgeon standing on the left side of the patient (**Fig. 2.1**). A CO_2 pneumoperitoneum is established using a pressure of 12–15 mmHg, either by Veress needle or by an open technique. A sub-umbilical trocar is introduced for a zero degree camera and two other 10–11 mm trocars are placed in the left and right subcostal region (**Fig. 2.2**). Firstly, inspection of the abdominal cavity is performed and the peritoneum is explored to identify peritoneal tumour spread. The visceral peritoneum, the left lobe of the liver, the anterior aspect of the stomach, lesser and greater omentum, and the spleen are inspected. The right side of the abdominal cavity is investigated by passing the camera beneath the falciform ligament. The Treitz ligament, mesenteric root and pancreatic head are exposed by moving the omentum and the transverse colon in front of the stomach. The mesocolon and duodenal curve can be evaluated for possible ingrowth of

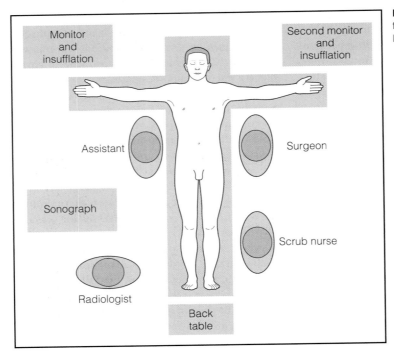

Figure 2.1 • Position in the operating theatre during laparoscopy and laparoscopic ultrasonography (LUS).

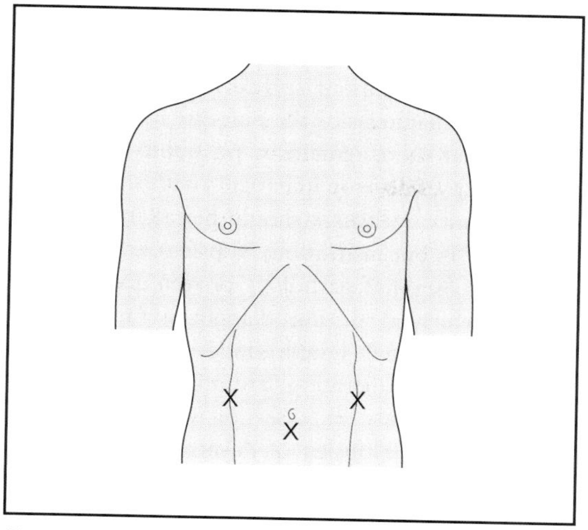

Figure 2.2 • Trocar placement for diagnostic laparoscopy and laparoscopic ultrasonography.

pancreatic tumour at this point. Better organ exposure during laparoscopy is obtained by placing the patient in reverse Trendelenburg position and tilting the table laterally from side to side. Because all trocars have sufficient diameter for introduction of the camera, inspection can be performed from different angles. This can be very helpful in evaluating liver tumours. The lesser sac can be opened to have a direct view on the pancreas and spleen, which can be important for the assessment of local ingrowth and suspicious lymph nodes at the coeliac axis in cases of pancreatic body and tail tumours.

Peritoneal lavage is performed subsequently for the inspection of the abdomen and prior to dissection or biopsy in order to prevent contamination of the lavage sample. Between 500 and 1500 mL of isotonic saline is instilled into the subhepatic space and dispersed by abdominal agitation. The fluid is drained through the left subcostal trocar and collected for cytological evaluation.

When histology-proven distant metastases or tumour ingrowth in the hepatoduodenal ligament or mesocolon are not found, laparoscopic ultrasonography is performed using either 10 mm-diameter rigid or flexible ultrasound probes. To ascertain an acoustic window, isotonic saline is instilled into the peritoneal cavity and the abdominal pressure can be decreased to 7–8 mmHg to improve contact with the liver surface.[3] We use a rigid 7.5 MHz linear array laparoscopic ultrasound (LUS) probe (UST-5522-7.5; Aloka Co., Tokyo, Japan) wrapped in a sterile polyethylene cover sheet, filled with sterile ultrasonic gel, to examine the liver, hepatoduodenal ligament, coeliac axis, gallbladder and pancreas as well as lymph nodes. The patient is scanned from multiple ports to evaluate the tumour from different angles. Biopsies of suspicious lesions are taken at the end of the procedure under direct laparoscopic vision or by laparoscopic ultrasound guidance using biopsy forceps (Fig. 2.3) (also in colour, see Plate 1, facing p. 20) or Tru-cut® (Travenol; Baxter Healthcare Corporation, Deerfield, IL, USA) and Rotex® (Ursus Konsult AB, Stockholm, Sweden) biopsy needles. In case of suspected liver cirrhosis, a visually guided biopsy of the liver, which may remain in situ following intended hepatic resection, is taken for histological investigation and grading of the cirrhosis. The abdominal cavity is decompressed and the wounds are closed in a standard fashion.[4]

SAFETY AND COMPLICATIONS

In general, diagnostic laparoscopy is a safe procedure with almost no mortality and low morbidity. Complications have been reported in 0.15–3% of cases, with a mortality of 0.05%.[5] In our prospective series of 420 patients, three patients (1%) had major complications, including anaphylactic shock, bile leakage after liver biopsy, and a small bowel perforation. Twelve patients (3%) had minor complications: four wound infections; two wound haematomas; three patients with undefined upper

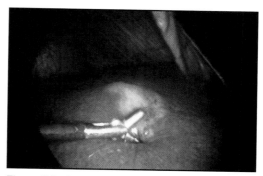

Figure 2.3 • Visual guided biopsy during laparoscopy. See also Plate 1, facing p. 20.

abdominal pain; one aspiration pneumonia; one urinary retention; and one incisional hernia. Although not observed in this series, it is known that biopsies from lesions in an inadequately drained liver segment may cause biliary leakage. Patients were discharged at a mean of 1.5 postoperative days. There was no mortality in this series.[6]

The most dangerous part of the procedure is probably the introduction of the first trocar or Veress needle because of the risk of vascular and bowel lesions. In a review of 2324 gynaecology patients, the overall complication rate was 0.22%, with more complications from the introduction of the Veress needle or trocar insertion than from the actual operative procedure itself.[7] The incidence of serious vascular lesions is extremely low (0.001–0.005%) but patients with such a complication have a mortality rate of up to 17%.

The incidence of vascular and bowel lesions increases when the patient has a history of a previous laparotomy, as is often the case in patients with secondary malignancies of the liver due to colorectal cancer. For these patients it is recommended to introduce the first trocar using an open procedure, such as with the Hasson® or TrocDoc trocar.[8] In a randomised controlled trial we showed that these open techniques are no more time consuming.[9] Therefore we now perform all laparoscopic procedures using an open technique to establish pneumoperitoneum. Although there remains a risk of delayed bowel injury due to diathermy injury, we believe that this procedure reduces the risk of perforating intra-abdominal organs or at least directly recognises such an injury when it occurs. In a series of more than 4500 patients, four of the ten bowel injuries were not recognised initially.[10]

Port-site metastases have been described rarely as a complication of diagnostic laparoscopy for intra-abdominal malignancies. In our series of 420 patients this was found in eight patients (2%) after a median period of 5 months after laparoscopy. All patients had advanced disease at the time the port-site metastases were discovered. These data are comparable to the study by Shoup et al., who reported 13 (0.8%) port-site metastases in 1650 patients undergoing diagnostic laparoscopy for upper gastrointestinal tract malignancies.[11] In their series the incidence was about the same for patients

who underwent a laparotomy. However, all patients in both series were in end stages of their disease, with peritoneal tumour spread in the abdomen at the time of diagnosis of the port-site metastases.

Given that there remains a possibility that port-site metastases develop in patients with small resectable tumours, measures should be taken to reduce this risk.[12] In our institution, biopsies of the primary tumour to establish pathology-proven diagnosis are never performed during diagnostic laparoscopy. Similarly, regional lymph nodes, which will be resected during operation, are not biopsied during laparoscopy. Only in cases of suspected distant metastases are biopsies of suspected lesions performed to prove unresectability. In such patients, the potential risk of port-site metastases is acceptable and does not influence the prognosis. Moreover, it is known from studies on laparoscopic colonic resections for malignancy that the expected danger of port-site metastases after this procedure is probably overestimated, since laparoscopic techniques and preventive methods have much improved.[13,14]

PANCREATIC AND PERIAMPULLARY CANCER

Unfortunately, pancreatic cancer still has a poor overall prognosis. The majority of patients with pancreatic cancer continue to present with advanced disease. Surgical resection is the only treatment modality with a chance of definitive cure. Surgical exploration can only be offered to about 10–20% of the patients, due to distant metastases and locally advanced disease at time of presentation. The development of endoscopic stenting to palliate jaundice in patients with periampullary cancer has made it unnecessary to explore all these patients and perform surgical bypass if the tumour is unresectable. Because pancreatic cancer tends to produce small liver and peritoneal metastases (**Fig. 2.4**) (also in colour, see Plate 2, facing p. 20) there has been great interest in performing diagnostic laparoscopy to try to prevent unnecessary open exploration in these patients.

CT scan and resectability

The widespread availability of spiral CT scan, and more recently the introduction of multislice spiral

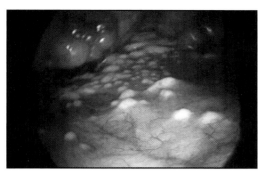

Figure 2.4 • Peritoneal metastases from pancreatic cancer. See also Plate 2, facing p. 20.

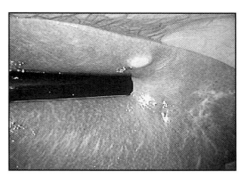

Figure 2.5 • Small liver metastases from pancreatic cancer during laparotomy. See also Plate 3, facing p. 20.

CT scan, have improved the possibilities for non-invasive staging of pancreatic cancer. Thinner slices, higher scanning speed, and the optimal use of contrast medium allow for the detection and characterisation of smaller lesions and produce more detailed information on the relationship of the primary tumour with surrounding structures. Unresectability can be determined with a high specificity (>90%), but sensitivity for the assessment of unresectability remains much lower (70%). This is caused mainly by the inability to characterise accurately very small liver lesions (**Fig. 2.5**) (also in colour, see Plate 3, facing p. 20) and peritoneal deposits as well as the inability to assess accurately the presence of subtle vascular invasion.

A recent review[15] stressed that the accuracy of laparoscopic staging is highly influenced by the pre-laparoscopic staging process. There is considerable variability of resectability rates in the published studies giving a different yield of laparoscopic staging. Moreover, in most series the information regarding the use of high-quality spiral CT scan is lacking.

Pisters et al.[15] stated that detection of occult metastatic disease should be less than 20% during laparoscopy otherwise the quality of prediagnostic imaging should be considered inadequate. **Table 2.1** summarises a number of studies from experienced centres in which the potential benefit of diagnostic laparoscopy in detection of metastases was evaluated during laparotomy after a high-quality spiral CT scan.[16–21]

Not only the quality of preoperative staging, but also the surgeons' attitude influences the resectability rate. At our institution we believe that gross ingrowth of a pancreatic tumour in the portal vein or superior mesenteric vein should be considered as a criterion for unresectability because it is associated with a dismal prognosis. The incidence of segmental venous resections for gross vascular

Table 2.1 • Peritoneal and/or liver metastases detected during laparotomy after high quality spiral CT scan

Author	Patients considered resectable	Resection rate (%)	Patients with metastases	Maximum % prevented
Steinberg et al.[16]	32	75	4	13
Friess et al.[17]	159	75	16	10
Rumstadt et al.[18]	194	89	9	5
Holzman et al.[19]	23	78	1	4
Spitz et al.[20]	118	80	18	15
Saldinger et al.[21]	68	76	3	4

Adapted from Pisters et al.[15]

involvement is currently only 3% in our centre.[22] In an earlier report from our institution the median survival after segmental venous resection was only 6 months.[23] A significantly better survival of 14 months is seen in the present series of patients with minimal vascular involvement and therefore only wedge resections but no extensive (segmental) resections and reconstructions are performed. This association between the extent of venous ingrowth and prognosis has also been shown by others.[24] The resectability rate and consequently the yield of diagnostic laparoscopy following spiral CT scan is totally different when compared to centres where vascular resections and reconstruction are frequently done for local tumour spread. Spitz et al. reported a series of 118 patients of whom only 2 (1%) were unresectable, whereas 25 patients (21%) underwent vascular resection and reconstruction for local ingrowth of tumour into a major vessel.[20]

Furthermore, in pancreatic cancer patients, studies that correlate CT findings with operative and histopathological findings have shown that the sensitivity and specificity of CT scan predicting unresectability is improved when thinner slices for scanning are used. Sensitivity and specificity were, respectively, 78% and 76% when 5 mm slices were used, compared with 91% and 90% respectively for a 3 mm slice thickness.[25,26] Additionally, it has been shown that a high predicted risk for unresectability with CT scan is associated with significantly poorer survival. In a study of 71 consecutive patients with potentially resectable pancreatic head cancer, Phoa et al. reported a median survival of 21 months for patients staged as resectable by CT scan compared to 9.7 months for the patients staged as unresectable. For the resected tumours survival was relatively poor if tumours were larger than 3 cm or if CT

signs of local unresectability were noted (hazard ratio 3.2).[27]

Improved radiological staging techniques, and in particular the routine use of high-quality spiral CT scan, has resulted in a better selection of patients. This, combined with a critical view to resectability and palliation of pancreatic tumours, has caused a decreased benefit of laparoscopic staging compared with our early experience. In **Table 2.2** the correlation between decline in benefit of diagnostic laparoscopy and the evolution of radiological staging modalities, especially for the improvements in CT scanning, is depicted.

The first report of laparoscopy in the management of pancreatic cancer from Cuschieri[1] described 73 consecutive patients. Fifty-one of these patients underwent laparotomy at the same time as the laparoscopic procedure. In this group 42 patients (82%) were correctly staged as having unresectable disease. In another early study, Warshaw et al.[28] reviewed the findings of 88 consecutive patients who had potentially curable pancreatic and periampullary cancer. Laparoscopy identified 22 (96%) of the 23 patients with distant metastases, and differentiation for the various tumour sites was made. Metastases were found in 15 (27%) of the 55 patients with pancreatic head cancer, 11 (65%) of the 17 patients with body and tail cancer, and one (6%) of the 17 patients with ampullary cancer. The first study in our institution to evaluate the additional value of laparoscopy in patients with a pancreatic head cancer was performed between 1993 and 1994.[29] The prelaparoscopy staging of 73 patients with potential resectable disease consisted of endoscopic retrograde cholangiopancreatography (ERCP), abdominal ultrasound with Doppler examination, and CT scan in the referring hospital

Table 2.2 • Influence of radiological imaging and time period on the yield of diagnostic laparoscopy for periampullary cancer in the Academic Medical Center (AMC)

	Period	Prevented laparotomy (%)	Radiological staging
Introduction	1993–94	19	Ultrasonography
Late laparotomy	1993–95	15	Ultrasonography + conventional CT scan
Randomised trial	1995–98	13	5-mm sliced spiral CT scan
Implementation study	1999–2001	9.5	3-mm sliced spiral CT scan

in the majority of the patients. A change in tumour stage was found in 29 patients (41%). This resulted in a change in therapy in 14 patients (25%) and a laparotomy was avoided in 17% of the patients. In the same period, the additional value of laparoscopy in patients with pancreatic head carcinoma varied widely in other studies between 18% and 82%, as shown in **Table 2.3**.[1–3,29–37]

While the most important objective in laparoscopy is to prevent an unnecessary laparotomy, a number of patients do need a late laparotomy for further palliation (e.g. bypass procedure for gastrointestinal obstruction) in a later stage of their disease. Therefore a further study focused on the overall efficacy of laparoscopy, defined as the early prevented laparotomies without the late laparotomies. In this study, 233 consecutive patients with upper gastrointestinal malignancies were included of whom 114 patients had a periampullary tumour. Laparotomy was avoided initially in 17 patients (15%) but 5 of these 17 patients (29%) needed a laparotomy for duodenal obstruction at a later stage of their disease.[38] This reduced, from 15% to 11%, the overall efficacy of laparoscopy in preventing unnecessary laparotomies. In a more recent study of 297 patients it was found that the yield of laparoscopy decreased to 13% (39 patients)[37] and other centres have reported similar findings (**Table 2.3**). The improvement of radiological staging techniques, including spiral CT and endoscopic and intravascular ultrasonography, has probably resulted in a better selection of patients.

Having recently abandoned the use of routine diagnostic and staging laparoscopy in patients with periampullary tumours in our institution, we investigated, in 186 consecutive patients, the value of only performing a high-quality spiral CT scan.[39] At laparotomy 63 patients (34%) had unresectable disease. Metastases were found in 29 patients (16%). Considering the previous accuracy of laparoscopy of 59%, the potential benefit was only 10%. We have, therefore, changed strategy to avoid routine preoperative staging laparoscopy and perform this only selectively.

Table 2.3 • Studies on the yield of diagnostic laparoscopy and detection of metastases in pancreatic and periampullary carcinoma

Author	Year	Patients	Metastases	Percentage
Warshaw et al.[2]	1986	57	17	30
Cuschieri[1]	1988	51	42	82
Murugiah et al.[30]	1993	12	6	50
Bemelman et al.[28]	1995	70	12	17
Fernandez-del Castillo et al.[31]	1995	89	16	18
John et al.[32]	1995	40	14	35
Pietrabissa et al.[33]	1996	21	9	43
Conlon et al.[3]	1996	108	39	39
Reddy et al.[34]	1999	109	29	27
Jimenez et al.[35]	2000	125	39	31
Brooks et al.[36]	2002	134	13	10
Van Dijkum et al.[37]	2003	297	39	13

Extended laparoscopy

Some authors have transformed staging laparoscopy in periampullary cancer to an extended procedure to imitate an open exploration so as to gain more information about the possible tumour invasion of retroperitoneal vessels.[3] In a series of 103 pancreatic cancers, examination was performed of the primary tumour, liver and porta hepatis, with division of the gastrohepatic omentum, inspection of the vena cava, caudate lobe, coeliac axis and lesser sac as well as examination of local tumour spread to the mesocolon, duodenum, jejunum and ligament of Treitz. Although the criteria of conlon et al. for unresectability are not accepted universally they found that in 14 patients (12%) this extension of the procedure identified unresectability. However, others have stated that this extensive procedure is time consuming and potentially dangerous.[35] Part of the time needed for the laparoscopic procedure could be regained when the therapeutic laparotomy is performed immediately after the laparoscopy during the same general anaesthesia. However, extended laparoscopy to assess local tumour extension into major vessels and biopsy for pathological examination at that point may lead to troublesome bleeding. Therefore, the addition of ultrasonography to the procedure to elucidate local tumour extension might increase the yield of diagnostic laparoscopy for local tumour ingrowth.

Laparoscopic ultrasonography

Laparoscopic ultrasonography has been introduced as an additional procedure to increase the detection of small intrahepatic liver metastasis (**Fig. 2.6**), to identify enlarged and suspicious lymph nodes, and to evaluate local ingrowth into the vascular structures. Some authors who found a high yield for this procedure have staged all liver lesions detected by ultrasonography without verification by pathological examination. Similarly, enlarged lymph nodes without biopsy or local suspected tumour ingrowth has been considered a finding of unresectability. It is our belief that these findings should only have therapeutic consequences when they are proven histopathologically. Metastases detected by laparoscopic ultrasonography that were not found during preoperative imaging are often too small for successful laparoscopic ultrasonographic-guided puncture to confirm the diagnosis histopathologically (**Fig. 2.7**). Interpretation of the literature on the additional value of laparoscopic ultrasonography is difficult due to differences in patient selection, success criteria and prelaparoscopic imaging techniques. The predictive value of local tumour ingrowth into major blood vessels is high with laparoscopic ultrasonography and it may therefore be useful in patients who show equivocal findings at spiral CT scanning. Most series do not give information on the additional value of laparoscopic ultrasonography after laparoscopic evaluation did not show unresectability. However, the additional value of laparoscopic ultrasonography on local ingrowth of pancreatic cancer that could be extracted from some studies is summarised in **Table 2.4**.[30,32,33,40–44] Nonetheless, patient selection in the various series makes it difficult to interpret the exact value of laparoscopic ultrasonography.

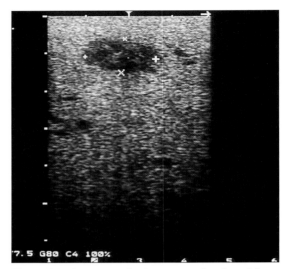

Figure 2.6 • Laparoscopic ultrasonography of small liver lesion.

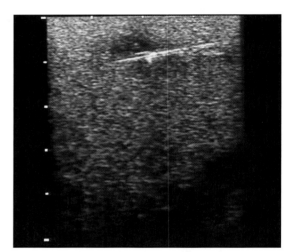

Figure 2.7 • Ultrasonographic guided biopsy of liver lesion.

We analysed the additional value of laparoscopic ultrasonography in 223 patients with a peri-ampullary cancer in terms of detection of metastases and/or local tumour ingrowth (**Fig. 2.8**), compared with radiological investigations and also whether these findings could be proven by pathological examination. In 17 patients metastases were found during laparoscopic ultrasonography, but most of these lesions were already found or suspected during external ultrasonography or CT scan. In only three

Table 2.4 • Additional value of laparoscopic ultrasonography on vascular tumour ingrowth in patients with periampullary cancer

Author	Year	Patients	Ingrowth on LUS*	Percentage
Murugiah et al.[30]	1993	8	2	25
John et al.[32]	1995	38	8	21
Pietrabissa et al.[33]	1996	21	4	19
van Delden et al.[40]	1996	48	12	25
Callery et al.[41]	1997	11	5	45
Minnard et al.[42]	1998	13	8	62
Catheline et al.[43]	1999	26	9	35
Taylor et al.[44]	2001	51	21	41

*Laparoscopic ultrasound.

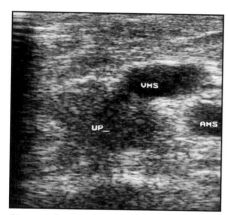

Figure 2.8 • Local ingrowth in the superior mesenteric vein (SMV) of pancreatic tumour visualised by laparoscopic ultrasonography. AMS = superior mesenteric artery; UP = tumour in uncinate process.

patients (1%) could these lesions be considered a new finding, and in only two patients was this confirmed pathologically. Detection of tumour ingrowth in major vessels was suspected in 22% but it was reported as a new finding in only 5%, and in none of the patients could biopsies be taken to prove the local ingrowth. It is, however, accepted that this is a limitation of any imaging modality which suggests the presence of vascular invasion. We do not consider laparoscopic ultrasonography useful in the work-up of patients with pancreatic carcinoma because of the demonstrated limited value of laparoscopic ultrasonography in the present study and the fact that about half the operation time is needed for this procedure.

Palliation

The evaluation of staging procedures is incomplete without the assessment of the consequences for the treatment in terms of improvement of outcome. Therefore we investigated the additional value of laparoscopy after complete radiological staging in terms of outcome in patients with histologically proven unresectable cancer and who underwent palliative treatment by endoscopic stent placement or surgical bypass. In this study, all patients with metastases diagnosed at laparoscopy were randomised. The primary endpoint for the diagnostic part of the study was prevention of laparotomy, and for the therapeutic part hospital-free survival. Laparoscopy detected histologically proven metastases in 39 of the 297 patients (13%). In another 13% of the patients unresectable disease was suspected but could not be proven with histological examination and therefore underwent exploration.[37]

It is known that percutaneous or endoscopic stent placement may, in fact, give the same long-term survival rate as traditional bypass surgery[45] and that most patients who are treated endoscopically do not need surgery later on.[46] However, the average hospital-free survival in our study was 94 days in the endoscopically treated patients, compared with an average hospital-free survival of 164 days after surgical palliative treatment. This study confirmed a limited benefit for laparoscopy in preventing laparotomy and more importantly no improved hospital-free survival after subsequent non-surgical palliation in patients with periampullary cancer.[37]

This study supports a role for laparoscopy in patients with periampullary cancer but only on a selective basis. Patients with a high risk of unresectability suspected on CT staging (such as equivocal or suspicious lesions detected at CT scan and that cannot be proven by percutaneous biopsy) or patients who are unlikely to benefit from surgical palliation could be selected for this staging procedure. For patients with pancreatic body and tail tumours, the yield of laparoscopy is much higher than for periampullary tumours.[6,18,47] On current information, there is no evidence to support the routine use of laparoscopy in the management of patients with periampullary and pancreatic cancer. The precise factors that might ensure an improvement in its selective use are yet to be determined.

PROXIMAL BILE DUCT TUMOURS

Generally, large gallbladder cancers are recognised easily by preoperative analysis or during laparoscopy. Characteristic findings at laparoscopy include an increased size of the gallbladder, a thickened whitish coloured wall, neovascularisation of the wall, omentum adherent to the gallbladder, and infiltration of tumour into the adjacent liver.[48] Early tumours, however, are often discovered incidentally and diagnosed after gallbladder removal. Additional liver bed resection and lymphadenectomy may be required in such cases. It is accepted that tumour dissemination during cholecystectomy may be minimised by removal of the gallbladder in a bag[49,50] or by conversion to an open procedure.[51] Nonetheless, in patients who have previously undergone cholecystectomy for incidental tumour and in advanced gallbladder cancer, laparoscopy may be useful to assess resectability. In advanced disease, histological confirmation of peritoneal or liver metastases may be required but in most cases this will be apparent prior to exploration.[52]

Proximal bile duct obstruction can be caused by proximal bile duct cancer or gallbladder cancer infiltrating the liver hilum. Differentiation between these two entities, and even from a benign lesion, might be difficult.[53] Hilar cholangiocarcinomas are often small and do not form a bulky mass, which makes them very difficult to visualise on any imaging modality. Occlusion of the portal venous system by hilar tumours is usually well seen at CT and magnetic resonance imaging (MRI), but limited tumour ingrowth in these vessels can be hard to determine. Moreover, accurate evaluation of the extent of intrahepatic tumour extension can be difficult without performing direct cholangiography (ERCP or percutaneous transhepatic cholangiography). Therefore, the surgeon dealing with malignant proximal bile duct obstruction is often faced with significant discrepancy between the findings of preoperative investigations and those visualised at the time of exploration. Tumours infiltrating the proximal bile ducts in particular tend to be unresectable and because palliation is preferably non-surgical these patients might benefit from laparoscopic staging to avoid unnecessary laparotomy.[54] Obviously, if intrahepatic biliary bypass surgery is the preferred method of palliation, as some centres have advocated, then there is no rationale for laparoscopic staging in these patients.[55]

Diagnostic and staging laparoscopy

Information on the additional value of diagnostic laparoscopy for malignant proximal bile duct obstruction is limited. In a pilot study from our institution incurable disease was diagnosed in 19 (40%) of the 47 patients by laparoscopy.[6] These results were explained, in part, by a change in diagnosis after laparoscopy. For example, a hilar stenosis can be caused by gallbladder cancer growing into the hepatoduodenal ligament and is therefore more likely to be unresectable than a primary bile duct tumour. Although on follow-up 15% of the patients who did not undergo exploratory laparotomy after laparoscopy required surgical palliation in a later stage,[38] laparoscopic staging still prevented a high percentage of unnecessary laparotomies in this patient population.

A more recent study of 110 consecutive patients in our institution has confirmed these data.[56] Laparoscopy revealed histologically proven incurable disease in 44 (41%) of patients. Of the 65 patients who underwent laparotomy, 35 patients (54%) were unresectable. Although in 41% of the cases laparotomy was avoided, laparoscopy could not assess the resectability correctly in 44% of cases.

These findings accord with a study from the Memorial Sloan Kettering Cancer Center[57] involving 100 patients with carcinoma of the extrahepatic biliary tree. Thirty-five patients (35%) were identified as unresectable during laparoscopy. Of the 65 patients who underwent laparotomy, a further 34 patients (52%) were unresectable resulting in an overall accuracy of 51% for detecting unresectable disease.

In both studies the yield of laparoscopy was greater for gallbladder cancer than for hilar cholangiocarcinoma. When using laparoscopy selectively, it is therefore suggested by several authors that this form of staging be undertaken in particular for gallbladder cancer.[58] In a further large series of 401 patients with hepatobiliary cancer, the highest yield for laparoscopy was also found in the group of patients with biliary cancers. However, this study also showed that the surgeons' preoperative impression of resectability was as important as the laparoscopic staging procedure.[59]

Laparoscopic ultrasonography

Laparoscopic ultrasonography has not been very useful in staging the local tumour spread of proximal bile duct cancer.[60] In our series of 35 patients, laparoscopic ultrasonography led to a change in diagnosis or tumour stage in 8 patients (23%). However, in only three patients (9%) was a laparotomy avoided due to the ultrasonography. In our more recent series of 110 proximal bile duct lesions, laparoscopic ultrasonography staged only one patient as unresectable.[56] These data are comparable to the findings of Vollmer et al.,[58] who described 2 of the 23 patients identified as unresectable (9%) as a result of the laparoscopic ultrasonography alone. The New York study confirmed that patients with unresectable disease most often had locally advanced tumours, but laparoscopic ultrasonography did not contribute to the assessment of resectability in these patients.[57] Additionally, it is believed that extensive biliary and vascular involvement can be assessed with high accuracy (91%) by external colour Doppler ultrasonography as well as thin-slice contrast-enhanced multislice CT.[61]

The additional value of laparoscopic ultrasonography is therefore too low to perform routinely in patients with proximal bile duct tumours.

Palliation

Although palliation of malignant proximal biliary obstruction is still controversial we prefer non-

surgical palliation and therefore laparoscopic staging has a potential yield.[62,63] In these patients, however, laparoscopic palliation is not used frequently despite innovative descriptions of its combined use with radiological and endoscopic guidance.[63]

 Current evidence suggests that laparoscopy is useful in avoiding unnecessary laparotomy in patients with proximal bile duct tumours and that it is most effective in the assessment of gall bladder cancer.

HEPATIC MALIGNANCIES

Diagnostic laparoscopy

Laparoscopy can be very useful in patients with hepatic malignancies because there is usually no indication for surgical palliation if curative resection is not possible. Diagnosis can often be established using radiological imaging such as ultrasonography, contrast-enhanced spiral CT scan, or MRI, which are becoming increasingly more accurate at detecting and characterising intrahepatic lesions. Shortcomings of these imaging techniques include a low sensitivity for detecting superficial liver lesions and peritoneal deposits, as well as a relatively low specificity in characterising small (<1 cm) intrahepatic lesions. These issues are particularly relevant in patients with cirrhosis, because it is difficult to detect lesions against the nodular, inhomogeneous background of cirrhosis, and because it is hard to differentiate malignant lesions from regenerative or dysplastic nodules. Nonetheless, MRI when used with liver contrast agents should improve these results in the near future. Laparoscopy can be used for examination of the abdominal cavity to rule out extrahepatic metastatic disease and can provide information on the hepatic status. Superficial liver lesions are easy to detect and even subcapsular deposits may be detected by forceps palpation. Evaluation of the degree of liver cirrhosis is very important prior to considering resection of hepatocellular carcinoma, and laparoscopic guided biopsies can be performed safely to assess the quality of the remaining liver even in the presence of a coagulation abnormality. Inabnet et al.[64] studied 58 biopsies in 22 consecutive patients with a prolonged prothrombin time, prolonged bleeding time, or thrombocytopenia. Only one patient (5%) required transfusion and laparotomy for haemostatic control. Most patients with secondary liver malignancies have previously undergone a laparotomy, making the visualisation of intra-abdominal organs more difficult due to adhesions. The failure rate of laparoscopy in these patients is reported as 5–15% in most series. It is important, therefore, to use an open technique for introduction of the first trocar. Unfortunately, some pitfalls remain in applying laparoscopy to the evaluation of liver malignancy. The nature of liver tissue and the relative ease with which iatrogenic injury can be caused by retraction and manipulation remain a concern.

In early reports of laparoscopic assessment of liver malignancy, a high percentage of prevented laparotomies was reported. Fourteen (48%) of 29 patients reported by Babineau et al.[65] with hepatic malignancies (12 primaries and 17 metastatic liver lesions) were shown to have unresectable disease at laparoscopy. Ten patients had metastatic disease and four had unsuspected cirrhosis. In the group of primary hepatic lesions, eight patients (67%) were unresectable and six patients (35%) in the group of secondary lesions had advanced disease. In another study by John et al.,[66] 52 consecutive patients with liver tumours were reviewed. In 23 (46%) patients the hepatic malignancy was demonstrated during laparoscopy. Extrahepatic disease was found in 18 patients, and 11 patients had bilobar disease. Four patients, who were thought to have primary liver malignancy, were shown to have unresectable metastases of a primary non-hepatic tumour. In this study, a significant reduction of unnecessary laparotomies was found in the group of patients in which laparoscopy was performed routinely. The resectability rate was 93% in this group, compared with 58% in the patients without laparoscopy and laparoscopic ultrasonography in the work-up before resection.

In a study from our institution during the same period, metastatic disease was found in 4 (40%) of the 10 patients with primary liver malignancy, and in 11 (33%) of the 33 patients with liver metastases following laparoscopy combined with laparoscopic ultrasonography.[6] The ability to detect and biopsy small peritoneal metastatic depositions together with ultrasonographic visualisation, has rendered this investigative combination an efficacious staging modality for liver malignancies and is part of the standard assessment of patients with hepatic malignancies in our hospital. However, it is likely that a more selective use of laparoscopy may increase the yield.

Laparoscopic ultrasonography

Laparoscopic ultrasonography appears particularly useful in the evaluation of liver lesions. Most studies reporting on the value of laparoscopy in primary and secondary liver malignancies have added this to their procedure. The gold standard for detecting secondary liver lesions is still intraoperative palpation and ultrasonography, but it has been demonstrated that laparoscopic ultrasonography detects these lesions effectively. Foley et al.[67] reached a sensitivity of 95% and specificity of 80% in pig livers, and a sensitivity of 80% and specificity of 91% in humans. Cuesta et al.[68] found additional information leading to a change in surgical approach in 20 of the 25 patients (80%) assessed by laparoscopic ultrasonography. However, the selection criteria employed may influence the treatment strategy in these patients. In a recent study in 84 consecutive patients, we found differences in the yield of laparoscopy combined with ultrasonography for primary ($n = 33$) and secondary ($n = 51$) liver malignancies.[69] Laparoscopy showed unresectability in 13 patients (39%) with primary malignancy and exploratory laparotomy showed that an additional 5 of the remaining 20 patients (25%) had unresectable disease. Laparoscopy demonstrated unresectability in 5 patients (12%) with colorectal liver metastasis ($n = 43$), and at laparotomy another 7 of the remaining 38 patients (18%) had unresectable disease. In five patients, from the latter group, laparoscopic ultrasonography could not be performed due to adhesions from earlier surgery. These data suggest that a more selective use of laparoscopic staging for the various hepatic malignancies may be appropriate.

Primary liver malignancy

Lo et al.[70] found 15 of 91 patients (16%) with primary liver cancer had unresectable tumours during laparoscopic evaluation whereas 9 patients

(12%) were not submitted to resection at laparotomy. Therefore an exploratory laparotomy was avoided in 63% of the unresectable patients. The procedure was accurate in assessing the quality of the liver remnant and the presence of intrahepatic metastases, but it was less sensitive in determining the presence of tumour thrombi in major vascular structures and the extent of local invasion, especially in large (>10 cm) tumours. The study by Ido et al.[71] clearly showed the value of laparoscopic ultrasonography in detecting and diagnosing small hepatocellular carcinomas. One hundred and thirty-four new nodules were visualised by laparoscopic ultrasonography in 64 (34%) of the 186 patients. Of these 134 nodules, 28 nodules in 23 patients were histologically diagnosed as hepatocellular carcinoma. New hepatocellular carcinoma lesions were detected by laparoscopic ultrasonography or guided needle aspiration in 23 (12%) of the 186 patients. Of these 23 patients, 18 had been diagnosed as solitary hepatocellular carcinoma before laparoscopy. Montorsi et al.[72] have confirmed these data and found new lesions of histologically proven hepatocellular carcinoma in 14 patients (22%). Even when preoperative staging includes a modern triphasic high-speed spiral CT, Foroutani et al.[73] demonstrated that laparoscopic ultrasonography was superior in detecting additional tumours. The ultrasonography confirmed all 201 tumours seen on CT scan and detected 21 additional tumours (9.5%) ranging in size from 0.3 to 2.7 cm in 11 patients (20%). These series and our recent study suggest that laparoscopic staging is useful in patients with primary liver malignancies since these tumours tend to be at high risk of being unresectable. The value of laparoscopic staging is doubled due to additional tumour detection and capacity to undertake guided biopsies to determine the quality of the liver remnant in cirrhotic patients.

Colorectal cancer liver metastases

There has been a change in the approach to the management of colorectal cancer liver lesions over the last decade and this has influenced the yield of laparoscopy in these patients. The indications for resection for metastases have changed towards a more aggressive approach for multiple (more than four) lesions as well as bilobar disease. The understanding of liver anatomy and familiarity with intraoperative ultrasonography has led to a segment-oriented approach in liver resections and made repeated resections possible. Furthermore, the use of local ablative techniques such as radio-frequency ablation in combination with resection has extended the possibilities for curative surgical treatment. These changes have meant that the only absolute limitations for curative resection include irresectable extrahepatic dissemination and the function of the liver remnant. Even the latter can be addressed by the use of portal vein embolisation to enlarge the liver remnant. All these recent improvements in liver surgery have increased the resectability rate of liver metastases.[74] These advances and improved imaging techniques such as high-quality spiral CT scans and MRI have reduced the possible yield of laparoscopy with ultrasonography in patients with secondary liver malignancy in recent years. Confirmation of this is provided by Gholghesaei et al.,[75] who reported a series of 59 patients in whom the yield of laparoscopy was 29%, with laparoscopic ultrasonography apparently not detecting more than CT scan. In an earlier study laparoscopic ultrasonography was shown to detect more liver metastases than CT scan[76] but in this report 8-mm sliced CT scans were used. Two lesions that were seen on laparoscopic ultrasonography were missed but might have been seen on thinner sliced CT scanning.

In a recent analysis of our own data, we found a decreased yield of laparoscopy in patients with secondary liver metastases.[69] We failed to perform proper examination in 11 of the 51 patients (20%) due to adhesions. Five out of 43 patients were correctly staged as unresectable giving a yield of 12% in this group. We detected 5 of the 12 patients (42%) with unresectable disease by laparoscopy and laparoscopic ultrasonography. The yield is considerably less compared to a previous study from our centre, in which 7 of 27 patients (26%) with colorectal liver metastases were prevented from undergoing an unnecessary laparotomy. Several series have reported variable success rates of 29–38% for laparoscopy in patients with secondary liver malignancy of colorectal cancer (**Table 2.5**).[6,65,66,70–73,75,77–79] Most of these series considered bilobar disease as an exclusion for resection, which

Table 2.5 • Studies on diagnostic laparoscopy in primary and secondary liver malignancy

Author	Year	Primary or secondary	Patients	Number unresectable (%)
Babineau et al.[65]	1994	Primary Secondary	12 17	8 (67) 6 (35)
John et al.[66]	1994	Primary/secondary	50	23 (46)
Lo et al.[70]	1998	Primary	91	15 (16)
Van Dijkum et al.[6]	1999	Primary Secondary	10 33	4 (40) 11 (33)
Ido et al.[71]	1999	Primary	186	64 (34)
Rahusen et al.[77]	1999	Secondary	50	18 (38)
Jarnagin et al.[78]	2000	Primary/secondary	104	26 (25)
Foroutani et al.[73]	2000	Primary Secondary	9 46	1 (11) 10 (22)
Montorsi et al.[72]	2001	Primary	70	14 (22)
Gholghesaei et al.[75]	2003	Secondary	59	17 (29)
Metcalfe et al.[79]	2003	Secondary	24	12 (50)

may have resulted in a higher yield for diagnostic laparoscopy than would have been found if modern resection criteria were used.

Nowadays, it would appear more appropriate to perform laparoscopy in a selective way in patients with colorectal cancer metastases. Jarnagin et al.[80] have described a clinical risk score that predicted survival after hepatic resection, and that was suitable in identifying the high-risk patients most likely to benefit from laparoscopy. In their series of 103 patients, occult unresectable disease was found in 12% of patients with a low score, but in 42% of patients with a high score, a significant increase. If laparoscopy had been used selectively for the patients with a high score, 57 laparoscopies would have been avoided. These data have been confirmed in a study of 73 patients by Metcalfe et al.,[79] who demonstrated that in the 24 patients selected to undergo diagnostic laparoscopy for colorectal metastases, the yield was 50% whereas in the group of 49 patients selected for direct surgical exploration 46 patients (94%) were resected. Although their selection criteria for laparoscopy were not very strict, they found that the likelihood of being unresectable is in part predicted by the disease-free interval and the number of hepatic metastases.

Non-colorectal cancer liver metastases

In a limited experience of eight patients with secondary non-colorectal liver malignancy, we detected unresectable disease in three patients (38%). Only one unresectable patient was missed by laparoscopic staging. A larger series of 30 consecutive patients with non-colorectal cancer metastases from the Memorial Sloan-Kettering Cancer Center showed a successfully completed laparoscopy in 80% of the patients.[81] Laparoscopy and ultrasonography staged 6 of the 30 patients (20%) as unresectable. Laparoscopy detected six of the nine patients (67%) with unresectable disease. The three patients with unresectable disease not found during laparoscopy were irresectable because of vascular involvement.

Laparoscopic treatment and palliation

Some recent studies have reported on the possibilities of laparoscopic treatment of liver tumours but, to date, most of these have included mainly benign tumours.[82] Gigot et al.[83] analysed the data of 37 patients with liver malignancies from several European centres, and small tumours located in the left lateral segments or in the anterior segments of the right lobe seem suitable for laparoscopic treatment. Surgery is seldom required for palliation of malignant liver tumours but occasionally endocrine liver tumours need to be resected for palliation.

Although results are not yet mature enough to establish long-term outcomes, there is increasing interest in local ablation with radiofrequency for the treatment of liver malignancies when resection is not possible.[84] Radiofrequency tumour ablation has been shown to be safe and effective in reducing tumour load in patients with primary and secondary liver tumours. Since radiofrequency ablation can be performed during laparoscopy and laparoscopic guided ultrasonography it seems appropriate to perform this procedure directly after the staging laparoscopy.[85] Long-term results of such an approach are awaited and it is appreciated that patients with extrahepatic disease diagnosed during laparoscopy are unsuitable for local ablative techniques.

Laparoscopic staging for hepatic malignancy has a higher yield for primary tumours, and improved criteria are required to better select patients with colorectal metastases for the procedure.

CYTOLOGY OF PERITONEAL LAVAGE

With the introduction of laparoscopic staging, lavage of the peritoneal cavity has often been added to the procedure.[86] Although peritoneal lavage is very easy to perform during laparoscopy, its exact value is still subject to debate. It is known that positive results of the lavage obtained during laparoscopic staging are often associated with metastatic disease,[31] and in gastric cancer patients it has been shown that patients with a positive cytology of their peritoneal washing (**Fig. 2.9**) (also in colour, see Plate 4, facing p. 20) had a worse prognosis then those who have not.[87] Free cancer cells found in the peritoneal lavage fluid are believed to be an indication of early seeding of peritoneal metastases, but the question remains whether it is of additional value to the diagnostic laparoscopy for the staging of intra-abdominal malignancies.

In the period 1992–97, diagnostic laparoscopy combined with peritoneal lavage was performed in 449 patients, of whom 362 had potential resectable HPB tumours.[88] Positive lavage was found in only 20 patients (6%), of whom 15 (75%) had already proven metastases during laparoscopy. Of the whole group, 236 patients had pancreatic or periampullary carcinoma but in only 7 patients with pancreatic tumours (3%)was lavage positive. Given that in five of these seven patients metastases had already been visualised during laparoscopy, peritoneal lavage resulted in an additional value of only two patients, or 0.9%. The sensitivity and specificity of lavage for detection of metastasis was 18% and 99% respectively.

Other studies on peritoneal cytology in pancreatic cancer are summarised in **Table 2.6**[86,88–93] and show positive cytology of 8–29%. None of the 15 patients with pancreatic cancer in the body and tail in our study had a positive lavage, whereas Warshaw found up to 40% positive cytology in this same group of patients.[86] Of the 39 patients with liver malignancy

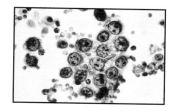

Figure 2.9 •
Peritoneal washing with malignant cells from pancreatic cancer. See also Plate 4, facing p. 20.

Table 2.6 • Peritoneal lavage during laparoscopic staging in patients with periampullary carcinoma

Author	Year	Patients	Positive cytology	Percentage
Warshaw[86]	1991	35	10	29
Lei et al.[89]	1994	36	3	8
Fernandez-del Castillo et al.[90]	1995	94	16	17
Van Dijkum et al.[88]	1998	236	7	3
Nakao et al.[91]	1999	74	22	29
Jimenez et al.[92]	2000	117	24	21
Konishi et al.[93]	2002	151	36	24

only two had positive lavage but one had already proven metastases. Of the 72 patients with proximal bile duct lesions 11 (15%) had positive lavage but only two did not have proven distant metastases. Surprisingly, one of these two patients had no malignancy at all, but was eventually diagnosed as primary sclerosing cholangitis and was therefore considered to represent a false-positive result of the peritoneal lavage.

Although a positive peritoneal lavage was associated significantly with a decreased median survival in our study this was not an independent predictor for survival in regression analysis.

 Therefore it is concluded that routine cytology of peritoneal lavage should not be performed because of the low additional benefit and limited prognostic value.

CONCLUSIONS

Laparoscopic staging for HPB tumours is only appropriate when non-surgical palliation is preferred for unresectable patients because the main objective of laparoscopic staging is the avoidance of an unnecessary laparotomy. Recent improvements in the quality of preoperative radiological imaging, especially of thin-sliced spiral CT scanning, has led to an accurate prediction of resectability of HPB tumours. These advances have decreased the yield of laparoscopy and laparoscopic ultrasonography for these tumours to a level where the routine use for staging is questionable. Only those tumours with a high chance of unresectability, such as proximal bile duct tumours, pancreatic body and tail tumours, and primary liver tumours, remain candidates for its standard use in the preoperative work-up. For other tumour locations a selective use of laparoscopic staging seems more appropriate.

Selection criteria to improve the success rate of laparoscopic staging are tumour related. For pan-

creatic cancers, criteria for selecting patients with high risk of occult metastases have been postulated by Pisters et al.:[15]

- larger primary tumours
- lesions in the neck, body and tail of the pancreas
- equivocal radiological findings suggestive of metastatic disease, such as low-volume ascites
- CT findings indicating possible carcinomatosis
- small hypodense regions suggesting hepatic metastases that are not amendable to percutaneous biopsy
- subtle clinical and laboratory findings suggesting advanced disease, e.g. increased CEA 19-9 levels
- severe back pain.

Laparoscopy for hepatic malignancies also seems valuable especially when used in a selective way. The yield for primary liver cancer is substantially higher than for secondary liver tumours such as colorectal cancer metastases. For this latter group, the criteria for resectability have changed to a more aggressive approach. Therefore, the yield of laparoscopic staging has decreased in recent years and better selection criteria for patients who might benefit from laparoscopy are needed. Clinical parameters, such as lymph-node-positive primary tumour, <1 year disease-free interval after colorectal cancer, >1 hepatic tumour, and largest tumour >5 cm, which are all predictors of survival,[94] seem to be relevant criteria for selecting patients who might benefit from laparoscopic staging.[80]

All the above mentioned criteria to improve the yield of laparoscopy are only feasible when preoperative radiological imaging is optimal. At present for HPB malignancy, this means a thin-sliced high-quality spiral CT scan.

Key points

Diagnostic laparoscopy is a safe staging method of which the yield is dependent on the location of the tumour, prelaparoscopy radiological staging and the criteria of success.

The yield of diagnostic laparoscopy for HPB malignancies should be measured by the avoidance of unnecessary laparotomies and is therefore only feasible when non-surgical palliation is preferred.

Laparoscopic staging should be performed routinely for patients with a high risk of unresectability, such as primary liver cancer, proximal bile duct tumours, and pancreatic body and tail tumours.

Laparoscopic staging of periampullary pancreatic cancer should not be performed routinely but in a selective way, preferably during the same session as the open exploration.

For colorectal cancer metastases improvements in resectability have decreased the yield of laparoscopic staging to a level that selection criteria should be identified for the use of this staging modality.

The additional value of laparoscopic ultrasonography is very low because of advances in preoperative imaging with high-quality CT scans. It is, however, helpful in characterisation of small intrahepatic lesions, which are suspicious and cannot be biopsied at ultrasound or CT, and it can find new and satellite lesions in primary liver malignancy

The yield of peritoneal lavage to detect metastatic disease is too low to warrant its routine use.

REFERENCES

1. Cuschieri A. Laparoscopy for pancreatic cancer: does it benefit the patient? Eur J Surg Oncol 1988; 14:41–4.

2. Warshaw AL, Tepper JE, Shipley WU. Laparoscopy in the staging and planning of therapy for pancreatic cancer. Am J Surg 1986; 151:76–80.

3. Conlon KC, Dougherty E, Klimstra DS et al. The value of minimal access surgery in the staging of patients with potentially resectable peripancreatic malignancy. Ann Surg 1996; 223:134–40.

Early report of the potential role of extended laparoscopy in 115 patients with potentially resectable peripancreatic malignancy.

4. Maartense S, Bemelman WA, Dunker MS et al. Randomized study of the effectiveness of closing laparoscopic trocar wounds with octylcyanoacrylate, adhesive papertape or poliglecaprone. Br J Surg 2002; 89:1370–5.

5. Boyd WP, Jr., Nord HJ. Diagnostic laparoscopy. Endoscopy 2000; 32:153–8.

6. Van Dijkum EJ, de Wit LT, van Delden OM et al. Staging laparoscopy and laparoscopic ultrasonography in more than 400 patients with upper gastrointestinal carcinoma. J Am Coll Surg 1999; 189:459–65.

7. Bateman BG, Kolp LA, Hoeger K. Complications of laparoscopy – operative and diagnostic. Fertil Steril 1996; 66:30–5.

8. Hasson HM, Rotman C, Rana N et al. Open laparoscopy: 29-year experience. Obstet Gynecol 2000; 96:763–6.

9. Bemelman WA, de Wit LT, Busch OR et al. Establishment of pneumoperitoneum with a modified blunt trocar. J Laparoendosc Adv Surg Tech A 2000; 10:217–8.

10. Schrenk P, Woisetschlager R, Rieger R et al. Mechanism, management, and prevention of laparoscopic bowel injuries. Gastrointest Endosc 1996; 43:572–4.

11. 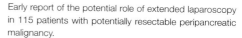 Shoup M, Brennan MF, Karpeh MS et al. Port site metastasis after diagnostic laparoscopy for upper gastrointestinal tract malignancies: an uncommon entity. Ann Surg Oncol 2002; 9:632–6.

Report of 1965 laparoscopic procedures for cancer demonstrating that the very small risk of port site recurrence (0.8%) cannot be used as an argument against laparoscopy in upper GI malignancy.

12. Tjalma WA. Laparoscopic surgery and port-site metastases: routine measurements to reduce the risk. Eur J Gynaecol Oncol 2003; 24:236.

13. Hubens G. Port site metastases: where are we at the beginning of the 21st century? Acta Chir Belg 2002; 102:230–7.

14. Lacy AM, Delgado S, Garcia–Valdecasas JC et al. Port site metastases and recurrence after laparoscopic colectomy. A randomized trial. Surg Endosc 1998;12:1039–42.

15. Pisters PW, Lee JE, Vauthey JN et al. Laparoscopy in the staging of pancreatic cancer. Br J Surg 2001; 88:325–37.

16. Steinberg WM, Barkin J, Bradley EL, III et al. Workup of a patient with a mass in the head of the pancreas. Pancreas 1998; 17:24–30.

17. Friess H, Kleeff J, Silva JC et al. The role of diagnostic laparoscopy in pancreatic and periampullary malignancies. J Am Coll Surg 1998; 186:675–82.

18. Rumstadt B, Schwab M, Schuster K et al. The role of laparoscopy in the preoperative staging of pancreatic carcinoma. J Gastrointest Surg 1997; 1:245–50.

19. Holzman MD, Reintgen KL, Tyler DS et al. The role of laparoscopy in the management of suspected pancreatic and periampullary malignancies. J Gastrointest Surg 1997; 1:236–44.

20. Spitz FR, Abbruzzese JL, Lee JE et al. Preoperative and postoperative chemoradiation strategies in patients treated with pancreaticoduodenectomy for adenocarcinoma of the pancreas. J Clin Oncol 1997; 15:928–37.

21. Saldinger PF, Reilly M, Reynolds K et al. Is CT angiography sufficient for prediction of resectability of periampullary neoplasms? J Gastrointest Surg 2000; 4:233–7.

22. van Geenen RC, ten Kate FJ, de Wit LT et al. Segmental resection and wedge excision of the portal or superior mesenteric vein during pancreatoduodenectomy. Surgery 2001; 129:158–63.

23. Allema JH, Reinders ME, van Gulik TM et al. Portal vein resection in patients undergoing pancreatoduodenectomy for carcinoma of the pancreatic head. Br J Surg 1994; 81:1642–6.

24. Nakao A, Harada A, Nonami T et al. Regional vascular resection using catheter bypass procedure for pancreatic cancer. Hepatogastroenterology 1995; 42:734–9.

25. Diehl SJ, Lehmann KJ, Sadick M et al. Pancreatic cancer: value of dual-phase helical CT in assessing resectability. Radiology 1998; 206:373–8.

26. Phoa SS, Reeders JW, Rauws EA et al. Spiral computed tomography for preoperative staging of potentially resectable carcinoma of the pancreatic head. Br J Surg 1999; 86:789–94.

27. Phoa SS, Reeders JW, Stoker J et al. CT criteria for venous invasion in patients with pancreatic head carcinoma. Br J Radiol 2000; 73:1159–64.

28. Warshaw AL, Gu ZY, Wittenberg J et al. Preoperative staging and assessment of resectability of pancreatic cancer. Arch Surg 1990; 125:230–3.

29. Bemelman WA, de Wit LT, van Delden OM et al. Diagnostic laparoscopy combined with laparoscopic ultrasonography in staging of cancer of the pancreatic head region. Br J Surg 1995; 82:820–4.

30. Murugiah M, Paterson-Brown S, Windsor JA et al. Early experience of laparoscopic ultrasonography in the management of pancreatic carcinoma. Surg Endosc 1993; 7:177–81.

31. Fernandez-del Castillo C, Rattner DW, Warshaw AL. Further experience with laparoscopy and peritoneal cytology in the staging of pancreatic cancer. Br J Surg 1995; 82:1127–9.

32. John TG, Greig JD, Carter DC et al. Carcinoma of the pancreatic head and periampullary region. Tumor staging with laparoscopy and laparoscopic ultrasonography. Ann Surg 1995; 221:156–64.

33. Pietrabissa A, Di Candio G, Giulianotti PC et al. Laparoscopic exposure of the pancreas and staging of pancreatic cancer. Semin Laparosc Surg 1996; 3:3–9.

34. Reddy KR, Levi J, Livingstone A et al. Experience with staging laparoscopy in pancreatic malignancy. Gastrointest Endosc 1999; 49:498–503.

35. Jimenez RE, Warshaw AL, Rattner DW et al. Impact of laparoscopic staging in the treatment of pancreatic cancer. Arch Surg 2000; 135:409–14.

36. Brooks AD, Mallis MJ, Brennan MF, Conlon KC. The value of laparoscopy in the management of ampullary, duodenal, and distal bile duct tumors. J Gastrointest Surg 2002; 6:139–45.

37. Nieveen van Dijkum EJ, Romijn MG, Terwee CB et al. Laparoscopic staging and subsequent palliation in patients with peripancreatic carcinoma. Ann Surg 2003; 237:66–73.

Large study on 287 consecutive patients with peripancreatic malignancy demonstrating a detection rate for laparoscopic staging of 35% and biopsy-proven irresectable disease in 13%. The study also suggested that there was no apparent gain for nonsurgical palliation.

38. Van Dijkum EJ, de Wit LT, van Delden OM et al. The efficacy of laparoscopic staging in patients with upper gastrointestinal tumors. Cancer 1997; 79:1315–9.

39. Tilleman EH, Kuiken BW, Phoa SS et al. Abolition of diagnostic laparoscopy for patients with a periampullary carcinoma; implementation of a new diagnostic strategy. Eur J Surg Oncol 2004; 30:658–62.

Author's own recent data suggesting that modern radiological imaging reduces the need for laparoscopic staging of periampullary cancer.

40. van Delden OM, Smits NJ, Bemelman WA et al. Comparison of laparoscopic and transabdominal ultrasonography in staging of cancer of the pancreatic head region. J Ultrasound Med 1996; 15:207–12.

41. Callery MP, Strasberg SM, Doherty GM et al. Staging laparoscopy with laparoscopic ultrasonography: optimizing resectability in hepatobiliary and pancreatic malignancy. J Am Coll Surg 1997; 185:33–9.

42. Minnard EA, Conlon KC, Hoos A et al. Laparoscopic ultrasound enhances standard laparoscopy in the staging of pancreatic cancer. Ann Surg 1998; 228:182–7.

43. Catheline JM, Turner R, Rizk N et al. The use of diagnostic laparoscopy supported by laparoscopic ultrasonography in the assessment of pancreatic cancer. Surg Endosc 1999; 13:239–45.

44. Taylor AM, Roberts SA, Manson JM. Experience with laparoscopic ultrasonography for defining tumour resectability in carcinoma of the pancreatic head and periampullary region. Br J Surg 2001; 88:1077–83.

45. Speer AG, Cotton PB, Russell RC et al. Randomised trial of endoscopic versus percutaneous stent insertion in malignant obstructive jaundice. Lancet 1987; 2:57–62.

46. Espat NJ, Brennan MF, Conlon KC. Patients with laparoscopically staged unresectable pancreatic adenocarcinoma do not require subsequent surgical biliary or gastric bypass. J Am Coll Surg 1999; 188:649–55.

   Follow-up of a large series of 155 laparoscopically staged patients with pancreatic cancer demonstrating that late reoperation for palliative surgical bypass is rarely necessary.

47. Fernandez-del Castillo C, Warshaw AL. Laparoscopy for staging in pancreatic carcinoma. Surg Oncol 1993; 2 (Suppl 1):25–9.

48. Chijiiwa K, Sumiyoshi K, Nakayama F. Impact of recent advances in hepatobiliary imaging techniques on the preoperative diagnosis of carcinoma of the gallbladder. World J Surg 1991; 15:322–7.

49. Contini S, Dalla VR, Zinicola R. Unexpected gallbladder cancer after laparoscopic cholecystectomy: an emerging problem? Reflections on four cases. Surg Endosc 1999; 13:264–7.

50. Sandor J, Ihasz M, Fazekas T et al. Unexpected gallbladder cancer and laparoscopic surgery. Surg Endosc 1995; 9:1207–10.

51. Wysocki A, Bobrzynski A, Krzywon J et al. Laparoscopic cholecystectomy and gallbladder cancer. Surg Endosc 1999; 13:899–901.

52. Kraas E, Frauenschuh D, Farke S. Intraoperative suspicion of gallbladder carcinoma in laparoscopic surgery: what to do? Dig Surg 2002; 19:489–93.

53. Gerhards MF, Vos P, van Gulik TM et al. Incidence of benign lesions in patients resected for suspicious hilar obstruction. Br J Surg 2001; 88:48–51.

54. Garner PD, Hall LD, Johnstone PA. Palliation of unresectable hilar cholangiocarcinoma. J Surg Oncol 2000; 75:95–7.

55. Jarnagin WR, Burke E, Powers C et al. Intrahepatic biliary enteric bypass provides effective palliation in selected patients with malignant obstruction at the hepatic duct confluence. Am J Surg 1998; 175:453–60.

56. Tilleman EH, de Castro SM, Busch OR et al. Diagnostic laparoscopy and laparoscopic ultrasound for staging of patients with malignant proximal bile duct obstruction. J Gastrointest Surg 2002; 6:426–30.

   Authors' study of 110 patients demonstrating that laparoscopy avoided unnecessary laparotomy in 41% of patients and concluding that the procedure should be performed routinely in assessing patients with potentially resectable tumour.

57. Weber SM, DeMatteo RP, Fong Y et al. Staging laparoscopy in patients with extrahepatic biliary carcinoma. Analysis of 100 patients. Ann Surg 2002; 235:392–9.

   Similar study in 100 patients with gall bladder and bile duct cancer supporting the use of laparoscopy.

58. Vollmer CM, Drebin JA, Middleton WD et al. Utility of staging laparoscopy in subsets of peripancreatic and biliary malignancies. Ann Surg 2002; 235:1–7.

59. D'Angelica M, Fong Y, Weber S et al. The role of staging laparoscopy in hepatobiliary malignancy: prospective analysis of 401 cases. Ann Surg Oncol 2003; 10:183–9.

   Study showing that one in five patients can be spared laparotomy by laparoscopic staging. Multivariate analysis showed that surgeon's preoperative impression of resectability is important.

60. van Delden OM, de Wit LT, Nieveen van Dijkum EJ et al. Value of laparoscopic ultrasonography in staging of proximal bile duct tumors. J Ultrasound Med 1997; 16:7–12.

61. Smits NJ, Reeders JW. Imaging and staging of biliopancreatic malignancy: role of ultrasound. Ann Oncol 1999; 10 (Suppl 4):20–4.

62. Gerhards MF, den Hartog D, Rauws EA et al. Palliative treatment in patients with unresectable hilar cholangiocarcinoma: results of endoscopic drainage in patients with type III and IV hilar cholangiocarcinoma. Eur J Surg 2001; 167:274–80.

63. Soulez G, Therasse E, Oliva VL et al. Left hepaticogastrostomy for biliary obstruction: long-term results. Radiology 1997; 204:780–6.

64. Inabnet WB, Deziel DJ. Laparoscopic liver biopsy in patients with coagulopathy, portal hypertension, and ascites. Am J Surg 1995; 61:603–6.

65. Babineau TJ, Lewis WD, Jenkins RL et al. Role of staging laparoscopy in the treatment of hepatic malignancy. Am J Surg 1994; 167:151–4.

66. John TG, Greig JD, Crosbie JL et al. Superior staging of liver tumors with laparoscopy and laparoscopic ultrasound. Ann Surg 1994; 220:711–9.

67. Foley EF, Kolecki RV, Schirmer BD. The accuracy of laparoscopic ultrasound in the detection of colorectal cancer liver metastases. Am J Surg 1998; 176:262–4.

68. Cuesta MA, Meijer S, Borgstein PJ et al. Laparoscopic ultrasonography for hepatobiliary and pancreatic malignancy. Br J Surg 1993; 80:1571–4.

69. de Castro SM, Tilleman EH, Busch OR et al. Diagnostic laparoscopy for primary and secondary liver malignancies: impact of improved imaging and changed criteria for resection. Ann Surg Oncol 2004; 11:522–9.

Authors' study of 84 consecutive patients over a six-year period demonstrating a greater role for laparoscopic staging of primary hepatic malignancy.

70. Lo CM, Lai EC, Liu CL et al. Laparoscopy and laparoscopic ultrasonography avoid exploratory laparotomy in patients with hepatocellular carcinoma. Ann Surg 1998; 227:527–32.

71. Ido K, Nakazawa Y, Isoda N et al. The role of laparoscopic US and laparoscopic US-guided aspiration biopsy in the diagnosis of multicentric hepatocellular carcinoma. Gastrointest Endosc 1999; 50:523–6.

72. Montorsi M, Santambrogio R, Bianchi P et al. Laparoscopy with laparoscopic ultrasound for pretreatment staging of hepatocellular carcinoma: a prospective study. J Gastrointest Surg 2001; 5:312–5.

73. Foroutani A, Garland AM, Berber E et al. Laparoscopic ultrasound vs triphasic computed tomography for detecting liver tumors. Arch Surg 2000; 135:933–8.

These authors conclude that laparoscopic ultrasonography was superior to triphasic CT imaging at detecting hepatic tumours.

74. Roh MS. Increasing the number of patients undergoing resection of colorectal liver metastases. Ann Surg Oncol 2000; 7:634–5.

75. Gholghesaei M, van Muiswinkel JM, Kuiper JM et al. Value of laparoscopy and laparoscopic ultrasonography in determining resectability of colorectal hepatic metastases. HPB 2003; 5:100–4.

76. Milsom JW, Jerby BL, Kessler H et al. Prospective, blinded comparison of laparoscopic ultrasonography vs. contrast-enhanced computerized tomography for liver assessment in patients undergoing colorectal carcinoma surgery. Dis Colon Rectum 2000; 43:44–9.

77. Rahusen FD, Cuesta MA, Borgstein PJ et al. Selection of patients for resection of colorectal metastases to the liver using diagnostic laparoscopy and laparoscopic ultrasonography. Ann Surg 1999; 230:31–7.

78. Jarnagin WR, Bodniewicz J, Dougherty E et al. A prospective analysis of staging laparoscopy in patients with primary and secondary hepatobiliary malignancies. J Gastrointest Surg 2000; 4:34–43.

79. Metcalfe MS, Close JS, Iswariah H et al. The value of laparoscopic staging for patients with colorectal metastases. Arch Surg 2003; 138:770–2.

80. Jarnagin WR, Conlon K, Bodniewicz J et al. A clinical scoring system predicts the yield of diagnostic laparoscopy in patients with potentially resectable hepatic colorectal metastases. Cancer 2001; 91:1121–8.

A scoring system that would have reduced the need for laparoscopy in 57 of 1103 patients being assessed for resection.

81. D'Angelica M, Jarnagin W, Dematteo R et al. Staging laparoscopy for potentially resectable non-colorectal, nonneuroendocrine liver metastases. Ann Surg Oncol 2002; 9:204–9.

82. Cherqui D. Laparoscopic liver resection. Br J Surg 2003; 90:644–6.

83. Gigot JF, Glineur D, Santiago AJ et al. Laparoscopic liver resection for malignant liver tumors: preliminary results of a multicenter European study. Ann Surg 2002; 236:90–7.

84. Curley SA. Radiofrequency ablation of malignant liver tumors. Ann Surg Oncol 2003; 10:338–47.

85. Topal B, Aerts R, Penninckx F. Laparoscopic radiofrequency ablation of unresectable liver malignancies: feasibility and clinical outcome. Surg Laparosc Endosc Percutan Tech 2003; 13:11–5.

86. Warshaw AL. Implications of peritoneal cytology for staging of early pancreatic cancer. Am J Surg 1991; 161:26–9.

87. Boku T, Nakane Y, Minoura T et al. Prognostic significance of serosal invasion and free intra-peritoneal cancer cells in gastric cancer. Br J Surg 1990; 77:436–9.

88. Van Dijkum EJ, Sturm PD, de Wit LT et al. Cytology of peritoneal lavage performed during staging laparoscopy for gastrointestinal malignancies: is it useful? Ann Surg 1998; 228:728–33.

Of 236 patients examined only 7 (3%) yielded positive cytology.

89. Lei S, Kini J, Kim K et al. Pancreatic cancer. Cytologic study of peritoneal washings. Arch Surg 1994; 129:639–42.

90. Fernandez-del Castillo CL, Warshaw AL. Pancreatic cancer. Laparoscopic staging and peritoneal cytology. Surg Oncol Clin N Am 1998; 7:135–42.

91. Nakao A, Oshima K, Takeda S et al. Peritoneal washings cytology combined with immunocyto-chemical staining in pancreatic cancer. Hepato-gastroenterology 1999; 46:2974–7.

92. Jimenez RE, Warshaw AL, Fernandez-del Castillo C. Laparoscopy and peritoneal cytology in the staging of pancreatic cancer. J Hepatobiliary Pancreat Surg 2000; 7:15–20.

93. Konishi M, Kinoshita T, Nakagohri T et al. Prognostic value of cytologic examination of peritoneal washings in pancreatic cancer. Arch Surg 2002; 137:475–80.

94. Fong Y, Fortner J, Sun RL et al. Clinical score for predicting recurrence after hepatic resection for metastatic colorectal cancer: analysis of 1001 consecutive cases. Ann Surg 1999; 230:309–18.

Three

Benign liver lesions

Rowan W. Parks and
O. James Garden

INTRODUCTION

Benign lesions of the liver are not uncommon and may be difficult to differentiate from primary and secondary hepatic tumours. Solid lesions may be identified as an incidental finding when radiological investigation is undertaken for unrelated intra-abdominal disease. Similarly, such lesions may be identified when coexistent hepatic pathology is present, and give rise to problems of diagnosis and management. Although these lesions may be of congenital origin, most are of unknown aetiology. They generally do not give rise to any symptoms but, since they are often slow growing, they may produce symptoms caused by mass effect. Less commonly, such lesions may give rise to acute symptoms because of necrosis, thrombosis, haemorrhage or rupture.

Routine liver function tests are invariably within normal limits in patients with benign hepatic pathology and are therefore of value in guiding the clinician towards a diagnosis of benign disease. Nonetheless, complications such as secondary haemorrhage and necrosis may be associated with increases in serum transaminase levels. Elevation in tumour markers such as carcinoembryonic antigen (CEA) or alpha-fetoprotein (AFP) and the development of paraneoplastic syndromes such as erythrocytosis, hyperglycaemia and hypercalcaemia are rarely observed with such benign pathology.

Characterisation of hepatic lesions is provided by imaging tests of the liver. Ultrasonography (US) and computed tomography (CT) are the cornerstones of diagnosis and often complement one another. More recently, magnetic resonance imaging (MRI) and positron emission tomography (PET) have shown promising results in the imaging of hepatic lesions. Abdominal ultrasonography will differentiate cystic forms from solid lesions, whereas CT using intravenous contrast and delayed imaging may detect the number and size of the lesions. Although hepatic angiography has been used in the past, it is not employed routinely in modern clinical practice to provide a specific diagnosis. Laparoscopy is used increasingly to allow direct visualisation of liver lesions and can be combined with laparoscopic ultrasonography to provide high-resolution images.

None of these tests will provide definitive histological diagnosis but the role of needle biopsy or aspiration of suspected hepatic lesions remains much debated. It is generally accepted that a biopsy is absolutely contraindicated for patients with suspected haemangioma, haemangioendothelioma and cysts suspected of being echinococcal in origin. In addition, it may be dangerous in patients with suspected hypervascular solid tumours to undertake either needle biopsy or fine-needle aspiration cytology. Such invasive investigation may be associated with haemorrhage, sampling error, misdiagnosis and needle-tract tumour seeding.

Tissue from a haemangioma may resemble fibrosis, and focal nodular hyperplasia may resemble cirrhosis. Needle samples of hepatic adenoma may be interpreted as normal tissue and may be difficult to differentiate from hepatocellular carcinoma. Percutaneous biopsy should only be performed in those patients who are not considered candidates for surgical intervention and only where the results of biopsy might influence further management. Despite extensive radiological imaging in an attempt to characterise a lesion, the final diagnosis may not be made until the lesion has been resected and the pathologist can undertake definitive examination of the resected tissue.

It is therefore apparent that the general surgeon should be thoroughly familiar with the gross appearance, clinical significance and natural history of these benign lesions as the treatment strategy may vary from simple observation (of focal nodular hyperplasia) to complex radical hepatic resection (of hepatocellular adenoma). Most symptomatic benign liver lesions are excised; however, hepatic resection, if performed without the proper indications, can prove hazardous.

CLASSIFICATION

Although a variety of benign liver tumours have been described, by far the majority are sufficiently rare that they can easily be labelled medical curiosities. A detailed description of these various lesions is beyond the scope of the current text but various benign pathologies, based on the cell of origin, are listed in **Box 3.1**. The majority of benign hepatic lesions encountered in clinical practice include hepatic cyst, haemangioma, liver cell adenoma, focal nodular hyperplasia and bile duct hamartoma. For completeness, a brief resume is provided of less common and miscellaneous lesions, including hepatic abscess, amoebic abscess and hydatid cyst, since these may give rise to diagnostic and management dilemmas.

HAEMANGIOMAS

Haemangiomas are the most common benign hepatic tumours of mesenchymal origin. Small capillary haemangiomas of the liver are more common than the larger cavernous haemangiomas and are

Box 3.1 • Classification of benign tumours of the liver

Epithelial tumours		

Hepatocellular:
  Nodular transformation
  Focal nodular hyperplasia
  Hepatocellular adenoma		

Cholangiocellular:
  Bile duct adenoma
  Biliary cystadenoma		

Mesenchymal tumours		

Tumours of adipose tissue:
  lipoma
  myelolipoma
  angiomyolipoma		

Tumours of muscle tissue: leiomyoma		
Tumours of blood vessels: infantile haemangioendothelioma		

haemangioma:
  hereditary haemorrhagic telangiectasia
  peliosis hepatis		

Tumours of mesothelial tissue: benign mesothelioma		
Mixed mesenchymal and epithelial tumours		
Mesenchymal hamartoma		
Benign teratoma		
Miscellaneous		
Adrenal rest tumour		
Pancreatic heterotopia		
Inflammatory pseudotumour		

From Ishak KG, Goodman ZD. Benign tumours of the liver. In: Berk JE (ed.) Bockus Gastroenterology, 4th edn. Philadelphia: WB Saunders, 1985.

often multiple. Small lesions are almost always asymptomatic and are usually an incidental finding; however, they may give rise to diagnostic difficulty in patients undergoing investigation for other hepatic pathology. Once accurate diagnosis has been made no further therapy is needed. Haemangiomas are probably of congenital origin rather than neoplastic and they do not undergo malignant transformation. The incidence of cavernous haemangioma of the liver in autopsy series varies considerably but has been reported to be as high as 8%. These lesions are considered the second most common hepatic tumour in the USA, exceeded only by hepatic metastases.[1] With the more widespread use of sensitive imaging studies of the upper abdomen, the identification of cavernous haemangiomas as an incidental finding will undoubtedly be more common. Cavernous haemangiomas may reach an enormous size, and lesions weighing up to 6 kg are well documented. Giant haemangiomas are defined as those 4 cm in diameter or greater.[2] Such haemangiomas are usually solitary, but multiple lesions have been described in about 10% of cases.[1] They may be associated with similar lesions in the skin and other organs. Lesions are usually evenly distributed throughout the liver and within the liver substance but large lesions situated peripherally may form a pedicle.

Pathology

Cavernous haemangiomas occur in all age groups but are seen most frequently in patients in the third to fifth decades of life. They are more common and more likely to become clinically manifest at a younger age in women, are more common with increasing parity, and may enlarge during pregnancy.[3-5] This indicates a possible role of female sex hormones in the development of hepatic haemangiomas, although an association with the oral contraceptive pill has not been proven. The aetiology of liver haemangiomas is still unclear but it is considered that they represent benign congenital hamartomas. These lesions appear to grow by progressive ectasia rather than hyperplasia or hypertrophy. At operation they appear as well-circumscribed, reddish-purple, hypervascular lesions, which may be multilobulated or have a smooth surface. There is a dissectable plane between the lesion and the normal liver parenchyma. When sectioned, the lesion will partially collapse due to the escape of blood, and it has a honeycombed cut surface. There may be gross evidence of thrombosis, fibrosis or calcification. Microscopically, haemangiomas are composed of cystically dilated vascular spaces, lined by endothelial cells and separated by fibrous septa of varying thickness. There is usually a clear plane between haemangioma and normal liver tissue as these lesions are usually encapsulated by a rim of fibrous tissue.

Clinical presentation

Most haemangiomas are asymptomatic until they exceed a diameter of 10 cm. Symptoms are often non-specific and include vague abdominal pain, abdominal fullness, early satiety, nausea, vomiting or fever. Rare presentations include obstructive jaundice, biliary colic, gastric outlet obstruction and spontaneous rupture. Although abdominal pain or discomfort is the most frequent indication for removing a liver haemangioma, it must be remembered that associated pathology may coexist and be the cause of the symptoms. Farges et al.[6] reported that 42% of the patients in their series had associated disorders, such as gallbladder disease, liver cysts, gastroduodenal ulcers or a hiatus hernia. The difficulty of attributing symptoms to the haemangioma is evidenced by the occasional persistence of symptoms after resection.[7]

Pain related to an uncomplicated haemangioma is most probably due to stretching or inflammation of Glisson's capsule. Occasionally, large lesions located in the left lobe of the liver may cause pressure effects on adjacent structures with resulting symptoms. Infarction or necrosis may account for the sudden onset of pain in some patients. Intra-abdominal haemorrhage due to spontaneous or traumatic rupture of haemangioma is a very rare complication.[5] A review of the literature published up to 1991 included only 28 reports of spontaneous, life-threatening haemorrhage due to liver haemangiomas, a minimal figure considering the prevalence of the tumour.[8] Thrombocytopenia and hypofibrinogenaemia have also been associated with cavernous haemangiomas of the liver (Kasabach–Merritt syndrome), and this effect may be related to consumption of coagulation factors.[1]

When a large haemangioma is present, the liver edge or a non-tender mass that descends with inspiration may be palpable. It is difficult to differentiate the consistency of a haemangioma from normal liver through the abdominal wall unless it has calcified or undergone thrombosis or fibrosis. Occasionally, a bruit is heard over a haemangioma, but this is a relatively non-specific finding. Liver function tests are normal in the patient presenting without complication.

Such lesions are generally hyperechoic on ultrasound examination (**Fig. 3.1**). Farges et al.[6] found

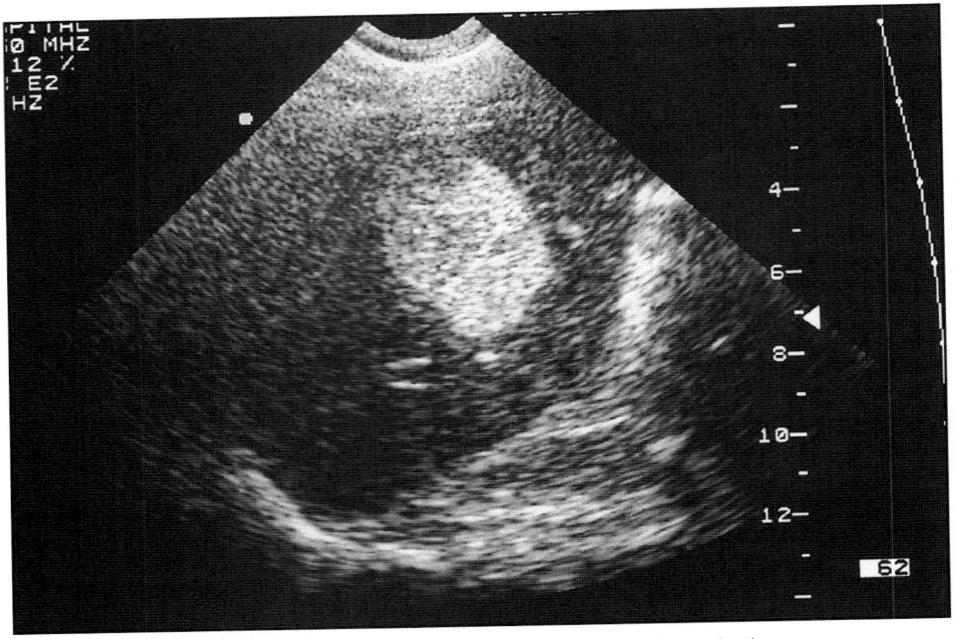

Figure 3.1 • Hyperechoic appearance of haemangioma on ultrasound examination.

the diagnosis to be established by ultrasonography alone in 80% of patients with haemangiomas smaller than 6 cm. However, this investigation alone cannot differentiate a haemangioma from hepato-cellular carcinoma, liver cell adenoma, focal nodular hyperplasia, or a solitary metastasis. CT has proven most useful in the diagnosis of haemangiomas.[9] Prior to intravenous contrast infusion, CT scan shows the haemangioma to consist of a well-demarcated hypodense mass. After the intravenous injection of contrast medium, serial scans will reveal a zone of progressive enhancement periph-erally that varies in thickness and often demon-strates an irregular margin (**Fig. 3.2**). The centre of the haemangioma remains hypodense and the overall lesion size does not change. Selective hepatic angiography shows a characteristic pattern consist-ing of normal-sized hepatic arteries without neo-vascularity or 'corkscrewing'. Typically there is rapid filling of the large blood-filled spaces of the haemangioma with contrast medium, producing the so-called 'cottonwool' appearance surrounding the feeding hepatic arteries. The CT findings are often sufficiently characteristic that the role for angiography in the diagnosis of cavernous haeman-

giomas is limited (**Fig. 3.3**).[9] Over the past decade MRI has emerged as a highly accurate technique for diagnosing and characterising liver haemangioma, with a reported 90% sensitivity, 95% specificity and 93% accuracy[10,11] (**Fig. 3.4**). Haemangiomas are typically very bright (light bulb sign) on T2-weighted images and show peripheral nodular enhancement on dynamic gadolinium-enhanced T1-weighted images.[12] Single-photon emisson CT (SPECT) using technetium-99m-labelled red blood cells has been shown to increase the spatial resolution of planar scintigraphy and has been shown to have a sensitivity and accuracy close to that of MRI.[13] In practice, a combination of these diagnostic modalities is preferred. Laparoscopy can also be of value[14] for lesions situated superficially where they can be recognised on gross examination and by gentle palpation, which reveals character-istic compressibility. In addition, this technique can be effectively combined with laparoscopic contact ultrasonography, which significantly adds to the diagnostic potential of laparoscopy alone.[15]

Needle biopsy of vascular liver lesions should not be performed. Diagnostic uncertainty is seldom a problem with cavernous haemangiomas, except in

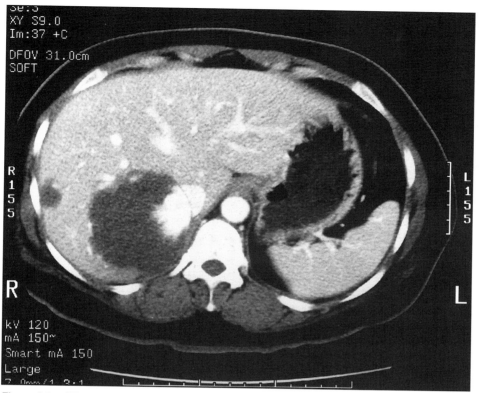

Figure 3.2 • CT scan demonstrating peripheral enhancement of a haemangioma after intravenous injection of contrast material.

lesions not large enough to show cavernous characteristics, which may necessitate diagnostic removal.

Management

A wide range of management strategies from observation to resection have been advocated for such lesions. The therapeutic modalities of hepatic arterial ligation, radiation therapy and corticosteroids have also been reported with limited success. Clearly, for patients in whom small lesions (i.e. <4 cm) have been detected as an incidental finding, simple reassurance should be given. For larger cavernous haemangiomas, consideration should be given to weighing the risk of operation against the natural history of untreated lesions. In a study assessing the natural history, Trastek et al.[5] followed-up 34 untreated patients who were observed for a maximum of 15 years. No patient had a lesion that bled, none reported abdominal

symptoms, and no patient had compromise of quality of life. A further report from the same group, when the observation period had been extended to 21 years (mean follow-up of 12.5 years), reported two patients with large symptomatic lesions of questionable resectability at initial presentation who remained symptomatic but with little documented growth of the haemangioma. The remainder were asymptomatic and there was no instance of rupture.[16] Two more recent longitudinal studies have supported the accepted view that asymptomatic giant haemangiomas of the liver can be managed safely by observation.[17,18]

Nichols et al.[16] reported the results of resection of cavernous haemangiomas in 41 patients. There were no operative deaths and the single postoperative complication was a wound infection.

Weimann et al.[19] reported a series of 69 patients who underwent surgery for liver haemangiomas; there were no postoperative deaths and the

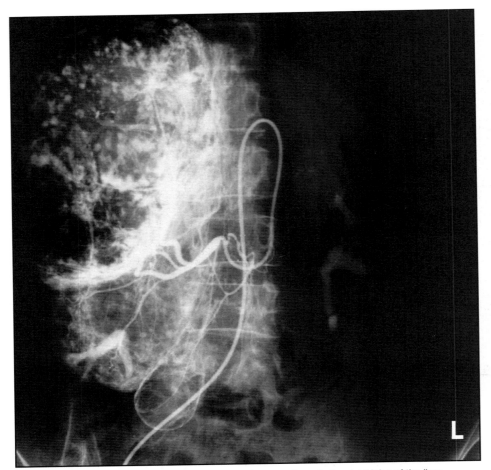

Figure 3.3 • Angiographic appearances of a giant haemangioma in the right lobe of the liver.

morbidity rate was 19%. Also in this series were 104 patients with haemangioma and 53 patients with focal nodular hyperplasia who were observed for a median of 32 months (range 7–132 months). There was no evidence of malignant transformation or tumour rupture in any of these patients. Therefore, safe resection of cavernous haemangiomas is possible; however, there is no evidence that asymptomatic patients should undergo resection since the risk of rupture is minimal.[6,20]

The indications for resection are therefore symptomatic lesions in patients with an acceptable surgical risk and cases where the nature of the lesion is not established despite preoperative investigation.

When treatment is indicated, surgical excision provides the only effective therapy. Reports of the effectiveness of hepatic arterial ligation are anecdotal. Arterial ligation or embolisation may, however, be considered for the temporary control of haemorrhage in exceptional circumstances in order to allow time for transfer of a patient for definitive management in a specialist centre. The benefits of radiation therapy in the treatment of cavernous haemangiomas have not been well documented and are inconsistent. Similarly, the effectiveness of corticosteroids in the treatment of haemangiomas is not well documented. It is possible that the success of non-resectional therapy, which has been ascribed to hepatic arterial ligation, radiation or steroids, may well be largely due to the naturally occurring spontaneous involution of these lesions.

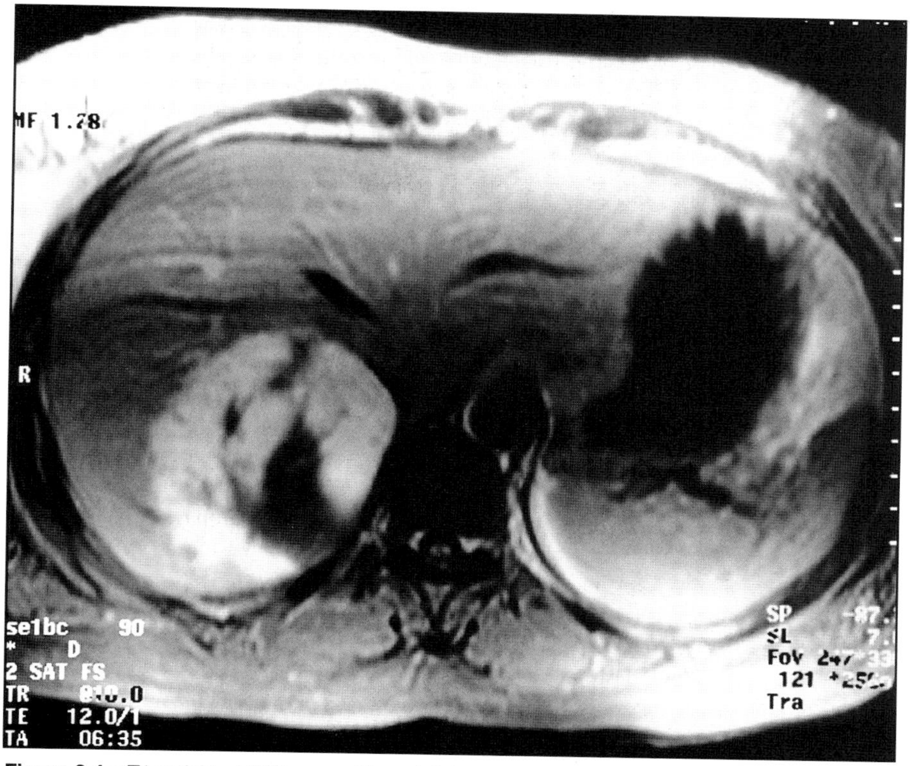

Figure 3.4 • T1 weighted MRI scan with gadolinium demonstrating the same haemangioma as in **Fig. 3.2**.

The choice of excision requires consideration of the size and anatomical location of the lesion. Haemangiomas can often be enucleated[21] to avoid loss of functional liver parenchyma, diminish blood loss and minimise postoperative bile leakage, although in some cases it may be wiser and safer to perform a formal anatomical liver resection. At enucleation, a plane between the lesion and the liver is easily found and this can be developed by blunt dissection. This can be facilitated by the use of the Cavitron ultrasonic surgical aspiration system (CUSA™) with concomitant control of the inflow vessels. Laparoscopic resection of liver haemangioma has been reported recently,[22] and orthotopic liver transplantation has also been used successfully to treat symptomatic patients with technically unresectable complicated giant haemangioma.[23]

Liver haemangioma rarely causes complications and resection should only be considered for symptomatic lesions.

LIVER CELL ADENOMA

Although liver cell adenoma requires differentiation from any solid hepatic lesion, it is often considered alongside focal nodular hyperplasia.[24]

Hepatic adenomas arise in otherwise normal liver and present as a focal abnormality or mass. The true prevalence of the disease is difficult to assess but 90% develop in women in the third to fifth decades of life.[25,26] These tumours were rarely reported before 1960, but their apparent increase in incidence since then corresponded with the introduction of oral contraceptives in the early 1960s. The causal relationship between liver cell adenoma and oral contraceptives was first suggested by Baum et al.[27] in 1973, and since then the oral ingestion of oestrogen has been strongly implicated in the pathogenesis of these tumours.[28] Ninety percent of patients with liver cell adenomas have used oral contraceptives and the annual incidence among oral contraceptive users has been reported to be 3–4 per

100 000 if the contraceptives are taken for more than 2 years. The risk of developing a liver cell adenoma increases with the dose and duration of use of the contraceptive preparation.[25] Furthermore, pregnancy has been associated with increased symptoms and an increased risk of complications in patients with liver cell adenomas.[25,29] The introduction of low-oestrogen-containing contraceptive preparations may result in a reduction in incidence, although adenomas are also associated with non-contraceptive oestrogen use, androgenic steroid use, diabetes, glycogen storage disease, galactosaemia and iron overload. This association implicates altered carbohydrate metabolism in the formation of liver cell adenomas.[30]

Pathology

Liver cell adenomas are usually solitary, round and occasionally encapsulated. Lesions are soft and smooth surfaced, but occasionally may be pedunculated. The cut surface has a pale-yellow fleshy appearance unless haemorrhage and necrosis produce discoloration. They are sharply demarcated from normal liver, although no fibrous capsule is present. Approximately 12–30% of these tumours are multiple, and if more than ten adenomas are present the condition is regarded as liver adenomatosis.[31] Liver adenomatosis may be a separate pathological entity from isolated liver cell adenoma as men and women are equally affected and there is usually no history of oral contraceptive usage.

Microscopically, the diagnosis is based on the findings of uniform masses of benign-appearing hepatocytes without ducts or portal triads. The hepatocytes appear paler than normal because of increased glycogen or fat content. Venous lakes (peliosis hepatis) are often seen.

There is debate as to whether liver cell adenomas are precancerous. Rooks et al.[25] reported the finding of hepatocellular carcinoma 5 years after resection of a liver cell adenoma, and other authors have recognised unequivocal areas of hepatocellular carcinoma adjacent to or within liver cell adenomas.[26,32,33] Also reported is the development of hepatocellular carcinoma several years after diagnosis of biopsy-proven benign liver cell adenoma.[30,34,35] These reports suggest that liver cell adenoma may be precancerous; however, Tao[36] concluded on histological grounds that liver cell adenoma was not a premalignant lesion, but that liver cell dysplasia was an irreversible premalignant condition that would progress to cancer.

Clinical presentation

Liver cell adenomas frequently present with abdominal pain caused by haemorrhage into the tumour or adjacent liver. A proportion of patients present acutely with severe abdominal pain due to intraperitoneal rupture and haemoperitoneum, which may be associated with hypovolaemic shock. Up to one-third of patients sense the presence of an abdominal mass. The remainder of adenomas are discovered incidentally at autopsy, laparotomy or during radiological assessment for another problem.

Although the clinical presentation may be suggestive of liver cell adenoma, definitive preoperative diagnosis may be difficult. Liver function tests are generally only abnormal in patients with associated tumour necrosis or haemorrhage. Anaemia may be present because of the tendency of these tumours to bleed. Ultrasound scan can detect small adenomas, which characteristically display a lesion of mixed echoity and heterogeneous texture. CT may show evidence of recent haemorrhage or necrosis. Lesions are generally hypodense prior to infusion of contrast medium and demonstrate a wide range of densities after intravenous contrast administration (**Fig. 3.5**). Liver cell adenomas often appear as well-demarcated, fat-containing or haemorrhagic lesions on MRI. If undertaken, selective visceral angiography shows a hypervascular tumour with irregular areas of hypovascularity secondary to haemorrhage or necrosis. Liver cell adenomas generally exhibit a peripheral blood supply. In young females, the differential diagnosis is normally with that of focal nodular hyperplasia. An isotope scan may be helpful in pointing towards a diagnosis of adenoma, which does not take up any isotope and therefore appears as a filling defect. Conventional radiological imaging may not be able to differentiate between liver cell adenoma and hepatocellular carcinoma; however, promising results have been reported with the use of positron emission tomography (PET) using fluorodeoxyglucose (FDG) to differentiate benign from malignant lesions.[37]

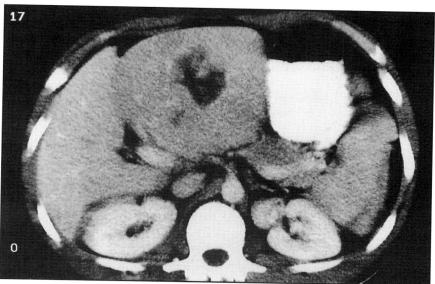

Figure 3.5 • CT scan of a liver cell adenoma.

Our own experience has shown that percutaneous needle biopsy or fine-needle aspiration cytology undertaken prior to referral is often misleading. Biopsy of these vascular tumours risks precipitating haemorrhage, and even an experienced histopathologist may experience difficulty in differentiating between liver cell adenoma and a well-differentiated hepatocellular carcinoma.

Management

In the symptomatic patient, surgical intervention will be required. A minority of patients will present with intraperitoneal bleeding, the cause of which might only be identified at laparotomy. Most deaths from liver cell adenomas are secondary to haemorrhage, with intraperitoneal bleeding carrying a 20% mortality rate in one series.[25] Hepatic arterial embolisation or packing might be considered to facilitate transfer of the patient to a specialist centre. Definitive control of bleeding is best achieved by formal hepatic resection. In some patients, haemorrhage may be contained within the liver or subcapsularly. If the patient remains haemodynamically stable, it may be prudent to defer elective surgical intervention to enable resolution of the haematoma, thereby enabling a more limited hepatic resection (Fig. 3.6).

For the asymptomatic patient, surgical intervention should still be considered. Several case reports document regression of liver cell tumours following cessation of oral contraceptives,[38,39] although this is not a consistent finding, and development of hepatocellular carcinoma in the site of adenoma regression has been reported.[34] Non-operative discrimination between liver cell adenoma and hepatocellular carcinoma is difficult. Furthermore, liver cell adenomas can harbour foci of tumour and may be premalignant lesions. They more commonly produce symptoms and may result in life-threatening haemorrhage. Therefore, hepatic resection should be considered in all patients with a suspected liver cell adenoma; however, each case must be individually evaluated and the risk of surgery weighed against the potential for future morbidity or mortality. Orthotopic liver transplantation has been described for unresectable benign liver tumours with severe symptoms and for patients with multiple adenomas.[19,40]

FOCAL NODULAR HYPERPLASIA

Focal nodular hyperplasia (FNH) is often difficult to differentiate from liver cell adenoma and for this

(a)

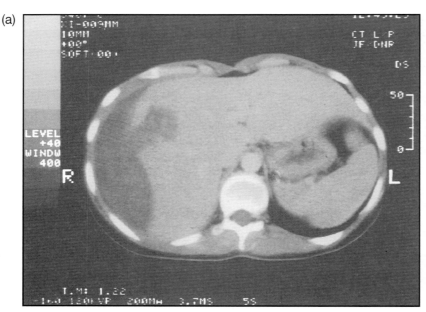

(b)

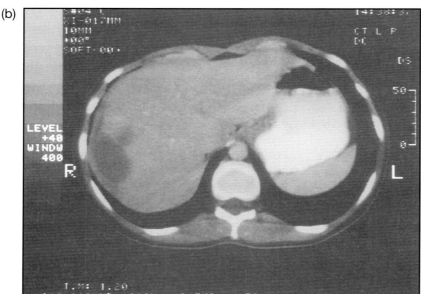

Figure 3.6 • **(a)** CT scan showing extensive subcapsular haematoma resulting from spontaneous haemorrhage into the liver. **(b)** CT scan taken two months later showing a reduction in the size of the haematoma. Contrast is now present within a small adenoma lying adjacent to the haematoma.

reason represents a substantial proportion of benign lesions submitted to hepatic resection (**Table 3.1**). The incidence of focal nodular hyperplasia has been increasing, although this is more likely to be related to improvements in abdominal imaging rather than a true increase in incidence. Many lesions are still found incidentally at laparotomy or autopsy. About 90% of cases occur in women, primarily in the second and third decades, although the condition may also afflict older women and a small number of men and children. The incidence of focal nodular hyperplasia does not appear to have increased since the introduction of oral contraceptives; however, some investigators have suggested that oral contraceptives may foster growth or increased vascularity of these lesions, and they have

Table 3.1 • Indications for 108 hepatic resections for benign disease in the Hepatobiliary Unit, Royal Infirmary, Edinburgh (October 1988–June 2003)

Aetiology	Number of patients
Cystic disease	29
Focal nodular hyperplasia	16
Haemangioma	15
Liver cell adenoma	10
Primary sclerosing cholangitis	7
Cystadenoma	6
Hepatic pseudotumour	6
Trauma	5
Liver abscess	5
Benign bile duct stricture	3
Intrahepatic calculi	2
Bile duct injury	2
Intrahepatic leiomyoma	1
Benign schwannoma	1
TOTAL	108

been implicated in the few cases that present with haemorrhage.

Pathology

Focal nodular hyperplasia has many similarities to liver cell adenoma and distinguishing between the two may be difficult. FNH consists of a firm lobulated localised lesion in an otherwise normal liver. These nodules are generally several centimetres in size and occasionally can grow much larger. Lesions are well circumscribed but have no capsule. On sectioning, there is generally a central scar with fibrous radiations, which account for the nodular and sometimes umbilicated appearance. Lesions are usually similar or slightly lighter in colour than adjacent normal hepatic parenchyma. Focal nodular hyperplasia is multifocal in up to 20% of cases and may coexist with haemangiomas in 5–10% of patients.[1]

Microscopically, FNH looks similar to cirrhosis, with regenerating nodules and connective tissue septa. The lesions consist of many normal hepatic cells mixed with bile ducts or ductules and divided by fibrous septa. The septa contain numerous bile ducts and a moderate, predominantly lymphocytic, infiltration, and there is usually some evidence of mild cholestasis.

Clinical features

FNH is a benign process that rarely causes symptoms but the main difficulty lies in differentiating this process from other hepatic lesions. Less than 10% of patients with FNH have symptoms, the most common being mild, vague right upper quadrant abdominal pain. Acute symptoms due to haemorrhage are exceptional.

Most imaging techniques used in isolation cannot reliably establish the diagnosis of FNH. Therefore, a combination of imaging modalities is preferred.[41] The appearances on ultrasound and CT are non-specific and on occasions the lesion may not be visualised (**Fig. 3.7**). Cholescintigraphy combined with either ultrasound or CT has been shown to have an 82% sensitivity and 97% specificity for diagnosing focal nodular hyperplasia.[19] A more invasive investigation, such as arteriography, is highly sensitive but lacks specificity and is now used infrequently for the diagnosis of focal nodular hyperplasia. The classical appearance on arteriography is that of a sharply delineated hypervascular mass with a single central artery and centrifugal filling of the vessels (spoke-wheel pattern). MRI may aid in diagnosis of focal nodular hyperplasia, and Cherqui et al. reported a 70% sensitivity and 98% specificity for MRI in detecting focal nodular hyperplasia.[42]

Management

Treatment of a patient with FNH depends essentially on the certainty of the diagnosis. In asymptomatic patients with the typical features of FNH unequivocally demonstrated by one or more radiological investigations, no further treatment is required. However, a malignant tumour will be found in up to 6% of patients with an undetermined, presumed benign lesion.[43]

Many surgeons believe that patients should be submitted to open or laparoscopic biopsy because of the difficulty in establishing a diagnosis pre-operatively and because of the dangers of needle

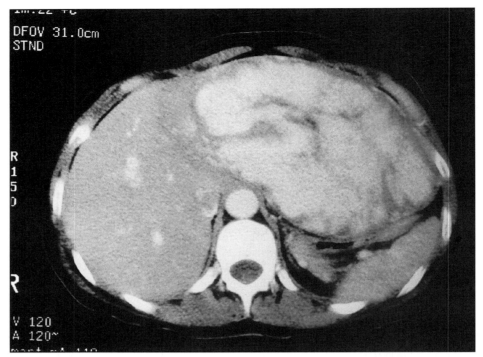

Figure 3.7 • CT scan demonstrating a large vascular lesion in the left lobe of the liver. Following resection, histopathology confirmed this to be a large area of focal nodular hyperplasia.

biopsy. Enucleation or resection should be undertaken if it can be performed with minimal morbidity for any lesion that is increasing in size, bleeding or unequivocally symptomatic.

Recent data on the natural history of FNH have been gathered by Kerlin et al.[26] Of 41 patients studied, 11 had lesions found incidentally at autopsy. Sixteen patients had open surgical biopsies of clinically apparent lesions, with the majority of the lesions left in situ. These patients were observed for up to 15 years, during which time none of the lesions bled or increased in size. Although it could be claimed that such lesions are best managed conservatively, a balanced approach is best adopted, with surgical excision being undertaken if this can be undertaken with minimal morbidity and mortality. Observation in selected patients may be considered if there is a significant risk of morbidity with surgical intervention.

Differentiation of adenoma and focal nodular hyperplasia may be difficult and resection of adenoma is considered appropriate because of the risk of misdiagnosis and malignant transformation.

NODULAR REGENERATIVE HYPERPLASIA (MACROREGENERATIVE NODULES)

This is a benign proliferative process in which the normal hepatic architecture is entirely replaced by diffuse regenerative nodules of hepatocytes. Autopsy reports suggest the prevalence of nodular regenerative hyperplasia (NRH) is approximately 2%. It predominantly occurs in older patients and is often associated with lymphoproliferative and rheumatological diseases or develops after organ transplantation.

The majority of patients are asymptomatic, are diagnosed incidentally and require no further treatment.[44] The most common physical findings are splenomegaly and hepatomegaly. A small percentage of patients may develop portal hypertension due to compression of intrahepatic portal radicles by the regenerating nodules, and present with variceal bleeding or ascites. Rarely, patients may develop hepatic failure and in some instances have undergone liver transplantation. Liver function tests are usually normal or slightly elevated, and the radiological features are relatively non-specific. The diagnosis of NRH is confirmed on the gross and histological findings of the liver. Macroscopically, the hepatic parenchyma is entirely replaced by nodules varying in size from 0.1 to 4 cm. The histological findings of NRH are regenerating hepatocytes separated by atrophic parenchyma, curvilinear compression of the central lobule, and absence of fibrous tissue or bands of scar tissue between the nodules. NRH may be suspected when a patient presents with symptoms of portal hypertension and a liver biopsy that fails to show cirrhosis or is interpreted as being normal. Confirmation may require open or laparoscopic liver biopsy. Liver cell dysplasia is a common finding in NRH and there are a small number of case reports of hepatocellular carcinoma developing in livers with NRH, leading some authors to suggest that NRH may represent a premalignant condition in some patients.

BILE DUCT ADENOMA (BILE DUCT HAMARTOMA)

Surgeons should be aware of bile duct adenomas since they are common and may be mistaken at operation as liver metastases. They do not manifest clinically but are incidental findings at laparotomy or autopsy.[45] Bile duct adenomas rarely exceed 1 cm in diameter and appear as raised greyish-white areas on the liver capsule. Histologically, they are composed of a mass of mature bile ducts surrounded by fibrous stroma, which blends indistinctly into the adjacent liver. They require to be distinguished from the nests of hyperplastic bile ducts that occur in focal nodular hyperplasia and also in undifferentiated adenocarcinomas of the biliary tract type.

The only clinical significance of the bile duct adenoma is its possible confusion at laparoscopy or laparotomy with metastatic carcinoma, cholangiocarcinoma or other focal hepatic lesions. When encountered, excisional biopsy should be performed to confirm the diagnosis.

HEPATIC PSEUDOTUMOURS

Hepatic pseudotumours may be considerable in size and can occur in any age group. These lesions are essentially overgrowths of chronic inflammatory tissue but may be mistaken for other neoplastic lesions of the liver.[46] The aetiology is not known but they may be secondary to thrombosis and infarction of a major vessel, represent a form of immune reaction, or result from resolution of an abscess. They appear as a hypodense lesion on CT, and may be either hyperechoic or hypoechoic on ultrasonography. Arteriography reveals a hypervascular mass. Such pseudotumours may require resection to prevent reactivation of infection. The clinical history and presentation are likely to point towards a diagnosis of pseudotumour.

MISCELLANEOUS BENIGN TUMOURS

Mesenchymal hamartomas are exceptional and probably of congenital origin. Such lesions are, therefore, most commonly described in infants under 12 months,[47] although a few have been described in adults.[48] Although they are entirely benign, hamartomas can compromise the liver and the individual by progressive enlargement and therefore these lesions should be resected. Microscopically, the tumour is characterised by a myxoid background of highly cellular embryonal mesenchyme, throughout which are found random groups of hepatic cells, bile ducts and multiple cysts, which may produce a honeycomb appearance. Recurrence following excision has not been reported.

Primary myxoma in the adult is exceptional.[47] Primary lipomas are rarely described in life but have been identified incidentally at post-mortem.[1] Other solid tumours include leiomyoma, mesothelioma and fibroma.[1] Benign teratoma of the liver has been reported but this generally occurs in children.[1,47]

LIVER ABSCESS

The incidence of pyogenic liver abscess has remained relatively constant over the past century despite earlier diagnosis and treatment of underlying causes and more aggressive antibiotic therapies. In recent years, the decrease in cases resulting from haematogenous spread from infected foci has been mirrored by an increase in cases secondary to hepatobiliary pathology. In almost half the patients reviewed in our own centre over a five-year period, biliary sepsis was the major predisposing factor.[49] In 20%

of patients, the presumed source of infection was from the portal route, but few cases were thought to have arisen from systemic infection. Hepatic abscesses secondary to ascending cholangitis are often multiple due to the distribution of the infecting organism along the biliary ductal system.[50]

Early reports implicated choledocholithiasis as the main causative factor; however, more recent series document malignant biliary obstruction as a more common aetiological factor.[49,51]

Infections within organs drained by the portal vein are dependent on the underlying illness. In the early literature, portal vein pyelophlebitis secondary to appendicitis was often associated with liver abscess formation, whereas diverticulitis, pancreatitis and diffuse peritonitis are now more frequently reported. Haematogenous spread from nongastrointestinal sources accounts for 10–20% of liver abscesses and has been reported most typically in association with bacterial endocarditis, other conditions associated with systemic bacteraemia such as urinary sepsis, pneumonia, osteomyelitis or following intravenous drug abuse. Liver abscesses may also occur due to direct extension into the liver parenchyma from a localised perforation of an adjacent viscus, particularly the gallbladder, colon, stomach or duodenum. In a significant percentage of patients (approximately 15–35%), the aetiology of hepatic abscess remains obscure (cryptogenic abscess) despite extensive clinical and pathological investigation.

Clinical presentation

Patients present with a spectrum of symptoms and signs, the most consistent being fever associated with malaise, anorexia, weight loss and upper abdominal pain. Jaundice is a feature in approximately 50% of cases. Laboratory studies typically reflect a systemic bacterial infection. Commonly reported findings are of leucocytosis, anaemia, hyperbilirubinaemia, hypoalbuminaemia and raised levels of acute-phase proteins. Ultrasonography is invariably diagnostic and will often demonstrate a fluid-filled cavity. There may be a hyperechoic wall, the presence of which is dependent on the chronicity of the abscess. CT may be useful to exclude the presence of other abscesses and to identify a primary source within the abdomen (**Fig. 3.8**). Magnetic resonance

cholangiography should be undertaken in patients with biliary symptoms, obstructive liver function tests or a dilated common bile duct, and can be combined with cross-sectional MRI to identify any hepatic parenchymal abnormality. Barium enema may be indicated to exclude a colonic source of portal pyaemia.

Management

The key to successful management is drainage of the purulent collection combined with the administration of appropriate antibiotic therapy, which is determined by the results of culture of blood and aspirated pus. Although virtually all pathogenic organisms have been identified, enteric organisms predominate. Polymicrobial infection is seen frequently when hepatic abscess is secondary to infection arising from within the drainage area of the portal venous system. Although antibiotic therapy as the sole treatment for hepatic abscess is rarely successful, prolonged systemic antibiotic administration may be the only option for patients with diffuse multiple microabscesses. In general, macroscopic hepatic collections require drainage of the purulent material. Over the past two decades, the introduction and refinement of percutaneous drainage techniques have dramatically altered the management of patients with pyogenic hepatic abscesses. There are no prospective randomised trials comparing non-operative techniques with open surgical drainage. However, percutaneous drainage has become the first-line therapeutic option in most centres for patients with single or multiple liver abscesses.[50,52–55] Abscess communication with the intrahepatic biliary tree does not prevent pyogenic collections being successfully treated by percutaneous techniques, although the period of drainage may be prolonged. The use of percutaneous aspiration combined with systemic antibiotics without drainage has been advocated by some groups but remains a controversial issue.[56,57]

There has been one randomised trial comparing percutaneous catheter drainage with percutaneous needle aspiration.[58] Percutaneous catheter drainage was successful in 100% of patients whereas aspiration was successful in only 60% of patients. However, higher success rates may have been achieved if repeated aspiration had been undertaken.

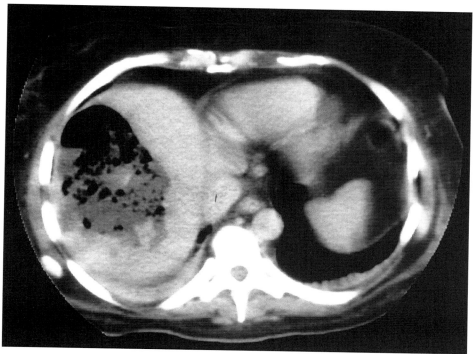

Figure 3.8 • Large liver abscess with air-fluid level in right lobe of liver.

Regular irrigation of drainage catheters reduces the risk of catheter blockage due to necrotic debris. Surgical drainage is usually reserved for patients who have failed percutaneous drainage, those who require surgical management of the underlying problem, and some patients with multiple macroscopic abscesses and others on steroids or with ascites. Liver resection is occasionally required for patients with liver abscess.[59] The indication is usually failed non-operative management, hepatolithiasis, intrahepatic biliary stricture or gross parenchymal destruction.

Effective decompression of the biliary tree is as important as abscess drainage where obstruction of the bile duct has contributed to the development of hepatic abscess. Following successful drainage of the abscess, antibiotic administration should be continued for a prolonged period (3–6 weeks) to assist in the complete eradication of infection.

Pyogenic liver abscess still carries a significant mortality. In our experience, one-third of patients will not survive admission to hospital, although this reflects the high proportion of patients developing hepatic abscess related to underlying malignancy and biliary obstruction.

AMOEBIC ABSCESS

This form of abscess is sufficiently common that it should be considered in the differential diagnosis of hepatic lesions. About 10% of the world's population is chronically infected with *Entamoeba histolytica*, although less than 10% of individuals are symptomatic.

Liver abscess is the most common extraintestinal manifestation of amoebiasis and is reported in 3–10% of affected patients. Males are more commonly affected than females, and the highest incidence is in the 20–50-year-old age group.[60]

The diagnosis is likely to be straightforward in areas where amoebiasis is endemic. It should be recognised, however, that the liver abscess may present many years after previous intestinal infection. Some 75–90% of abscesses are in the right lobe, and involvement of the left lobe usually indicates more advanced disease. Rupture occurs in 2–17% of cases and usually occurs into the peritoneal cavity, but rupture can occur into the pleural cavity, the bronchial tree or the pericardium. Signs and symptoms of amoebic liver abscess are the same as for pyogenic abscess. On ultrasound and CT scanning, the boundaries of the abscess are generally poorly defined (**Fig. 3.9**). Patients with amoebic liver abscess virtually always have serum antiamoebic antibodies, which can be detected by an indirect haemagglutination test or an enzyme-linked immunosorbent assay (ELISA) technique. Percutaneous aspiration produces a sterile and odourless fluid, which is described as having the appearance of 'anchovy paste'. Routine percutaneous aspiration is now regarded as superfluous in the management of amoebic liver abscess unless serology is inconclusive, a therapeutic trial with antiamoebic drugs is deemed inappropriate (as in pregnancy), or rupture is suspected to be imminent.

A preliminary diagnosis can be made on the basis of a dramatic clinical response to metronidazole, which should be commenced empirically in endemic areas.[60]

If clinical symptoms do not resolve within 48–72 hours of treatment, an incorrect diagnosis or a secondary bacterial infection should be suspected. Percutaneous aspiration may be beneficial for patients in whom medical treatment has failed. Percutaneous catheter drainage is indicated rarely as the abscess contents are often viscous and bacterial superinfection may occur. Open surgical drainage is indicated in complicated cases and in those who fail to respond to conservative therapy.

In a meta-analysis of 3081 patients with amoebic liver abscess the mortality rate was 4% compared with a mortality rate of 46% in patients with pyogenic liver abscess.[61]

HYDATID CYST

Echinococcus infection is a zoonosis that can give rise to liver lesions. These collections are better classified as cysts rather than abscesses because the organism is almost entirely determined by the hepatic environment and little host inflammatory reaction is present. An intense fibrous reaction around the lesion is characteristic but there is no epithelial lining to the cyst. The incidence of *Echinococcus granulosus* is in decline but sporadic cases are reported in Europe, Australia, New Zealand, South America, Asia and Africa. The prevalence of human echinococciasis is directly related to contact with dogs and sheep. *Echinococcus multilocularis*,

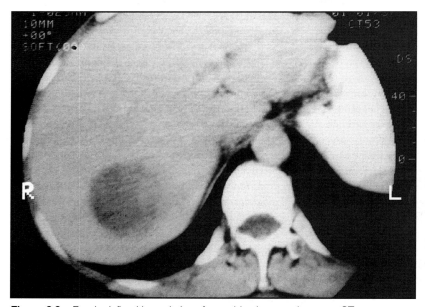

Figure 3.9 • Poorly defined boundaries of amoebic abscess shown on CT scan.

or alveolar hydatid disease, is much less common, although it is a much more dangerous condition. It pursues a more invasive course than the more common form of the disease but is fortunately confined to specific areas of the USA and Europe.

Hydatid cysts are most commonly unilocular and may grow as large as 20 cm. The cyst wall is about 5 mm thick and consists of an external laminated hilar membrane (ectocyst layer) and an internal enucleated germinal layer (endocyst layer), which is responsible for production of the colourless hydatid fluid, brood capsules and daughter cysts. Brood capsules are small cellular masses and together with caleareous bodies form 'hydatid sand'. About 70% of lesions are in the right lobe and 15% in the left, with both lobes involved in approximately 15% of cases.

Clinical presentation

Many infections are probably contracted during childhood and lie latent for many years, often until complications occur. Clinical symptoms of echinococcal cystic disease are often insidious but there is usually a history of contact with dogs or sheep. Distension of the liver capsule may produce right upper quadrant pain. Jaundice is infrequent but may be due to extrinsic biliary compression or due to rupture into the biliary tree leading to obstruction by cystic debris. Secondary bacterial infection of the cyst occurs in approximately 10% of cases. Liver function tests are generally abnormal and eosinophilia is present in up to one-third of patients.

Echinococcal disease may occasionally mimic a primary liver tumour or metastatic disease. Serology may be helpful in establishing a diagnosis. Plain abdominal radiographs may reveal a calcified cyst wall. Ultrasound and CT scanning may demonstrate septa, 'hydatid sand' or daughter cysts within the main cyst cavity, which are important signs for differentiating hydatid from other benign liver cysts (**Figs 3.10** and **3.11**). Percutaneous aspiration and drainage should be avoided because of the risk of dissemination or anaphylaxis.

Management

Once the diagnosis has been established, surgery is generally required as the natural history of viable hydatid cysts is one of growth and potential complications. Significant morbidity and mortality may result from rupture into the peritoneal or thoracic cavity or the development of a bronchobiliary fistula. Surgery might best be avoided in elderly frail patients with small, asymptomatic calcified cysts. Treatment with an oral anthelmintic agent, such as mebendazole or albendazole, to minimise the risks of hydatid spread at surgery or reduce the incidence of postoperative recurrence, has been advocated by some authors, although there remains considerable doubt as to its efficacy. Aspiration of the hydatid cyst with instillation of scolicidal agents, such as hypertonic saline, silver nitrate, chlorhexidine,

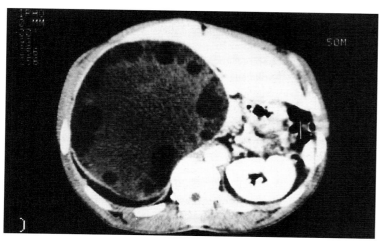

Figure 3.10 • Hydatid cyst with multiple peripheral daughter cysts within the main cyst cavity.

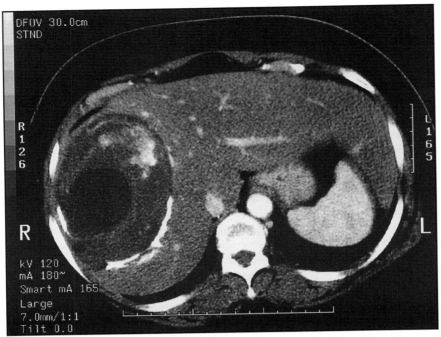

Figure 3.11 • Hydatid cyst with calcified cyst wall and a few peripheral daughter cysts.

cetrimide, hydrogen peroxide, formalin or alcohol, has generally been abandoned because of the risk of anaphylaxis or the risk of developing sclerosing cholangitis if a bile duct communication is present. These have been generally replaced by peroperative cover with an anthelmintic agent.

The main principle of surgical treatment is to eradicate the parasite, prevent intraoperative spillage of cyst contents and obliterate the residual cavity.[62] At operation, the operating field is generally packed off with swabs soaked in hypertonic saline. After decompression of the hydatid cyst, the cyst and contents are shelled out by peeling the endocyst off the host ectocyst layer. The fibrous host wall of the residual cavity should be carefully examined for any bile leakage from biliary–cyst communications, which are then sutured. The residual cyst cavity can be marsupialised, packed with omentum or plicated.[63] Pericystectomy is advocated by some but should preserve those portions of the cyst wall that come into contact with major blood vessels, which can be identified by intraoperative ultrasonography. For smaller, more peripheral lesions, formal hepatic resection may be considered, particularly if a diagnostic dilemma remains. The mortality for surgery of hydatid disease should be low and confined to

complicated disease. In a series of 505 patients, Milicevic reported a mortality rate of 1.5% and a morbidity rate of 30%.[63]

SIMPLE CYSTS OF THE LIVER

Non-parasitic cystic disease of the liver can result from a congenital malformation of the intrahepatic bile ducts. These cysts may be single, multiple or diffuse (polycystic liver disease). Simple cysts contain serous fluid and do not communicate with the intrahepatic biliary tree. Small cysts are surrounded by normal liver tissue, although as these enlarge, there may be displacement and atrophy of adjacent hepatic tissue. A large cyst may occupy an entire lobe of the liver and result in compensatory hypertrophy of the residual liver. Such simple cysts have no septa and are unilocular. Microscopically, they are lined by a single layer of cuboidal or columnar epithelial cells, which resemble those of biliary epithelium. Simple cysts have a prevalence of about 3.6%.[64] The female to male ratio is 4:1 in asymptomatic cases, but rises to 10:1 in symptomatic or complicated simple cysts.[65] Huge cysts almost exclusively affect women over the age of 50 years.

Clinical presentation

The vast majority of simple cysts are asymptomatic and are discovered incidentally. A small percentage of large cysts may cause abdominal pain or discomfort, and occasionally a mass can be palpated in the right hypochondrium. Other symptoms may include anorexia, early satiety or vomiting. Complications are rare; however, acute onset of pain may result from intracystic haemorrhage, rupture, torsion or infection. Obstructive jaundice is uncommon, but may be caused by external compression of the biliary tree.[66] Likewise, portal hypertension has been reported as a consequence of portal vein compression.[67]

Diagnosis can be made on the basis of abdominal ultrasonography, which demonstrates a circular anechoic area with a well-defined boundary with the liver. No wall is evident and posterior acoustic enhancement arises because of the accentuation of the ultrasound waves beyond the cyst. Internal acoustic shadowing may result from intracystic haemorrhage; however, the presence of cyst wall nodules or solid intracystic components must be considered neoplastic and treated as such. Ultrasound examination of the kidneys is useful to exclude the presence of polycystic disease. Further diagnostic investigation is rarely required, although where intervention is contemplated, CT will provide more accurate anatomical localisation and exclude the presence of other cysts. Cysts appear as well-rounded water-dense lesions without septa (**Fig. 3.12**). Intravenous contrast enhancement will confirm the avascularity of these lesions. Scintigraphy and angiography are not required to make a diagnosis. Where complications such as haemorrhage occur, the simple cyst may appear relatively thick-walled and may contain cystic debris. In such instances, serological tests should be undertaken to exclude parasitic infection. It should be borne in mind that calcification is absent in simple cysts but may be present with hydatid cysts.

MANAGEMENT

There has been much recent debate regarding the management of simple liver cysts. Asymptomatic simple cysts require no treatment; however,

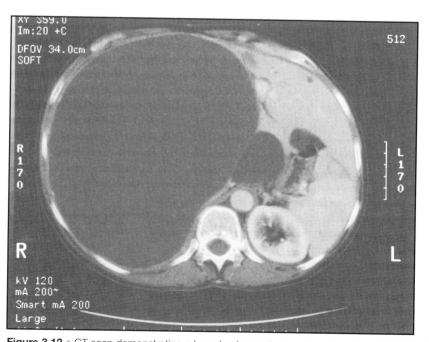

Figure 3.12 • CT scan demonstrating a large benign cyst occupying the entire right lobe of the liver. At least two further cysts are seen in the caudate and left lobes of the liver. Note the normal left kidney. This patient underwent successful laparoscopic deroofing of the cyst.

symptomatic or complicated simple cysts may require intervention. Percutaneous aspiration risks introducing infection and does not provide definitive therapy.[68] However, Gigot and colleagues have advocated this technique as a diagnostic test for patients with questionable symptoms.[69] Aspiration followed by percutaneous instillation of sclerosant agents has shown promising results in reducing symptomatic and radiological cyst recurrence.[70] Open deroofing of simple liver cysts has, in the past, been the established conventional treatment. Total cystectomy is not required and may be hazardous because, unlike hydatid disease, there is no plane of dissection between the cyst and the liver. In recent years, laparoscopic deroofing of such solitary cysts has been advocated. This technique was first described in 1991,[71] and is associated with higher patient acceptability and shorter postoperative stay compared with open surgical techniques.

In a recent comprehensive review of 21 papers on the laparoscopic management of hepatic cysts, Klingler et al. reported 61 laparoscopic deroofing procedures with an overall morbidity rate of 10%.[72]

Even at open surgery, deroofing of large centrally placed cysts may not prevent reconstitution of the cyst with recurrence of symptoms. In such patients, we would now advocate more radical resection, which does not generally involve substantial sacrifice of functioning hepatic parenchyma.

POLYCYSTIC LIVER DISEASE (PCLD)

Adult polycystic kidney disease is frequently associated with multiple liver cysts, which are macroscopically and microscopically similar to simple cysts of the liver. However, in this condition the liver cysts are multiple when present and may extensively replace both lobes of the liver. In addition to the macroscopic cysts, there are usually numerous microscopic cysts and clusters of multiple bile ductules, designated as von Meyenburg complexes. The condition is an autosomal dominant disorder and carries a much more sinister prognosis because of the risk of chronic renal failure. There is an increased prevalence associated with increasing age and the female sex.[73]

Clinical presentation

In most patients with adult polycystic kidney disease, the liver cysts are clinically silent. The commonest symptoms, if present, are related to increase in liver size and include abdominal discomfort and respiratory compromise. An abdominal mass will be present in three-quarters of patients. There are rarely signs of cholestasis, liver failure or portal hypertension, and liver function tests are usually normal. Both ultrasonography and CT will demonstrate multiple fluid-filled cysts with well-defined margins in the liver and the kidneys (**Fig. 3.13**). Liver cysts increase in size slowly and complications are uncommon. Rupture and bacterial infection are reported to be more common with immunosuppression following kidney transplantation.[74]

Management

Asymptomatic patients require no treatment. Percutaneous aspiration of cysts and instillation of sclerosant rarely produce satisfactory long-term relief of symptoms. Surgical deroofing or fenestration according to the technique described by Lin et al.[75] is the most widely used treatment modality for symptomatic patients but must be extensive and radical to achieve satisfactory results. Some have suggested that laparoscopic deroofing may provide good relief of symptoms.[76] However, in our own series this technique was associated with a high recurrence rate.[65] Recent evidence suggests that a more aggressive open surgical approach involving resection of the liver may provide longer-lasting relief of symptoms[77,78] but it should be appreciated that hepatic resection is difficult in such patients and is associated with a significant morbidity rate. Nonetheless, extensive resection with associated deroofing of hepatic cysts may allow the abdomen to better accommodate the enlarged residual liver. Surgical intervention is often associated with transient but massive ascites in the postoperative period.[79] Liver transplantation may be indicated in selected patients with hepatic failure.[80]

CYSTADENOMA

Cystadenoma of the liver is rare, but it has a strong tendency to recur and has a malignant potential.

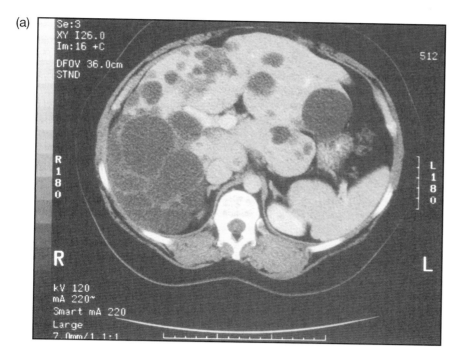

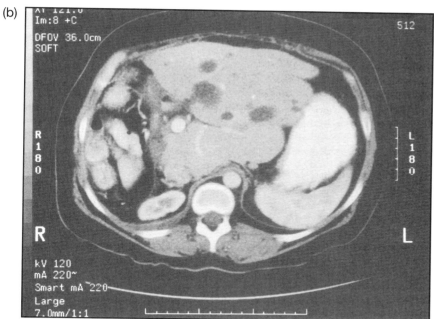

Figure 3.13 • **(a)** Contrast-enhanced CT scan demonstrating the presence of multiple cysts within the liver and kidneys. Note the predominance of large cysts within the right lobe of the liver. **(b)** CT scan taken 1 month following right hepatectomy and deroofing of the residual cyst in the same patient.

It is usually solitary and mainly affects women over 40 years of age. Cystadenomas are often multiloculated and may measure up to 20 cm in diameter. Histologically, the locules are mostly lined by a single layer of cuboidal or columnar cells; however, in areas the epithelium may form papillary projections. The presenting features are similar to other mass-forming hepatic pathologies, namely abdominal discomfort, anorexia, nausea and abdominal swelling. A large hepatic mass may be palpable. Liver function tests are usually normal. Diagnosis is based on ultrasonography and CT (**Fig. 3.14**). The ultrasound characteristics are of a large, anechoic, fluid-filled area with irregular margins. Internal echoes may be seen due to septa

or papillary projections from the cyst wall. CT scanning provides more accurate localisation, but may be less sensitive than ultrasonography for demonstrating the thin septations. Other imaging modalities are rarely indicated. Cystadenomas grow very slowly. Complications include biliary obstruction, intracystic haemorrhage, bacterial infection, rupture, recurrence after partial excision and the transformation into cystadenocarcinoma. This may be suspected radiologically by the presence of large projections into the cyst lobules and septal calcification.[81] Cystadenoma of the liver, even if asymptomatic, must be treated by complete excision.

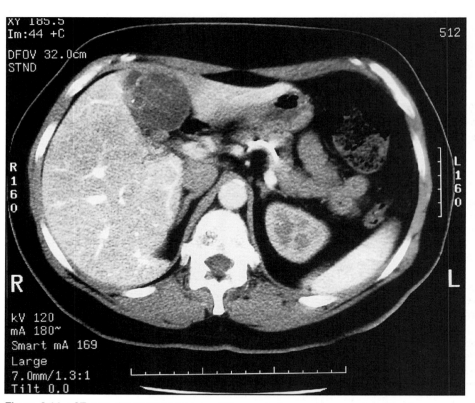

Figure 3.14 • CT scan demonstrating septa within a cystadenoma in segment 4 of the liver.

Key points

Successful management of patients with benign solid or cystic lesions of the liver requires accurate diagnosis and thorough knowledge of the natural history.

Inappropriate investigation may give rise to morbidity and compromise definitive management.

Modern liver resection for benign lesions can now be undertaken with minimal morbidity and mortality because of increasing centralisation of expertise and improved operative techniques.

A better understanding of the prognosis of unresected haemangioma, focal nodular hyperplasia and liver cell adenoma has made it possible to consider a more conservative approach in management.

Patients with symptomatic lesions or lesions that have the potential for further growth, complications or malignant transformation should undergo surgical treatment.

Careful consideration must be given to the risk of hepatic resection against the possible morbidity or mortality from observation.

REFERENCES

1. Ishak KG, Rabin L. Benign tumors of the liver. Med Clin North Am 1975; 59:995–1013.

2. Adam YG, Huvos AG, Fortner JG. Giant hemangiomas of the liver. Ann Surg 1970; 172:239–45.

3. Schwartz SI, Husser WC. Cavernous hemangioma of the liver: a single institution report of 16 resections. Ann Surg 1987; 205:456–65.

4. Sewell JH, Weiss K. Spontaneous rupture of hemangioma of the liver. Arch Surg 1961; 83:105–9.

5. Trastek VF, van Heerden JA, Sheedy PF et al. Cavernous hemangiomas of the liver: resect or observe? Am J Surg 1983; 145:49–53.

6. Farges O, Daradkeh S, Bismuth H. Cavernous hemangiomas of the liver: are there any indications for resection? World J Surg 1995; 19:19–24.

   Longitudinal study of 163 patients with cavernous haemangioma of the liver describing their natural history, diagnosis and management.

7. Bornman PC, Terblanche J, Blumgart RL et al. Giant hemangiomas: diagnostic and therapeutic dilemmas. Surgery 1987; 101:445–9.

8. Yamamoto T, Kawarada Y, Yano T et al. Spontaneous rupture of haemangioma of the liver: treatment with transcatheter hepatic arterial embolisation. Am J Gastroenterol 1991; 86:1645–9.

9. Johnson CM, Sheedy PF, Stanson AW et al. Computed tomography and angiography of cavernous hemangiomas of the liver. Radiology 1985; 138: 115–21.

10. Birnbaum BA, Weinreb JC, Mengibow AJ, et al. Definitive diagnosis of hepatic hemangiomas: MR imaging versus Tc-99m labelled red blood cell SPECT. Radiology 1990; 176:95–102.

11. Choi BI, Shin YM, Chung JW et al. MR findings of hepatic cavernous hemangioma after intraarterial infusion of iodized oil. Abdom Imaging 1994; 16:507–11.

12. Mahfouz AE, Hamm B, Taupitz M et al. Hypervascular liver lesions: differentiation of focal nodular hyperplasia from malignant tumours with dynamic gadolinium-enhanced MR imaging. Radiology 1993; 186:133–42.

13. Krause T, Hauenstein K, Studier-Fischer B et al. Improved evaluation of technetium-99m-red blood cell SPECT in haemangioma of the liver. J Nucl Med 1993; 34:375–80.

14. Grieco MB, Miscall BG. Giant haemangiomas of the liver. Surg Gynecol Obstet 1978; 147:783–7.

15. Yamagata M, Kanematsu T, Matsumata T et al. Management of haemangioma of the liver: comparison of results between surgery and observation. Br J Surg 1991; 78:1223–5.

16. Nichols FC, van Heerden JA, Weiland LH. Benign liver tumors. Surg Clin North Am 1989; 69:297–314.

17. Pietrabissa A, Giulianotti P, Campatelli A et al. Management and follow-up of 78 giant haemangiomas of the liver. Br J Surg 1996; 83:915–18.

18. Terkivatan T, Vrijland WW, Den Hoed PT et al. Size of lesion is not a criterion for resection during management of giant liver haemangioma. Br J Surg 2002; 89:1240–4.

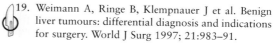

19. Weimann A, Ringe B, Klempnauer J et al. Benign liver tumours: differential diagnosis and indications for surgery. World J Surg 1997; 21:983–91.

   Review of 437 patients with benign liver tumours from a single institution. The aims of the study were to evaluate a noninvasive diagnostic algorithm to identify haemangioma and FNH, and to clarify the indications for surgery after considering the results from surgery and observation.

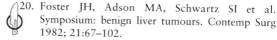

20. Foster JH, Adson MA, Schwartz SI et al. Symposium: benign liver tumours. Contemp Surg 1982; 21:67–102.

   Consensus publication following a symposium on benign liver tumours.

21. Baer HU, Dennison AR, Mouton W et al. Enucleation of giant hemangiomas of the liver. Ann Surg 1992; 216:673–6.

22. Cunningham JD, Katz LB, Brower ST et al. Laparoscopic resection of two liver hemangiomata. Surg Laparosc Endosc 1995; 5:277–80.

23. Longeville JH, de-la-Hall P, Dolan P et al. Treatment of a giant haemangioma of the liver with Kasabach–Merritt syndrome by orthotopic liver transplant, a case report. HPB Surg 1997; 10:159–62.

24. Nagorney DM. Benign hepatic tumors: focal nodular hyperplasia and. hepatocellular adenoma. World J Surg 1995; 19:13–18.

   Review of experience from Mayo Clinic regarding the management of 21 patients with FNH and 24 patients with hepatic adenoma with good overview of the literature.

25. Rooks JB, Ory HW, Ishak KG et al. Epidemiology of hepatocellular adenoma: the role of oral contraceptive use. J Am Med Assoc 1979; 242:644–8.

26. Kerlin P, Davis GL, McGill DB et al. Hepatic adenoma and focal nodular hyperplasia: clinical, pathologic and radiologic features. Gastroenterology 1983; 84:994–1002.

27. Baum JK, Bookstein JJ, Holtz F et al. Possible association between benign hepatomas and oral contraceptives. Lancet 1973; 2:926–9.

28. Fechner RE. Benign hepatic lesions and orally administered contraceptives. A report of seven cases and a critical analysis of the literature. Hum Path 1977; 8:255–68.

29. Kent DR, Nissen ED, Nissen SE et al. Effect of pregnancy on liver tumour associated with oral contraceptives. Obstet Gynecol 1978; 51:148–51.

30. Leese T, Farges O, Bismuth H. Liver cell adenomas: a 12 year surgical experience in a specialist hepatobiliary unit. Ann Surg 1988; 208:558–64.

31. Chiche L, Dao T, Salame E et al. Liver adenomatosis: reappraisal, diagnosis, and surgical management: eight new cases and review of the literature. Ann Surg 2000; 231:74–81.

32. Ferrell LD. Hepatocellular carcinoma arising in a focus of multilobular adenoma. Am J Surg Pathol 1993, 17:525–9.

33. Scott FR, El-Rafaie A, More L et al. Hepatocellular carcinoma arising in an adenoma: value of Qbend 10 immunostaining in diagnosis of liver cell carcinoma. Histopathology 1996; 28:472–4.

34. Gordon SC, Reddy KR, Livingstone AS et al. Resolution of a contraceptive steroid-induced hepatic adenoma with subsequent evolution into hepatocellular carcinoma. Ann Int Med 1986; 105:547–9.

35. Gyorffy EJ, Bredfeldt JE, Black WC. Transformation of hepatic cell adenoma to hepatocellular carcinoma

due to oral contraceptive use. Ann Int Med 1989; 110:489–90.

36. Tao LC. Oral contraceptive-associated liver cell adenoma and hepatocellular carcinoma: cytomorphology and mechanism of malignant transformation. Cancer 1991; 68:341–7.

37. Delbeke D, Martin WH, Sandler MP et al. Evaluation of benign vs malignant hepatic lesions with positron emission tomography. Arch Surg 1998; 133:510–16.

38. Edmondson HA, Reynolds TB, Henderson B et al. Regression of liver cell adenomas associated with oral contraceptives. Ann Int Med 1977; 86:180–2.

39. Steinbrecker WP, Lisbona R, Huang SN et al. Complete regression of hepatocellular adenoma after withdrawal of oral contraceptives. Dig Dis Sci 1981; 26:1045–50.

40. Tepetes K, Selby R, Webb M et al. Orthoptic liver transplantation for benign hepatic neoplasms. Arch Surg 1995; 130:153–6.

41. Welch TJ, Sheedy PJ, Johnson CM et al. Focal nodular hyperplasia and hepatic adenoma: comparison of angiography, CT, US, and scintigraphy. Radiology 1985; 156:593–5.

42. Cherqui D, Rahmouni A, Charlotte F et al. Management of focal nodular hyperplasia and hepatocellular adenoma in young women: a series of 41 patients with clinical, radiological, pathological correlations. Hepatology 1995; 22:1674–81.

43. Belghiti J, Pateron D, Panis Y et al. Resection of presumed benign liver tumours. Br J Surg 1993; 80:380–3.

   Study of 51 patients treated surgically for presumed benign liver tumours to compare preoperative and final pathological diagnosis and to determine if surgical resection was justified.

44. Trotter JF, Everson GT. Benign focal lesions of the liver. Clin Liver Dis 2001; 5:17–42.

45. Allaire GS, Rabin L, Ishak KG. Bile duct adenoma: a study of 152 cases. Am J Surg Pathol 1988; 12:708–15.

46. Shek TWH, Ng IOL, Chan KW. Inflammatory pseudotumor of the liver: Report of four cases and review of the literature. Am J Surg Pathol 1993; 17:231–8.

47. Foster JH, Berman M. Solid liver tumors. Philadelphia: WB Saunders, 1977.

48. Grases PJ, Matos-Villalobos M, Arcia-Romero F et al. Mesenchymal hamartoma of the liver. Gastroenterology 1979; 76:1466–9.

49. Rintoul R, O'Riordain MG, Laurenson IF et al. The changing management of pyogenic liver abscess. Br J Surg 1996; 83:215–18.

50. Chou FF, Sheen-Chen SM, Chen YS et al. Single and multiple pyogenic liver abscesses: clinical course, etiology and results of treatment. World J Surg 1997; 21:384–9.

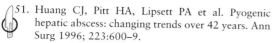

51. Huang CJ, Pitt HA, Lipsett PA et al. Pyogenic hepatic abscess: changing trends over 42 years. Ann Surg 1996; 223:600–9.

    Analysis of 233 patients with pyogenic liver abscesses managed over a 42-year period documenting changes in the aetiology, diagnosis, bacteriology, treatment and outcome.

52. Farges O, Leese T, Bismuth H. Pyogenic liver abscess: an improvement in prognosis. Br J Surg 1988; 75:862–5.

53. Branum GD, Tyson GS, Branum MA et al. Hepatic abscess: Changes in etiology, diagnosis and management. Ann Surg 1990; 212:655–62.

54. Chu KM, Fan ST, Lai EC et al. Pyogenic liver abscess: an audit of experience over the past decade. Arch Surg 1996; 131:148–52.

55. Pearce NW, Knight R, Irving H. Non-operative management of pyogenic liver abscess. HPB 2003; 5:91–95.

56. Stain SC, Yellin AE, Donovan AJ et al. Pyogenic liver abscess: modern treatment. Arch Surg 1991; 126:991–6.

57. Giorgio A, Tarantino L, Mariniello N et al. Pyogenic liver abscesses: 13 years of experience in percutaneous needle aspiration with US guidance. Radiology 1995; 195:122–4.

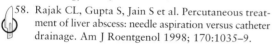

58. Rajak CL, Gupta S, Jain S et al. Percutaneous treatment of liver abscess: needle aspiration versus catheter drainage. Am J Roentgenol 1998; 170:1035–9.

    Randomized trial of 50 patients with liver abscesses showing that percutaneous catheter drainage was more effective than needle aspiration.

59. Strong RW, Fawcett J, Lynch SV et al. Hepatectomy for pyogenic liver abscess. HPB 2003; 5:86–90.

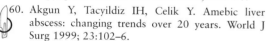

60. Akgun Y, Tacyildiz IH, Celik Y. Amebic liver abscess: changing trends over 20 years. World J Surg 1999; 23:102–6.

    Study comparing outcome of conservative treatment of amoebic abscesses with metronidazole and percutaneous drainage with a historical group of patients who underwent surgical drianage

61. Pitt HA. Surgical management of hepatic abscesses. World J Surg 1990; 14:498–504.

    A meta-analysis of 3081 patients with amoebic abscess.

62. Agaoglu N, Turkyilmaz S, Arslan MK. Surgical treatment of hydatid cysts of the liver. Br J Surg 2003; 90:1536–41.

63. Milicevic M. Hydatid disease. In: Blumgart LH (ed.) Surgery of the liver and biliary tract, 3rd edn. London:WB Saunders, 2000; pp. 1167–204.

    Report of 818 patients with hydatid cysts.

64. Huang JF, Chen SC, Lu SN et al. Prevalence and size of simple hepatic cysts in Taiwan: community- and hospital-based sonographic surveys. Kao-Hsiung I Hsueh Ko Hseuh Tsa Chih (Kaohsiung Journal of Medical Sciences) 1995; 11:564–7.

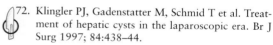

65. Martin IJ, McKinley AJ, Currie EJ et al. Tailoring the management of nonparasitic liver cysts. Ann Surg 1998; 228:167–72.

    Report of 38 patients who underwent a total of 48 operations for symptomatic hepatic cysts of mean diameter of 12 cm, with a mean follow-up of 41 months.

66. Lai ECS, Wong J. Symptomatic nonparasitic cysts of the liver. World J Surg 1990; 14:452–6.

67. Johnstone AJ, Turnbull LW, Allan PL et al. Cholangitis and Budd–Chiari syndrome as complications of simple cystic liver disease – a case report. HPB Surg 1993; 6:223–8.

68. Saini S, Mueller PR, Ferucci JT, Jr et al. Percutaneous aspiration of hepatic cysts does not provide definitive therapy. Am J Roentgenol 1983; 141:559–60.

69. Gigot JF, Legrand M, Hubens G et al. Laparoscopic treatment of nonparasitic liver cysts: adequate selection of patients and surgical technique. World J Surg 1996; 20:556–61.

70. Montorsi M, Torzilli G, Fumagalli U et al. Percutaneous alcohol sclerotherapy of simple hepatic cysts. Results from a multicentre survey in Italy. HPB Surgery 1994; 8:89–94.

71. Paterson-Brown S, Garden OJ. Laser assisted laparoscopic excision of liver cyst. Br J Surg 1991; 78:1047.

72. Klingler PJ, Gadenstatter M, Schmid T et al. Treatment of hepatic cysts in the laparoscopic era. Br J Surg 1997; 84:438–44.

    Review of 21 papers on laparoscopic management of hepatic cysts.

73. Milutinovic J, Failkow PJ, Rudd TG et al. Liver cysts in patients with autosomal dominant polycystic kidney disease. Am J Med 1980; 68:741–4.

74. Bourgeois N, Kinnaert P, Vereerstraeten P et al. Infection of hepatic cysts following kidney transplantation in polycystic disease. World J Surg 1983; 7:629–31.

75. Lin TY, Chen CC, Wang SM. Treatment of non-parasitic disease of the liver: a new approach to therapy of the polycystic liver. Ann Surg 1968; 168:921–7.

76. Morino M, De Giuli M, Festa V et al. Laparoscopic management of symptomatic non-parasitic cysts of the liver: indications and results. Ann Surg 1994; 219:157–64.

77. Henne-Bruns D, Klomp HJ, Kremer B. Non-parasitic liver cysts and polycystic liver disease:

results of surgical treatment. Hepatogastroenterology 1993; 40:1–5.

78. Que F, Nagorney DM, Gross JB, Jr et al. Liver resection and cyst fenestration in the treatment of severe polycystic liver disease. Gastroenterology 1995; 108:487–94.

79. Farges O, Bismuth H. Fenestration in the management of polycystic liver disease. World J Surg 1995; 19:25–30.

80. Starzl TE, Reyes J, Tzakis A et al. Liver transplantation for polycystic liver disease. Arch Surg 1990; 125:575–7.

81. Korobkin M, Stephens DH, Lee JKT et al. Biliary cystadenoma and cystadenocarcinoma: CT and sonographic findings. Am J Roentgenol 1989; 153:507–11.

Four

Primary malignant tumours of the liver

Olivier Farges and
Jacques Belghiti

With the exception of hepatocellular carcinoma (HCC), which is one of the most common malignancies, primary tumours of the liver are relatively rare in adults. HCC arises from hepatocytes and is closely linked to cirrhosis, which is its main aetiological factor. This tumour is the subject of considerable epidemiological and management interest due to its rising incidence and the development of innovative treatments such as liver transplantation and percutaneous ablation. Intrahepatic cholangiocarcinoma (ICCA) arises from the peripheral intrahepatic biliary radicles and is the second most frequent primary liver tumour. Primary tumours can also arise from mesodermal cells, and include angiosarcoma, epithelioid haemangio-endothelioma and sarcoma, but they are extremely rare and will be only briefly discussed.

HEPATOCELLULAR CARCINOMA

HCC accounts for 90% of all primary liver malignancy and its incidence is rising. It is the fifth most common neoplasm, accounting for more than 5% of all cancers, and is also the third most common cause of cancer-related death.[1] There is evidence that its incidence is rising in many areas of the world, and the numbers of new cases and of cancer-related deaths are each estimated to be 500 000 per

year. It usually occurs in male patients, on a background of chronic liver disease and in particular viral cirrhosis. HCC is therefore a major cause of death in high endemic areas of hepatitis B virus (HBV) or hepatitis C virus (HCV) infection. In patients with HCC, the death rate due to cancer is 50–60% while hepatic failure and gastrointestinal bleeding due to the underlying liver disease are responsible for approximately 30% and 10% of the deaths respectively.[2] HCC was classically diagnosed at an advanced stage and associated with a poor prognosis but there has been considerable progress in the diagnosis and treatment of this tumour over the past 10 years. HCC may now be identified at an early stage, particularly through the screening of high-risk patients. Control of HCC nodules may be achieved successfully by surgical resection and by percutaneous treatment. The precise role of each treatment is currently being evaluated and will depend on the morphological features of the tumour and the functional status of the non-tumorous liver. These treatments, however, share a high incidence of tumour recurrence due to the persistence of the underlying cirrhosis, which represents a pre-neoplastic condition. Liver transplantation may seem a logical alternative treatment but has its own limitations, including tumour recurrence, the limited availability of grafts, and its cost. The most exciting areas of progress are the control of HBV or HCV, the prevention of carcinogenesis in patients with chronic liver disease, and the development of adjuvant therapies.

Incidence of HCC

One of the most important epidemiological characteristics of HCC is its considerable geographical variation. The world age-adjusted incidence in men is 14.9 per 100 000.[3] It is greater than 20 cases per 100 000 inhabitants in the sub-Saharan and western coastal Africa as well as in eastern and southeastern Asia and in particular Korea, Hong Kong, Thailand, Japan and China. The incidence may be as high as 99 per 100 000 in Mongolian men. South European countries (Italy, Spain and France) and more generally Mediterranean countries also have a fairly high incidence of 11–20 cases per 100 000. North European countries, such as the UK and Germany, have a lower risk, of 5–10 cases per 100 000. Scandinavia, the USA and Canada traditionally have an even lower risk, of less than 5 cases per 100 000. The age-adjusted incidence in women is two to four times less than in men but the geographical variation is comparable.

These striking geographical variations in incidence are closely related to the presence of environmental factors,[4] the most important of which is viral cirrhosis. Hepatitis B (HBV) and hepatitis C (HCV) viruses are the main risk factors of HCC; although their respective contributions differ in different areas of the world, together they account for three-quarters of all cases (Table 4.1). HCC usually develops 20–40 years after the viral contamination but cofactors may account for variations in the tumour evolution.

The second epidemiological characteristic of HCC is its rising incidence. This was first documented in the USA, where the incidence doubled between the late 1970s and the early 1990s,[5] currently reaching 3 cases per 100 000. A comparable increase has also been recently registered in Canada, Australia, Japan and various European countries. The recent epidemic of HCV infection probably accounts for a large part of this increase, which is anticipated to persist during the next two or three decades despite a reduction in the risk of HCV contamination. Alternative explanations include aging of the population, increased detection, and improved survival of cirrhotic patients.

Table 4.1 • Relative frequencies of serological markers of viral infection in HCC patients

Country	Anti-HCV +ve HBsAg ±ve (%)	Anti-HCV –ve HBsAg +ve (%)	Anti-HCV +ve and/or HBsAg +ve (%)
Europe			
Italy, Spain, France	50–75	10–25	80–95
Germany, Switzerland	25–50	15–25	50
USA	25–45	10–30	30–70
Asia			
Taiwan, Hong Kong	10–40	50–80	80–95
Japan	60–75	15–25	70–95
South Africa	20–30	35–50	60–70

+ve, positive; –ve, negative; ±ve, positive or negative. Adapted from Ref. 4.

Risk factors of HCC

CIRRHOSIS

Chronic liver disease is the predominant risk factor for the development of HCC, with 80–90% of all HCC arising in patients with cirrhosis or extensive fibrosis. It is not clear whether this association is an effect of the regenerative process or the direct effect of the underlying cause of cirrhosis. The risk of tumour development varies with the type of cirrhosis; the highest risks are reported for cirrhosis related to chronic viral hepatitis, whereas lower risks are associated with other forms of cirrhosis such as primary biliary cirrhosis. Multiple risk factors (in particular viral coinfections, alcohol ingestion and obesity) are, however, increasingly identified in individual patients. The largest population at risk of chronic liver diseases and therefore HCC are patients with insulin resistance (worldwide prevalence 10%), high alcohol consumption (10%), HBV infection (5%), HCV infection (3%), and genetic haemochromatosis (0.5%).

Once cirrhosis is established, the predictors of tumour development are male gender, age (probably a surrogate for the duration of the underlying liver disease), disease severity and high liver cell proliferation activity. Other risk factors that may act in concert include alcohol consumption, obesity and aflatoxin B1 intake.

HBV INFECTION

The carcinogenic potential of HBV infection has been established from both epidemiological observation and biological studies. Areas of high prevalence for chronic HBV infection (Asia and Africa) also have the highest incidence of HCC. Conversely, vaccination campaigns against the HBV in high endemic areas such as Taiwan have resulted in a decrease in HBsAg (hepatitis B surface antigen) prevalence among children from 10% to 1%, and have been associated with a 60% decrease in the incidence of HCC.[6] On the biological side, there is evidence that HBV-DNA sequences integrate into the genome of malignant hepatocytes and can be detected in the liver tissues of patients with HCC despite the absence of classical HBV serological markers. HBV specific protein may also interact with liver genes. HBV is therefore a direct risk factor for HCC and can occur in patients without cirrhosis.

The risk of HBV-associated HCC increases with age at infection, level of viral replication, duration of infection and severity of the underlying hepatitis.[7] HBV infection acquired early in life or during pregnancy (vertical transmission), as is the case in highly endemic areas of HBV, often becomes persistent. In Taiwan, for example, the risk of HCC in men chronically infected with HBV is 102 times greater than the risk for non-carriers. HCC typically involves individuals aged 40 years or younger, at a symptomatic phase. In contrast, the risk of HCC is lower in the Western world, where infection is acquired at a later stage through sexual or parenteral routes (horizontal transmission) and carries only a 5% risk of chronicity. In these areas, case–control studies have demonstrated that chronic HBV carriers have a 5–15-fold increased risk of HCC compared with the general population.[8]

Viral replication (as evidenced by the presence of hepatitis B e antigen, HBeAg) further increases this risk. In HBsAg-positive patients, those with HBeAg have a 60 times greater risk of developing HCC than HBsAg-negative patients, whereas the relative risk is 9 times for non-replicating patients.[7] The risk of malignant transformation also correlates with the severity of the underlying liver disease. The annual incidence of HCC is 0.5% in patients with chronic hepatitis and 2% in cirrhotic patients, but figures as high as 7% have been reported. Alcohol and aflatoxin exposure also increase the risk of HCC formation in HBV-positive patients. Vaccination against HBV is probably the most effective mean of decreasing the incidence of HBV-related HCC.

HCV INFECTION

A wealth of epidemiological data has accumulated linking HCV infection to HCC,[9] and the expansion of HCV infection probably accounts for the increased incidence of HCC observed over the past ten years.[5] This is particularly so in Western countries, with up to 70% of HCC patients having anti-HCV antibodies in their serum. The mean time for developing HCC following HCV infection is approximately 30 years.[10,11] Hence, although the incidence of HCV infection has decreased through screening of blood products, it is estimated that the incidence of HCC will continue to increase by 60–120% during the next two decades.[12]

Case–control studies have shown that the risk of HCC is increased 17-fold among HCV-infected patients.[7] As with HBV, the risk of HCC correlates with the severity of the hepatitis, age, and male gender, and duration of the disease. The annual incidence of HCC is 0.4% for unselected HCV carriers with persistently high alanine aminotransferase (ALT) values, and ranges between 3% and 8% in cirrhotic patients. Patients with high transaminase levels are at increased risk of progression to cirrhosis and of developing HCC. The influence of the viral genotype on the risk of HCC is more controversial. HCV-related HCC is very rare before the age of 40 in the absence of cofactors. The incidence subsequently increases linearly to peak in patients aged 70–75 years in the Western world.[5] A synergistic role of high body mass index, alcohol, HBV and HIV coinfection in the development of HCV-related cirrhosis and HCC has also been demonstrated and may in part explain the epidemiological and clinical heterogeneity of the tumour. In HIV-positive patients, the prevalence of HCV infection in Europe and the USA is 35%, and even higher rates have been reported in drug-users.[13] Cirrhosis and HCC occur 15–20 years earlier than in patients infected by HCV alone.

Conversely, HCV coinfection increases the risk of progression to AIDS.

The mechanism of HCV-related HCC is still not very clear. Replicating HCV-RNA and virus-specific protein expression has been detected in the infected livers but no genomic integration into the host chromosomal DNA has been documented. Furthermore, the great majority of patients with HCV-related HCC have cirrhosis, suggesting that it is the presence of cirrhosis that is crucial for the development of this tumour. HCV-associated HCC has nevertheless also been reported in non-cirrhotic patients, although considerably less frequently than for HBV, indicating that it could also have a mutagenic effect. The core and NS3 proteins of HCV are likely oncogenic candidates.

Because anti-HCV vaccination is not available, prevention of HCV infection and of progression of chronic HCV infection to cirrhosis through antiviral treatments is the only means to reduce the incidence of HCV-related HCC. Responders to interferon therapy seem to be at a lower risk than non-responders.[14] Abstinence from alcohol is also strictly recommended.

HCV-related HCC occurs in Western countries in patients aged 60 years or more,[5] with increased transaminase levels, and associated conditions such as obesity and diabetes. These issues are important restrictive factors in the choice of treatment (see below).

OTHER VIRAL INFECTIONS

Infection with the hepatitis delta virus (HDV) is found in patients who are also infected with HBV. Despite HDV coinfection being associated with a faster progression to cirrhosis, there are no epidemiological data supporting an increased risk of HCC development related to HDV infection. Similarly, hepatitis A virus (HAV) and hepatitis E virus (HEV) infection cause neither chronic hepatitis nor HCC.

ALCOHOL

Heavy (>50–70 g/day) and prolonged alcohol ingestion is a classical risk factor. The risk of HCC is increased by 13 times in comparison to those who abstain. Its relative role should, however, probably be reassessed in view of the high incidence (75%) of HCV infection in HCC patients presumed to have 'alcoholic' cirrhosis.[15] It is estimated that it accounts

for 10% (Asia) to 20% (Europe and North America) of HCC. However, alcohol is such an important and frequent cofactor in the development of HCV- or HBV-related HCC[16] that it is, at least to some extent, involved in most HCC. The overall male predominance of HCC may be related in part to more frequent alcohol use in men.

NON-ALCOHOLIC FATTY LIVER DISEASE (NAFLD)

NAFLD (liver steatosis in the absence of alcohol ingestion) has recently been recognised as being one of the most common causes of liver disease in the USA[17] (and other Western countries). It is frequently associated with type 2 diabetes and morbid obesity but may also be observed in lean individuals. It may progress to liver cirrhosis in up to 5% of the cases, and represents a significant and increasing percentage of cryptogenic cirrhosis due to the rising prevalence of obesity. There is also recent evidence that it may progress to HCC and, as for alcohol, favour the development of HCC in HCV patients.[18]

AFLATOXIN

Aflatoxin B1 has also long been associated with the development of HCC because areas with a large consumption of this toxin coincide with areas of high incidence of HCC (Asia and sub-Saharan Africa). Aflatoxin is ingested in food as a result of contamination of imperfectly stored staple crops by *Aspergillus flavus*. It is thought to induce HCC through mutation of the tumour suppressor gene p53. Although some studies suggest that it is an independent risk factor,[19,20] others suggest that it could be a cocarcinogen only in patients with HBV infection. HCC in this setting frequently develops in a non-cirrhotic liver.

METABOLIC LIVER DISEASE AND HCC

The relative risk for the development of HCC in haemochromatosis with cirrhosis is greater than 200 and rises with increasing age.[21] The cancer develops in highly iron-overloaded patients whether they have been de-ironed or not, and HCC may also develop within fibrotic livers before cirrhosis develops.[22] The annual incidence, once cirrhosis has occurred, is estimated to be 5%. An increased risk of HCC is recognised in some other forms of metabolic liver disease such as alpha-1-antitrypsin deficiency, porphyrias, cutanea tarda tyrosinaemia and especially hypercitrullinaemia. Glycogenosis type IV, hereditary fructose intolerance and Wilson disease may also develop HCC but with a lower risk. There is evidence that iron and copper overload in haemochromatosis and Wilson disease generate, respectively, oxygen/nitrogen species and unsaturated aldehydes that cause mutations in the p53 tumour suppressor gene.

ADENOMA, CONTRACEPTIVES AND ANDROGENS

Adenoma complicating type I glycogenosis and related to anabolic steroids or androgens may transform into HCC within non-cirrhotic livers. Fanconi disease may also be complicated by HCC, especially if it has been treated by steroids. The risk of transformation of adenomas secondary to contraceptives and oestrogen treatments is real[23] but probably less than 10%. It is, however, the main rationale for removing all adenomas. The risk of malignant transformation of polyadenomatosis also exists but it is even lower.[24]

Pathology of HCC and of nodular lesions in chronic liver disease

Cirrhotic livers contain a variety of nodular lesions, including benign macroregenerative nodules, dysplastic nodules (DNs) and HCC,[25] in addition to the other benign conditions that may be present in normal livers. DNs, which represent the preneoplastic condition of HCC,[26] are defined as a nodular region of less than 2 cm in diameter with dysplasia but without definite histological criteria of malignancy. Encapsulation, necrosis and haemorrhage are not seen. Low-grade DNs are around 1 cm in diameter and slightly yellowish. Their morphological separation from large regenerative nodules is almost impossible but both have a very low probability of becoming malignant. High-grade DNs are less common, slightly larger nodules (up to 2 cm) and characterised by increased cell density with an irregular thin-trabecular pattern and occasionally unpaired arteries. These lesions are often difficult to differentiate from highly differentiated HCC. Because they may contain distinct foci of well-differentiated HCC they are considered as precancerous lesions and become malignant in a

third of cases.[27] It must be appreciated that lesions smaller than 2 cm may also represent HCC, some of which have already disseminated. Tumour invasion into the portal vein and intrahepatic metastases are found in 25% and 10%, respectively, of such lesions. These features help in identifying the malignant nature of these early HCCs but molecular analysis will probably become the optimum tool in the future.

Nodules larger than 2 cm are seldom regenerative or dysplastic nodules and usually correspond to HCC.[25] One of the characteristics as they increase in size and become malignant is the appearance of non-triadal arteries, which account for their hypervascularisation on imaging studies. Macroscopically, HCC may be polychromic as a result of intratumoral haemorrhage, the presence of bile, of steatotic foci or of necrosis. They can be stratified into three types:

- unifocal expansive type
- infiltrating type
- multifocal (diffuse) type.

The unifocal type present as a soft solid mass; the infiltrating type are frequently less differentiated with ill-defined margins; and the multifocal or diffuse type have multiple, minute, indistinct nodules present throughout the liver. Tumour nodules may be surrounded by a distinct fibrous capsule. This capsule, present in 80% of resected HCC, has a variable thickness, may or may not be complete, and is frequently infiltrated by tumour cells. Extracapsular microscopic invasion by tumour cells is influenced by the size of the tumour; it is present in one-third of tumours smaller than 2 cm in diameter, as compared with two-thirds of those with a larger diameter.[2] Tumours are multiple in more than 50% of cases on imaging studies. Multiple tumours are due either to multifocal carcinogenesis or to the intrahepatic dissemination through portal vein invasion. Microscopically, HCC exhibits variable degrees of differentiation. Very well-differentiated HCC can resemble normal hepatocytes and the trabecular structure may reproduce a near normal lobar architecture so that histological diagnosis by biopsy may occasionally be very difficult.[25] HCC can also be stratified by the four-stage Edmondson classification, characterised in particular by increasing cytonuclear atypia. The fibrolamellar variant has distinct epidemiological, histopathological and prognostic characteristics and will be discussed separately in this chapter.

HCC have a great tendency to spread locally and to invade blood vessels, particularly the portal vein. Portal vein invasion is influenced by the type of HCC, the differentiation and the size of the tumour. The rate of portal invasion is higher in cases of expansive type, in poorly differentiated HCC and in large tumours.[28] Whatever the treatment it must be emphasised that the presence of portal invasion is the most important predictive factor associated with recurrence. The tumour thrombus has its own arterial supply, mainly from the site of the original venous invasion. Once HCC invades the portal vein, tumour thrombi grow rapidly in both directions, and in particular towards the main portal vein. The consequences of this mode of extension are twofold. First, tumour fragments are spread throughout the liver as the thrombus crosses segmental branches. Second, once the tumour thrombus has extended into the main portal vein, there is a high risk of complete portal vein thrombosis and increased portal hypertension. This accounts for the frequent presentation of these patients with fatal rupture of oesophageal varices, or liver decompensation including ascites, jaundice and encephalopathy. Invasion of hepatic veins is possible, although less frequent. The thrombus eventually extends into the suprahepatic vena cava or the right atrium. Hepatic vein invasion is associated with a high risk of lung metastases. More rarely, HCC may also invade the biliary tract and give rise to jaundice or haemobilia. Mechanisms of HCC-induced biliary obstruction include:

- intraductal tumour extension
- obstruction by a fragment of necrotic tumour debris
- haemorrhage of the tumour resulting in haemobilia
- metastatic lymph node compression of major bile ducts in the porta hepatis.

The rate of invasion of the first branch portal vein or portal trunk, hepatic vein trunk or inferior vena cava (IVC), and bile duct are 9, 2 and 1.5%, respectively.[2]

When present, metastases are most frequently found in the lung; other locations by decreasing order of frequency are: adrenal glands, bones, lymph nodes, meninges, pancreas, brain and kidney. Large size of the tumour, bilobar disease and poor differentiation are risk factors for metastatic disease.

HCCs have been classified according to either the Tumour Node Metastasis (TNM) staging or Okuda classification; the TNM staging has been modified repeatedly because of its poor prognostic accuracy. For the tumour classification, the latest proposals[29,30] take into account the number (single or multiple) and size of the nodules as well as the presence of vascular invasion. It has a better prognostic prediction but requires the pathological analysis of the resected specimen (**Table 4.2**).

Clinical presentation

The severity of the clinical findings depends on the stage of the tumour, on the functional status of the non-tumorous liver and whether patients are submitted or not to a screening programme. In developed countries, a growing number of tumours

Table 4.2 • UICC TNM classification of primary liver cancer, 5th edition

Stage	Tumour	Lymph node	Metastasis
I	T1	N0	M0
II	T2	N0	M0
IIIa	T3	N0	M0
	T1, 2, 3	N1	M0
IVa	T4	Any N	M0
IVb	Any T	Any N	M1

Primary tumour. Tx: cannot be assessed. T0: no evidence of primary tumour. T1: solitary tumour ≤2 cm, no vascular invasion. T2: solitary tumour ≤2 cm with vascular invasion; or multiple tumours, one lobe ≤2 cm, no vascular invasion; or solitary tumours >2 cm, without vascular invasion. T3: solitary tumour >2 cm, with vascular invasion; or multiple tumours, one lobe ≤2 cm, with vascular invasion; or multiple tumours, one lobe >2 cm, with/without vascular invasion. T4: multiple tumours, more than one lobe; or any tumour(s) invading major branch of portal or hepatic veins or invasion of adjacent organs other than gallbladder, or perforation of visceral peritoneum.
Lymph nodes. Nx: cannot be assessed. N0: no regional lymph node metastases. N1: regional lymph node metastases.
Metastasis. Mx: cannot be assessed. M0: no distant metastases. M1: distant metastases.

are discovered at an early asymptomatic stage as a result of either screening programmes (see below) or of incidental findings of abnormal imaging or biochemical abnormalities on routine checkup or during the investigation of unrelated diseases. As tumours increase in size, they may become symptomatic resulting in abdominal pain associated with a variable degree of malaise, weight loss, asthenia, anorexia and fever. These symptoms may be acute as a result of tumour extension or complication.

Spontaneous rupture of HCC occurs in 5–15% of patients.[31] This complication is observed particularly in patients with superficial or protruding tumours. Ruptured HCC should be suspected in patients with a known HCC or cirrhosis presenting with acute epigastric pain as well as in Asian or African men who develop an acute abdomen or signs of a haemoperitoneum. Minor rupture manifests as abdominal pain or haemorrhagic ascites, and hypovolaemic shock is only present in about half of the patients. Portal vein invasion may manifest as upper gastrointestinal bleeding or acute ascites as a result of increased portal pressure. Invasion of hepatic veins or IVC may result in pulmonary embolism or sudden death.

Clinical symptoms resulting from biliary invasion or haemobilia are present in 2% of the patients. Possible paraneoplastic syndromes associated with HCC include polyglobulia, hypercalcaemia and hypoglycaemia. Finally, in patients with underlying liver disease, a sudden onset or worsening of ascites or liver decompensation may be the first evidence of HCC formation.

In patients with normal livers, HCC is usually diagnosed at an advanced stage, but the presentation of symptoms in these patients does not preclude curative treatment. In contrast, the presence of symptoms in cirrhotic patients has a clear detrimental impact on outcome.

Clinical examination may only reveal large or superficial tumours. There may be clinical signs of cirrhosis, in particular ascites, a collateral circulation, umbilical hernia, hepatomegaly and splenomegaly.

Liver function tests and tumour markers

Liver function test impairment is usually non-specific and tends to reflect either the underlying liver pathology (cirrhosis or chronic active hepatitis) or the presence of a space-occupying lesion (resulting in an increase in alkaline phosphatase or gamma-glutamyl transpeptidase). Because most HCCs develop within a cirrhotic liver and since HCCs on normal livers are usually large, normal liver function tests are exceptional. Jaundice is most frequently the result of liver decompensation but may be due to biliary or portal vein invasion.

Serum alpha-fetoprotein (AFP) is the most widely recognised serum marker of HCC. It is secreted during fetal life but the residual levels are very low in the adult (0–20 ng/mL). It may increase in HCC patients and serum levels greater than 500 ng/mL can be considered as an indicator of an HCC with a 95% confidence. These levels may rise to 10 000 ng/mL or more in 5–10% of HCCs. Although the influence of AFP on prognosis overall is controversial, very high levels are usually correlated with tumour aggressiveness and vascular invasion. This marker, however, lacks sensitivity and specificity. AFP is normal in 40% of patients.[2] The sensitivity of a cut-off value greater than 200 is less than 50%. Thirty percent of patients with chronic active hepatitis but without an HCC have a moderately increased AFP. This usually correlates with the degree of histological activity and raised levels of transaminase, and it may therefore fluctuate. Tumours other than HCC can also be associated with an increased AFP level but these are very rare (hepatoid gastric tumours, neuroendocrine tumours). Alternative serum markers for HCC, such as des-gamma-carboxy prothrombin, have not come into common practice as it is highly dependent on the size of the tumour and is only superior in patients with tumours larger than 5 cm.[32]

Morphological studies

The aims of imaging in the context of HCC are:

1. to screen high-risk patients;
2. to identify small lesions (only these may be accessible to treatment with some long-term benefit);
3. to differentiate HCC from other space-occupying lesions;
4. to select the appropriate treatment.

The number of lesions, their size and extent, the presence of daughter nodules or of vascular invasion along with extrahepatic spread and the presence of an underlying liver disease are critical in choosing the most appropriate treatment. These aims may, to some extent, be achieved by ultrasonography (US), computed tomography (CT), magnetic resonance imaging (MRI), angiography or a combination of these. The accuracy of all these techniques has improved considerably over the past five years.

Ultrasound

Ultrasound (US) is the first-line investigation because of its low cost, high availability and high sensitivity in identifying a focal liver mass. With dedicated equipment in experienced hands, US may currently identify 85–95% of lesions of 3–5-cm diameter and 60–80% of lesions of 1 cm. Typically, small HCCs are hypoechoic and homogeneous. They cannot therefore be differentiated from regenerating or dysplastic nodules. As they increase in size, they may become either hypo- or hyper-echoic but most importantly heterogeneous. A hypo-echoic peripheral rim corresponds to the capsula. The infiltrating type is usually very difficult to identify in a grossly heterogeneous cirrhotic liver. Besides echogenicity, the accuracy of US in the diagnosis of HCC depends on the dimension and location of the tumour, as well as on the experience of the operator. A tumour of diameter 1 cm can be visualised if it is deeply located, whereas the same lesion located on the surface can easily be missed. Similarly, tumours located in the upper liver segments or on the edge of the left lateral segment may also be missed. Tumours discovered at an advanced stage despite surveillance are frequently located at these sites. Obesity may also prevent accurate exploration of the liver. Doppler US may demonstrate the presence of a feeding artery and/or draining veins. US is also very accurate in identifying vascular or biliary invasion as well as indirect evidence of cirrhosis such as segmental atrophy, splenomegaly, ascites or collateral veins. Tumour thrombosis, as opposed to cruoric thrombosis, is associated with enlargement of the vascular lumen, and an arterial signal may be detected by duplex Doppler. This portal vein invasion is an important clue to the diagnosis of HCC as it is exceptional in other malignancies.

To improve this accuracy, a role for contrast agents in ultrasound is being actively pursued. Agents that may prove useful rely on increasing the echo intensity by adding a substance with an acoustic impedance different from that of normal tissue. Several types of agents have been studied, and include the infusion of free gas bubbles into the hepatic vessels.[33]

Computed tomography

Computed tomography (CT) is much more accurate than US in identifying HCCs and their lobar or segmental distribution, particularly with the development of helical and multislice spiral CT scanners.[34] Spiral CT should be done without contrast and during the arterial (25–50 s), portal (60–65 s) and equilibrium (130–180 s) phases after contrast administration. In addition, it is useful for identifying features of underlying cirrhosis, accurately measuring liver and tumour volumes, and assessing extrahepatic tumour spread. HCCs are usually hypodense. Spontaneous hyperdensity is usually associated with iron overload. The most specific features are an early uptake of contrast media with a mosaic shape pattern. During the portal phase, the density diminishes sharply. However, HCCs may show variable vascularity depending on tumour grade. The capsule, when present, is best seen at the portal or late phase as an enhanced thickening at the periphery. Vascular invasion of segmental branches may also be identified. Fatty infiltration presenting as a hyperdensity within the tumour is seen in 2–20% of the patients. Intra-tumoral arterioportal fistula may present as an early enhancement of portal branches or as a triangular area distal to the tumour with a contrast enhancement different from that of the adjacent parenchyma. Arterioportal fistulas are seen frequently in cirrhotic patients without HCC as infracentimetric hypervascular subcapsular lesions and should not be mistaken for an HCC.

Magnetic resonance imaging

Magnetic resonance imaging (MRI) tends to be more accurate than the other imaging techniques in differentiating HCC from other liver tumours, especially when they are larger than 2 cm. As for CT, the technique of MRI should be accurate with T1- and T2-weighted images and with an early, intermediate and late phase following contrast injection of gadolinium. The characteristics of an

HCC are the mosaic shape structure and the presence of a capsule. HCCs classically are hypo-intense on T1-weighted images and hyperintense on T2-weighted images but these characteristics are present in only 54% of patients. The second most frequent features are hypointensity on both T1 and T2 images, accounting for 16% of HCCs, mainly when they are less than 1.5 cm. Hyperintensity on T1-weighted images is also possible, and associated with fatty, copper or glycogen infiltration of the tumour. Additional contrast agents are currently under evaluation.

Arteriography

The improvement in the accuracy of CT and MRI have considerably reduced the diagnostic usefulness of angiography. It is nevertheless still widely used as part of arterial chemoembolisation. HCC is typically hypervascular but some HCCs may be avascular or appear so due to necrosis, bleeding or vascular occlusion. Other features of angiography include arterioportal or arteriovenous shunting as well as portal vein involvement.

Arteriography is usually coupled with Lipiodol injection, which is retained selectively for a prolonged period of time by the tumour. On a CT performed 4 weeks later, the retained Lipiodol is radiodense and reveals the tumour as a high-density area. However, nodular uptake within the liver is not specific for HCC, since all hypervascular liver tumours, including focal nodular hyperplasia, adenoma, angioma and metastatic lesions, will retain Lipiodol. False-negative results may be observed in cases of avascular, necrotic or fibrotic tumours or if not all areas of the liver have been perfused with Lipiodol because of catheter malposition or vascular interruption. Because the sensitivity of CT Lipiodol does not seem to be greater than that of spiral CT (in contrast to conventional CT) it has almost been abandoned.

Accuracy of imaging techniques

CT and MRI with contrast enhancement have the highest accuracy (>80%) in the diagnosis of HCC. Both techniques can be combined occasionally to ascertain the diagnosis (see below). Comparison with the pathological analysis of explanted livers of transplant candidates, however, shows that both techniques lose accuracy in the assessment of extension of the disease. For any technique, additional intrahepatic tumours, especially those less than 1 cm, are not diagnosed preoperatively in 30% of cases, which is an important limitation in the selection of transplant candidates (see below). MRI angiography with 2-mm thin section is currently considered the most accurate technique, with a sensitivity of 100% for nodules more than 20 mm, 89% for nodules 10–20 mm, and 34% for nodules <10 mm.[35]

Diagnosis of HCC

Although the differential diagnosis of HCC includes a number of non-neoplastic conditions and malignant tumours, the key challenge is the differentiation of HCC from macroregenerative nodules or borderline nodules within a cirrhotic liver. MRI is currently the most reliable in differentiating regenerating nodules from HCC, and nodules larger than 2 cm are seldom macroregenerative or borderline nodules.

The diagnostic criteria have recently been established by a panel of experts.[36] If the nodule is less than 1 cm on US, the probability that it is an HCC is 50%; the other imaging techniques are unlikely to reliably confirm the diagnosis and the accuracy of liver biopsy is also low. It is therefore reasonable, from a clinical point of view, to repeat the US at 3-month intervals until the lesion becomes larger than 1 cm. An early HCC may occasionally take more than a year to grow to this size. If the nodule is larger than 2 cm, the probability that it is an HCC is much greater, and confirmation of the diagnosis is mandatory. In patients with cirrhosis, the diagnosis of HCC can be established if either two coincident imaging techniques (US, spiral CT, MRI or angiography) demonstrate the presence of arterial hypervascularisation of the lesion or if the hypervascular mass is associated with a serum AFP greater than 400 ng/mL. Biopsy is recommended if the size of the mass is between 1 and 2 cm.

Requirement for histological study

Pathological confirmation of HCC can be obtained by cytology, histology or a combination of these (by order of increasing accuracy). A routine biopsy is not indicated in cirrhotic patients when the diagnosis has been achieved by imaging techniques and/or AFP measurements (see above). The decision to perform a biopsy should also take into account the clinical impact of the result as well as the potential drawbacks of the technique. Liver biopsy is limited by its potential complications of haemorrhage and pain. Furthermore, percutaneous needle biopsy of HCC may occasionally be responsible for neoplastic seeding as well as vascular spread. The incidence of needle tract seeding after either percutaneous biopsy or percutaneous ethanol injection is, however, 1–5%.[37] Furthermore, tumoral involvement is generally limited to subcutaneous tissues at the site of puncture. These cutaneous metastases have a slow progression, and it is possible to perform local excision without significant changes in the survival of those patients.[38] Even if the proportion of false positives for the diagnosis of HCC with current imaging techniques is low, the risk of needle tract seeding is balanced by the risk of pursuing an aggressive treatment such as resection or transplantation in a patient without malignancy. In the future, biopsy of the tumour and the non-tumorous liver may also provide a molecular profiling of the disease and help plan screening or treatment. Finally, one should be aware that there is a 30–40% false-negative rate of fine-needle biopsy and that a negative result should therefore never rule out malignancy.[37]

Natural history of HCC and staging systems

The natural history of HCC is traditionally considered particularly grim, based on the analysis of historical controls whose advanced tumour stage made them unsuitable for any form of treatment. In these patients, the life expectancy was measured in weeks. This uniformly poor prognosis has, however, been questioned over the past 10 years. The estimation of HCC doubling times are quite variable, ranging between 27 and 605 days, with a mean value of 200 days.[39] Furthermore, the prognosis of untreated patients who are not all end-stage at the time of presentation[39–41] is better than anticipated, with 2- and 3-year survival ranges of 40–56% and 13–28%, respectively. Survival in these patients is influenced by the presence of cancer-related symptoms (such as a declined performance status or presence of weight loss or anorexia), of an invasive tumour phenotype (such as portal invasion or extrahepatic spread of the tumour), as well as the severity and evolutivity of the cirrhosis. In asymptomatic patients without a tumoral invasion pattern, the spontaneous 3-year survival may be as high as 50%.[41]

These observations have important implications in the evaluation of uncontrolled trials. The efficacy of a given treatment in particular cannot be properly assessed if the follow-up is too short. They are also important in the design of controlled trials. Stratification based on these criteria is probably necessary when evaluating palliative treatments, as evidenced, for example, by studies on chemoembolisation (see below).

The better knowledge of this natural history has led several groups, over the past five years, to compute prognostic models aiming at predicting the survival of a given patient based on simple criteria.[42–44] The main characteristics of these studies are outlined in **Table 4.3**. They are based on the prospective follow-up of large, unselected population samples, the treatment for which was

Table 4.3 • Main studies used to compute prognostic models of HCC

Origin	Study period	No. of patients	Surgery (%)	PEI* (%)	TACE† (%)	Supportive care (%)
Italy (CLIP)[42]	1990–92	435	3	32	17	42
France (GRETCH)[43]	1990–92	761	7	3	20	53
China (CUPI)[44]	1996–98	926	10	–	–	58

*Percutaneous ethanol injection; †transarterial chemoembolisation.

Table 4.4 • Main variables retained in prognostic models. The numbers refer to the score given to each variable. A total score is obtained by adding each individual score. In the CLIP score, the median survivals according to the score in the initial[42] and prospective validations[45] were: score 0: 36–42 months; score 1: 22–32 months; score 2: 8–16 months; score 3: 4–7 months, score 4 or above: 1–3 months

	GRETCH		CLIP		CUPI	
Tumour morphology			Multinodular extension <50%	1	TNM I and II	−3
			Multinodular extension >50%	2	TNM III	−1
					TNM IV	0
	Portal thrombosis	1	Portal thrombosis	1		
Tumour biology	AFP >35 ng/mL	2	AFP >400 ng/mL	1	AFP >500 ng/mL	3
Liver function	Bilirubin >50 µmol/L	3	Child–Pugh A	0	Bilirubin <34 µmol/mL	0
	Alk. phosph. >2N*	2	Child–Pugh B	1	Bilirubin 34–51 µmol/mL	3
			Child–Pugh C	2	Bilirubin >51 µmol/mL	4
					Alk. phosph. >200 IU/L	3
General status	Karnofsky index <80	3			Asymptomatic	−4
Score range	0 to 11		0 to 6		−7 to 12	

*2N = twice normal.

not uniform. Approximately half received supportive care alone while the other half underwent surgery, percutaneous treatment, or arterial embolisation. These studies therefore provide a rough estimate of the proportion of HCC patients whose tumours are accessible to surgery or percutaneous treatment in a given country.

The variables recorded at the time of prognosis that proved independent in the multivariate analysis differed between studies but reflect the extension of the tumour, the liver function tests and the performance status (**Table 4.4**). Although these variables still have limitations, and for some require external validation, they proved more accurate in predicting outcome than unidimensional systems such as the TNM, Child–Pugh index, Karnofsky index or performance status used alone.

Screening for HCC

Screening for liver cancer is used routinely in countries where effective therapeutic interventions are available despite the usual lack of randomised controlled trials or hard evidence that these programmes are cost-effective. The reason for this is that HCC fulfils most of the criteria required for a surveillance or screening programme to be justified. HCC is common in highly endemic areas (and its incidence is growing in others) and it is associated with a high mortality. Furthermore, the survival is extremely poor by the time patients present with symptoms related to the tumour, and the population at risk is clearly defined (i.e. cirrhotic patients). Acceptable screening tests of low morbidity and high efficacy exist that allow the tumour to be recognised in the latent/early stage. Finally, effective treatments exist in selected patients.

The two most common tests used for screening of HCC are ultrasonography and serum AFP measurements. Their limits have been outlined above. This applies particularly to AFP, which most clinicians consider to be of little or no use for screening. However, the regular increase of AFP in patients who have a normal AFP at baseline should prompt the performance of a CT or MRI scan if US is negative.

The optimal interval of surveillance is related to the tumour growth rate. Available data suggest that the time taken for an undetectable lesion to grow to 2 cm is about 4–12 months, and that it takes 5 months for the most rapidly growing HCC to reach 3 cm. Because surgical or percutaneous treatments are best performed on tumours <3 cm, screening programmes are therefore usually performed at 6-month intervals. However, there does not appear to be a difference in terms of feasibility of treatment and survival between patients who have semiannual and annual surveillance,[46] with the latter being the most cost-effective strategy. No randomised trial has directly addressed this issue.

There are several limitations to screening programmes. Of patients presenting with HCC, 20–50% have previously undiagnosed cirrhosis and would therefore escape surveillance. Access to medical care is a serious limitation in highly endemic areas as well as compliance with regular follow-up in developed countries, where 50% of patients with alcoholic cirrhosis drop out from surveillance over a 5-year period. The reliability of US is highly dependent on the performance of the radiologist, and the cost and invasiveness of CT scan or MRI, which are less operator dependent, make them unsuitable as screening tools.

> Surveillance of at-risk patients is being used increasingly at a 6-month interval with ultrasound and AFP estimation to detect HCC at an early stage.
>
> Surveillance for HCC should be considered in high-risk groups such as those with established cirrhosis due to HBV, HCV and haemochromatosis. Male patients with alcohol-related cirrhosis who are abstaining from alcohol or likely to comply with treatment should also be considered.
>
> If surveillance is offered, ultrasound is recommended as a screening tool whereas CT and MRI are most useful in confirming the diagnosis. Liver biopsy is recommended in selected cases only.

The impact of screening programmes on patient management and survival is still controversial[47] although the most recent studies tend to indicate that they increase the chance of successful treatment and improve survival. Some workers have found that although 50–75% of tumours detected by screening were unifocal and 3 cm or less in size, this did not translate into comparable resection rates. In contrast, in the only prospective randomised controlled study involving more than 17 000 HBV patients from Shanghai, surgical resection could be performed in 70% of the screened patients compared with 0% of the non-screened patients.[48] The 1-year survival was 88% in the former and zero in the latter. The discrepancies between the earlier and the most recent studies might be related to improvement in US and medical treatment but also to the causative agent of the HCC or area of the world where the study was performed. As outlined previously, most HCCs in China are related to early HBV infection and therefore occur in relatively young patients with less severe underlying liver disease. Similar large-scale investigations are therefore required in different countries.

Although screening is recommended in cirrhotic patients, the current trend has to take into account the available treatment options when deciding whether or not to screen a patient. Screening of Child C patients is, for example, inappropriate if they are not potential liver transplant candidates. Screening of Child B patients might also be controversial as resection is usually contraindicated and there is no evidence yet that treatment of the tumour, apart from transplantation, will improve survival. A better identification of risk factors for HCC will probably also allow a more selective screening and therefore improve its cost-effectiveness.

Treatment options

Treatment of HCC may rely on liver transplantation, partial liver resection, percutaneous destruction or chemoembolisation. Apart from transplantation, all these options share the drawback of not treating the underlying liver disease when it is present. Hence, the risk of recurrence is particularly high whatever the treatment in the cirrhotic patient. In patients with normal livers, the ideal treatment that should be considered first is liver resection, but this treatment should be delayed if the tumour is complicated by haemorrhage. However, HCC in normal liver accounts for only a small proportion of HCCs. In patients with cirrhosis, the choice is more difficult and should take into account the age of the patient, the extension of the tumour and the presence of impaired liver function. Using appropriate selection criteria, liver transplantation, liver resection, percutaneous treatment and chemoembolisation have, in decreasing order, the greatest efficacy but, in increasing order, the greatest feasibility and should be considered in this order. The proportion of patients undergoing radical treatment is highly variable around the world, even in developed countries.

HCC IN NORMAL LIVERS

The indication for treatment is least controversial in patients with no or only very mild coexisting fibrosis.

However, this does not preclude the presence of some risk factors such as HBV infection, genetic haemochromatosis, alcohol ingestion and steatosis.[49] HCCs are usually large but solitary in this setting; they occur in relatively young patients, and the non-tumorous liver has a high regenerating capacity. Surgical resection, through major hepatectomies, is associated with mortality, morbidity and transfusion rates less than 1%, 15% and 30%, respectively.[50] The 5-year survival is greater than 50%,[51,52] and no other treatment equals these results. In practice, percutaneous treatments are not performed due to the large size of the tumour. Liver transplantation is associated with a risk of early mortality close to 10%, a need for long-term immunosuppression, and has long-term results no different from those of resection.[51] Transplantation has been performed with poor results in the past in patients with tumours judged unresectable. Follow-up is of the utmost importance to detect recurrence at an early stage. Recurrence should be treated by repeat resection whenever possible. A small group of patients may benefit from transplantation if their recurrence is confined to the liver and not accessible to a repeat resection.

LIVER RESECTION OF HCC IN CIRRHOTIC PATIENTS

Cirrhosis three limitations are several to resection of HCC.

1. The tumour is multifocal in 20–60% of cirrhotic livers at the time of diagnosis whereas liver resection, as a rule, can only be considered in patients with unifocal tumours.
2. Furthermore, cirrhosis is an important risk factor for the development of postoperative complications.
3. Tumour recurrence. The incidence of in-hospital death following liver resection in cirrhotic patients was around 10% until recently due to the poor functional reserve of the liver and its impaired ability to regenerate, which resulted in a high incidence of liver failure.[53] This risk has progressively decreased to 0–5% over the past 10 years[54,55] due to improved patient selection and surgical expertise, although the risk of postoperative complications is still higher than in patients with normal livers.

The predominant risk factors for postoperative liver failure are the patient's Child grade[56] and the extent of resection. Any resection is contraindicated in patients who are grade C at the time of surgery, and only limited resection is possible in patients who are grade B. However, even in grade A cirrhotic patients with apparently normal serum bilirubin and prothrombin time and no ascites, the risk of liver surgery is increased. A spectrum of additional risk factors for liver incompensation in these Child A patients have been identified in different areas of the world. They include high indocyanine green (ICG) retention at 15 minutes,[57] serum transaminase level greater than twice the normal upper range,[58] or evidence of portal hypertension.[59] Transjugular measurement of portal hypertension is an invasive procedure that is not used routinely. Indirect evidence of portal hypertension includes previous history of variceal bleeding or ascites, presence of oesophageal varices, platelet count lower than 100×10^9/L, or a radiologically visible porto-systemic shunt. These three additional risk factors probably overlap, at least in part. When these factors are present, large resections should be considered with extreme caution and normally can only be performed in 10–15% of HCC patients.

Because the risk of postoperative liver failure is in part related to the inability of the remnant liver to regenerate, there has been considerable interest during the past 5 years in the optimal management of the remnant liver. This includes, in particular, more selective use of inflow occlusion[60] and avoiding excessive mobilisation of the liver during surgery.[61] Similarly, when a major hepatectomy is contemplated, preoperative portal vein embolisation (PVE) of the lobe to be resected is performed with increasing frequency in order to increase the volume of the remnant liver. When a right hepatectomy is contemplated, the right portal vein is percutaneously injected, under ultrasonographic guidance, with glue or ethanol. This induces an atrophy of the right liver within 2–6 weeks and hypertrophy of the left future remnant liver as assessed by CT scan volumetry.[62] A prospective controlled trial has shown that preoperative PVE caused approximately a 50% reduction in risk of postoperative complications and in-hospital stay.[63] However, this occurs only if PVE induces hypertrophy of the contralateral lobe, which might not take place if the portal pressure is too high or if porto-systemic shunts are present. PVE can therefore also be viewed as a way of testing the ability of the liver to regenerate.

The last important issue is whether the extent of resection influences outcome. Limited resections are the preferred option in many centres because they are associated with a reduced risk of postoperative liver failure. There is, however, growing evidence that anatomical resections, removing both the tumour and the adjacent segments that have the same portal tributaries, are associated with improved patient and disease-free survival compared with limited resections.[64,65]

The largest series of resected patients comes from the Liver Cancer Study Group in Japan, which has reported 1-, 3-, 5- and 10-year survival rates of 85%, 64%, 45% and 21% respectively in 6785 cirrhotic patients treated by hepatic resection between 1988 and 1999.[2] Comparable results have been reported by other groups worldwide (**Table 4.5**), with no differences between Western and Asian studies.[81] Survival rates as high as 60% at 5 years may be achieved in Child grade A patients with well-encapsulated tumours of 2 cm diameter or less.

RECURRENCE FOLLOWING RESECTION OF HCC

Tumour recurrence is the major cause of death following resection of HCC both in cirrhotic and non-cirrhotic livers, although it is much more frequent in the former than in the latter. The frequency of tumour recurrence in cirrhotic patients is estimated at 40% within the first year, 60% at 3 years and around 80% at 5 years. However, it is virtually constant if follow-up is extended beyond 10 years as the precursor condition (cirrhosis) persists after surgery.[82] Alternative mechanisms of recurrence include seeding of tumour cells as a result of surgical manipulation and pre- or intra-operative incomplete staging.

Recurrence within the liver is multifocal in 50% of the patients and is associated with distant metastasis in 15%, especially in the lungs, bones or adrenal gland.[83] Extrahepatic recurrence without simultaneous intrahepatic recurrence is infrequent in cirrhotic livers. Variables that have been found to be associated significantly with a greater incidence of recurrence are:[84]

- presence and severity of the underlying cirrhosis
- the presence of more than one nodule
- tumour of more than 5 cm diameter
- lack of a capsule
- moderately or poorly differentiated HCC
- presence of daughter nodules
- venous invasion
- infiltrating rather than expansive tumour
- insufficient cancer-free margin
- intraoperative blood transfusion.

The relative weight of each of these parameters is difficult to assess because most overlap. It is, for example, generally accepted that the incidence of portal vein invasion and intrahepatic metastasis correlate with the tumour size. However, tumour factors, in particular multinodularity and vascular invasion, tend to account for most of the early recurrences whereas late recurrences are mainly related to the activity of the underlying liver disease.[65]

Strategies to prevent recurrence in randomised controlled trials have been recently reviewed.[85] Preoperative chemoembolisation fails to reduce the risk of recurrence and has even been reported to be associated with a poorer survival. Adjuvant chemoembolisation or systemic chemotherapy add no benefit although chemoembolisation with ^{131}I-labelled lipiodol has shown promising results. Similarly, interferon, adaptive immunotherapy and retinoids may prove beneficial in the future if the recent initial trials are confirmed. For the present, the best way to improve survival is to monitor resected patients regularly as some may benefit from the treatment of recurrence if it is confined to the liver.[86] This treatment may rely on re-resection, transarterial chemoembolisation, percutaneous treatment or even liver transplantation. The risk and outcome of a repeat resection appears comparable to that of a first hepatectomy.[87,88]

LIVER TRANSPLANTATION

HCC is the only tumour for which transplantation plays a significant role, and this is the most attractive therapeutic option because it removes both detectable and undetectable tumour nodules together with all the preneoplastic lesions that are present in the cirrhotic liver. In addition, it simultaneously treats the underlying cirrhosis and prevents the

Table 4.5 • Results after curative surgical resection of HCC in Asian series, and in European and America series

References	Study period	No. of patients	Cirrhosis (%)	Diameter <5 cm (%)	In-hospital mortality (%)	1-year survival (%)	3-year survival (%)	5-year survival (%)
Asian series								
Nagasue et al. 1993[56]	1980–90	229	77	75	11	80	51	26
Kawasaki et al. 1995[66]	1990–93	112	68	83	2	92	79	–
Takenada et al. 1996[67]	1985–93	280	52	–	2	88	70	50
Chen & Jeng 1997[68]	1983–94	382	45	40	4	71	52	46
Makuuchi et al. 1998[69]	1990–97	352	–	–	10	92	73	47
Poon et al. 2001[70]	1989–94	136	50	29	13	68	47	36
	1994–99	241	43	45	2	82	62	49
Shimozawa & Hanazaki 2004[71]	1987–2001	135	71	100	2	95	73	55
European and American series								
Franco et al. 1990[72]	1983–88	72	100	60	7	68	51	–
Castells et al. 1993[73]	1987–91	33	100	100	9	81	44	–
Vauthey et al. 1995[74]	1970–92	106	33	17	6	–	–	41
Nagorney & Gigot 1996[75]	–	120	22	–	8	82	44	31
Mazziotti et al. 1998[76]	1983–98	229	100	59	5	85	63	41
Llovet et al. 1999[77]	1989–97	77	100	75	–	85	62	51
Belghiti et al. 2002[78]	1990–99	300	82	47	6	81	57	37
Ercolani et al. 2003[79]	1983–99	224	100	81	3	83	63	42
Cha et al. 2003[80]	1990–2001	164	40	4	–	79	51	40

development of postoperative or distant complications associated with portal hypertension and liver failure.

Liver transplantation was performed initially in patients in whom partial liver resection could not be contemplated due to the high number and/or large size of their tumours. HCC in these early days (the 1980s) accounted for almost 40% of liver transplantation indications in Europe. The results were disappointing, with a high rate of recurrence within the first month or year post transplant.[89] Furthermore, the use of immunosuppressive treatments accelerated markedly the course of recurrence.[90] The survival curve was therefore clearly lower than for the other indications of transplantation (30% vs. 70% at 5 years). Although a 30% 5-year survival is a fair result for a malignancy, the donor shortage resulted in high mortality rates for patients on liver transplantation waiting lists. Such patients anticipated a better outcome, and this has led to the consensus that transplantation should not be proposed for cirrhotic patients with large or multifocal HCCs.

On the other hand, the outcome in patients transplanted with an HCC incidentally discovered by pathological examination of the explanted liver is extremely favourable, with a small incidence of tumour recurrence and survival comparable to patients transplanted without malignancy.[91] These observations have therefore led several groups to

analyse retrospectively their results as a function of tumour extension. It was found that limited tumour involvement – defined by the presence of a single tumour less than 5 cm or the presence of two or three tumours less than 3 cm in patients with no vascular invasion and no extrahepatic disease (the so-called Milan criteria) – was associated with a much better outcome.[92,93] With the adoption of these criteria by the United Network for Organ Sharing (UNOS), the 5-year survival has increased in the USA from 25% in the period 1987–91 to 61% in the period 1997–2001.[94] These good results have been reproduced by others worldwide with 5-year survival currently ranging between 60 and 75% (**Table 4.6**). However, because of these strict oncological limitations, less than 5–10% of HCC patients are potential transplant candidates, and HCC currently accounts for only 10% of all liver transplantations. Although there have been successful attempts to broaden these indications,[95,96] they are still strictly applied in most centres. Tumour staging is therefore crucial in the preoperative evaluation. Although imaging techniques have improved, the number of small nodules is underestimated in 70% of the patients, and macroscopic vascular invasion and satellite nodules are present in 5% and 40% of patients fulfilling the Milan criteria. There is therefore considerable interest in the development of new markers of recurrence following transplantation and in particular tumour differentiation,

Table 4.6 • Results of liver transplantation for HCC in patients with cirrhosis reported in the 1990s using restrictive carcinological criteria

Study	No. of patients	1-year survival (%)	3-year survival (%)	5-year survival (%)
Mazzaferro et al. 1996[93]	48	90	75	–
Figueras et al. 1997[98]	38	82	79	75
Llovet et al. 1999[77]	87	82	69	69
Jonas et al. 2001[99]	120	90	77	71
Yao et al. 2001[100]	60	90	–	75
Adam et al. 2001[101]	195	80	66	60
Margarit et al. 2002[102]	103	81	66	58
Moya et al. 2002[103]	104	74	–	63
Vivarelli et al. 2002[104]	106	–	–	64
De Carlis et al. 2003[105]	121	–	–	62

microscopic vascular invasion and proliferation activity.

No randomised controlled trial has compared liver resection and transplantation. Retrospective studies on the two techniques are difficult to compare because there is generally a greater proportion of Child B and C patients and of small and multiple tumours in transplantation groups. Nevertheless, survival following transplantation appears greater than after partial liver resection (**Tables 4.5 and 4.6**). Similar results were observed when focusing on Child A patients.[97] However, several additional limitations of liver transplantation exist that should be taken into account when interpreting these results.

Liver transplantation is not readily available or not available at all in high endemic areas of HCC. Moreover, for cadaveric liver transplantation, the average time from listing to transplantation has become longer than 10–12 months due to donor shortage in Europe and the USA. It is therefore not uncommon for patients to be excluded from the waiting list due to disease progression. The 6- and 12-month cumulative drop-out from the waiting list has been estimated to be 7–15% at 6 months and 25% at 12 months.[106] Hence, in Barcelona, on an intention to treat basis, the 2-year survival was 84% after transplantation but 54% from the time of listing.[77] Similarly, the UCSF group reported a 73% 5-year survival after transplantation but a 73% 2-year survival from the time of listing.[106] In both series, the results of resection compared favourably with those of transplantation. Suggested strategies to overcome this limitation include increasing the donor pool through the use of marginal donors, prioritising HCC patients in the transplantation waiting list, and limiting tumour progression during the waiting period by trans-arterial chemoembolisation (TACE), percutaneous treatments or partial liver resection. The efficacy of these systems has yet to be validated. Living-related transplantation is another option in patients with an anticipated long waiting time, but only 25% of candidates have a potential donor relative and there is an inherent risk of mortality (0.5%) in the donor.

The third limitation in considering transplantation is that not all patients with an HCC fulfilling the criteria are potential transplant candidates. Age above 60–65 years is a contraindication in many centres due to donor shortage, although outcome of liver transplantation in selected older patients is not very different from that of younger patients. This is a serious limitation to transplantation for HCV-related HCC in the Western world as more than 50% of these patients are 60 years or more. In patients with an HBV-DNA replication or persistent alcohol consumption, transplantation is contraindicated as cirrhosis is likely to recur within the graft. In contrast, HCV infection is not a contraindication although graft failure due to recurrence is a rising problem.

TRANSARTERIAL CHEMOEMBOLISATION (TACE) OF HCC

The rationale for treating HCC by arterial embolisation is that, in contrast to the liver paren-chyma, this neoplasm receives almost 100% of its blood supply from the artery. When the artery is obstructed, the tumour experiences an ischaemic insult that results in extensive necrosis. Several agents may be used to achieve this, including gelfoam, starch microspheres and metallic coils. Injection of iodised oil has been combined to improve the efficacy of embolisation of the tumour arterial supply. Iodised oil (Lipiodol), which is hyperdense on CT scan, is cleared from the normal hepatic parenchyma but retained in malignant tumours for periods ranging from several weeks to over a year. This accumulation, which is not associated with significant adverse effects, may be used for targeting cytotoxic drugs by increasing their concentration in the tumour cells. Cytotoxic drugs employed in this selective form of chemo-therapy (chemoembolisation) include 5-fluorouracil (5-FU), doxorubicin, mitomycin C, epirubicin or cisplatin and iodine-131. Contraindications for TACE include liver decompensation, biliary obstruction, bilioenteric anastomosis, impaired kidney function and portal vein thrombosis, as a simultaneous arterial embolisation may lead to liver necrosis. However, the latter contraindication is relative provided the patient has compensated liver disease and the embolisation is performed selectively on a limited tumour volume.

In patients with good liver function, arterial embolisation is usually well tolerated. In contrast, a pre-embolisation abnormal serum bilirubin or prothrombin time is associated with a risk of liver decompensation, especially if the dosage of chemo-therapy is not modified. The mortality associated with this procedure ranges between 0 and 2% in Child A patients[107–109] but is 8% and 37% in Child grade B and C patients, respectively.[110] Overall, more than 75% of the patients develop a post-embolisation syndrome characterised by fever, abdominal pain, nausea and raised serum transaminase level. These symptoms, which are not prevented by antibiotics or anti-inflammatory drugs, are self-limiting and last for less than 1 week. A most severe form requiring prolonged hospitalisation is observed in 15%. The postembolisation syndrome, which was attributed to the tumour necrosis, seems to be in fact related to injury of the non-tumorous liver, with a higher rate of fever and cytolysis in patients with minor fibrotic changes.[111] This tends to become less severe as the procedures are repeated. More severe complications occur in less than 5% of patients and include, in decreasing order of frequency: cholecystitis or gallbladder infarction, gastric or duodenal wall necrosis, and acute pancreatitis.[111] These are probably related to the inadvertent migration of embolisation material in the cystic, pyloric or gastroduodenal artery, and they have became less frequent with the use of supraselective embolisation. Ulcer prophylaxis should therefore be routine, and an ultrasound scan performed if pain or fever persists. Hepatic abscess formation is rare but is the rationale for excluding from embolisation patients with a bilioenteric anastomosis. An early CT scan may show the presence of gas in the tumour, which is more frequently due to the inadvertent injection of air during the procedure than an anaerobic superinfection.

The efficacy of TACE is assessed by a dynamic CT scan (performed usually 1 month after TACE) as:

1. a decrease in tumour diameter;
2. a dense uptake of lipiodol by the tumour;
3. a decrease in tumour vascularity;
4. the absence of new tumours.

These features do not necessarily evolve in parallel. A decrease in tumour size may, for example, be associated with persistent vascularisation (i.e. residual tumour) whereas compact lipiodol uptake without residual vascularisation may indicate complete tumour necrosis despite no significant decrease in size. Case–control studies have shown that TACE is associated with a decrease in tumour size in 50–80% of patients, and with a significant

delay in tumour progression and vascular invasion.[110,112,113] Similarly, many surgical studies have reported an approximate 20% rate of complete tumour necrosis in the resected specimens of patients treated preoperatively by TACE. Furthermore, TACE provides effective symptomatic relief of pain in the majority of patients.[110]

The clinical efficacy of intra-arterial and conservative treatments has been compared in seven randomised controlled trials, including a total of 516 patients who were further included into a meta-analysis. Initial trials failed to demonstrate significant improved survival despite antitumoral effect.[109,114–116] These were, however, criticised for having included patients with advanced tumour stage and poor hepatic function. More recently, two excellent trials focusing on patients with unresectable HCC, but applying stricter selection criteria by excluding patients with diffuse neoplasm and severe liver failure, have shown significant survival advantage with an active re-treatment schedule.[117,118] These results have been confirmed by meta-analysis.[119] TACE is therefore a validated treatment option in selected patients. Variables associated with improved survival following TACE, besides treatment response, are a hypervascular HCC at baseline,[120] a compact uptake of lipiodol within the tumour,[121] and the repetition of the procedures.

Although this treatment has been used routinely for more than 20 years and the technique of the procedure has evolved significantly to become more selective, there is no good evidence for the best chemotherapeutic agent and the optimum retreatment strategy. TACE is usually repeated at fixed intervals (2 to 3 months) until an arbitrarily planned number of courses is reached, technical difficulties are encountered or the patient dies. Discontinuation is, however, reasonable if there is either progression despite two procedures or, conversely, if there is evidence of complete tumour necrosis. A long-term side effect of repeated TACE is the progressive development of distal arterial injuries that precludes the performance or efficacy of subsequent courses.

PERCUTANEOUS LOCAL ABLATIVE THERAPY

Loco-regional therapies are those percutaneous treatment modalities that allow the injection of a damaging agent directly into the tumour or the application of an energy source. Damaging agents include chemicals such as ethanol or acetic acid, radioactive isotopes such as yttrium-90 microspheres, or hyperthermic agents such as saline, water or chemotherapeutic agents. Energy sources either aim at increasing temperature by radiofrequency, microwave or interstitial laser photocoagulation or, alternatively, at decreasing temperature (cryoablation). Among these numerous techniques, ethanol injection and radiofrequency are the most widely used.

These methods have common advantages and limitations. On the one hand they are minimally invasive, preserve the uninvolved liver parenchyma, have no systemic side effects, and avoid the mortality and morbidity of major hepatic surgery. On the other hand, they can only be performed in patients with small tumours confined to the liver. Only tumours less than 5 cm are likely to be successfully treated. The presence of multiple tumours (more than three) is also a limitation because of the need for repeated punctures. In addition, multiple tumours are either the result of multifocal carcinogenesis or vascular extension, and a focal treatment is therefore unlikely to be very effective. Other contraindications include gross ascites (because it will prevent adhesions between the liver and the abdominal wall and hence favour intraperitoneal bleeding), coagulopathy that cannot be corrected, and obstructive jaundice (due to the risk of abscess formation or bile peritonitis). A common requirement for percutaneous treatments is the need to clearly visualise the tumour by US. Hence, isoechoic HCC or tumours located in the upper part of segments 4, 7 and 8 may occasionally be unsuitable for treatment, although intraoperative radiofrequency may overcome this limitation. Finally, whichever technique is used, the needle should not enter the tumour directly but pass through the hepatic parenchyma so as to prevent intraperitoneal bleeding or seeding of tumour cells. This may prove impossible for some superficial or protruding tumours.

Percutaneous ethanol injection (PEI)

PEI was introduced in the 1980s and has rapidly gained wide popularity because of its high antitumoral efficacy coupled with its relatively simple and inexpensive application. Absolute ethanol is injected through a fine needle into the tumour, causing dehydration and necrosis of cells as well as thrombosis of small blood vessels. The procedure is undertaken with US guidance, and ethanol is injected until the whole tumour becomes hyperechoic. The fact that HCCs are relatively soft in comparison to the surrounding liver parenchyma promotes the diffusion of the ethanol within the tumour, in particular when it is encapsulated. The drawback is that PEI is unlikely to create a safety margin of ablation in the liver parenchyma surrounding the nodule where satellite nodules may be present. Ethanol injections are repeated if contrast enhancement persists on CT.[122] PEI can also be combined with TACE, and the combination is more effective than TACE alone (for large tumours)[123] or PEI alone (for small lesions)[124] in patients with unresectable HCC.

Following PEI, side effects occur in less than a third of patients and include pain and fever. A transient rise in transaminase levels is common. Complications are rare and result from the passage of ethanol into the bile ducts (resulting in cholangitis) or the portal radicles (resulting in thrombosis). The mortality rate associated with this procedure is minimal and it can usually be performed on an outpatient basis.

Consensus is currently lacking on the ideal method of PEI – using either a single or repeated injections. With large tumours and in cases of recurrence, PEI should be repeated. Although HCCs (up to 10 cm) may be treated successfully by PEI, it has become clear that the smaller the tumour, the greater is the probability of achieving a complete response.[125] The rate of complete tumour necrosis is 90–100% in HCCs smaller than 2 cm, 70% in those of 3 cm, and 50% in HCCs of 5 cm.[126,127] The 5-year survival rate in Child grade A patients with HCCs less than 5 cm ranges between 47 and 51% at 5 years. However, recurrence within the liver exceeds 50% at 2 years and ranges between 65 and 98% at 5 years.[128] Although no prospective controlled trial has compared PEI and surgical resection, several studies have shown that the long-term outcome could be comparable for small tumours. PEI, which is associated with a lower early risk, should be preferred in Child grade B patients with solitary HCCs less than 3 cm.

Radiofrequency (RF)

RF, first described in 1993, exploits the conversion of electromagnetic energy into heat. It is done through a needle electrode (15–18G) with an insulated shaft and a non-insulated tip, which is positioned into the tumour under US guidance. The patient is made into an electric circuit by placing grounding pads on his or her thighs. The radio-frequency emitted from the tip causes ionic agitation and frictional heat, which leads to cell death from coagulation necrosis. The objective is to maintain a 55–100°C temperature throughout the entire target volume for a sufficient period of time. Due to the relatively slow thermal conduction from the electrode, the duration of the procedure depends on the tumour diameter and is longer (20–90 minutes) than with PEI. Because it is also more painful, the procedure is generally performed under general anaesthesia.

As for PEI, the main limitation to RF is tumour size. With the conventional monopolar RF, the diameter of coagulation is limited to 1.6 cm. Larger diameters (up to 4 cm) can be achieved with more complex electrode geometry, such as J-hooked needles that are advanced within the tumour after locating the tip of the electrode in the tumour. Other approaches consist of injecting saline into the lesion during treatment to cool the electrode tip. Monitoring the impedance is important because excessive heating results in tissue charring, increased tissue impedance and decreased energy absorption. Finally, simultaneous occlusion of the arterial supply increases the diameter of induced necrosis. This is the rationale for recent trials combining chemoembolisation and RF in patients with larger tumours (5 cm). Another limitation specific to RF is the proximity of large vessels, such as major portal branches, hepatic veins or the inferior vena cava, because the continuous blood flow may prevent adequate heating. Moreover, RF of tumours adjacent to the biliary confluence may result in biliary damage.

RF achieves at least the same necrotic response as PEI but in fewer sessions (1.5 vs. 4). For tumours larger than 3 cm, the rate of complete necrosis is higher with RF than with PEI, and a recent controlled trial demonstrated improved recurrence-free survival rates.[129] Despite this better local tumoral control, a survival benefit of RF over PEI has not been clearly demonstrated. Treatment response is assessed by CT scan or MRI no sooner than 1 month after the procedure. RF may result in a rim of fibrotic tissue (hypervascular at the late phase of MRI or CT scan) at the periphery of the tumour, which should not be mistaken for residual tumour tissue.

The main drawback of RF compared to PEI, besides increased cost, is a higher rate of complications. In a recent literature review, the mortality was 0.5% and the morbidity was 9%.[130] These include, in particular, abscess formation, perforation of adjacent organs and intraperitoneal bleeding. It is therefore contraindicated in patients with bilioenteric anastomosis or superficial tumours, particularly those located close to the right colon. The latter contraindication can be overcome by performing the RF under laparoscopy and separating these adjacent organs from the tumour. Another potential problem is tumour seeding, which seems more frequent than after PEI because of the larger needle diameter. Risk factors include subcapsular location and poor histological differentiation of the tumour. Coagulating the needle tract while removing the needle may reduce this risk.

OTHER PALLIATIVE TREATMENTS

Systemic and regional chemotherapy of HCC

Systemic chemotherapy has very limited value as a primary treatment modality for HCC, and only a small number of patients will obtain meaningful palliation. Several randomised controlled trials have assessed the role of systemic chemotherapy by the intravenous route – using either single agents (doxorubicin, cisplatin, mitomycin C, 5-fluorouracil) or combined agents – on tumour progression and survivals. These trials have described an overall partial response rate of less than 20%, with a negligible complete response rate.[119] Therefore, there is no rationale for using chemotherapy in unresectable HCC outside of clinical trials.

Radiation therapy of HCC

External beam radiation therapy has been of limited value in treating HCC because the tumour is relatively radioresistant whereas the normal liver parenchyma is very radiosensitive. Maximum tolerance of the normal liver to irradiation is generally accepted to be between 2500 and 3000 Gy. Above these values, the risk of radiation hepatitis increases quickly and is associated with a mortality rate close to 50%. In addition, it is difficult to protect the surrounding organs such as the colon, duodenum and kidney.

Greater interest has therefore been placed on targeted therapy with intravenously administered radioactive iodine-131. The injection of radio-isotopes directly into the hepatic artery offers the advantage of increased delivery of isotope within the tumour and decreased systemic toxicity. This technique can be used in patients with portal vein thrombosis and may result in the disappearance of the thrombus. In this setting, a controlled trial has shown that intra-arterial injection of ^{131}I-iodised oil was associated with a 6-month survival rate of 48% as compared with 0% in a control group receiving only medical support.[131]

Antiandrogen treatment

Both antiandrogenic and antioestrogenic treatments have been used as a palliative treatment of HCC. Results with antiandrogens have been disappointing.[119] There has been more interest regarding the use of antioestrogenic treatment with tamoxifen. Results of controlled studies are controversial but, overall, this treatment has no impact on 1-year survival.[119]

Treatment of complicated HCC

HCC with portal vein invasion is associated with a dismal prognosis, with a median survival of 4 months. Most patients with this condition are unsuitable for any form of treatment. A very small proportion of patients with good general condition, preserved liver function and limited tumour extension can benefit from treatment options including surgical resection of the tumour and the thrombus, TACE, targeted radiotherapy or US-guided injection of chemotherapy or alcohol within the thrombus.

A ruptured HCC should not always be considered as a contraindication to treatment. Without any treatment, the mortality of this complication is close to 100%. The primary aim of treatment is to stop the bleeding because ascites and/or impaired coagulation usually prevent spontaneous haemostasis. Several methods of emergency haemostasis have been advocated, including TACE, hepatic artery ligation, local control through suture plication, or packing and resection of the tumour.[132] It is very difficult to compare the results of various treatments since some patients experienced tumour rupture

with a 'terminal' presentation including multiple tumours, portal thrombosis and liver insufficiency. Initial haemostasis by TACE may allow subsequent hepatectomy after complete evaluation of the extent of the cancer and functional liver reserve. Although rupture of HCC may be associated with peritoneal seeding of tumour cells, this should not be regarded as a contraindication to subsequent radical treatment. Data available from the literature indicate that the 1-year survival of patients undergoing second-stage hepatectomy is 40%, and long-term survival has been reported.

FIBROLAMELLAR CARCINOMA

Fibrolamellar carcinoma (FLC) is a rare variant of HCC,[49] with several pathological and clinical features distinct from that of HCC. It is most frequently observed in the Western hemisphere, where it accounts for less than 2% of hepatocellular carcinoma. These tumours occur at a younger age than HCC (between 20 and 35 years) and, in contrast to classical HCC, there is no apparent relationship with gender. Most importantly, FLC rarely occurs on a background of chronic liver disease and occurs more commonly in the left lobe. The most common presenting symptoms are a palpable mass, abdominal pain, weight loss, malaise and anorexia. AFP levels are raised in less than 15% of the patients. FLC usually presents as a large solitary hypervascular liver mass with a central hypodense region due to central necrosis or fibrosis. Calcification is present in 65% of the patients. Histology demonstrates deeply eosinophilic, polygonal neoplastic cells surrounded by a dense, layered fibrous stroma.

Although the natural history of FLC is ill-defined, these tumours are usually considered as having a relatively better prognosis than HCC. However, it is still unclear whether the histology alone, the absence of underlying chronic liver disease or the greater resectability rate account for this better prognosis. Prolonged survival has been reported even in patients with advanced tumour stage and metastatic spread. The 5-year survival following resection ranges between 40 and 65%.[133,134] Because intrahepatic recurrence is frequently observed and these tumours are slow growing, transplantation has been proposed as an alternative in rare cases of unresectable FLC arising in a normal liver. When possible, resection is preferred to transplantation, since long-term results are comparable.[133] If resection is considered, simultaneous lymphadenectomy of the hepatic pedicle may be recommended.

> Patients with a single small HCC (≤5 cm) or up to three lesions (≤3 cm) should be referred for assessment for consideration of hepatic resection or liver transplantation.
>
> Hepatic resection should be considered as primary therapy in any patient with HCC and a non-cirrhotic liver.
>
> Non-surgical therapy should only be used where surgical therapy is not possible. Percutaneous ethanol injection and radiofrequency ablation have been shown to produce necrosis of small HCCs, and both treatments are best suited to peripheral lesions measuring less than 3 cm in diameter.
>
> Chemoembolisation can produce tumour necrosis and has been shown to improve survival in highly selected patients with good liver reserve.

INTRAHEPATIC CHOLANGIOCARCINOMA

Intrahepatic cholangiocarcinoma (ICCA) is a rare malignant tumour arising from the peripheral intra-hepatic biliary radicles and has only relatively recently been identified as a separate entity with specific pathological and radiological features. In the USA the incidence is approximately 3 per million.[135] Although ICCA and HCC may coincide, this is extremely rare. As with HCC, there is also evidence that the incidence of this tumour is increasing.[135,136] The majority of patients with ICCA have a normal underlying liver, although up to 30% may have some evidence of underlying fibrosis and/or risk factors such as HCV infection. Other risk factors include Caroli disease, sclerosing cholangitis, Thorotrast exposure, parasitic infestation and hepatolithiasis. The Liver Cancer Study Group of Japan proposed a gross classification of ICCA into three types on the basis of the macroscopic finding of the cut surface of the tumour: mass forming, which is the commonest type; periductal infiltrating; and intraductal growth type.[137] Owing

to its intrahepatic location, the tumour rarely produces early symptoms and is generally discovered at an advanced stage.[138] Therefore, the presentation of ICCA is similar to other intrahepatic malignancies and includes abdominal pain and weight loss. The serum alkaline phosphatase level is usually elevated. Jaundice is infrequent and occurs at a late stage as a result of extrinsic compression of the hepatic confluence by the tumour. Serum tumour markers such as carcinoembryonic antigen, CA19-9 and CA125, may be elevated.

Imaging findings of ICCA consist of a large fibrous non-encapsulated heterogeneous tumour, associated with narrowing of portal adjacent veins and a retraction of the liver capsule.[139] Because it has a marked fibrotic content, the tumour is enhanced only at the late phase of injection. As the tumour grows, satellite nodules frequently develop in the vicinity of the tumour, or in the contralateral lobe. When superficial, these satellite nodules may not be visible on imaging, which is a rationale for staging laparoscopy. This tumour also has a greater propensity to invade lymph nodes of the hepatic pedicle and to produce peritoneal metastases. In contrast to HCC, this tumour does not invade the lumen of the portal veins but may encase them producing segmental liver atrophy. Localised dilatation of intrahepatic bile ducts is also possible.

Percutaneous liver biopsies yield a diagnosis of adenocarcinoma. An endoscopy is therefore frequently performed to rule out a diagnosis of liver metastases. Immunostaining with CK7 (positive in ICCA) and CK20 (positive in colon metastases) may be helpful. Because ICCAs are generally discovered at an advanced stage, the resectability rate is low and in some series only 30% of these patients have resectable tumours.[140] At the time of surgery, mean tumour size varies from 6 to 10 cm and the lesion is often centrally located.[138] Most of these tumours can therefore only be removed by major hepatectomies. The postoperative mortality rate ranges in most series between 3 and 7%.

Surgery is the best option for patients with ICCA.[141] The overall 5-year survival rate following resection varies between 25% and 50%, the best results coming from Asian series. These differences may be explained by differences in the gross anatomy of intrahepatic cholangiocarcinoma. Intraductal ICCAs, which are rare in Western countries, have a better long-term prognosis, and the mass-forming type has a better prognosis than the infiltrating type.[142,143] The worse prognosis of the infiltrating type is due to its spread along Glisson's capsule and the high incidence of lymph node involvement.

The presence of satellite nodules, often correlated with tumour size and with metastatic lymph nodes, is the predominant prognostic factor. A 5-year survival rate for patients without satellite nodules or positive lymph nodes can be observed in 35% of cases. Few patients with one or the other features survive for more than 3 years. Intrahepatic recurrences are the most common cause of death. These recurrences are not accessible to any form of treatment, in contrast to hepatocellular carcinoma. Liver transplantation is usually not considered as an effective therapy for ICCA since the 5-year survival is less than 30%.

EPITHELIOID HAEMANGIOENDOTHELIOMA (EHE)

EHE is a rare tumour that develops from the endothelial cells lining the sinusoids and progresses along the sinusoids, hepatic venules and portal vein branches. The neoplastic cells have an epithelioid or a dendritic shape but their vascular origin is identified by antibodies against factor VIII-related antigen or other endothelial markers. The stroma of this tumour has a myxoid appearance, which may become fibrotic. Calcification is identified on abdominal radiograph or CT scans in 10–30% of the patients.

The tumour usually develops in young adults but no risk factors have been identified. It does not generally arise on a background of chronic liver disease although an association with cirrhosis or nodular regenerative hyperplasia is reported.[144] The tumour usually has a multifocal distribution in the liver, and 20% of the patients have lung (or more rarely bone) metastases at the time of diagnosis.

MRI is the most reliable radiological investigation[145] but is not specific and a biopsy is mandatory to confirm the diagnosis. It is, however, important to be aware that EHE can occasionally be very difficult to differentiate from other tumours

(such as cholangiocarcinoma or angiosarcoma) due to the epithelioid shape of the tumour cells and the dense fibrotic stroma.

The natural history is highly variable and prolonged survival of more than 10 years has been reported without any treatment.[146] However, 20% of patients are dead within 2 years of diagnosis, and 20% survive more than 5 years.[147] Although the potentially lengthy clinical course following diagnosis favours resection, partial hepatectomy is rarely feasible due to the invariable multifocal involvement of the liver. Total liver resection (i.e. liver transplantation) has been performed in a limited number of patients, some of whom had metastasis at the time of transplantation. The actuarial survival after transplantation is 82% at 2 years and 43% at 5 years, with most of the deaths being due to tumour recurrence although metastatic tumour regression has been described after transplantation.[148] There is no evidence that liver transplantation improves the prognosis of these patients. The current shortage of liver grafts and the prolonged waiting time may dictate that liver transplantation is only indicated in very selected patients. Chemotherapy, chemo-embolisation or radiotherapy do not appear to be effective.

ANGIOSARCOMA

Angiosarcomas are the most frequent sarcomas of the liver but they remain rare tumours representing less than 1% of primary liver malignancies. The tumour develops from endothelial cells lining the hepatic sinusoids, and grows along sinusoids, hepatic venules and portal vein branches. Disruption of hepatic plates may result in the development of cavities filled with tumour debris or clotted blood, which favours the invasion of hepatic and portal veins. These tumours have ill-defined borders and typically involve the entire liver.

There is a clear association of angiosarcoma with prior exposure of the patient to thorium dioxide (Thorotrast, a contrast medium used in radiology during the first half of the 20th century), arsenicals or vinyl chloride (used in the manufacture of plastics).[149] An association with androgenic anabolic steroids, oestrogens, oral contraceptives, phenelzine and cupric acid has also been reported. Overall, up to 50% of angiosarcomas are associated with previous exposure to a chemical carcinogenic agent. These risk factors may account for the male predominance (gender ratio of 3:1) and the age at the time of diagnosis (50–70 years). About 20% of patients with angiosarcoma have cirrhosis. The result of imaging studies is variable.[150]

Angiosarcomas are rapidly growing tumours and, because they are frequently discovered at a late stage, median survival is 6 months. Death may result from liver failure or from intraperitoneal bleeding due to rupture of the tumour. Bleeding is favoured by the hypervascularisation of the tumour by thrombocytopenia as part of a consumption coagulopathy or by liver failure. Prolonged survival beyond 7 years has, however, been reported.[151] It is, therefore, reasonable to attempt resection (whenever possible) and to administer adjuvant chemotherapy. Liver transplantation has not been associated with survival beyond 3 years due to tumour recurrence, and is therefore not indicated in patients with angiosarcoma. Radiation therapy may have some value in this particular tumour.

Other sarcomas, besides angiosarcoma, include in particular leiomyosarcoma, and resection should be attempted if feasible.[152]

PRIMARY HEPATIC LYMPHOMA

Although malignant lymphoma frequently involves the liver, primary hepatic lymphomas are rare.[153] Gross examination reveals a single large tumour mass or multiple small masses with a diffuse hepatic involvement in about 10% of cases. Most primary hepatic lymphomas are classified as diffuse large-cell lymphomas of B-cell lineage. Some cases of

primary hepatic lymphomas associated with AIDS or with chronic liver disease have been reported.

Since primary lymphoma of the liver may not necessarily represent disseminated disease, resection should be considered, when possible, in addition to chemotherapy.

• **Key points**

The incidence of HCC is rising.

Its development is closely linked to the presence of an underlying liver disease. Viral infection or coinfection, alcohol ingestion and excessive weight are frequently implicated in its development.

The annual incidence of HCC, once cirrhosis has developed, ranges between 2% and 7%.

Surveillance of cirrhotic patients is recommended to detect HCC at an early stage provided treatment is feasible

US is recommended as a screening tool while CT scan and MRI are most useful to confirm the diagnosis. Liver biopsy is recommended in selected cases.

Liver transplantation is the treatment of choice in cirrhotic patients with limited tumour involvement.

Liver resection is the treatment of choice in patients with normal livers and is indicated in cirrhotic patients with preserved liver function, no severe portal hypertension and no associated active hepatitis.

Percutaneous treatments are effective in patients with small tumours.

Selective chemoembolisation is effective in selected patients with preserved liver function.

REFERENCES

1. Parkin DM, Bray F, Ferlay J et al. Estimating the world cancer burden: GLOBOCAN 2000. Int J Cancer 2001; 94:153–6.

2. Ikai I, Itai Y, Okita K et al. Report of the 15th follow-up survey of primary liver cancer. Hepatol Res 2004; 28:21–9.

3. Ferlay J, Bray F, Pisani P et al. GLOBOCAN 2000/Cancer incidence, mortality and prevalence worldwide, version 1.0. IARC Cancer Base N°5. Lyon: IARC, 2001.

4. Caselmann WH, Alt M. Hepatitis C virus infection as a major risk factor for hepatocellular carcinoma. J Hepatol 1996; 24:61–6.

5. El Serag HB, Andrew C. The increasing incidence of hepatocellular carcinoma in the United States. N Engl J Med 1999; 340:745–50.

   Study documenting the increasing incidence of HCC in the USA.

6. Chang MH, Chen CJ, Lai MS et al. Universal hepatitis B vaccination in Taiwan and the incidence of hepatocellular carcinoma in children. Taiwan Childhood Hepatoma Study Group. N Engl J Med 1997; 336:1855–9.

Study documenting the reduction in HBV carriers and HBV-related cirrhosis following the introduction of a vaccination programme in Taiwan.

7. Yang HI, Lu SN, Liaw YF et al. Hepatitis B e antigen and the risk of hepatocellular carcinoma. N Engl J Med 2002; 347:168–74.

8. DonatoF, Boffetta P, Puoti M. A meta-analysis of epidemiological studies on the combined effect of hepatitis B and C virus infection in causing hepatocellular carcinoma. Int J Cancer 1998; 75:347–54.

9. DiBisceglie AM. Hepatitis C and hepatocellular carcinoma. Hepatology 1997; 26:34S–8.

10. Kiyosawa K, Sodeyama T, Tanaka E et al. Interrelationship of blood transfusion, non-A, non-B hepatitis and hepatocellular carcinoma: analysis by detection of antibody to hepatitis C virus. Hepatology 1990; 12:671–5.

11. Tong MJ, el-Farra NS, Reikes AR et al. Clinical outcomes after transfusion-associated hepatitis C. N Engl J Med. 1995; 332:1463–6.

12. Salomon JA, Weinstein MC, Hammitt JK et al. Empirically calibrated model of hepatitis C virus infection in the United States. Am J Epid 2002; 156:761.

Study investigating the anticipated increase in the incidence of HCV-related HCC.

13. Verucchi G, Calza L, Manfredi R et al. Human immunodeficiency virus and hepatitis C virus coinfection: epidemiology, natural history, therapeutic options and clinical management. Infection 2004; 32:33–46.

14. Yoshida H, Shiratori Y, Moriyama M et al. Interferon therapy reduces the risk for hepatocellular carcinoma: national surveillance program of cirrhotic and noncirrhotic patients with chronic hepatitis C in Japan. IHIT Study Group. Inhibition of Hepatocarcinogenesis by Interferon Therapy. Ann Intern Med 1999;131:174–81.

15. Bruix J, Barrera JM, Calvet X et al. Prevalence of antibodies to hepatitis C virus in Spanish patients with hepatocellular carcinoma and hepatic cirrhosis. Lancet 1989; 2:1004–6.

16. Yamauchi M, Nakahara M, Maezawa Y et al. Prevalence of hepatocellular carcinoma in patients with alcoholic cirrhosis and prior exposure to hepatitis C. Am J Gastroenterol 1993; 88:39–43.

17. Marrero JA, Fontana RJ, Su GL et al. NAFLD may be a common underlying liver disease in patients with hepatocellular carcinoma in the United States. Hepatology 2002; 36:1349–54.

18. Regimbeau JM, Colombat M, Mognol P et al. Obesity and diabetes as a risk factor for hepatocellular carcinoma. Liver Transpl 2004;10:S69–73.

19. Peers FJ, Bosch FX, Kaldor JM et al. Aflatoxin exposure, hepatitis B virus and liver cancer in Swaziland. Int J Cancer 1987; 39:545–53.

20. Chen CJ, Wang LY, Lu SN et al. Elevated aflatoxin exposure and increased risk of hepatocellular carcinoma. Hepatology 1996; 24:38–42.

21. Niederau C, Fischer R, Sonnenberg A et al. Survival and causes of death in cirrhotic and in non-cirrhotic patients with primary hemochromatosis. N Engl J Med 1985; 313:1256–9.

22. Deugnier YM, Olivier L, Turlin B et al. Liver pathology in genetic hemochromatosis: a review of 135 homozygous cases and their bioclinical correlations. Gastroenterology 1993; 102:2050–9.

23. Leese T, Farges O, Bismuth H. Liver cell adenomas. A 12-year surgical experience from a specialist hepatobiliary unit. Ann Surg 1988; 208:558–64.

24. Chiche L, Dao T, Salame E et al. Liver adenomatosis: reappraisal, diagnosis, and surgical management: eight new cases and review of the literature. Ann Surg 2000; 231:74–81.

25. International working party. Terminology of nodular hepatocellular lesions. Hepatology 1995; 22:983–93.

26. Borzio M, Fargion S, Borzio F et al. Impact of large regenerative, low grade and high grade dysplastic nodules in hepatocellular carcinoma development. J Hepatol 2003; 39:208–14.

27. Takayama T, Makuuchi M, Hirohashi S et al. Malignant transformation of adenomatous hyperplasia to hepatocellular carcinoma. Lancet 1990; 336:1150–3.

28. Washington K. Pathology of primary and secondary liver tumors. In: Clavien PA (ed.) Malignant liver tumours. Malden, MA: Blackwell Science, 1999; pp. 3–26.

29. Poon RT, Fan ST. Evaluation of the new AJCC/UICC staging system for hepatocellular carcinoma after hepatic resection in Chinese patients. Surg Oncol Clin N Am 2003; 12:35–50.

30. Vauthey J, Lauwers G, Esnaola N et al. Simplified staging for hepatocellular carcinoma. J Clin Oncol 2002; 20:1527–36.

31. Yeh CN, Lee WC, Jeng LB et al. Spontaneous tumour rupture and prognosis in patients with hepatocellular carcinoma. Br J Surg 2002; 89:1125–9.

32. Weitz IC, Liebman HA. Des-gamma-carboxy (abnormal) prothrombin and hepatocellular carcinoma: a critical review. Hepatology 1993; 18:990–7.

33. Choi BI. The current status of imaging diagnosis of hepatocellular carcinoma. Liver Transplantation 2004; 10:S20–5.

34. Murakami T, Kim T, Takahashi S et al. Hepatocellular carcinoma: multidetector row helical CT. Abdom Imaging 2002; 27:139–46.

35. Burrel M, Llovet JM, Ayuso C et al. MRI angiography is superior to helical CT for detection

of HCC prior to liver transplantation: an explant correlation. Hepatology 2003; 38:1034–42.

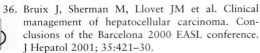

36. Bruix J, Sherman M, Llovet JM et al. Clinical management of hepatocellular carcinoma. Conclusions of the Barcelona 2000 EASL conference. J Hepatol 2001; 35:421–30.

    Summary of the guidelines established by a panel of European experts on the management of HCC.

37. Durand F, Regimbeau JM, Belghiti J et al. Assessment of the benefits and risks of percutaneous biopsy before surgical resection of hepatocellular carcinoma. J Hepatol 2001; 35:254–8.

38. Koffi E, Moutardier V, Sauvanet A et al. Wound recurrence after resection of hepatocellular carcinoma. Liver Transpl Surg 1996; 2:301–4.

39. Ebara M, Ohto M, Shinagawa T et al. Natural history of hepatocellular carcinoma smaller than three centimeters complicating cirrhosis. A study in 22 patients. Gastroenterology 1986; 90:289–98.

40. Barbara L, Benzi G, Gaiani S et al. Natural history of small untreated hepatocellular carcinoma in cirrhosis: a multivariate analysis of prognostic factors of tumour growth rate and patient survival. Hepatology 1992; 16:132–7.

41. Llovet JM, Bustamante J, Castells A et al. Natural history of untreated nonsurgical hepatocellular carcinoma: rationale for the design and evaluation of therapeutic trials. Hepatology 1999; 29:62–7.

42. CLIP. A new prognostic system for hepatocellular carcinoma: a retrospective study of 435 patients: the Cancer of the Liver Italian Program (CLIP) investigators. Hepatology 1998; 28:751–5.

43. Chevret S, Trinchet JC, Mathieu D et al. A new prognostic classification for predicting survival in patients with hepatocellular carcinoma. J Hepatol 1999; 31:133–41.

44. Leung TW, Tang AM, Zee B et al. Construction of the Chinese University prognostic index for hepatocellular carcinoma and comparison with the TNM staging system, the Okuda staging system, and the cancer of the liver Italian program staging system: a study based on 926 patients. Cancer 2002; 94:1760–9.

45. The Cancer of the Liver Italian Program (CLIP) Investigators. Prospective validation of the CLIP score: a new prognostic system for patients with cirrhosis and hepatocellular carcinoma. Hepatology 2000; 31:840–5.

46. Trevisani F, De Notariis S, Rapaccini G et al. Semiannual and annual surveillance of cirrhotic patients for hepatocellular carcinoma: effects on cancer stage and patient survival (Italian experience). Am J Gastroenterol 2002; 97:734–44.

47. Yuen MF, Lai CL. Screening for hepatocellular carcinoma: survival benefit and cost-effectiveness. Ann Oncol 2003; 14:1463–7.

48. Yang B, Zhang B, Xu Y et al. Prospective study of early detection for primary liver cancer. J Cancer Res Clin Oncol 1997; 123:357–60.

49. Bralet MP, Regimbeau JM, Pineau P et al. Hepatocellular carcinoma occurring in nonfibrotic liver: epidemiologic and histopathologic analysis of 80 French cases. Hepatology 2000; 32:200–4.

50. Belghiti J, Hiramatsu K, Benoist S et al. Seven hundred forty-seven hepatectomies in the 1990s: an update to evaluate the actual risk of liver resection. J Am Coll Surg 2000; 191:38–46.

51. Iwatsuki S, Starzl TE, Sheahan DG et al. Hepatic resection versus transplantation for hepatocellular carcinoma. Ann Surg 1991; 214:221–9.

52. Chang CH, Chau GY, Lui WY et al. Long-term results of hepatic resection for hepatocellular carcinoma originating from the noncirrhotic liver. Arch Surg 2004; 139:320–5.

53. Nagasue N, Yakaya H, Kohno H. Human liver regeneration after major hepatic resection. A study of normal liver and livers with chronic hepatitis and cirrhosis. Ann Surg 1987; 206:30.

54. Fan ST, Lo CM, Liu CL et al. Hepatectomy for hepatocellular carcinoma: toward zero hospital deaths. Ann Surg 1999; 229:322–30.

    Large single-centre experience documenting reduced operative mortality with better selection and increasing experience.

55. Makuuchi M, Sano K. The surgical approach to HCC: our progress and results in Japan. Liver Transplantation 2004; 10:S46–52.

56. Nagasue N, Kohno H, Chang YC et al. Liver resection for hepatocellular carcinoma. Results of 229 consecutive patients during 11 years. Ann Surg 1993; 217:375–84.

57. Makuuchi M, Kosuge T, Takayama T et al. Surgery for small liver cancers. Semin Surg Oncol 1993; 9:298–304.

58. Noun R, Jagot P, Farges O et al. High preoperative serum alanine transferase levels: effect on the risk of liver resection in Child grade A cirrhotic patients. World J Surg 1997; 21:390–4.

59. Bruix J, Castells A, Bosch J et al. Surgical resection of hepatocellular carcinoma in cirrhotic patients: prognostic value of preoperative portal pressure. Gastroenterology 1996, 111:1018–22.

60. Belghiti J, Noun R, Malafosse R et al. Continuous versus intermittent portal triad clamping for liver resection. Ann Surg 1999; 229:369–75.

61. Belghiti J, Guevara OA, Noun R et al. Liver hanging maneuver: a safe approach to right hepatectomy without liver mobilization. J Am Coll Surg. 2001; 193:109–11.

62. Abdalla EK, Hicks ME, Vauthey JN. Portal vein embolization: rationale, technique and future prospects. Br J Surg 2001; 88:165–75.

63. Farges O, Belghiti J, Kianmanesh R et al. Portal vein embolization before right hepatectomy: prospective clinical trial. Ann Surg 2003; 237:208–17.

64. Regimbeau JM, Kianmanesh R, Farges O et al. Extent of liver resection influences the outcome in patients with cirrhosis and small hepatocellular carcinoma. Surgery 2002; 131:311–17.

65. Imamura H, Matsuyama Y, Tanaka E et al. Risk factors contributing to early and late phase intrahepatic recurrence of hepatocellular carcinoma after hepatectomy. J Hepatol 2003; 38:200–7.

   A recent in-depth analysis of the risk factors for recurrence after resection of HCC.

66. Kawasaki S, Makuuchi M, Miyagawa et al. Results of hepatic resection for hepatocellular carcinoma. World J Surg 1995; 19:31–4.

67. Takenada K, Kawahara N, Yamamoto K et al. Results of 280 liver resections for hepatocellular carcinoma. Arch Surg 1996; 131:71–6.

68. Chen MF, Jeng LB. Partial hepatic resection for hepatocellular carcinoma. J Gastroenterol Hepatol 1997; 12:S329–34.

69. Makuuchi M, Takayama T, Kubota K et al. Hepatic resection for hepatocellular carcinoma – Japanese experience. Hepatogastroenterology 1998; 45:1267–74.

70. Poon RT, Fan ST, Lo CM et al. Improving survival results after resection of hepatocellular carcinoma: a prospective study of 377 patients over 10 years. Ann Surg 2001; 234:63–70.

71. Shimozawa N, Hanazaki K. Long term prognosis after hepatic resection for small hepatocellular carcinoma. J Am Coll Surg 2004; 198:356–65.

72. Franco D, Capussotti L, Smadja C et al. Resection of hepatocellular carcinomas. Results in 72 European patients with cirrhosis. Gastroenterology 1990; 98:733–8.

73. Castells A, Bruix J, Bru C et al. Treatment of small hepatocellular carcinoma in cirrhotic patients: a cohort study comparing surgical resection and percutaneous ethanol injection. Hepatology 1993; 18:1121–6.

74. Vauthey JN, Klimstra D, Franceshi D et al. Factors affecting long-term outcome after hepatic resection for hepatocellular carcinoma. Am J Surg 1995; 169:28–35.

75. Nagorney DM, Gigot JF. Primary epithelial hepatic malignancies: etiology, epidemiology and outcome after subtotal and total hepatic resection. Surg Oncol Clin North Am 1996; 5:283–300.

76. Mazziotti A, Grazi GL, Cavallari A. Surgical treatment of hepatocellular on cirrhosis: a Western experience. Hepatogastroenterology 1998; 45:1281–7.

77. Llovet JM, Fuster J, Bruix J. Intention-to-treat analysis of surgical treatment for early hepatocellular carcinoma: resection versus transplantation. Hepatology 1999; 30:1434–40.

78. Belghiti J, Regimbeau JM, Durand F et al. Resection of hepatocellular carcinoma: a European experience on 328 cases. Hepatogastroenterology 2002; 49:41–6.

79. Ercolani G, Grazi GL, Ravaioli M et al. Liver resection for hepatocellular carcinoma on cirrhosis: univariate and multivariate analysis of risk factors for intrahepatic recurrence. Ann Surg 2003; 237:536–43.

80. Cha C, Fong Y, Jarnagin WR et al. Predictors and patterns of recurrence after resection of hepatocellular carcinoma. J Am Coll Surg 2003; 197:753–8.

81. Pawlik T, Esnoala NF, Vauthey JN. Surgical treatment of hepatocellular carcinoma: similar long term results despite geographic variations. Liver Transplantation 2004; 10:S74–80.

82. Belghiti J, Panis Y, Farges O et al. Intrahepatic recurrence after resection of hepatocellular carcinoma complicating cirrhosis. Ann Surg 1991; 214:114–7.

83. Chen MF, Hwang TL, Jeng LB et al. Postoperative recurrence of hepatocellular carcinoma. Arch Surg 1994; 129:738–42.

84. Shimada M, Takenaka K, Gion T et al. Prognosis of recurrent hepatocellular carcinoma: a 10-year surgical experience in Japan. Gastroenterology 1996; 111:720–6.

85. Schwartz JD, Schwartz M, Mandeli J et al. Neoadjuvant and adjuvant therapy for resectable hepatocellular carcinoma: review of the randomised clinical trials. Lancet Oncol 2002; 3:593–603.

86. Poon RTP, Fan ST, Lo CM et al. Intrahepatic recurrence after curative resection of hepatocellular carcinoma. Long-term results of treatment and prognostic factors. Ann Surg 1999; 229:216–22.

87. Farges O, Regimbeau JM, Belghiti J. Aggressive management of recurrence following surgical resection of hepatocellular carcinoma. Hepatogastroenterology 1998; 45:S1275–80.

88. Minagawa M, Makuuchi M, Takayama T et al. Selection criteria for repeat hepatectomy in patients with recurrent hepatocellular carcinoma. Ann Surg 2003; 238:703–10.

89. Ringe B, Pichlmayr R, Wittekind C et al. Surgical treatment of hepatocellular carcinoma: experience with liver resection and transplantation in 198 patients. World J Surg 1991; 15:270–85.

90. Iwatsuki S, Gordon RD, Shaw BW et al. Role of liver transplantation in cancer therapy. Ann Surg 1985; 202:401–7.

91. Penn I. Hepatic transplantation for primary and metastatic cancers of the liver. Surgery 1991; 110:726–35.

92. Bismuth H, Chiche L, Adam R et al. Liver resection versus transplantation for hepatocellular carcinoma in cirrhotic patients. Ann Surg 1993; 218:145–51.

93. Mazzaferro V, Regalia E, Doci R et al. Liver transplantation for the treatment of small hepatocellular carcinomas in patients with cirrhosis. N Engl J Med 1996; 334:693–9.

   Study investigating the influence of the so-called Milan criteria on the results of liver transplantation for HCC.

94. Yoo HY, Patt CH, Geschwind JF et al. The outcome of liver transplantation in patients with hepatocellular carcinoma in the United States between 1988 and 2001: 5-year survival has improved significantly with time. J Clin Oncol 2003; 21:4329–35.

95. Yao FY, Ferrell L, Bass NM et al. Liver transplantation for hepatocellular carcinoma: comparison of the proposed UCSF criteria with the Milan criteria and the Pittsburgh modified TNM criteria. Liver Transplantation 2002; 8:765–74.

96. Cillo U, Vitale A, Bassanello M et al. Liver transplantation for the treatment of moderately or well-differentiated hepatocellular carcinoma. Ann Surg 2004; 239:150–9.

97. Bigourdan JM, Jaeck D, Meyer N et al. Small hepatocellular carcinoma in Child A cirrhotic patients: hepatic resection versus transplantation. Liver Transplantation 2003; 9:513–20.

98. Figueras J, Jaurrieta E, Valls C et al. Survival after liver transplantation in cirrhotic patients with and without hepatocellular carcinoma: a comparative study. Hepatology 1997; 25:1485–9.

99. Jonas S, Bechstein WO, Steinmuller T et al. Vascular invasion and histopathologic grading determine outcome after liver transplantation for hepatocellular carcinoma in cirrhosis. Hepatology 2001; 33:1080–6.

100. Yao FY, Ferrell L, Bass NM et al. Liver transplantation for hepatocellular carcinoma: expansion of the tumor size limits does not adversely impact survival. Hepatology 2001; 33:1394–403.

101. Adam R, Azoulay D, Castaing D et al. Long-term results of transplantation for hepatocellular carcinoma with or without cirrhosis: 15 years' experience at Paul Brousse hospital. In: Kitajima M, Shimazu M et al. (eds) Current issues in liver and small bowel transplantation, 9. Berlin: Springer, 2001; pp. 135–44.

102. Margarit C, Charco R, Hidalgo E et al. Liver transplantation for malignant diseases: selection and pattern of recurrence. World J Surg 2002; 26:257–63.

103. Moya A, Berenguer M, Aguilera V et al. Hepatocellular carcinoma: can it be considered a controversial indication for liver transplantation in centers with high rates of hepatitis C? Liver Transplantation 2002; 8:1020–7.

104. Vivarelli M, Bellusci R, Cucchetti A et al. Low recurrence rate of hepatocellular carcinoma after liver transplantation: better patient selection or lower immunosuppression? Transplantation 2002; 74:1746–51.

105. De Carlis L, Giacomoni A, Lauterio A et al. Liver transplantation for hepatocellular cancer: should the current indication criteria be changed? Transpl Int 2003; 16:115–22.

106. Yao FY, Bass NM, Nikolai B et al. Liver transplantation for hepatocellular carcinoma: analysis of survival according to the intention-to-treat principle and dropout from the waiting list. Liver Transplantation 2002; 8:873–83.

107. Bruix J, Castells A, Montanya X et al. Phase II study of transarterial embolisation in European patients with hepatocellular carcinoma: need for controlled trials. Hepatology 1994; 20:643–50.

108. Jeng KS, Ching HJ. The role of surgery in the management of unusual complications of transcatheter arterial embolisation for hepatocellular carcinoma. World J Surg 1988; 12:362–8.

109. Groupe d'étude et de traitement du carcinome hépatocellulaire. A comparison of lipiodol chemoembolisation and conservative treatment for unresectable hepatocellular carcinoma. N Engl J Med 1995; 332:1256–61.

110. Bismuth H, Morino M, Sherlock D et al. Primary treatment of hepatocellular carcinoma by arterial chemoembolisation. Am J Surg 1992; 163:387–94.

111. Paye F, Farges O, Dahmane M et al. Cytolysis following chemoembolisation for hepatocellular carcinoma. Br J Surg 1999; 86:176–80.

112. Vetter D, Wenger JJ, Bergier JM et al. Transcatheter oily chemoembolisation in the management of advanced hepatocellular carcinoma in cirrhosis: results of a Western comparative study in 60 patients. Hepatology 1991; 13:427–33.

113. Stefanini GF, Amorati P, Biselli M et al. Efficacy of transarterial targeted treatments on survival of patients with hepatocellular carcinoma. Cancer 1995; 75:2427–34.

114. Lin DY, Liaw YF, Lee TY et al. Hepatic arterial embolisation in patients with unresectable hepatocellular carcinoma – a randomised controlled trial. Gastroenterology 1988; 94:453–6.

115. Pelletier G, Roche A, Ink O et al. A randomised trial of hepatic arterial chemoembolisation in patients with unresectable hepatocellular carcinoma. J Hepatol 1990; 11:181–4.

116. Bruix J, Llovet JM, Castells A et al. Transarterial embolization versus symptomatic treatment in patients with advanced hepatocellular carcinoma: results of a randomized controlled trial in a single institution. Hepatology 1998; 127:1578–83.

117. Lo CM, Ngan H, Tso WK et al. Randomized controlled trial of transarterial lipiodol chemoembolization for unresectable hepatocellular carcinoma. Hepatology 2002; 35: 1164–71.

    First two studies demonstrating a survival benefit following chemoembolisation of HCC.

118. Llovet JM, Real MI, Montana X et al. Arterial embolisation or chemoembolisation versus symptomatic treatment in patients with unresectable hepatocellular carcinoma: a randomised controlled trial. Lancet 2002; 359:1734–9.

119. Llovet JM, Bruix J. Systematic review of randomized trials for unresectable hepatocellular carcinoma: chemoembolization improves survival. Hepatology 2003; 37:429–42.

120. Katyal S, Oliver JH, Peterson MS et al. Prognostic significance of arterial phase CT for prediction of response to transcatheter arterial chemoembolization in unresectable hepatocellular carcinoma: a retrospective analysis. AJR 2000; 175:1665–72.

121. Lee HS, Kim KM, Yoon JH et al. Therapeutic efficacy of transcatheter arterial chemoembolization as compared with hepatic resection in hepatocellular carcinoma patients with compensated liver function in a hepatitis B virus-endemic area: a prospective cohort study. J Clin Oncol 2002; 20:4459–65.

122. Livraghi T, Benedini V, Lazzaroni S et al. Long-term results of single session PEI in patients with large hepatocellular carcinoma. Cancer 1998; 83:48–57.

123. Tanaka K, Nakamura S, Numata K et al. Hepatocellular carcinoma: treatment with percutaneous ethanol injection and transcatheter arterial embolisation. Radiology 1992; 185:457–60.

124. Koda M, Murawaki Y, Mitsuda A et al. Combination therapy with transcatheter arterial chemoembolization and percutaneous ethanol injection compared with percutaneous ethanol injection alone for patients with small hepatocellular carcinoma: a randomized control study. Cancer 2001; 92:1516–24.

125. Vilana R, Bruix J, Bru C et al. Tumour size determines the efficacy of percutaneous ethanol injection for the treatment of small hepatocellular carcinoma. Hepatology 1992; 16:353–7.

126. Livraghi T, Giorgio A, Marin G et al. Hepatocellular carcinoma and cirrhosis in 746 patients: long term results of percutaneous ethanol injection. Radiology 1995; 197:101–8.

127. Lencioni R, Pinto F, Armillotta N et al. Long-term results of percutaneous ethanol injection therapy for hepatocellular carcinoma in cirrhosis: a European experience. Eur Radiol 1997; 7:514–19.

128. Livraghi T. Percutaneous ablation of early hepatocellular carcinoma. In: Arroyo V, Bosch J, Bruguera M et al. (eds) Treatment of liver diseases. Barcelona: Masson, 1999; pp. 337–54.

129. Lencioni RA, Allgaier HP, Cioni D et al. Small hepatocellular carcinoma in cirrhosis: randomized comparison of radio-frequency thermal ablation versus percutaneous ethanol injection. Radiology 2003; 228:235–40.

130. Mulier S, Mulier P, Ni Y et al. Complication of radiofrequency coagulation of liver tumors. Br J Surg 2002; 89:1206–22.

131. Raoul JL, Guyader D, Bretagne JF et al. Randomised controlled trial for hepatocellular carcinoma with portal vein thrombosis versus medical support. J Nucl Med 1994; 35:1782–7.

132. Leung KL, Lau WY, Lai PBS et al. Spontaneous rupture of hepatocellular carcinoma. Arch Surg 1999; 134:1103–7.

133. Belghiti J, Durand F, Farges O. Transplantation for liver tumours. In: Clavien PA (ed.) Malignant liver tumors. Malden, MA: Blackwell Science, 1999; pp. 189–97.

134. Ringe B, Wittekind C, Weimann A et al. Results of hepatic resection and transplantation for fibrolamellar carcinoma. Surg Gynecol Obstet 1992; 175:299–305.

135. Patel T. Increasing incidence and mortality of primary intrahepatic cholangiocarcinoma in the United States. Hepatology 2001; 33:1353–7.

136. Wood R, Brewster DH, Fraser LA et al. Do increases in mortality from intrahepatic cholangiocarcinoma reflect a genuine increase in risk? Insights from cancer registry data in Scotland. Eur J Cancer 2003; 39:2087–92.

137. Yamasaki S. Intrahepatic cholangiocarcinoma: macroscopic type and stage classification. J Hepatobiliary Pancreat Surg 2003; 10:288–91.

138. Valverde A, Bonhomme N, Farges O et al. Resection of intrahepatic cholangiocarcinoma. A Western experience. J Hepatobiliary Pancreat Surg 1999; 6:122–7.

139. Lim JH. Cholangiocarcinoma: morphologic classification according to growth pattern and imaging findings. Am J Roentgenol 2003; 181:819–27.

140. Nagorney DM, Donohue JH, Farnell MB et al. Outcomes after curative resections of cholangiocarcinoma. Arch Surg 1993; 128:871–7.

141. Khan SA, Davidson BR, Goldin R et al. Guidelines for the diagnosis and treatment of cholangiocarcinoma: consensus document. Gut 2002; 51(suppl 6):VI1–VI9.

142. Chen MF, Jan YY, Chen TC. Clinical studies of mucin-producing cholangiocellular carcinoma: a study of 22 histopathology proven cases. Ann Surg 1998; 227:63–9.

143. Tajima Y, Kuroki T, Fukuda K et al. An intraductal papillary component is associated with prolonged survival after hepatic resection for

intrahepatic cholangiocarcinoma. Br J Surg 2004; 91:99–104.

144. Ishak KG, Sesterhenn IA, Goodman ZD et al. Epithelioid hemangioendothelioma of the liver: a clinicopathologic and follow-up study of 32 cases. Hum Pathol 1984; 15:839–52.

145. Lyburn ID, Torreggiani WC, Harris AC et al. Hepatic epithelioid hemangioendothelioma: sonographic, CT, and MR imaging appearances. Am J Roentgenol 2003; 180:1359–64.

146. Makhlouf HR, Ishak KG, Goodman ZD. Epithelioid hemangioendothelioma of the liver: a clinicopathologic study of 137 cases. Cancer 1999; 85:562–82.

147. Uchimura K, Nakamuta M, Osoegawa M et al. Hepatic epithelioid hemangioendothelioma. J Clin Gastroenterol 2001; 32:431–4.

148. Marino IR, Todo S, Tzakis AG et al. Treatment of hepatic epithelioid hemangioendothelioma with liver transplantation. Cancer 1988; 62:2079–84.

149. Weinman MD, Chopra S. Tumours of the liver, other than primary hepatocellular carcinoma. Gastroenterol Clin North Am 1987; 16:627–50.

150. Koyama T, Fletcher JG, Johnson CD et al. Primary hepatic angiosarcoma: findings at CT and MR imaging. Radiology 2002; 222:667–73.

151. Locker GY, Doroshow JH, Zwelling LA et al. The clinical features of hepatic angiosarcoma: a report of four cases and a review of the English literature. Medicine 1979; 58:48–64.

152. Poggio JL, Nagorney DM, Nascimento AG et al. Surgical treatment of adult primary hepatic sarcoma. Br J Surg 2000; 87:1500–5.

153. Aozasa K, Mishima K, Ohsawa M. Primary malignant lymphoma of the liver. Leuk Lymphoma 1993; 10:353–7.

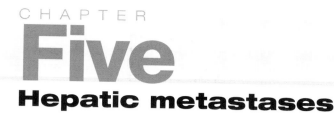

CHAPTER Five

Hepatic metastases

Thomas J. Hugh, Paula Ghaneh and
Graeme J. Poston

INTRODUCTION

The liver is one of the commonest sites for meta-static spread of tumours, particularly for those originating in the gastrointestinal tract. In autopsy studies of patients who die of malignant disease, hepatic metastases are found in up to 36% of cases, with the most frequent primary sites being colon and rectum, bronchus, pancreas, breast, stomach and 'primary of unknown origin'.[1] The prognosis of untreated hepatic metastases is generally very poor, especially when derived from oesophageal, stomach, pancreas, colorectal, or breast primary tumours. If left untreated, the majority of patients will succumb to their disease within 12 months of diagnosis.[2,3] There has been a steady increase in the number of patients developing gastrointestinal cancer over the past three to five decades,[4,5] but metastatic disease is now being detected at an earlier stage due to improvements in imaging techniques and screening programmes, as for breast cancer. Thus for the growing number of patients with metastatic disease, aggressive therapy may be an option.

This chapter examines the aetiology and modes of presentation of hepatic metastases, and describes the relevant investigations and management options of this condition, with a particular emphasis on surgical resection. The various non-surgical treatments and novel therapies, which are at the pre-clinical or clinical stage, will be discussed as they may have future application in patients with advanced disease.

AETIOLOGY AND PATHOPHYSIOLOGY OF HEPATIC METASTASES

Almost half of all patients who die of cancer of the stomach, pancreas or breast are found to have liver metastases at autopsy; with endometrial tumours, metastatic spread to the liver occurs in approximately 40% of cases. Liver metastases may be present in as many as 35% of patients with colorectal cancer at the time of operation, and another 8–30% will be found to have liver metastases on subsequent follow-up.[6] The 5-year survival following an apparently curative resection of a colorectal primary tumour is only 50%, and the liver is the most frequent site of relapse.[7]

The predilection for metastases to develop in the liver is partly related to the fact that the liver receives the portal drainage of the gastrointestinal tract, from where tumour cells can embolise via the mesenteric veins.[8] However, less than 0.1% of circulating tumour cells survive the mechanical trauma and host defence mechanisms encountered during their passage through the vascular and lymphatic vessels, and those that do develop into a metastasis are a selected subpopulation.[9] This subpopulation is more homogeneous compared to the primary tumour since they are a clonal expansion of a few highly metastatic cells that have arrested in the capillary beds of the liver.[10] The process of invasion and metastasis of a malignant cell involves a series of linked, sequential steps necessitating detachment from the primary tumour, invasion of the extracellular matrix and subsequent reattachment and independent growth in the new environment.[11] This involves a large number of factors, such as adhesion molecules, proteases (matrix metalloproteinases), growth factors and angiogenic factors. Adhesion molecules such as E-cadherin have been shown to play an important role in colorectal tumour cell invasion,[12] as well as integrins, which are receptors for extracellular matrix proteins. The complex interactions of tumour cells with the lining endothelial and lymphatic cells are, in part, what determines their final organ distribution.[13] Also, tumour cells 'recognise' tissue-specific motility factors, which direct their movement and invasion properties.[14] The complete explanation as to why a cancer cell leaves the circulation at a specific organ is not known but is thought to involve a homing receptor on the cancer cell and an addressin on the endothelial cell.[15]

In several experimental tumour models of liver metastasis, it has been shown that metastatic cells first come into contact with, and implant in, the portal endothelium, within a limited portion of the sinusoid.[16] From here, tumour cells may break off into a portal radical and reseed close to the initial lesion or may spread by periportal lymphatic pathways. Such satellite formation close to a large liver metastasis is common with secondary tumours of the liver. Also, approximately 10% of patients with colorectal cancer who are candidates for liver resection are found to have spread to extrahepatic lymph nodes, highlighting the importance of this mode of spread, which, if found, excludes the possibility of cure.[17]

The right lobe of the liver is involved with metastases more frequently than the left lobe, although the reasons for this remain unclear as there is no gross difference of either arterial or portal venous blood received by each lobe.[18] It may be that this reflects the fact that the right lobe is usually larger than the left lobe, but it may also be a consequence of portal vein 'streaming' resulting in

tumour emboli preferentially entering the right portal vein branches. Approximately one-third of patients with colorectal liver metastases will have disease limited to one lobe, whereas multiple deposits throughout the liver are more commonly seen in patients with breast, oesophageal, gastric and pancreatic cancer and are indicative of a more widespread metastatic process.[19,20]

Although there are no lymphatic channels draining directly to the liver from the gastrointestinal tract, a metastatic deposit may arise by sequential lymphatic spread from draining lymph nodes. Tumour cells that invade lymphatics may also spread haematogenously via venolymphatic communications or directly via the thoracic duct.[21] Certainly, liver metastases develop in the absence of lymph node involvement, and presumably this occurs via the haematogenous route. Some large metastases do not demonstrate spread to local periportal lymph nodes even in the presence of extensive disease within the liver.[22]

Macroscopically, liver metastases are usually more lightly coloured and firmer to palpation than the surrounding normal liver tissue. They enlarge by concentric growth with extension in all directions, and surface lesions may show central umbilication, probably as a result of infarction when the tumour outgrows its blood supply. A liver metastasis may attain an enormous size, sometimes occupying much of the liver and may occasionally spread to adjacent structures, such as the diaphragm, by penetrating the usually unyielding Glisson's capsule.

PRESENTATION OF HEPATIC METASTASES

Liver metastases detected at the time of presentation of primary disease are termed **synchronous metastases**; those detected after presentation are termed **metachronous metastases**. The aim of a thorough preoperative work-up and routine follow-up after resection of a primary tumour is to identify metastases as early as possible in order to select patients who might benefit from further surgery, adjuvant or palliative chemotherapy and exclude those for whom such treatment might not be helpful.

Small lesions within the liver are usually asymptomatic and are difficult to detect with conventional imaging techniques. Patients with advanced disease usually present with a combination of upper abdominal discomfort, weight loss and general malaise. Pain may be due to unremitting rapid growth of large metastases, and is referred occasionally to the right shoulder. Central necrosis and infarction of a metastasis may also cause pain and pyrexia but these are usually only transient symptoms. Hepatomegaly is indicative of advanced disease and may occasionally be accompanied by fulminant hepatic failure if the metastases are rapidly growing. Evidence of advanced liver failure, such as jaundice, ascites and occasionally portal hypertension, are late signs and are indicative of an extremely poor prognosis.

In patients with carcinoid, the first presentation may be with the carcinoid syndrome, characterised by diarrhoea, flushing and wheezing due to excessive secretion of serotonin and tachykinin peptides from the hepatic metastases.

INVESTIGATION OF HEPATIC METASTASES

There is still no consensus concerning the long-term follow-up of patients who have had colonic surgery and are at risk for liver metastases. Follow-up data suggest that the average disease-free survival time between primary operation and recurrence is one and a half years.[23]

Depending on institution there may be regular measurements of tumour markers, such as carcino-embryonic antigen (CEA), and/or regular ultrasound. CEA levels can be useful for follow-up but can be misleading if solely relied upon for diagnosis. CEA levels can be increased in other benign and malignant diseases of the liver and gastrointestinal tract, and therefore this assay can suffer from low specificity. In one study CEA levels were found to be complementary to history and physical examination in the diagnosis of liver metastases.[24] Serum levels of alkaline phosphatase, aspartate amino-transaminase, glutamyl transferase and, occasionally, alpha-fetoprotein may be increased in the presence of liver metastases.[25] There are a variety of imaging modalities available, and their use is dictated by the local availability of equipment and level of expertise (**Table 5.1**).

Transabdominal ultrasound (TUS)

TUS is the most widespread and useful test available. It is inexpensive and non-invasive and is good at distinguishing solid from cystic lesions. It is operator dependent for scan interpretation. It has a sensitivity of 94% for lesions over 2 cm in size, but this drops to 56% for lesions of less than 1 cm.[33]

Computed tomography (CT)

Contrast-enhanced computed tomography (CE-CT) using multislice CT scanners may allow for more detailed definition of smaller (≤1 cm) lesions compared with TUS. CE-CT scan achieves an accuracy of 80–93% for lesions over 1 cm, and this falls to 68% for lesions smaller than 1 cm.[34]

CT scan arterial portography (CTAP) involves selective catheterisation of the superior mesenteric artery (SMA) followed by bolus contrast injection and CT scanning of the liver during the portal phase. The necessity to perform angiography in order to deliver the contrast agent has restricted its use, although CTAP is particularly helpful for detecting lesions less than 5 mm in diameter, and may allow precise localisation of the tumour within the hepatic segments.[35]

In a prospective evaluation of the accuracy of preoperative imaging in patients undergoing liver resection for colorectal metastases, Yamaguchi et al.[36] have shown that CTAP was significantly better than ultrasound, contrast CT or hepatic angiography in detecting metastases less than 10 mm in diameter. In a comparison of the different CT scan modalities in 109 patients with various hepatic tumours, Karl et al.[37] demonstrated that CTAP was significantly more sensitive than either delayed or conventional CT in assessing the distribution of intrahepatic disease. Besides being invasive, the other major limitation of CTAP is the number of false-positive findings caused by defects of perfusion from flow artefacts.[38]

Typical liver metastases are hypodense on CT scanning (**Fig. 5.1**) but may be surrounded by a hyperdense ring due to contrast uptake in the compressed surrounding parenchyma. Unenhanced CT scanning may detect hepatic metastases but some are only seen after contrast enhancement.

Table 5.1 • Comparison of imaging modalities in hepatic metastases

Study	Year	Number	Method*	Sensitivity (%)	Specificity (%)
Rafaelsen et al.[26]	1995	295	TUS IOUS	70 97	– –
Moran et al.[27]	1995	60	TUS CTAP IOUS	70 95 98	– – –
Carter et al.[28]	1996	73	TUS CT IOUS	75 95 77	100 92 100
Delbeke et al.[29]	1997	52	PET CE-CT CTAP	92 78 80	– – –
Valls et al.[30]	1998	35	CE-CT CTAP	76 74	– –
Bunk et al.[31]	1998	60	CE-CT TUS Doppler	78 77 86	– – –
Helmberger et al.[32]	1999	46	CE-CT MRI SPIO MRI	96 93 97	48 71 88

*CE-CT = contrast-enhanced computed tomography; CTAP = computed tomography during arterial portography; IOUS = intraoperative ultrasound; MRI = magnetic resonance imaging; PET = positron emission tomography; SPIO MRI = ferumoxide enhanced MRI; TUS = transabdominal ultrasound.

Occasionally a metastasis may appear dense due to haemorrhage or calcification, and if there is extensive central necrosis they may also appear cystic. Most liver metastases are hypovascular and therefore may be distinguished from hypervascular lesions such as hepatocellular carcinomas, adenomas and focal nodular hyperplasia. CE-CT remains the most useful and reproducible procedure at present for the routine detection of liver metastases and extrahepatic disease.

Magnetic resonance imaging (MRI)

The exact role of MRI in the detection of liver metastases is rapidly evolving. It is non-invasive, and with the evolution of advanced machines with modern pulse sequences and tissue-specific contrast agents the sensitivity and specificity have improved in the range of 80–95%.[32] MRI scans of liver metastases are characterised by a prolonged relaxation time in T1 and T2. On T1-weighted images,

metastatic lesions appear hypointense, sometimes associated with a 'doughnut' appearance, whereas T2-weighted images tend to be hyperintense compared to the surrounding normal liver parenchyma.[35,39] Ferumoxide-enhanced MRI was found to be superior to unenhanced MRI at detecting lesions of less than 1 cm after inconclusive CE-CT scanning.[32] One study found that MRI had an accuracy equivalent to CTAP for liver lesion detection.[40] Although MRI is near universally available, the cost of these enhanced MRI techniques probably precludes its routine use as a screening tool for metastases in the follow-up of primary colorectal cancer. However, it is extremely useful in characterising equivocal suspicious lesions detected by cheaper modalities in these patients.

Positron emission tomography (PET)

PET scanning initially showed much promise as a technique for detecting liver metastases. The scan

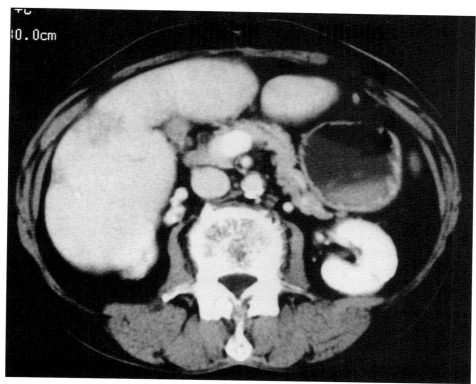

Figure 5.1 • Typical CT appearance of a solitary resectable colorectal liver metastasis.

relies on the uptake of fluorodeoxyglucose (FDG), which is high in the liver and in tumour deposits. PET scanning has been used in the detection of pancreatic metastases, and was found to have an accuracy of 90%.[41] In one study PET demonstrated a higher accuracy than CE-CT or CTAP in identifying both intrahepatic and extrahepatic disease for colorectal metastases.[29] PET-CT is not yet widely available but may prove to be the investigation of choice for detecting occult recurrence of disease in patients with a rising tumour marker, yet no obvious lesion in the liver (or elsewhere) on routine CT or MRI.

Colour flow Doppler

Hepatic flow scintigraphy and duplex colour ultrasound scanning allow measurement of the hepatic perfusion index (HPI), which has been used to detect liver metastases; the HPI is altered in patients with metastases as a result of a relatively increased hepatic arterial flow and decreased portal venous flow.[42,43] Duplex Doppler ultrasound is a more reliable means of measuring the HPI (Doppler perfusion index, or DPI) than dynamic scintigraphy and is particularly attractive because it is non-invasive.[43] Leen et al.[44] have shown that patients with colorectal cancer who have a raised DPI are more likely to develop hepatic metastases than those with a normal DPI. In their hands, the sensitivity, accuracy, and negative predictive rate of DPI for detecting colorectal liver metastases is 100%, 86% and 100% respectively. These results are generally better than those achieved by either standard CT, transabdominal US, or palpation at laparotomy,[44] and appear to be superior to Dukes staging in predicting survival from colorectal cancer,[45] although the technique has been slow to be adopted by others. Doppler imaging also appears to show a higher sensitivity for the detection of infiltration of hilar structures.[46] This technique relies on experienced practitioners but is again non-invasive and is relatively inexpensive.[47] The main drawback to all the preoperative imaging modalities is the failure to detect small liver lesions less than 10 mm and extra-hepatic spread and in particular to the peritoneum. It is these occult metastases that have the most significant impact on long-term survival.[48] Lastly, it is our experience that the early reports of this technique have proved extremely difficult to repro-duce in the hands of less experienced investigators. Therefore, as the quality of other imaging modalities improves then this technique will largely be abandoned.

Intraoperative ultrasound (IOUS)

Several studies have confirmed that intraoperative ultrasound is highly sensitive and specific for detecting liver metastases compared with pre-operative ultrasound, CT scan, or palpation at laparotomy.[26,49]

Previously undetected lesions may be seen and, prior to resection of known lesions, it is possible to clearly delineate anatomical landmarks in relation to the tumour. Intraoperative ultrasound may also be useful for identifying lesions deep within the liver, particularly those less than 10 mm in diameter,[50] and these findings may tip the balance against a curative resection. Anatomical variations that may make the resection more difficult, such as accessory hepatic veins or common origins of the portal pedicles, may also be identified.[50] Additional liver metastases may be found in as many as 33% of patients with lesions detected by preoperative imaging,[51] and in those with negative preoperative scans a further 5% will be found to have occult disease.[52]

Laparoscopy and laparoscopic ultrasound (LUS)

The benefits of laparoscopy and LUS are similar to those at open operation and IOUS. This allows for peritoneal inspection, and assessment of liver paren-chyma, extrahepatic disease and vessel invasion. The obvious benefit is the avoidance of unnecessary laparotomy and improved organisation of theatre time. A recent study confirmed that for patients in whom it was possible to perform laparoscopy, the combination of diagnostic laparoscopy and LUS significantly improved the selection of candidates for curative resection.[53]

These approaches are the subject of continuing studies to assess the potential benefits of each approach so that an optimal investigation pathway can be formulated. Prospective trials comparing these imaging modalities are still needed. At present most institutions will initially use TUS and CE-CT as the first line. At operation LUS or IOUS will be performed.

Biopsy

We would not advocate the routine biopsy of liver lesions as part of the diagnostic process for patients who are thought to have potentially resectable lesions. This is because of the danger of peritoneal seeding, therefore biopsy is not recommended if a patient is being considered for curative surgery. Indeed, it is the experience of some liver surgeons that biopsy of colorectal liver metastases (by whatever modality: peroperative at colectomy; laparoscopic; and/or percutaneously under US/CT guidance) may decrease the chance of cure after hepatectomy by as much as 50% (M. Rees, personal communication 2004).

The optimum means of assessing liver involvement by colorectal metastases is based generally on local expertise and availability of imaging modalities. There is increasing evidence that contrast-enhanced computed tomography using multislice imaging is the most useful for the routine detection and staging of liver metastases in extrahepatic disease. Magnetic resonance imaging is yet to be adopted generally for staging of hepatic metastases, and the precise role of positron emission tomography has yet to be determined.

There is evidence that percutaneous biopsy of liver tumours may be associated with extrahepatic dissemination of tumour.

STAGING

The extent of liver involvement by metastatic tumour is an important determinant of long-term survival,[54] and hence accurate staging of liver metastases may provide a guide to the likelihood of success following surgical intervention. Also, staging systems allow meaningful comparisons of treatments for liver metastases by classifying patients into matched groups. Several staging systems for liver metastases from colorectal carcinomas have been proposed, and the prognostic significance of each system has been evaluated although, unfortunately, no single system is universally accepted.

A staging system, modified from the International Union Against Cancer (UICC) and The American Joint Committee on Cancer (AJCC) recommendations for primary hepatobiliary tumours, has been proposed (**Table 5.2**).[55] In this system tumour size, tumour distribution, number of metastatic lesions, and the extent of extrahepatic disease are incorporated. In an analysis of 204 patients who underwent potentially curative hepatic resection for metastatic colorectal cancer in Pittsburgh, Gayowski et al.[55] confirmed that stage I and II cases (unilobar solitary tumours of any size, or unilobar multiple tumours of 2 cm or smaller without nodal disease or direct invasion) had an overall 5-year survival of 61%, while those with stage III, IVa and IVb (unilobar disease with multiple lesions greater than 2 cm, bilobar involvement, and nodal involvement

Table 5.2 • Staging and survival of hepatic colorectal metastases (adapted from Gayowski et al. Surgery 1994; 199:502–8)

	Staging		**5-year survival (%)**	
Stage I	mT1	N0	M0	61
Stage II	mT2	N0	M0	61
Stage III	mT3	N0	M0	28
Stage IVa	mT4	N0	M0	20
Stage IVb	Any mT	N1	M0,M1	0
		N0,N1	M1	

mT1 = solitary <2 cm. mT2 = solitary >2 cm, unilobar; or multiple <2 cm, unilobar. mT3 = multiple >2 cm, unilobar. mT4 = solitary or multiple, bilobar, invasion of major branch of portal or hepatic veins or bile ducts. N0 = no lymph nodes; N1 = abdominal lymph node. M0 = no metastatic disease; M1 = extrahepatic metastases or direct invasion to adjacent organs.

or extrahepatic disease, respectively) had overall 5-year survivals of 28%, 20% and 0%, respectively. Despite the fact that stage III and IV disease was generally associated with a poor outcome, a small percentage of patients with stage IV disease were still alive and disease free 5 years after resection, suggesting that patients should not always be rejected for surgery on the basis of stage of liver metastases alone.

NATURAL HISTORY OF UNTREATED LIVER METASTASES

The two most important factors known to influence the survival of patients with untreated liver metastases are the extent of hepatic involvement at the time of diagnosis and the histological grade of the primary tumour. Other factors that indicate a poor outlook in untreated patients are the presence of abnormal liver function tests, spread of tumour to extrahepatic sites, and primary tumours that are not resected.[56] Thus, in untreated patients, tumour burden is the major determinant of outcome, and patients with solitary metastases usually live longer than those with multiple, bilobar disease.[57] However, prolonged follow-up of untreated patients, even with solitary hepatic metastases, has confirmed that survival beyond 5 years is rare. This is in contrast to results from most series of hepatic resection for colorectal metastases, where 5-year survival rates are approximately 25–35% and where 10- and even 20-year survivors following resection have been documented.[58]

The natural history of liver metastases in untreated patients has been studied, and tumour doubling times for these metastases have been shown to be between 50 and 95 days.[59] By assuming that a tumour requires approximately 30 tumour volume doublings to reach 1 cm in diameter it has been estimated that the subclinical phase of a liver metastasis (i.e. from metastatic implantation to clinical appearance) may be 2.5–5 years.[59] This suggests that survival rates may be improved if liver metastases are detected much earlier.

Overt liver metastases sometimes appear years after apparently successful resection of the primary tumour. This long delay in the development of clinically detectable metastases suggests that in such patients host defence mechanisms have induced tumour dormancy following initial treatment.

Survival of patients with hepatic colorectal metastases at 5 years is exceptional.

RESECTION OF HEPATIC METASTASES

At the present time hepatic resection offers the only chance of long-term survival for patients with liver metastases. In 1963, Woodington and Waugh[60] published their experience of resection of colorectal metastases at the Mayo Clinic, and demonstrated that a 20% 5-year survival was possible for selected patients, and these results were confirmed by an early experience of liver resection for metastases from a variety of gastrointestinal primary tumours.[61]

In 1976 Wilson and Adson[62] reported a further series of liver resections for colorectal metastases from the Mayo Clinic, with follow-up data extending to 23 years. They documented a 5-year survival of 28% and recommended aggressive surgical treatment of apparent solitary lesions (**Fig. 5.2**).

Most data concerning resection of liver metastases come from patients with colorectal cancer because isolated (1–3 unilobar) liver metastases occur more frequently than in other cancers. Therefore, in the early series only 7–10% of all patients with colo-

rectal liver metastases benefited from resection. This figure represents a very small proportion of the total number of patients with colorectal cancer. It has been estimated that in the USA some 5000 patients each year might be suitable for resection of their liver metastases by these resection criteria[63] and, extrapolated to the UK, this figure would barely exceed 1000 patients annually. There is still a degree of nihilism among clinicians regarding the treatment of patients with hepatic metastases, although there is now ample evidence that survival may be improved by resection of isolated hepatic metastases from renal, adrenal and carcinoid tumours, as well as those from colorectal cancer.[64]

The current success of liver resection is due to major advances in metabolic, haemodynamic, and respiratory support as well as to developments in surgical technique. The need for detailed knowledge of liver anatomy as a prerequisite for liver resection has been emphasised by Starzl et al.[65] Better understanding of liver inflow and outflow control to reduce intraoperative blood loss and the use of intraoperative ultrasound, ultrasonic dissection, argon beam coagulation, and topical haemostatic agents have all contributed to accurate segmental resection with minimal postoperative morbidity or mortality.

Resection of hepatic metastases, with acceptable blood loss and transfusion requirements, is accomplished by controlling the hilar structures,

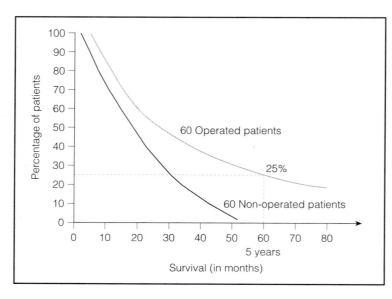

Figure 5.2 • One hundred and twenty colorectal cancer patients with a similar number of liver metastases and extent of disease. Comparative survival curves of two cohorts of patients who presented in the 1960s and 1970s to the Mayo Clinic. Half of the patients declined surgery (none survived 5 years), and their survival is compared to those who underwent liver resection. From Wilson SM, Adson MA. Archives of Surgery 1976; 111:330–34. With permission of the American Medical Association.

with or without the use of the Pringle manoeuvre, and extrahepatic control of the hepatic veins. Placing the patient in the Trendelenburg position and maintaining a low central venous pressure have also been shown to reduce the likelihood of bleeding during the resection.[66]

Morbidity and mortality after resection

Because the long-term survival benefit of liver resection for metastases is relatively small (33% survival 5 years after hepatectomy), the risks of surgery assume great significance. Perioperative morbidity should be low and the perioperative mortality must be less than the anticipated 5-year survival rate. In the larger series of patients undergoing resection of colorectal liver metastases, reported operative mortality rates vary from 0 to 8%. Most patients have a postoperative stay of 10–12 days, and operative morbidity rates range from 10 to 39%.[55,57,63,67,68] In a review of morbidity and mortality after hepatic resection of colorectal liver metastases, Doci et al.[68] noted that intra-abdominal sepsis was the most frequent 'major' complication and pulmonary infection or atelectasis was the most frequent 'minor' complication reported. A large residual cavity is often left after partial hepatectomy and this may fill with blood or bile and, combined with sloughing of devitalised tissue at the resection line, may lead to intra-abdominal infection.[68] Simultaneous hepatectomy and gastrointestinal resection with anastomosis during 'one-stage' procedures may lead to postoperative intra-abdominal infection. Elias et al. have examined this issue in a retrospective study of 53 patients with colorectal cancer, and showed that postoperative complications could be minimised by thoroughly preparing the bowel preoperatively and by using a defunctioning colostomy to protect low anastomoses.[69]

Most postoperative complications after liver resection can be managed without re-operation, and percutaneous drainage of perihepatic collections and endoscopic stenting of biliary leaks are now routine.[70]

Excessive bleeding during hepatic resection is thankfully a very rare but major complication associated with a perioperative mortality as high as 17%.[71] However, the introduction of newer technology – low central venous pressure (CVP) anaesthesia, ultrasonic dissectors, intraoperative ultrasound, argon beam coagulator and fibrin glue – has improved control of haemorrhage although surgeons must still be familiar with the established techniques of finger fracture and hepatic vascular isolation.

Hepatic failure occasionally occurs following liver resection for metastases and is often a lethal complication.[68]

The probability of postoperative hepatic failure depends on the volume and function of the residual liver, and there is evidence that a preoperative estimate of a post-resection liver volume of at least 35% is predictive of a good outcome.[72]

As a general rule, the larger the liver resection, the greater the probability of postoperative complications. Therefore, hepatic metastases should ideally be removed with a satisfactory clear margin, preferably by segment-orientated resections, but at the same time sparing as much normal liver as possible.

Most of the larger published series of resection of liver metastases report a gradual improvement in perioperative mortality rates over time as experience and technical skill with resection have developed and, as such, there is general agreement that liver resection is most safely performed by surgeons in specialised units.[70]

Survival following resection

Hepatic resection offers the only chance of cure from certain metastases confined to the liver, although significant survival benefit is only seen if resection is performed with minimal morbidity and mortality. The reported overall 5-year survival rates following hepatic resection of colorectal metastases range from 6 to 52% (**Table 5.3**).

A few series have extensive follow-up data and are able to document actual survival figures,[57,63,70] but most long-term figures are predicted from early survival curves. Many of these studies do not take perioperative deaths into account when calculating survival data and thus tend to distort the true survival picture.

A survival plateau is noted about 5 years after resection of liver metastases.[82,83] These patients

Table 5.3 • Survival rates following hepatic resection for colorectal liver metastases

Study	Year	Number	Morbidity (%)	Mortality (%)	Median survival (months)	Actuarial survival rate (%) 3-year	5-year
Gayowski et al.[55]	1994	204	–	0	33	43	32
Scheele et al.[70]	1995	434	16	4	33	43	39
Nordlinger et al.[73]	1996	1568	–	2.3	–	44	28
Jamieson et al.[74]	1997	280	–	–	–	–	27
Taylor et al.[75]	1997	123	–	0	–	–	34
Rees et al.[76]	1997	89 radical*	6	1	–	–	37
		18 palliative	–	–	–	–	6
Bakalakos et al.[77]	1998	301	–	1	21	–	–
Elias et al.[78]	1998	269	–	2	–	–	25
Ambiru et al.[79]	1999	168	–	3.5	–	42	26
Yazaki et al.[80]	1999	154	–	–	–	41	27
		14 radical IVC*	25	6	–	33	22
Nagashima et al.[81]	1999	64	–	–	–	55	47

*Radical = radical inferior vena cava resection.

subsequently have a similar life expectancy to a matched non-cancer cohort.[82] Ten-year survival rates after hepatic resection for colorectal metastases are approximately 24%,[70,82] and some even report 20-year survival rates approaching 20%.[70]

There has never been a controlled trial to address the question of resection versus non-resection or conservative treatment of potentially resectable colorectal liver metastases. Therefore, these figures for survival after resection need to be compared with survival rates of untreated, historical controls. Studies of the natural history of untreated liver metastases have revealed that a minority of patients with limited disease may live for long periods without treatment, and this group offers the most realistic comparison with patients undergoing liver resection.[54] Even though some of these patients have 'favourable' tumour biology, possibly allowing prolonged survival without treatment, long-term survival beyond 5 years is rare without liver resection.[54] This compares to overall 5-year survival rates of 25–35% reported in most series following resection of colorectal liver metastases. However, overall survival figures may give an overoptimistic impression of the curative benefit of resection, and

a substantial percentage of patients may remain alive but with recurrent disease. In a large multi-institutional study of liver resections for colorectal metastases, overall 5-year survival was 32% but only 24% of patients were disease free.[84] Despite the frequency of relapse following surgery, the natural history of the disease is probably altered by hepatic resection, as evidenced by the unusual sites of colorectal cancer recurrence that occur in these patients, such as in the lungs.[83] Aggressive surgical approaches have been used in patients with metastases involving the inferior vena cava resulting in 22% 5-year survival rates in a highly selected group of patients.[80] The development of pulmonary metastases as well as hepatic metastases may not preclude potentially curative surgery. Patients have undergone resection of disease in both organs; in one study the operative mortality was 0% and median survival was 19 months.[85] This approach may be suitable for a highly selected group of patients with hepatic and pulmonary metastases.[86]

 Although no controlled data are available, it is accepted that duration of survival is improved following curative resection of colorectal liver metastases.

Prognostic factors

A variety of factors have been shown to influence survival following liver resection. These markers should be used when assessing individual patients to arrive at a reasonable management plan and to avoid unnecessary surgery. Many studies have used univariate analysis of these factors to determine their prognostic significance although this may be misleading because of the influence of the multiple factors involved in liver resection. Therefore, only data obtained from studies that examined the various prognostic factors by multivariate analysis are considered.

NUMBER AND DISTRIBUTION OF METASTASES

There is no significant difference in long-term outcome following resection of one, two or three metastases.

Some authors advise against resection if there are four or more lesions because, in their experience, long-term survival is rare.[87] However, Scheele et al.[70] describe patients with up to five randomly distributed metastases who have survived more than 5 years after complete resection, and argue that the limiting factor to the number of lesions that can be resected is whether it is technically possible to remove all of the tumour (**Fig. 5.3**).[70]

In a series of hepatic resections from Pittsburgh, survival was adversely affected by the presence of more than three metastases although 20% of the patients in this group still survived to 5 years.[55] These authors, and others, suggest that the presence of multiple metastases should not be an absolute contraindication to resection.[55,70,88,89]

Multivariate analyses of the number of metastases resected has shown this to be a significant factor for long-term survival in some[55,87–89] but not all studies.[70,88,89] Most of these reports also show that the distribution of metastases to one or both lobes of the liver does not affect prognosis. It is therefore reasonable to consider resection for more than three metastases if the procedure can be done with a low risk of liver failure. This is particularly the case where a cluster of similar-sized metastases (suggestive of a common tumour embolic event) has clearly occurred in a segment or lobe, and the residual liver is disease free. It is debatable whether the presence of satellite metastases has any impact on survival,[70] although some studies have shown worse survival for patients with satellite nodules.[79]

RESECTION MARGINS

There is considerable debate concerning the ideal resection margin of healthy liver tissue that must be obtained around the metastasis to maximise the benefit of resection. Data from the Registry of

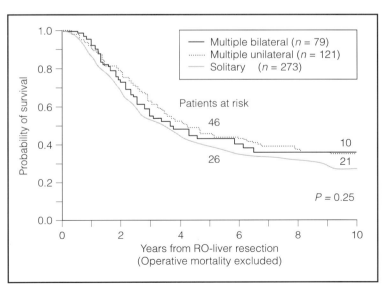

Figure 5.3 • Comparison of long-term survival following resection of colorectal liver metastases from solitary, multiple unilateral, and multiple bilateral disease. From Scheele J., Stang R. World Journal of Surgery 1995; 19:59–71. With permission of Springer-Verlag ©.

Hepatic Metastases, a multi-institutional database of liver resections, showed that a margin greater than 1 cm was associated with a 45% 5-year survival, but only 23% survived 5 years if the margin was less. However, this factor was not found to be statistically significant as information on margin size was not available for many cases.[90]

Conventional teaching advocates a margin of at least 10 mm clear of microscopic disease, and this is supported by the results from several series that document a significantly poorer overall and disease-free 5-year survival in patients with margins less than 10 mm,[71,87] particularly if closely related to contralateral vascular structures.

However, this teaching is challenged by others who argue that strict adherence to obtaining a margin of 10 mm may not be important (**Fig. 5.4**).[70] Furthermore, a margin that may appear to be adequate during resection, may be reported subsequently as inadequate by the pathologist, who may note microscopic involvement of resection margins. It may also be possible to destroy a field of liver parenchyma adjacent to the resection margin with either argon beam coagulation or wide-field cryotherapy to a depth of several millimetres. The presence of a microscopic fibrous pseudocapsule surrounding the metastasis has been associated with better long-term survival.[79]

Protagonists of generous resection margins cite evidence of a higher incidence of hepatic recurrence associated with narrow margins. This may reflect the extent of liver involvement, necessitating a greater resection with tight margins to preserve residual liver function. It is our experience that when disease recurs in the liver it is more often at some site distant from the original resection line, and we assume it is most likely to have arisen in undetected micrometastases present at the time of original liver resection. Therefore, ideally, a resection margin of at least 10 mm should be attempted, judged by intraoperative ultrasonography, but if this is not technically possible, narrow margins should not be an absolute contraindication to resection.

SIZE OF METASTASES

Clearly the size of a metastasis is related to its 'age', or time since onset of the malignant process. Larger liver metastases have usually been present for a longer time than smaller lesions. Metastases of differing sizes are probably indicative of showers of tumour emboli occurring at different times.

In several large studies metastases greater than 5 cm were associated with poorer survival than smaller metastases,[67,71,91] although multivariate analysis of this factor in other studies has failed to show an influence on survival.[87]

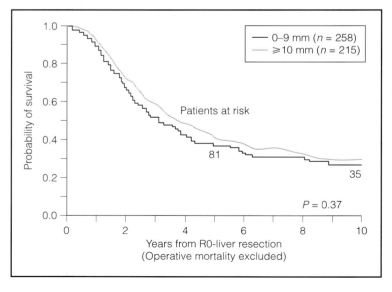

Figure 5.4 ▪ Impact of resection margin (<10 mm versus ≥10 mm) of resected colorectal liver metastases on long-term survival. From Scheele J., Stang R. World Journal of Surgery 1995; 19:59–71. With permission of Springer-Verlag ©.

In some situations, extended (and occasionally non-anatomical) resections are required to remove very large deposits. Usually these resections are dictated by the extent and number of deposits and are indicative of a more aggressive malignant process with a poorer outcome, regardless of intervention. In the specific situation of a giant solitary metastasis, tumour biology is such that the capacity for multiple metastases may well be limited, and therefore outcome may be good after resection. In a recent study patients with lesions larger than 6 cm had a significantly worse prognosis than those with smaller lesions.[92]

SYNCHRONOUS VERSUS METACHRONOUS DISEASE

There is controversy over the value of resection of liver metastases found synchronously with the primary lesion. Several studies have documented poorer outcome in patients who undergo resection of synchronous metastases and, conversely, better survival in patients with disease-free intervals of one or more years after resection of their primary tumours.[67,71] This may reflect better tumour biology in lesions detected at a later date since it is likely that these deposits were present, but undetectable at the time of resection of the primary lesion. In interpreting data concerning the benefits of resection of metachronous versus synchronous metastases, consideration should be given to progress in methods of earlier detection (see above).

However, several other studies used multivariate analysis to show that the prognosis after resection is not dependent on the time of detection of metastatic disease.[87,89,93,94] Therefore, if patients have potentially resectable synchronous metastases and are otherwise well, they should be considered for hepatectomy after they have been appropriately staged.

RESECTION IN THE PRESENCE OF EXTRAHEPATIC METASTASES

The presence of extrahepatic disease significantly reduces the likelihood of long-term survival[71,87] and is usually a contraindication to liver resection. Palliation of symptoms may be attained by resection of a large tumour but, in most cases, this has no beneficial effect on survival.[70] However, there are certain circumstances where long-term survival has been achieved after liver resection in the presence of extrahepatic disease. Patients with resectable pulmonary or adrenal gland metastases may survive for more than 5 years after a successful liver resection, although most will develop further recurrence during that time.[95] Anecdotal reports cite successful resection of solitary cerebral metastases after resection of liver metastases, but there are no verifiable 5-year survival data to support such interventions. The series of Scheele described above found that survival was poor in patients with extrahepatic disease who underwent hepatic resection, with only 3 of 73 patients surviving after 10 years.[70] There are some instances, however, where patients with extrahepatic disease could be considered for resection with potentially curative intent. These cases include direct diaphragmatic invasion, resectable local hepatic recurrence, and resectable lung metastases that are readily resectable and few in number.[96]

Occasionally a subcapsular hepatic metastasis appears to invade an adjacent structure (mostly the diaphragm). This attachment is usually fibrotic and probably represents an inflammatory response to the tumour.[97] If frozen-section analysis of the area is clear of malignant disease then the outcome after resection is similar to that without extrahepatic attachment.

Recent data suggest that if pulmonary colorectal metastases are resectable then as many as 35% of patients are alive 5 years later.[98] These authors suggest that factors that adversely influence outcome after thoracotomy include: preoperative CEA levels; number of metastases resected; grade of primary tumour; and presence of non-resectable disease elsewhere.

PORTAL LYMPH NODE INVOLVEMENT

Hepatic pedicle lymph node involvement may be present in 20–30% of patients with hepatic metastases, and almost none of these patients survives 5 years after hepatectomy.[67,99] Some studies suggest benefit from radical excision of nodes in the region of the hepatic pedicle[71] although this is not practised widely.

In a study of 126 patients who underwent complete resection of metastases, it was found that 28% of patients had tumour infiltration of lymph nodes from the hepatoduodenal ligament. The 3- and

5-year survival rates were 48% and 22%, respectively, for patients without nodal involvement, but only 3% and 0%, respectively, for lymph node-positive patients.[100] Presently, there is only one reported single long-term survivor of resection for colorectal metastases who had positive portal nodal involvement.[101] Therefore, if at the time of surgery, histopathological examination of frozen-section tissue confirms portal nodal involvement, patients should not generally be considered for resection.

TYPE OF RESECTION

Simple 'shelling out' of metastases is associated with higher recurrence rates than formal resections, which remove a margin of normal liver tissue.[67,91] In addition, non-segmental resection may compromise the vascularity of adjacent residual liver tissue and may be technically more difficult.[67,102] Consequently hepatic segmentectomy is preferable for small, localised lesions unless this increases the risk of postoperative liver failure.

Multivariate analysis in several studies has shown that anatomical resections have a significant survival benefit over lesser procedures,[70] although these findings have not been confirmed in other studies.[71,87]

It is important that all tumour is removed with an adequate margin, and for larger tumours this may be difficult with non-anatomical wedge excisions. Clearly, for small, awkwardly located lesions (such as at the apex of segment 8 in the axilla of the right and middle hepatic veins), local resection might be preferable to formal hemihepatectomy, in which a whole, healthy lobe may need to be sacrificed for a small deposit. A diligent search for other metastases should be carried out using intraoperative ultrasound before attempting to 'wedge out' an apparently superficial tumour nodule. For larger metastases or multiple deposits, standard anatomical resections based on Couinaud segments should ensure adequate margins.[67,70] If more radical procedures (right and left trisegmentectomy) are necessary to obtain adequate clearance the prognosis is poorer.[100] Patients who require an extended (one lobe plus one or two segments of the other lobe) resection to obtain clearance are likely to have more disease than those with tumour confined to one anatomical lobe. However, there are 5-year survivors following extended hepatectomy, and

therefore this criterion alone should not preclude a patient from resection.

PATIENT AGE

In the multi-institutional study by Hughes[90] the patient's age was shown significantly to influence the outcome after resection of liver metastases although this relationship has not been observed in other studies.[70,71,88]

It is reasonable to base the decision to offer liver resection to patients on biological rather than chronological age as it has been shown that there is no difference in perioperative mortality or morbidity between elderly and young patients following hepatectomy.[103] The major determinant of success in the elderly (>80 years of age) is the volume of residual liver (since liver adaptation following resection diminishes with age), and fitness for general anaesthesia. In large studies age has not been shown to be a prognostic factor.

GENDER

It has been suggested that males have a poorer survival than females after resection of liver metastases,[105] although most studies do not confirm this.[71,93,88–91] This should therefore not be a factor in the decision whether or not to offer liver resection to patients.

OPERATIVE BLOOD LOSS

Major operative blood loss has been related to a poorer prognosis following partial hepatectomy for colorectal metastases.[93,106] Obviously, this finding may be confounded by the fact that larger tumours are likely to be associated with greater blood loss during resection. Some authors have shown that perioperative transfusion requirements were not an independent prognostic factor in survival.[55] Blood loss is not a factor that can be taken into account preoperatively when selecting patients for resection.

SITE OF PRIMARY TUMOUR

Several groups have noted that the site of the primary tumour was an independent predictor of survival in patients with colorectal liver metastases.[56,107] Rougier et al.[56] have demonstrated that in patients whose liver metastases are left untreated (or received palliative chemotherapy), those whose primary tumours arose in the right colon fared worse than those whose primary developed elsewhere in the colon or rectum.

Younes et al.[107] confirmed these findings in patients who underwent resection of the liver metastases, although a contradictory finding was reported by Jatzko et al.,[6] who noted that patients with rectal tumours had a worse survival than patients with colon tumours. Whether these results reflect later presentation of right-sided disease or higher local recurrence rates of rectal cancers is speculative. In most series, however, the site of the primary colorectal cancer has not been shown to influence the long-term outcome following hepatectomy for liver metastases.[55,70,71,108]

GRADE OF PRIMARY TUMOUR

Some authors have noted that patients with histologically high-grade primary tumours have poorer survival after resection of liver metastases.[70] This is not surprising as the grade of the primary tumour is known to influence survival after resection of the primary tumour, independent of whether liver metastases are present. However, in other studies multivariate analysis of the grade of primary tumour has not been found to be an independent predictor of survival.[55,87,109]

The majority of liver metastases are either moderately or poorly differentiated and are likely to have arisen from similarly differentiated primary tumours. Since we would not advocate tumour biopsy prior to hepatectomy, in order to reduce the risk of tumour spill (the liver resection is the biopsy), then such information regarding differentiation of the metastasis is not available preoperatively. Regardless, there are survivors who are disease free 5 years after resection of poorly differentiated liver metastases.

STAGE OF PRIMARY TUMOUR

Several authors have reported a statistical correlation between the stage of primary tumour and outcome after hepatectomy,[54,67,71,88,89] although others have not recorded this relationship.[55,87,93]

Tumours that have the capacity to invade and metastasise to lymphatics are clearly more aggressive than those without this potential and, conceivably may bypass the liver, by spreading to pre-aortic lymph nodes and beyond to the thoracic duct and systemic circulation. Although there may be a correlation between primary tumour stage and survival, the relationship is not strong enough to preclude liver resection for patients with more advanced primary tumours.

CARCINOEMBRYONIC ANTIGEN (CEA)

Several studies have shown that an increased preoperative serum level of CEA is an independent predictor of poor survival in patients who undergo hepatectomy.[71,107] One study showed that patients with CEA ≤30 ng/mL are more likely to be resectable and have the longest survival.[109]

A scoring system has been developed based on data from 1568 patients who underwent liver resection. The 2- and 5-year survival were affected by age, size of largest metastasis or CEA level, stage of primary tumour, disease-free interval, number of liver nodules and resection margin.[73] These factors were identified through univariate and multivariate analysis and it may be that this system can be used for further prospective validation.

 There is no consensus on which factors predict survival following hepatic resection but it is accepted that no residual disease should be left behind following attempted resection of colorectal metastases.

CONTRAINDICATIONS TO LIVER RESECTION

Resection may be considered in patients fit enough to tolerate general anaesthesia, with no major comorbidity and normal liver function. Absolute contraindications for resection of colorectal liver metastases have not been clarified, but most would agree that patients should not be offered resection if they have uncontrolled primary disease or such widespread intrahepatic involvement that the residual liver function after resection would be inadequate. Most authorities would agree that presently it would be safe to resect up to 70% of a healthy (non-cirrhotic) liver for colorectal metastases. Relative contraindications include situations where resection of a hepatic metastasis is not performed easily, such as those involving the caudate lobe (segments 1 and 9), or tumours invading the inferior vena cava. Tumour involvement of the portal vein confluence would also limit the potential curability

Table 5.4 • Changing criteria for resection of colorectal liver metastases

Traditional selection criterion	Current view	
No more than 3 metastases	Patients with >3 metastases have poorer prognosis but may still benefit from/be cured by resection	
Unilobar disease	Bilateral disease not a barrier to resectability	
Small tumours (<5 cm in diameter)	Patients with large tumours (>7 cm) in diameter have poorer prognosis but may still benefit from/be cured by resection	
Metachronous detection of metastases	Synchronous detection not a contraindication to resectability	
Dukes A or B primary tumours only	Patients with Dukes stage C primary have poorer prognosis but may still benefit from/be cured by resection	
Resection margin >1 cm required	1 mm resection margin may be acceptable; radical (R0) resection not possible except for palliation	
No extrahepatic disease	Exceptions for isolated lung metastases, resectable local hepatic recurrence, direct diaphragmatic invasion	
Not patients >65 years	Patients >70 years eligible for resection	
No portal nodal involvement	Criterion remains valid	

of the resection. Bilobar distribution of metastases or size of metastases are relative contraindications and do not necessarily limit resectability.

In summary, despite the persisting contra-indications of R0 or curative resection (portal nodal involvement and most presentations of extrahepatic disease), the overall trend has been towards a much more inclusive philosophy in the resection of colorectal liver metastases. This paradigm shift in defining resectability criteria for these patients has already demonstrated a doubling in resection rates from the previous 10% to 20% of all patients with colorectal liver metastases in the centres that have adopted this approach.[55,70,73,110,111] Unless liver resection is highly unlikely to have any prospect of saving or significantly prolonging the patient's life, it should be considered because it offers patients with metastatic colorectal cancer their only chance of long-term survival (**Table 5.4**).

RE-RESECTION OF LIVER METASTASES

Recurrence may occur in up to 65% of patients following liver resection for metastases, the most common site being in the liver.[71] Approximately 20% of these patients have liver-only recurrence

and hence may be suitable for re-resection. Intra-hepatic recurrence after resection of metastases may arise from inadequate clearance of tumour or may be due to residual micrometastatic disease else-where in the liver. In a large multicentre study from the French Association of Surgery, 23% of patients underwent repeat hepatectomy following resection of colorectal liver metastases. Recurrent disease occurred in the opposite side of the liver in more than a third of cases.[71] Repeat hepatectomy is often more difficult than the initial procedure because of dense adhesions and because the liver parenchyma may be more friable or fibrotic. Surprisingly, reported mortality and morbidity rates after repeat liver resection of metastases are similar to those reported after initial hepatectomy.[112] Survival figures from the larger series of repeat hepatic resection of colorectal metastases are also similar to those achieved after the first procedure (**Table 5.5**). As with the initial resection, the presence of extra-hepatic disease or incomplete tumour clearance are associated with a poorer outcome.[112]

The majority of patients who develop recurrence following hepatic resection of colorectal metastases relapse within 2 years of surgery; aggressive surveil-lance with regular serum CEA levels, abdominal and chest CT or conventional ultrasound following resection may improve the detection of recurrent

Table 5.5 • Survival following repeat hepatectomy for colorectal metastases

Study	Year	Re-resection/ total resection	Median survival (months)	Actuarial survival rate (%)		
				1-year	3-year	5-year
Adam et al.[96]	1997	64/243	–	–	60	42
Chu et al.[113]	1997	10/74	16	78	–	23
Kin et al.[114]	1998	15/67	–	–	42	21
Yamamoto et al.[115]	1999	90	–	–	48	31

disease.[112] In patients who do develop recurrence it seems reasonable to consider these lesions in the same way as the first metastasis and offer re-resection to patients based on operative risk and probable survival.

It has been shown that for a small number of patients who are suitable for repeat hepatectomy following previous resection of colorectal liver metastases, the operative risk and survival prospects are similar to those in patients following initial hepatectomy.

RESECTION OF NON-COLORECTAL HEPATIC METASTASES

Improvements in perioperative mortality of major hepatic resection have led to a more liberal application of this procedure for metastatic disease. Hepatic resections of metastases from non-colorectal primary tumours have occasionally been reported although all have involved relatively small numbers of patients.[64] Resection of non-colorectal liver metastases is not performed routinely because widespread hepatic infiltration occurs more frequently with non-colorectal liver metastases. In a review of the literature on hepatic resection for non-colorectal, non-neuroendocrine metastases, Schwartz suggested that resection of confined liver metastases arising from primary renal cell carcinomas, Wilms' tumours, and adrenocortical carcinomas may improve long-term survival. Five-year survival rates following partial hepatectomy for these metastases are equivalent to those achieved following resection of colorectal metastases, and it seems reasonable, therefore, to offer resection to patients with resect-able lesions who can tolerate surgery.[64] However, experience with metastases from other non-colorectal primary tumours would indicate that there is no survival advantage in performing liver resection although palliation of symptoms from bulky metastases may be achieved by resection in selected patients.[64]

Elias et al.[116] have reported a series of 21 patients who underwent hepatectomy for liver metastases from breast carcinoma. Preoperative and postoperative chemotherapy were also used for many of these patients, which makes interpretation of the survival data difficult. They reported an overall 5-year survival rate of 24% from commencement of combined therapy, although only 9% of patients were alive 5 years after surgery. Unsuspected metastases were found at laparotomy in 22% of patients, and the authors conceded that hepatectomy for metastases from breast carcinoma was mainly a cytoreductive procedure that did not prolong survival.[116]

Hepatic resection of metastases from soft-tissue sarcomas has been reported, most commonly from primary visceral leiomyosarcomas. The experience of the Memorial Sloan-Kettering Cancer Center suggests that patients with retroperitoneal leiomyosarcomas are most at risk of metastasising to the liver whereas sarcomas of the extremity rarely spread in this fashion. In 14 patients who underwent hepatic resection all developed recurrent disease, which was mainly within the liver, and there were no 5-year survivors. These authors conclude that resection of hepatic metastases from primary sarcomas is only indicated if it is feasible to completely remove all tumour from the liver and, even if this is undertaken, survival beyond 5 years is rare.[117]

True isolated metastatic deposits from gastric or gallbladder adenocarcinomas are rare, and there are few reported long-term survivors in patients who have undergone resection of metachronous hepatic metastases. However, some authors suggest that isolated metastatic deposits of gastric cancer may be resected, with a chance of cure, if the original primary tumour showed no evidence of serosal invasion, lymphatic or vascular involvement.[118]

Isolated reports of liver resection of metastases from gynaecological, pancreatic and oesophageal primary tumours would suggest there is little survival benefit from this procedure.[64]

Hepatic resection of metastatic neuroendocrine tumours, such as carcinoids and VIPomas, have been performed on the basis that these tumours are slowly growing and clinical symptoms are known to correlate directly with tumour bulk. Several studies have reported excellent palliation of symptoms and even long-term survivors after this procedure.[119,120]

CHEMOTHERAPY

Palliative chemotherapy

Even nowadays, the majority of patients with liver metastases are unsuitable for resection and chemotherapy offers the only hope of palliation. It is not possible to cure patients with liver metastases by using chemotherapy, but symptom palliation and prolonged survival has been reported for patients with disseminated disease.[121]

In the past, chemotherapy has been administered systemically or regionally via the hepatic artery or portal vein. The most widely used agent for systemic treatment of colorectal liver metastases for many years was the antimetabolite, 5-fluorouracil (5-FU). This agent is a prodrug that is metabolised by cells to active cytotoxic species that can inhibit the key enzyme, thymidylate synthase. In patients given 5-FU alone an objective tumour response is seen in only 5–18% of cases,[122] although this has had little effect on survival. Folinic acid (leucovorin) may be combined with 5-FU to enhance overall cytotoxicity by promoting its transformation into fluoro-deoxyuridine monophosphate (F-dUMP). Mean response rates are approximately 30%, with median

survivals of approximately 12 months, which is significantly better than seen in untreated patients or those treated with 5-FU alone.[123]

Other systemic chemotherapeutic agents proven to be as effective as 5-FU combined with folinic acid include Tomudex and capecitabine.[120] However, although easier to administer than 5-FU–folinic acid, Tomudex is of no greater efficacy and has now largely been abandoned. Capecitabine is an analogue of 5-FU that is as effective as systemic 5-FU–folinic acid when taken orally and will supersede systemic 5-FU in future regimens.

A large variety of cytotoxic agents have been used in single and combination approaches, and the advantages of each approach are currently being assessed in phase II and III trials. Newer agents such as irinotecan (topoisomerase I inhibitor) have demonstrated improved 1-year survival compared with the 'standard' 5-FU regimen.[125]

Cytotoxic agents are administered regionally due to the fact that hepatic metastases exclusively derive their blood supply from the hepatic artery. Regional perfusion of established liver metastases allows delivery of high doses of chemotherapeutic agents directly to the tumour while avoiding high systemic levels since much of the drug will be eliminated by the liver.[126] The two most frequently used agents for hepatic artery infusion (HAI) are 5-FU and FUDR (5-fluoro-2-deoxyuridine).[118] HAI is usually indicated in patients with unresectable hepatic metastases that are confined to the liver. Preoperative angiography will identify variations in arterial anatomy, especially a right hepatic artery arising from the superior mesenteric artery. At laparotomy, a catheter is inserted and fixed at the proximal end of the gastroduodenal artery. A cholecystectomy is usually required to avoid subsequent chemical cholecystitis. Satisfactory liver perfusion may be confirmed intraoperatively by injecting fluorescein or methylene blue through the subcutaneous port of the catheter. Implantable constant infusion devices connected to inert, siliconised catheters can be used and allow longer, more tolerable infusions than previously possible with external pump devices.

Response rates of intra-arterial chemotherapy have appeared higher than those seen with systemic chemotherapy although only one study has documented marginal survival benefit over systemic chemotherapy.[127] Allen-Mersh et al.[128] demonstrated that hepatic artery infusion of FUDR also contributes to improved quality of life.

HAI has been studied in combination with systemic chemotherapy for the treatment of unresectable colorectal metastases, but has not been shown to be superior to HAI alone.[129]

Complications of regional chemotherapy are not uncommon. These include biliary sclerosis, chemical hepatitis, arterial thrombosis, infections, catheter displacement, gastroduodenal inflammation and peritonitis. The addition of dexamethasone to the hepatic artery infusion may reduce the toxicity of regional chemotherapy and possibly increase response rates, although the mechanism of these actions is unclear. Close monitoring of liver function tests is necessary when patients undergo hepatic artery infusion, and abnormalities, particularly a rising bilirubin, are usually indicative of hepatotoxicity, requiring cessation of treatment.[130] In an attempt to improve the results of regional chemotherapy some authors have used vasoactive agents, such as angiotensin or vasopressin, to try to alter the pharmacokinetics of bolus HAI 5-FU although there is no evidence this significantly alters survival. Synchronous primary tumour resection and regional hepatic chemotherapy have been reported and shown to be well tolerated.[131]

Adjuvant chemotherapy

A randomised trial comparing two groups of patients undergoing hepatic resection with one group receiving adjuvant 5-FU and folinic acid was commenced under the auspices of the European Organisation for Research and Treatment of Cancer (EORTC). Unfortunately it ended prematurely without having shown any survival benefit for the adjuvant group (B. Nordlinger, personal communication). The use of HAI as adjuvant therapy is an attractive prospect for delivering high doses of cytotoxic agents to the tumour. Local response rates have been high using this method. The effect on long-term survival has been encouraging in retrospective studies. One study compared survival of 78 patients who had HAI with 30 patients who had portal vein infusion and 66 patients who had resection alone. The HAI group had significantly prolonged disease-free and overall survival.[132]

It is estimated that after surgery for colorectal liver metastases, relapse will occur in 60–70% of patients.[96,112] The 5-year survival rates after surgical resection in advanced disease have historically been about 35% for patients with one or two liver metastases at resection and 14% for those with three or more,[82] although as previously stated, presentation with three or more metastases should not necessarily be taken as a contraindication to resection.

Effective postoperative therapy after resection of metastases may reduce the recurrence rate and prolong survival.[133] However, the optimal strategy for chemotherapy after liver resection is still under investigation. Recently, there has been particular interest in HAI. A Memorial Sloan-Kettering study of chemotherapy following liver resection compared standard systemic chemotherapy based on 5-FU–folinic acid (leucovorin) with a regimen consisting of systemic 5-FU–folinic acid alternating with hepatically infused FUDR.[95,132–135] The regimen incorporating HAI was more effective in terms of overall survival, which was 86% at 2 years in the patients who received HAI compared with 72% in patients who received systemic therapy only ($P = 0.03$). At 5 years, actuarial survival in the HAI group was 61%, compared with 49% in the systemic therapy group. HAI also benefited patients in terms of progression-free survival, with 2-year actuarial survival figures of 57% for the regimen incorporating HAI and 42% for systemic therapy only ($P = 0.07$), and median durations of progression-free survival of 37.4 months and 17.2 months, in the HAI and systemic therapy groups, respectively.

As might be expected, the benefits of HAI were especially pronounced with regard to hepatic progression. The 2-year actuarial survival free of hepatic progression was 90% in the HAI group and 60% in the systemic therapy group ($P <0.001$). Median hepatic progression-free survival in the systemic-only therapy group was 42.7 months, while at the time of publication the median hepatic progression-free survival had not been reached in the systemic therapy group. Overall, hepatic progression occurred in some 23% of patients treated with HAI but in 68% of those treated with systemic therapy.

The main limitation of HAI was that while the addition of HAI reduced the recurrence of liver metastases, there was no reduction in the incidence of metastases elsewhere in the body. Lung metastases, for instance, were observed in 20.3% of HAI-treated patients in the first 2 years of treatment, compared with 20.7% of those receiving systemic therapy. The incidence of recurrence at most other non-hepatic sites was similar. Thus, although HAI does increase both 2- and 5-year survival as well as progression-free survival, and has a marked effect on the occurrence of liver metastases, these benefits appear to be tempered by a failure to reduce the incidence of metastases elsewhere in the body. Although HAI undoubtedly provides better local control of metastatic spread, there is clearly a need for improved systemic therapies, and for the development of regimens in which the efficacy of systemic exposure is sustained alongside the periodic use of HAI.

The next logical step in the development of postoperative chemotherapy for metastatic colorectal cancer may therefore be the combination of HAI with a new and more potent systemic regimen. To this end, a phase II clinical study is now in progress through the North Central Cancer Treatment Group (NCCTG), with the participation of the National Surgical Adjuvant Breast and Bowel Program (NSABP), in which patients with resected liver-only metastases are being treated with hepatic infusions of FUDR alternating with a systemic regimen consisting of oxaliplatin and capecitabine, a combination that has similar antitumour efficacy to oxaliplatin plus 5-FU–folinic acid. Postoperative therapy based on this combination of agents is likely to reduce further the rate of recurrence after the resection of metastases.

Cytoreductive chemotherapy

The development of a neoadjuvant chemotherapy approach is a consequence of two key developments. First and most importantly, new, more effective chemotherapeutic agents have recently become available for the treatment of colorectal cancer. The most important of these in the context of liver resection is oxaliplatin, which when used in combination with established 5-FU–folinic acid-based therapy substantially increases the rate and degree of tumour response. In consequence, the ability of neoadjuvant chemotherapy to downsize liver

metastases and enable resection to take place has been enhanced in many patients whose tumours were initially inoperable. In addition, innovative techniques in postoperative chemotherapy following resection promise to reduce the risk of recurrence.

In tandem with the development of more effective cytoreductive chemotherapy, surgery for patients with colorectal liver metastases has in recent years been applied in a wider range of clinical circumstances. Many presentations of hepatic metastasis that would previously have been considered unsuitable for surgery are now considered amenable to resection. In addition, the practice of re-resecting subsequent metastases has become more established as a viable life-prolonging and in some cases, life-saving procedure.

This conjunction of more effective chemotherapy and a more enterprising approach to liver surgery has expanded significantly the population of patients with metastatic colorectal cancer in whom treatment with curative intent can be attempted. This new approach carries the potential for significantly prolonged survival, and the chance of cure, to a group of patients for whom the prognosis would previously have been uniformly bleak.

The only potential therapy offering long-term survival for patients with colorectal metastases considered unresectable at presentation is therefore cytoreductive chemotherapy. A key study of the benefits of neoadjuvant therapy followed by resection for initially unresectable liver metastases was reported in 1996 by Bismuth and colleagues, with 5-year survival data emerging in 2002.[73,111,136] In this investigation, a large series of 872 patients with initially unresectable colorectal liver metastases were treated with neoadjuvant therapy based on oxaliplatin (25 mg/m^2/day), chronomodulated 5-FU (700–2000 mg/m^2/day) and folinic acid (300 mg/m^2/day) for 4–5 days on a 3-week treatment cycle. Of a total of 872 patients, 171 (19.6%) were immediately eligible for curative resection. The remaining 701 patients were treated with oxaliplatin-based neoadjuvant therapy, and 95 (13.6%) achieved a response sufficient to permit curative resection. The overall resectability rate was therefore increased from 20% to 30% by this neoadjuvant regimen. At the time of publication of the study, 87 of the patients who were resected after neoadjuvant therapy had completed 5 years of follow-up, of whom 34 (39%) were alive and 19 (22%) had no evidence of disease. The authors noted that this level of response and survival was similar to that achieved following primary liver resection (**Figs 5.5** and **5.6**).

Although these results are impressive, it is notable that they were achieved with a moderate dose of oxaliplatin (25 mg/m^2 daily maximum, totalling 125 mg/m^2 per 3-week cycle) and with only moderate doses of chronomodulated 5-FU–folinic acid. A series of further studies has investigated whether the resectability rate can be improved using

alternative therapeutic regimens. A recent North Central Cancer Treatment Group (NCCTG) study investigated neoadjuvant treatment of advanced colorectal cancer in 44 patients with unresectable liver-only metastases.[137] These patients were treated with the FOLFOX-4 regimen, based on a standard 85 mg/m^2 dose of oxaliplatin and high-dose continuous 5-FU–folinic acid, until the best response was achieved, with resection then carried out if possible. Interim results presented at the ASCO meeting in 2001 revealed that of 28 patients evaluable, 9 had sufficient tumour shrinkage to permit

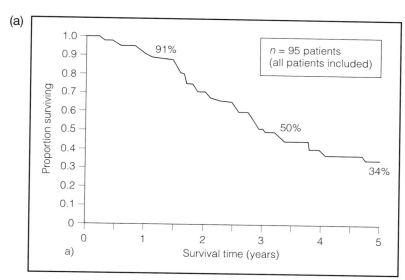

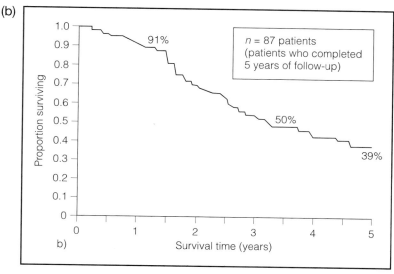

Figure 5.5 • Long-term survival of patients with initially deemed inoperable colorectal liver metastases following downstaging to operability using oxaliplatin-based chemotherapy. **(a)** All patients included ($n = 95$); **(b)** patients who completed 5 years of follow-up ($n = 87$). From Adam R et al. Annals of Surgical Oncology 2001; 8(4):347–53. With permission of Lippincott, Williams & Wilkins.

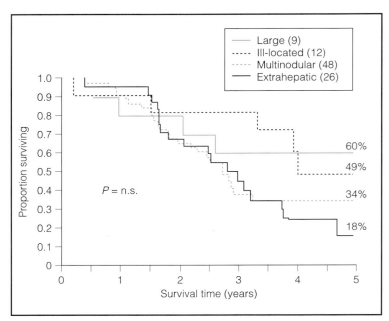

Figure 5.6 • Long-term survival of patients with colorectal liver metastases deemed initially inoperable following downstaging with chemotherapy according to reasons for initial unresectability. From Adam R et al. Annals of Surgical Oncology 2001; 8(4):347–53. With permission of Lippincott, Williams & Wilkins.

surgery with 8 having a complete resection, suggesting a resectability rate in initially non-resectable tumours of about 29%, substantially higher than the 13.6% reported in the Bismuth study (although this study included lung metastases).

Similar results were reported in a study of 151 patients with metastatic colorectal cancer confined to the liver but unresectable at presentation.[138] Treatment with chronomodulated chemotherapy based on oxaliplatin plus 5-FU–folinic acid resulted in tumour shrinkage of more than 50% in 89 patients (59.6%), and enabled surgery to be carried out in 77 patients (51%). Complete resection was achieved in 58 patients (38%). Among the 77 patients who were operated upon, median overall survival was 48.8 months, 5-year survival was 50% and 7-year survival was 30%. All these patients would have been expected to die in less than 5 years had surgery not been carried out after successful neoadjuvant chemotherapy. Lastly, a recently reported crossover trial compared an oxaliplatin-based regimen (FOLFOX) to an irinotecan-based regimen (FOLFIRI) in 222 clearly non-resectable patients when the primary end point was time to progression. Twenty-one (19%) of the patients who received FOLFOX as first-line therapy achieved sufficient tumour regression to be considered suitable

for liver resection, and R0 resection was achieved in 13 (61%) of these 21 patients (**Fig. 5.7**).[139]

These findings indicate that the use of oxaliplatin-based chemotherapy in a neoadjuvant setting will permit resection in a significant number of patients with initially unresectable hepatic metastases. The maximum resectability rate achievable using oxaliplatin-based chemotherapy is likely to be considerably higher than was observed in the Bismuth study. With aggressive treatment, including high-dose continuous infusion of 5-FU–folinic acid plus oxaliplatin at a dose of 85 mg/m^2 or higher, resectability rates of approximately 40% appear to be possible. This strategy therefore has the potential to increase substantially the proportion of patients with advanced disease who become eligible for surgery (**Fig. 5.8**).

There is concern that patients with hepatic metastases of colorectal cancer are treated with palliative chemotherapy without consideration of whether curative resection can be attempted. This approach is no longer tenable, and the possibility of curative intervention should now be considered in most patients with metastatic colorectal cancer confined entirely or almost entirely to the liver. With this new strategy, the key contemporary developments in surgery and chemotherapy for

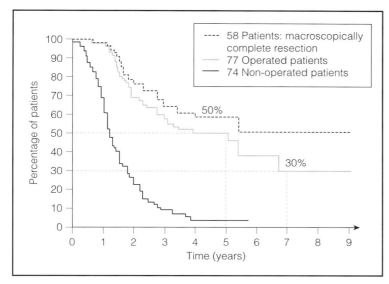

Figure 5.7 • Comparison of survival of 151 patients initially deemed unresectable who subsequently received oxaliplatin-based chemotherapy: long-term survival of those who came to resection versus those who did not downstage to resectability. From Giacchetti S et al. Annals of Oncology 1999; 10(6):663–69. With permission of Oxford University Press.

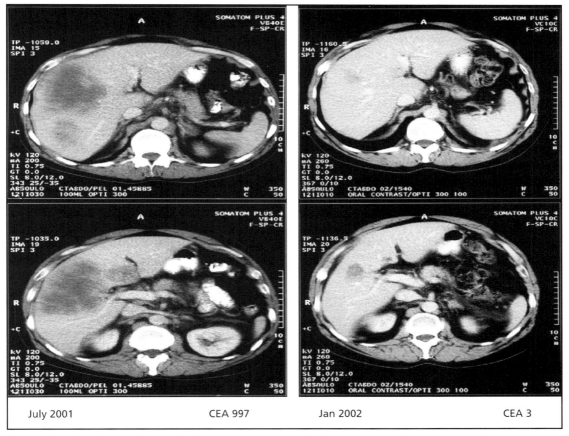

Figure 5.8 • Downstaging of colorectal liver metastases to resectability using oxaliplatin-based chemotherapy.

colorectal liver metastases are brought together into an integrated, combined modality framework. Patients with colorectal metastases that are considered unresectable or marginally resectable at presentation are placed on cytoreductive therapy. Patients with resectable metastases proceed directly to surgery or undergo neoadjuvant tumour-reducing chemotherapy according to their specific presentation. Patients placed on neoadjuvant chemotherapy are monitored regularly and those whose tumours become resectable are given surgery. All patients who receive curative resections are given postoperative chemotherapy. Patients continue to be monitored and are considered for serial resections if hepatic recurrences occur.

Following the results of studies that addressed adjuvant HAI chemotherapy after hepatectomy, an important priority is to assess the role of combined neoadjuvant and adjuvant systemic chemotherapy in resectable disease. Early results using 5-FU-based regimens of adjuvant chemotherapy proved disappointing.[133,140] Therefore, the hypothesis that neoadjuvant and adjuvant oxaliplatin-based chemotherapy may be of benefit to those patients undergoing liver resection for liver-only disease defined as resectable by 'classical' criteria (as outlined above) is now being examined in the EPOC study. In this study patients are randomised to either surgery alone or surgery preceded by 3 months of neoadjuvant chemotherapy (oxaliplatin with 5-FU-folinic acid), followed by a further 3 months of adjuvant chemotherapy after surgery. This study was launched in Europe in mid-2001, and at the time of writing the target of 330 patients necessary for the study had been recruited. The study endpoints include overall survival and disease-free survival, in addition to time to progression and operability rates at the time of liver surgery.

Based on available data, neoadjuvant therapy should include a combination of oxaliplatin, a fluoropyrimidine such as 5-FU, and folinic acid (leucovorin). A high-dose strategy should be used, such as the FOLFOX2 or FOLFOX7 regimen, since this is likely to achieve the largest and most rapid tumour response. At the present time it is debatable if the metastases continue to respond to neoadjuvant treatment beyond the stage at which resection becomes possible, that treatment should be continued to improve prognosis after surgery.

However, surgery should not be delayed if the response is tailing off or stable disease has been achieved. If the EPOC study confirms an improved survival benefit of neoadjuvant oxaliplatin-based chemotherapy for these patients, then certainly one of the next studies must be a comparison of fixed-time neoadjuvant chemotherapy versus neoadjuvant chemotherapy that continues prior to surgery for as long as the tumours continue to regress.

While the most appropriate strategy for postoperative chemotherapy is still being investigated, a very promising approach appears to be to combine HAI and systemic chemotherapy. A trial is now in progress to investigate the use of FUDR administered by HAI plus systemic therapy based on 5-FU-folinic acid plus oxaliplatin. A potent form of systemic therapy is necessary alongside HAI to reduce the risk of distant metastatic recurrence.

The success of a combined modality approach will depend ultimately on a productive collaboration between clinical oncologists and surgeons. A multidisciplinary team approach with surgical and oncological involvement can now achieve prolonged survival, and in some cases complete recovery, in a group of patients who would previously have been considered beyond the reach of curative intervention.

 There is increasing evidence that a bimodal approach employing new adjuvant oxaliplatin-based chemotherapy and liver resection is associated with prolonged survival in a group of patients who were previously thought not to be candidates for curative resection of colorectal liver metastases.

Chemoembolisation

This involves the selective injection into the hepatic artery of a combination of cytotoxic drugs with an occluding agent such as gelfoam or starch microspheres. The aims of this treatment are to combine two forms of local treatment, namely acute ischaemia and chemotherapy, and localise the chemotherapy in the liver. Experimental and clinical work has suggested that embolisation may promote arterial perfusion of underperfused metastases and at the same time block the arterioles to the healthy liver, the effect being to enhance cytotoxicity.[126] However, there is no evidence that this form of treatment confers any significant survival benefit over regional chemotherapy alone in patients with colorectal liver metastases.

ABLATIVE OR DESTRUCTIVE THERAPIES

Cryotherapy

Hepatic cryotherapy using at laparotomy insulated probes containing liquid nitrogen has been used successfully by several groups to treat liver metastases.[141–143] Its role in the treatment of colorectal liver metastases remains to be identified, and the indications for its use have not been defined clearly. Cryotherapy may be indicated in patients with non-resectable liver metastases. The presence of extrahepatic disease is generally considered a contraindication, and in patients with multiple hepatic deposits cryotherapy is usually only undertaken in patients with less than ten metastases. CEA levels have been shown to fall following cryotherapy of colorectal liver metastases and may be used as a guide to effective control of disease.[143] Several groups have reported no deaths following hepatic cryotherapy,[141,144] although others have documented postoperative deaths due to uncontrollable coagulopathy and subsequent multisystem organ failure.[142] Reported complications following this procedure include hepatic bleeding, thrombocytopenia, hypothermia, myoglobinuria, pleural effusions, acute tubular necrosis, hepatic abscess and bile duct injury.[142,144]

Cryotherapy may be useful to treat small lesions in the contralateral lobe during resection of a large metastasis. There are reports of cryo-assisted hepatic resection of metastases, which allows controlled resections with well-defined margins, thereby maximising preservation of functional parenchyma.[145] A number of non-randomised studies have assessed long-term survival after cryotherapy in a total of 1000 patients.[146] Median survival times range from 26 to 32 months and 5-year survival is 13.4%.[147–152] Low preoperative CEA, small (<3 cm) tumours and no extrahepatic disease have been associated with a favourable outcome following cryotherapy.[149] The size of lesion may be a limiting factor for cryotherapy. One study

showed that treatment of more than 5–6 deposits was not beneficial.[150] Follow-up data have shown that there is a recurrence at the cryosite in 33% of cases. It has been recommended that it is necessary to freeze a surrounding margin of 1 cm of normal liver tissue to reduce local recurrence rates.[151] Minimally invasive techniques using laparoscopic cryotherapy have been developed to treat these patients.[152]

As yet, no randomised trials have compared cryotherapy with best supportive care or chemotherapy regimens. However, although still practised in a number of centres, cryotherapy is now being abandoned, largely because of the high risk of treatment-related complications and also because of the need for a traditional, open operative approach.

Cryotherapy and regional chemotherapy

A retrospective study of 38 patients examined the effect of combined hepatic cryotherapy and regional chemotherapy in patients with colorectal liver metastases.[147] This suggested that patients who had more than 3 months of hepatic artery chemotherapy (5-FU–folinic acid) following hepatic cryotherapy had a longer survival compared with those who did not receive this treatment. Phase I and II trials are currently being conducted to examine this issue further.

Ethanol and interstitial radiotherapy

Other cytoreductive techniques that produce controlled hepatic destruction include ethanol injection and interstitial radiotherapy. The aim of these treatments is to palliate patients with unresectable liver metastases. They have the advantage of being performed percutaneously, but the disadvantage of not being able to visualise and therefore control the scale of tissue destruction by intraoperative ultrasound.

Percutaneous alcohol injection has been used to treat unresectable colorectal liver metastases but usually produces only partial responses, and early recurrence of tumour is common. Although this technique has been shown to be safe for treating liver metastases, pain following the injection has been reported, and because of poor response rates there is little to commend this form of treatment.[153] Radioactive implants have been used to treat gross residual disease or to sterilise known positive margins following hepatic resection of colorectal metastases, although early resection margin recurrence, as well as distant recurrence commonly occurs.[154] Selective internal radiation (SIR) of hepatic metastases involves embolising radioactive microspheres into the hepatic arterial circulation. Recently this technique has been shown, in an animal model, to have a potential role as an adjuvant treatment for patients who are at high risk of developing liver metastases.[155]

Interstitial laser

Another technique that has been studied is magnetic resonance-guided laser-induced thermotherapy (LITT). This is a minimally invasive approach that utilises the effect of the Nd YAG laser on tumour tissue. Online monitoring via magnetic resonance (MR) thermometry results in extremely precise monitoring and targeting. Early results show few side effects and a high tumour control rate. The median survival in a recent study of patients who had undergone MR-guided LITT for colorectal liver metastases was 39 months.[156]

Radiofrequency ablation

Percutaneous or laparoscopic US-guided radiofrequency tissue ablation (RFA) of liver metastases can produce a response rate of 67%.[157–167] Needle electrodes for RFA are thin (15G) and are easily introduced into tumour tissue without significant harm to the surrounding normal liver. RFA has proven to be an extremely safe procedure, with complication rates of less than 10%.[157–167]

Up to now, local tumour ablative techniques have mainly been used in patients with unresectable disease. In these patients tumour ablative therapy was used either alone or in combination with hepatic resection, in which case the hepatectomy dealt with the main tumour mass and unresectable small-volume residual tumour was treated with destructive therapy. Using this combined approach, most reported series describe 1- and 2-year survival rates of 80% and 60%, respectively.[141,146] Some

have claimed that these results are better than chemotherapy alone, which historically reports 1-year and 2-year survival rates of around 60% and 30%, respectively.[121–125]

There are no prospective randomised trials showing any therapeutic advantage for any of these destructive therapies over chemotherapy alone in non-resectable disease confined to the liver. Although many studies show effective responses after destructive therapy, the precise impact of local tumour ablative therapy on survival in colorectal liver metastases remains unclear. Hence, the superior results of local ablative treatment of liver metastases compared to chemotherapy alone, as reported in the literature, may be due to patient selection. However, despite this lack of grade one evidence, the US Food and Drug Administration (FDA) licensed the use of RFA for the treatment of unresectable liver tumours in 2001. The British National Institute for Clinical Excellence (NICE) is presently arguing for the need of such evidence to support the generalised use of RFA in the UK. Such a trial (Chemotherapy + Local ablation versus Chemotherapy, or CLOCC) has now commenced across Europe under the auspices of the EORTC (Trial 40004) to address the role of RFA in the treatment of non-resectable colorectal liver metastases.

TRANSPLANTATION

Pichlmayr et al.[168] have demonstrated that liver transplantation may have a role in the treatment of selected patients with liver metastases from neuroendocrine primary tumours. A recent study demonstrated 2- and 5-year survival of 60 and 47%, respectively.[169] However, in the limited number of patients with a variety of non-neuroendocrine hepatic metastases who have undergone liver transplantation, no survivors beyond 3 years have been documented. These results are in agreement with the data from the Cincinnati Transplant Tumor Registry, where early recurrence following transplantation occurred in 59% of patients with liver metastases from a variety of primary tumours.[170] Most authors agree that because of the high probability of recurrence there is no role, at present, for liver transplantation in the treatment of non-neuroendocrine hepatic metastases.

NOVEL THERAPIES

Treatments aimed at reversing the depression of host defences in the perioperative period may reduce the dissemination of disease that invariably occurs after hepatectomy and thereby improve the long-term results of surgery.

Interleukin 2 (IL-2) has been used as a neoadjuvant therapy in patients with resectable colorectal liver metastases.[171] In a recent randomised multicentre study comparing the combination of chemotherapy and IL-2 with chemotherapy alone, a higher response rate was observed in the combination group. However, interleukin has now been largely abandoned in the treatment of advanced colorectal cancer.[172]

Targeting of liver metastases with monoclonal antibodies recognising specific antigens within tumour cells has also been investigated.[173] The major difficulty associated with this technique is the poor specificity of the antibodies, which can be directed at cells within normal tissue. Studies have so far failed to produce encouraging results. Immunisation with vaccines is another approach to treatment.[174] In a phase II clinical trial, Schlag et al.[174] immunised 23 patients with autologous, irradiated, metastasis-derived tumour cells following resection of their colorectal liver metastases. After a follow-up of 18 months only 61% of the immunised group developed recurrence as compared with 87% in the group treated by resection alone.[174] Preclinical studies of autologous tumour vaccine expressing granulocyte/macrophage colony-stimulating factor (GM-CSF) have been encouraging,[175] but prospective randomised trials are required to further evaluate this form of treatment. New therapies that exploit the molecular mechanisms of cancer are currently under preclinical and clinical evaluation. Antiangiogenic agents such as TNP470 have been used in early clinical trials, and gene therapy approaches are being developed to increase the selectivity and efficacy of treatment.[176,177]

Key points

An increasing proportion of patients are suitable for potentially curative liver resection for hepatic metastases.

The long-term survival and morbidity and mortality associated with hepatic resection for colorectal metastases have improved considerably.

Improvements in chemotherapy regimens, new methods of physical tumour ablation and novel therapies are currently undergoing assessment with the aim of increasing patient survival without sacrificing their quality of life.

REFERENCES

1. Willis RA. The spread of tumours in the human body. London: Butterworths, 1973.

2. Bengtsson I, Carlsson G, Hafstrom L et al. Natural history of patients with untreated liver metastases from colorectal cancer. Am J Surg 1981; 141:586–9.

3. Foster JH, Lundy J. Liver metastases. Curr Probl Surg 1981; 18:158–204.

4. HMSO. Great Britain Office of Population Censuses and Surveys: Cancer Statistics. London: HMSO, 1998.

5. Blot WJ, Devesa SS, Fraumeni JF Jr. Continuing climb in rates of esophageal adenocarcinoma. An update. JAMA 1993; 270:1320.

6. Jatzko GR, Lisborg PH, Stettner HM et al. Hepatic resection for metastases from colorectal carcinoma – a survival analysis. Eur J Cancer 1995; 31A:41–6.

7. Gordon NLM, Dawson AA, Bennett B et al. Outcome in colorectal adenocarcinoma – two 7-year studies of a population. Br Med J 1993; 307:707–10.

8. Fisher ER, Turnbull RB. The cytological demonstration and significance of tumor cells in the mesenteric venous blood in patients with colorectal carcinoma. Surg Gynecol Obstet 1955; 100:102–8.

9. Fidler IJ. Metastasis: quantitative analysis of distribution and fate of tumor emboli labelled with

1,5-iodo-2-deoxyuridine. J Natl Cancer Inst 1970; 45:773–82.

10. Poste G, Fidler IJ. The pathogenesis of cancer metastasis. Nature 1980; 283:139–46.

11. Nigam AK, Pignatelli M, Boulos PB. Current concepts in metastasis. Gut 1994; 35:996–1000.

12. Pignatelli M, Liu D, Nasim MM et al. Morpho-regulatory activities of E-cadherin and beta-1 integrins in colorectal tumour cells. Br J Cancer 1992; 66:629–34.

13. Naito S, Giavazzi R, Fidler IJ. Correlation between the in vitro interaction of tumor cells with an organ environment and metastatic behavior in vivo. Invasion Metastasis 1987; 7:16–29.

14. Nicolson GL, Dulski KM. Organ specificity of metastatic tumour colonisation is related to organ-selective growth properties of malignant cells. Int J Cancer 1986; 38:289–94.

15. Jiang WG, Puntis MC, Hallett MB. Molecular and cellular basis of cancer invasion and metastasis: implications for treatment. Br J Surg 1994; 81:1576–90.

16. Barberaguillem E, Alonsovarona A, Vidalvanaclocha F. Selective implantation and growth in rats and mice of experimental liver metastasis in acinar zone one. Cancer Res 1989; 49:4003–10.

17. August DA, Sugarbaker PH, Schneider PD. Lymphatic dissemination of hepatic metastases – implications for the follow-up and treatment of patients with colorectal cancer. Cancer 1985; 55:1490–4.

18. Holbrook RF, Rodriguezbigas MA, Ramakrishnan K et al. Patterns of colorectal liver metastases according to Couinaud's segments. Dis Colon Rectum 1995; 38:245–8.

19. Cady B, Stone MD. The role of surgical resection of liver metastases in colorectal carcinoma. Semin Oncol 1991; 18:399–406.

20. Pickren JW, Tsukada Y, Lane WW. Liver metastasis: analysis of autopsy data. In: Weiss L, Gilbert HA (eds) Liver metastasis. Boston: GK Hall Medical Publishers, 1982; pp. 219–305.

21. Fisher B, Fisher ER. The interrelationship of hematogenous and lymphatic tumor cell dissemination. Surg Gynecol Obstet 1966; 122:791–8.

22. Dworkin MJ, Earlam S, Fordy C et al. Importance of hepatic artery node involvement in patients with colorectal liver metastases. Clin Pathol 1995; 48:270–2.

23. Sato T, Konishi K, Yabusgita K et al. The time interval between primary colorectal carcinoma resection to occurrence of liver metastases is the most important factor for hepatic resection. Analysis of total course following primary resection of colorectal cancer. Int Surg 1998; 83:340–2.

Useful study analysing the timing of hepatic recurrence of tumour following primary resection of colorectal cancer.

24. Balalakos EA, Burak WE, Young DC et al. Is carcinoembryonic antigen useful in the follow-up management of patients with colorectal liver metastases? Am J Surg 1999; 177:2–6.

25. Huguier M, Lacaine F. Hepatic metastases in gastrointestinal cancer – diagnostic value of biochemical investigations. Arch Surg 1981; 116:399–401.

26. Rafaelsen SR, Kronborg O, Larsen C et al. Intra-operative ultrasonography in detection of hepatic metastases from colorectal cancer. Dis Colon Rect 1995; 38:355–60.

27. Moran BJ, O'Rourke N, Plant GR et al. Computed tomographic portography in pre-operative imaging of hepatic neoplasms. Br J Surg 1995; 82:669–71.

28. Carter R, Hemingway D, Cooke TG et al. A prospective study of six methods for detection of colorectal liver metastases. Ann R Coll Surg Engl 1996; 78:27–30.

29. Delbeke D, Vitola JV, Sandler MP et al. Staging recurrent metastatic colorectal carcinoma with PET. J Nuclear Med 1997; 38:1196–201.

30. Valls C, Lopez E, Guma A et al. Helical CT versus CT arterial portography in the detection of hepatic metastases of colorectal carcinoma. Am J Roentgenol 1998; 170:1341–7.

31. Bunk A, Stoelben E, Konopke R et al. Clinical significance of the colour Doppler imaging in pre-operative investigation for surgery of the liver. Ultraschall Der Medizin 1998; 19:202–12.

32. Helmberger T, Gregor M, Holzknecht N et al. Comparison of dual-phase helical CT with native and ferumoxide enhanced magnetic resonance imaging in detection and characterisation of focal liver lesions. Radiology 1999; 39:678–84.

33. Sheu JC, Sung JL, Chen DS et al. Ultrasonography of small hepatic tumours using high resolution linear array real time instruments. Radiology 1984; 150:797–802.

34. Helmberger T, Rau H, Linke R et al. Hepatic metastases: diagnosis and staging. Chirurgie 1999; 70:678–84.

35. Tubiana JM, Deutsch JP, Taboury J et al. Imaging of hepatic colorectal metastases: diagnosis and resectability. In: Nordlinger B, Jaeck D (eds) Treatment of hepatic metastases of colorectal cancer. Paris: Springer-Verlag, 1992; pp. 55–69.

36. Yamaguchi A, Ishida T, Nishimura G et al. Detection by CT during arterial portography of colorectal cancer metastases to liver. Dis Colon Rectum 1991; 34:37–40.

37. Karl RC, Morse SS, Halpert RD et al. Preoperative evaluation of patients for liver resection – appropriate CT imaging. Ann Surg 1993; 217:226–32.

38. Soyer P, Lacheheb D, Levesque M. False positive CT portography – correlation with pathological findings. Am J Roentgenol 1993; 160:285–9.

   Three prospective studies demonstrating the accuracy of CTAP in assessing hepatic involvement by tumour.

39. Launois B, Landen S, Heautot JF. Colorectal metastatic liver tumours. In: Terblanche J (ed.) Hepatobiliary malignancy. Its multidisciplinary management. London: Edward Arnold, 1994; pp. 271–300.

40. Semelka RC, Cance WG, Marcos HB et al. Liver metastases: comparison of current MR techniques and spiral CT during arterial portography for detection in 20 surgically staged cases. Radiology 1999; 213:86–91.

41. Nakamoto Y, Higashi T, Sakahara H et al. Contribution of PET in the detection of liver metastases from pancreatic tumours. Clin Radiol 1999; 54:248–52.

42. Leveson SH, Wiggins PA, Giles GR et al. Deranged liver blood flow patterns in the detection of liver metastases. Br J Surg 1985; 72:128–30.

43. Leen E, Goldberg JA, Robertson J et al. Detection of hepatic metastases using duplex color doppler sonography. Ann Surg 1991; 214:599–604.

44. Leen E, Angerson WJ, Wotherspoon H et al. Detection of colorectal liver metastases – comparison of laparotomy, CT, US, and doppler perfusion index and evaluation of postoperative follow-up results. Radiology 1995; 195:113–16.

45. Leen E, Angerson WG, Cooke TG et al. Prognostic power of doppler perfusion index in colorectal cancer: correlation with survival. Ann Surg 1996; 223:199–203.

46. Bunk A, Stoelben E, Konopke R et al. Clinical significance of the colour Doppler imaging in pre-operative investigation for surgery of the liver. Ultraschall Der Medizin 1998; 19:202–12.

47. Shuman WP. Liver metastases from colorectal carcinoma – detection with doppler US-guided measurements of liver blood flow past, present, future. Radiology 1995; 195:9–10.

48. Finlay IG, McArdle CS. Occult hepatic metastases in colorectal carcinoma. Br J Surg 1986; 73:732–5.

49. Hagspiel KD, Neidl KFW, Eichenberger AC et al. Detection of liver metastases: comparison of super-paramagnetic iron oxide-enhanced and unenhanced MR imaging at 1.5 T with dynamic CT, intra-operative US, and percutaneous US. Radiology 1995; 196:471–8.

   Prospective study confirming that enhanced MR imaging and intraoperative US are highly sensitive and specific for detecting hepatic metastases.

50. Castaing D. The role of intraoperative ultrasound in the surgical treatment of hepatic metastases of colorectal origin. In: Nordlinger B, Jaeck D (eds) Treatment of hepatic metastases of colorectal cancer. Paris: Springer-Verlag, 1992; pp. 71–3.

51. Paul MA, Mulder LS, Cuesta MA et al. Impact of intraoperative ultrasonography on treatment strategy for colorectal cancer. Br J Surg 1994; 81:1660–3.

52. Soyer P, Elias D, Zeitoun G et al. Surgical treatment of hepatic metastases – impact of intraoperative sonography. Am J Roentgenol 1993; 160:511–14.

53. Foley EF, Kolecki RV, Schirmer BD. The accuracy of laparoscopic ultrasound in the detection of colo-rectal liver metastases. Am J Surg 1998; 176:262–4.

54. Wagner JS, Adson MA, Vanheerden JA et al. The natural history of hepatic metastases from colo-rectal cancer – a comparison with resective treatment. Ann Surg 1984; 199:502–8.

55. Gayowski TJ, Iwatsuki S, Madariaga SR et al. Experience in hepatic resection for metastatic colo-rectal cancer – analysis of clinical and pathological risk factors. Surgery 1994; 116:703–11.

56. Rougier P, Milan C, Lazorthes F et al. Prospective study of prognostic factors in patients with unresected hepatic metastases from colorectal cancer. Br J Surg 1995; 82:1397–400.

57. Adson MA, Vanheerden JA, Adson MH et al. Resection of hepatic metastases from colorectal cancer. Arch Surg 1984; 119:647–51.

58. Scheele J, Stangl R, Altendorfhofmann A. Hepatic metastases from colorectal carcinoma – impact of surgical resection on the natural history. Br J Surg 1990; 77:1241–6.

   Three studies that document poor survival prospects for untreated hepatic metastases and define particularly poor prognostic criteria. The latter study contrasts this out-come with the longer-term survival that can be achieved with hepatic resection in selected patients.

59. Finlay IG, Meek D, Brunton F et al. Growth rate of hepatic metastases in colorectal carcinoma. Br J Surg 1988; 75:641–4.

60. Woodington GF, Waugh JM. Results of resection of metastatic tumors of the liver. Am J Surg 1963; 105:24–9.

61. Flanagan L, Foster JH. Hepatic resection for metastatic cancer. Am J Surg 1967; 113:551–7.

62. Wilson SM, Adson MA. Surgical treatment of hepatic metastases from colorectal cancers. Arch Surg 1976; 111:330–4.

63. Steele G, Bleday R, Mayer RJ et al. A prospective evaluation of hepatic resection for colorectal carcinoma metastases to the liver – gastrointestinal tumor study group protocol-6484. J Clin Oncol 1991; 9:1105–12.

   Frequently cited studies highlighting survival advantages for patients undergoing hepatic resection for colorectal metastases.

64. Schwartz SI. Hepatic resection for noncolorectal nonneuroendocrine metastases. World J Surg 1995; 19:72–5.

65. Starzl TE, Iwatsuki S, Shaw BW et al. Left hepatic trisegmentectomy. Surg Gynecol Obstet 1982; 155:21–7.

66. Cunningham JD, Fong Y, Shriver C et al. 100 consecutive hepatic resections – blood loss, transfusion, and operative technique. Arch Surg 1994; 129:1050–6.

Prospective study evaluating important aspects of hepatic resection for colorectal metastases.

67. Hughes KS, Rosenstein RB, Songhorabodi S et al. Resection of the liver for colorectal carcinoma metastases – a multi-institutional study of long-term survivors. Dis Colon Rectum 1988; 31:1–4.

68. Doci R, Gennari L, Bignami P et al. Morbidity and mortality after hepatic resection of metastases from colorectal cancer. Br J Surg 1995; 82:377–81.

69. Elias D, Detroz B, Lasser P et al. Is simultaneous hepatectomy and intestinal anastomosis safe? Am J Surg 1995; 169:254–60.

70. Scheele J, Stang R, Altendorfhofmann A et al. Resection of colorectal liver metastases. World J Surg 1995; 19:59–71.

Large single-centre experience demonstrating improvement in perioperative mortality rates over time. The authors also argue that curative resection rather than number of metastases is an important determinant of outcome. High-grade primary colorectal tumours have a poorer survival after resection of hepatic metastases.

71. Nordlinger B, Jaeck D, Guiget M et al. Surgical resection of hepatic metastases: multicentric retrospective study by the French Association of Surgery. In: Nordlinger B, Jaeck D (eds) Treatment of hepatic metastases of colorectal cancer. Paris: Springer-Verlag, 1992; pp. 129–61.

72. Soyer P, Roche A, Elias D et al. Hepatic metastases from colorectal cancer: influence of hepatic volumetric analysis of surgical decision making. Radiology 1992; 184:695–7.

Prospective study indicating that the probability of postoperative hepatic failure depends on the volume and function of the residual liver.

73. Nordlinger B, Guiguet M, Vaillant J-C et al. Surgical resection of colorectal carcinoma metastases to the liver. A prognostic scoring system to improve case selection, based on 1568 patients. Cancer 1996; 77:1254–62.

Selection of patients for hepatic resection may be improved by taking into account patient age, size of metastasis, CEA level, stage of primary tumour, disease-free interval, number of hepatic nodules and resection margin.

74. Jamieson RL, Donohue JH, Nagorney DM et al. Hepatic resection for metastatic colorectal cancer results in cure for some patients. Arch Surg 1997; 132:505–10.

75. Taylor M, Forster J, Langer B et al. A study of prognostic factors for hepatic resection for colorectal metastases. Am J Surg 1997; 173:467–71.

76. Rees M, Plant G, Bygrave S. Late results justify resection for multiple hepatic metastases from colorectal cancer. Br J Surg 1997; 84:1136–40.

77. Bakalakos EA, Kim JA, Young DC et al. Determinants of survival following hepatic resection for metastatic colorectal cancer. World J Surg 1998; 22:399–405.

78. Elias D, Cavalcanti A, Sabourin JC et al. Results of 136 curative hepatectomies with a safety margin of less than 10 mm for colorectal metastases. J Surg Oncol 1998; 69:88–93.

79. Ambiru S, Miyazaki M, Isono T et al. Hepatic resection for colorectal metastases – analysis of prognostic factors. Dis Colon Rectum 1999; 42:632–9.

The presence of a fibrous pseudocapsule may be associated with a better outcome.

80. Yazaki M, Ito H, Nakagawa K et al. Aggressive surgical resection for hepatic metastases involving the inferior vena cava. Am J Surg 1999; 177:294–8.

81. Nagashima I, Oka T, Hamada C et al. Histopathological prognostic factors influencing long-term prognosis after surgical resection for hepatic metastases from colorectal cancer. Am J Gastroenterol 1999; 94:739–43.

82. Adson MA. Resection of liver metastases: when is it worthwhile? World J Surg 1987; 11:511–20.

83. Steele G, Ravikumar TS. Resection of hepatic metastases from colorectal cancer. Ann Surg 1989; 210:127–38.

84. Hughes KS, Scheele J, Sugarbaker PH. Surgery for colorectal cancer metastatic to the liver optimising the results of treatment. Surg Clin North Am 1989; 69:339–59.

85. Regnard JF, Grunenwald D, Spaggiari L et al. Surgical treatment of hepatic and pulmonary metastases from colorectal cancers. Ann Thoracic Surg 1998; 66:214–18.

86. Lehnert T, Knaebel M, Dück M et al. Sequential hepatic and pulmonary resections for metastatic colorectal cancer. Br J Surg 1999; 86:241–3.

87. Ekberg H, Tranberg KG, Andersson R et al. Determinants of survival in liver resection for colorectal secondaries. Br J Surg 1986; 73:727–31.

Substantial study advising against resection for four or more metastases.

88. Fortner JG, Silva JS, Golbey RB et al. Multivariate analysis of a personal series of 247 consecutive patients with liver metastases from colorectal cancer. Treatment by hepatic resection. Ann Surg 1984; 199:306–16.

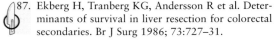

89. Doci R, Gennari L, Bignami P et al. 100 patients with hepatic metastases from colorectal cancer treated by resection – analysis of prognostic determinants. Br J Surg 1991; 78:797–801.

90. Hughes KS. Resection of the liver for colorectal carcinoma metastases – a multi-institutional study of indications for resection. Surgery 1988; 103:278–88.

91. Scheele J, Stangl R, Altendorfhofmann A et al. Indicators of prognosis after hepatic resection for colorectal secondaries. Surgery 1991; 110:13–29.

92. Irie T, Itai Y, Hatsuse K et al. Does resection of small liver metastases from colorectal cancer improve survival of patients? Br J Radiology 1999; 72:246–9.

93. van Ooijen B, Wiggers T, Meijer. Hepatic resections for colorectal metastases in the Netherlands – a multi-institutional 10-year study. Cancer 1992; 70:28–34.

Frequently cited references that have looked at a number of factors determining long-term survival following hepatic resection for colorectal metastases.

94. Lise M, Dapian PP, Nitti D et al. Colorectal metastases to the liver – present status of management. Dis Colon Rectum 1990; 33:688–94.

95. Kemeny N, Huang Y, Cohen A et al. Hepatic arterial infusion of chemotherapy after resection of hepatic metastases from colorectal cancer. N Engl J Med 1999; 341:2039–48.

96. Adam R, Bismuth H, Castaing D et al. Repeat hepatectomy for colorectal liver metastases. Ann Surg 1997; 225:51–60.

97. Bradpiece HA, Benjamin IS, Halevy A et al. Major hepatic resection for colorectal liver metastases. Br J Surg 1987; 74:324–6.

98. Kangmatsu Y, Kato T, Hirai T et al. Preoperative probability model for predicting survival after resection of pulmonary metastases from colorectal cancer. Brit J Surg 2004; 91:112–20.

99. Ekberg H, Tranberg KG, Andersson R et al. Pattern of recurrence in liver resection for colorectal secondaries. World J Surg 1987; 11:541–7.

100. Beckurts KT, Holscher AH, Thorban S et al. Significance of lymph node involvement at the hepatic hilum in the resection of colorectal liver metastases. Br J Surg 1997; 84:1081–4.

101. Rodgers MS, McCall JL. Surgery for colorectal liver metastases with hepatic lymph node involvement: a systematic review. Br J Surg 2000; 87:1142–55.

102. Franco D, Smadja C, Kahwaji F et al. Segmentectomies in the management of liver tumors. Arch Surg 1988; 123:519–22.

103. Iwatsuki S, Esquivel CO, Gordon RD et al. Liver resection for metastatic colorectal cancer. Surgery 1986; 100:804–10.

104. Fong Y, Blumgart LH, Fortner JG et al. Pancreatic or liver resection for malignancy is safe and effective for the elderly. Ann Surg 1995; 222:426–37.

105. Holm A, Bradley E, Aldrete JS. Hepatic resection of metastasis from colorectal carcinoma: morbidity, mortality, and pattern of recurrence. Ann Surg 1989; 209:428–34.

106. Stephenson KR, Steinberg SM, Hughes KS et al. Perioperative blood transfusions are associated with decreased time to recurrence and decreased survival after resection of colorectal liver metastases. Ann Surg 1988; 208:679–87.

Operative blood loss may be an adverse prognostic factor in terms of long-term survival.

107. Younes RN, Rogatko A, Brennan MF. The influence of intraoperative hypotension and perioperative blood transfusion on disease-free survival in patients with complete resection of colorectal liver metastases. Ann Surg 1991; 214:107–13.

108. Cady B, Stone MD, McDermott WV et al. Technical and biological factors in disease-free survival after hepatic resection for colorectal cancer metastases. Arch Surg 1992; 127:561–9.

109. Balalakos EA, Burak WE, Young DC et al. Is carcinoembryonic antigen useful in the follow-up management of patients with colorectal liver metastases? Am J Surg 1999; 177:2–6.

110. Fong Y, Cohen AM, Fortner JG et al. Liver resection for colorectal metastases. J Clin Oncol 1997; 15:938–46.

111. Bismuth H, Adam R, Levi F et al. Resection of initially unresectable liver metastases from colorectal cancer following systemic chemotherapy. Ann Surg 1996; 224:509–22.

112. Wanebo HJ, Chu QD, Avradopoulos KA et al. Current perspectives on repeat hepatic resection for colorectal carcinoma: A review. Surgery 1996; 119:361–71.

113. Chu QYD, Vezeridis MP, Avradopoulos KA et al. Repeat hepatic resection for recurrent colorectal cancer. World J Surg 1997; 21:292–6.

114. Kin T, Nakajima Y, Kanehiro H et al. Repeat hepatectomy for recurrent colorectal metastases. World J Surg 1998; 22:1087–91.

115. Yamamoto J, Kosuge T, Shimada K et al. Repeat liver resection for recurrent colorectal liver metastases. Am J Surg 1999; 178:275–81.

116. Elias D, Lasser PH, Montrucolli D et al. Hepatectomy for liver metastases from breast cancer. Eur J Surg Oncol 1995; 21:510–13.

117. Jaques DP, Coit DG, Casper ES et al. Hepatic metastases from soft tissue sarcoma. Ann Surg 1995; 221:392–7.

Five-year survival following hepatic resection for metastases from primary sarcoma is rare.

118. Ochiai T, Sasako M, Mizuno S et al. Hepatic resection for metastatic tumours from gastric cancer – analysis of prognostic factors. Br J Surg 1994; 81:1175–8.

119. Barney T, Mentha G, Roth AD et al. Results of surgical resection of liver metastases from non-colorectal primaries. Br J Surg 1998; 85:1423–7.

120. Lindell G, Ohlsson B, Saarela A et al. Liver resection of non-colorectal secondaries. J Surg Oncol 1998; 69:66–70.

Long-term survival may be possible following hepatic resection for metastatic neuroendocrine tumour.

121. Scheithauer W, Rosen H, Kornek G-V et al. Randomised comparison of combination chemotherapy plus supportive care with supportive care alone in patients with metastatic colorectal cancer. Br Med J 1993; 306:2–5.

Randomized controlled trial demonstrating improved duration of survival with combination chemotherapy.

122. Rougier P, Lasser L, Elias D. Chemotherapy of hepatic metastases of colorectal origin (systemic and local, in palliative or adjuvant treatment). In: Nordlinger B, Jaeck D (eds) Treatment of hepatic metastases of colorectal cancer. Paris: Springer-Verlag, 1992; p. 1092.

123. Kerr D, de Takats PG. Chemotherapy for gastrointestinal cancer: teaching old drugs new tricks. Cancer 1995; 1:3–7.

124. Cunningham D, Zalcberg JR, Rath U et al. 'Tomudex' (ZD1694): results of a randomised trial in advanced colorectal cancer demonstrate efficacy and reduced mucositis and leucopenia. The 'Tomudex' Colorectal Cancer Study Group. Eur I Cancer 1995; 31A:1945–54.

Tomudex has a similar efficacy to 5-FU in the treatment of advanced colorectal carcinoma.

125. Rougier P, Van-Cutsen E, Bajetta E et al. Randomised trial of irinotecan versus fluorouracil by continuous infusion after fluorouracil failure in patients with metastatic colorectal cancer. Lancet 1998; 352:1407–12.

The new topoisomerase I inhibitor, irinotecan, improved 1-year survival in advanced colorectal carcinoma.

126. Ridge JA, Bading IR, Gelbard AS et al. Perfusion of colorectal hepatic metastases – relative distribution of flow from the hepatic artery and portal vein. Cancer 1987; 59:47–53.

127. Rougier P, Laplanche A, Huguier M et al. Hepatic arterial infusion of floxuridine in patients with liver metastases from colorectal carcinoma: long-term results of a prospective randomised trial. Clin Oncol 1992; 10:1112–18.

Randomized control trial demonstrating a marginal 1-year survival benefit for irresectable hepatic metastases.

128. Allen-Mersh TG, Earlam S, Fordy C et al. Quality of life and survival with continuous hepatic artery floxuridine infusion for colorectal liver metastases. Lancet 1994; 344:1255–60.

129. Wagman LD, Kemeny MM, Leong L et al. A prospective, randomised evaluation of the treatment of colorectal cancer metastatic to the liver. J Clin Oncol 1990; 8:1885–93.

The addition of systemic chemotherapy to selective hepatic arterial infusion chemotherapy resulted in a marginal survival benefit.

130. Kemeny NE. Regional chemotherapy of colorectal cancer. Eur J Cancer 1995; 31A:2039–48.

131. Dasappa V, Ross WB, King DW et al. Primary resection and synchronous regional hepatic cryotherapy or cryotherapy for colorectal cancer with liver metastases. Int J Colorectal Dis 1996; 11:38–41.

132. Ambiru S, Miyazaki M, Ito H et al. Adjuvant regional chemotherapy after hepatic resection for colorectal liver metastases. Br J Surg 1999; 86:1025–31.

133. Khayat D, Gil-Delgado M, Antoine EC et al. The role of irinotecan and oxaliplatin in the treatment of advanced colorectal cancer. Oncology (Huntington) 2001; 15:415–29.

134. Rudroff C, Altendorfmann A, Stangl R et al. Prospective randomised trial on adjuvant hepatic artery infusion chemotherapy after R0 resection of colorectal liver metastases. Langenbecks Arch Surg 1999; 384:243–9.

135. Lorenz M, Muller HH, Schramm H et al. Randomised trial of surgery versus surgery followed by adjuvant hepatic arterial infusion with 5-fluorouracil and folinic acid for liver metastases of colorectal cancer. German Cooperative on liver metastases. Ann Surg 1998; 228:756–62.

Two randomized controlled trials demonstrating no difference in long-term survival with hepatic arterial chemotherapy.

136. Adam R, Avisar E, Ariche A et al. Five year survival following hepatic resection after neoadjuvant therapy for non-resectable colorectal liver metastases. Ann Surg Oncol 2001; 8: 347–353.

137. Alberts SR, Horvath W, Donohue JH et al. Oxaliplatin, f-FU and leucovorin for patients with liver only metastases from colorectal cancer: a North Central Cancer Treatment Group phase II study. Proc Am Soc Clin Oncol 2001: 20:129a (abstract 511).

138. Giacchetti S, Itzhaki M, Gruia G et al. Long-term survival of patients with unresectable colorectal cancer liver metastases following infusional chemotherapy with 5-fluorouracil, leucovorin, oxaliplatin and surgery. Ann Oncol 1999; 10:663–9.

139. Tournigand C, Louvet C, Quinaux E et al. FOLFIRI followed by FOLFOX versus FOLFOX followed by

FOLFIRI in metastatic colorectal cancer: final results of a phase III study. Proc Am Soc Clin Oncol 2001; 20:124a (abstract 494).

140. Lorenz M, Staib-Sebler E, Koch B et al. The value of post-operative arterial infusion following curative liver resection. Anticancer Res 1997; 17(5B):3825–33

141. Ravikumar TS, Kane R, Cady B et al. A 5-year study of cryosurgery in the treatment of liver tumors. Arch Surg 1991; 126:1520–4.

142. Weaver MI, Atkinson D, Zemel R. Hepatic cryosurgery in treating colorectal metastases. Cancer 1995; 76:210–14.

143. Preketes AP, King J, Caplehorn JRM et al. CEA reduction after cryotherapy for liver metastases from colon cancer predicts survival. Aust NZ J Surg 1994; 64:612–14.

144. Morris DL, Horton MD, Dilley AV et al. Treatment of hepatic metastases by cryotherapy and regional cytotoxic perfusion. Gut 1993; 34:1156–7.

145. Polk W, Fong YM, Karpeh M et al. A technique for the use of cryosurgery to assist hepatic resection. J Am Coll Surg 1995; 180:171–6.

146. Seifert JK, Junginger T, Morris DL. A collective review of the world literature on hepatic cryotherapy. J R Coll Edin 1998; 141–54.

147. Weaver ML, Ashton JG, Zemel R. Treatment of colorectal liver metastases by cryotherapy. Semin Surg Oncol 1998; 14:163–70.

148. Hewitt PM, Dwerryhouse SJ, Zhao J et al. Multiple bilobar liver metastases: cryotherapy for residual lesions after liver resection. J Surg Oncol 1998; 67:112–6.

149. Seifert JK, Morris DL. Prognostic factors after cryotherapy for hepatic metastases from colorectal cancer. Ann Surg 1998; 228:201–8.

150. Sheen AJ, Poston GJ, Sherlock DJ. Cryotherapeutic ablation of liver tumours. Brit J Surg 2002; 89:1396–1401.

151. Seifert JK, Morris DL. Indicators of recurrence following cryotherapy for hepatic metastases from colorectal cancer. Br J Surg 1999; 86:234–40.

152. Iannitti DA, Heniford T, Hale J et al. Laparoscopic cryoablation of hepatic metastases. Arch Surg 1998; 133:1011–15.

153. Amin Z, Bown SG, Lees WR. Local treatment of colorectal liver metastases – a comparison of interstitial laser photocoagulation and percutaneous alcohol injection. Clin Radiol 1993; 48:166–71.

154. Armstrong JG, Anderson LL, Harrison L. Treatment of liver metastases from colorectal cancer with radioactive implants. Cancer 1994; 73:1800–4.

155. Burton MA, Gray BN. Adjuvant internal radiation therapy in a model of colorectal cancer-derived hepatic metastases. Br J Cancer 1995; 71:322–5.

156. Vogl TJ, Mack MG, Muller PK et al. Interventional MR: interstitial therapy. Eur Radiol 1999; 9:1479–87.

157. Solbiati L, Ierace T, Goldberg SN et al. Percutaneous US-guided radio-frequency tissue ablation of liver metastases: treatment and follow-up in 16 patients. Radiology 1997; 202:195–203.

158. Solbiati I, Goldberg SN, Ierrace T et al. Hepatic metastases: percutaneous radiofrequency ablation with cooled tip electrodes. Radiology 1997; 205:367–73.

159. Bilchik AJ, Wood TF, Allegra D et al. Cryosurgical ablation and radiofrequency ablation for unresectable hepatic malignant neoplasms: a proposed algorithm. Arch Surg 2000; 135:657–64.

160. Elias D, Goharin A, Otmany A et al. Usefulness of intraoperative radiofrequency thermoablation of liver tumours associated or not with hepatectomy. Eur J Surg Oncol 2000; 26:762–9.

161. Curley SA, Izzo F, Delrio P et al. Radiofrequency ablation of unresectable primary and metastatic hepatic malignancies. Ann Surg 1999; 230:1–8.

162. Wood TF, Rose DM, Chung M et al. Radiofrequency ablation of 231 unresectable hepatic tumors: indications, limitations and complications. Ann Surg Oncol 2000; 7:593–600.

163. Jiao LR, Hansen PD, Havlik R et al. Clinical short-term results of radiofrequency ablation in primary and secondary liver tumors. Am J Surg 1999; 177:303–6.

164. Pearson AS, Izzo F, Fleming RY et al. Intraoperative radiofrequency ablation or cryoablation for hepatic malignancies. Am J Surg 1999; 178: 592–9.

165. Siperstein A, Garland A, Engle K et al. Local recurrence after laparoscopic radiofrequency thermal ablation of hepatic tumors. Ann Surg Oncol 2000; 7:106–13.

166. Goldberg SN, Gazelle GS, Compton CC et al. Treatment of intrahepatic malignancy with radiofrequency thermal ablation: radiologic-pathologic correlation. Cancer 2000; 88:2452–63.

167. Kainuma O, Asano T, Aoyama H et al. Combined therapy with radiofrequency thermal ablation and intra-arterial infusion chemotherapy for hepatic metastases from colorectal cancer. Hepatogastroenterology 1999; 46:1071–77.

168. Pichlmayr R, Weimann A, Oldhafer K et al. Role of liver transplantation in the treatment of unresectable liver cancer. World J Surg 1995; 19:807–13.

169. Lehnert T. Liver transplantation for metastatic neuroendocrine carcinoma. An analysis of 103 patients. Transplantation 1998; 66:1307–12.

170. Penn I. Hepatic transplantation for primary and metastatic cancers of the liver. Surgery 1991; 110:726–35.

171. Elias D, Farace F, Triebel F et al. Phase I–II randomised study on prehepatectomy recombinant interleukin-2 immunotherapy in patients with metastatic carcinoma of the colon and rectum. J Am Coll Surg 1995; 2:1303–10.

172. Okuno K, Yasutomi M, Kon M et al. Intrahepatic interleukin-2 with chemotherapy for unresectable liver metastases: a randomised multicentre trial. Hepatogastroenterology 1999; 46:1116–21.

Trials demonstrating a better response to treating resectable colorectal liver metastases with a combination of chemotherapy and IL-2.

173. Welt S, Divgi CR, Scott AM et al. Antibody targeting in metastatic colon cancer: A phase I study of monoclonal antibody F19 against a cell-surface protein of reactive tumour stromal fibroblasts. J Clin Oncol 1994; 12:1193–1203.

174. Schlag P, Manasterski M, Gerneth T et al. Active specific immunotherapy with Newcastle-disease-virus-modified autologous tumour cells following resection of liver metastases in colorectal cancer – 1st evaluation of clinical response of a phase II trial. Cancer Immunol Immunother 1992; 35:325–30.

175. Suh KW, Plantodosi S, Yazdi HA et al. Treatment of liver metastases from colon carcinoma with autologous tumour vaccine expressing granulocyte-macrophage colony stimulating factor. J Surg Oncol 1999; 72:218–24.

176. Humphreys M, Ghaneh P, Greenhalf W et al. Regional delivery of a retroviral vector expressing the E. coli cytosine deaminase gene and systemic treatment with 5-fluorocytosine suppresses growth of colorectal liver metastases in a model system. Br J Cancer 1999; 80:24.

177. Kooby PA, Carew JF, Haltermann MW et al. Oncolytic viral therapy for human colorectal cancer and liver metastases using a multi-mutated herpes simplex virus type-1 (G207). FASEB J 1999; 13:1325–34.

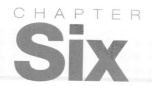

CHAPTER

Six

Portal hypertension

John A.C. Buckels, Geoffrey H. Haydon and
Simon P. Olliff

INTRODUCTION

The management of portal hypertension, once the
remit of surgeons, has evolved into a true multidisciplinary discipline. The majority of patients are
now managed successfully by medical and radio-
ogical treatments, although surgery still has a
distinct role for selected patients. These are chiefly
those with extrahepatic portal hypertension and
those suitable for liver transplantation, which can
cure both the complications and the underlying liver
disease. Portal hypertension itself does not require
treatment, but intervention is indicated when the
risk of bleeding from varices is present or when
complications, such as actual variceal haemorrhage
or the formation of ascites, occur. The management
of many patients commences with a herald variceal
bleed, which requires effective therapy before a plan
can be made for longer-term treatment. A significant choice of options is now available, many of
which are evidence-based. These include:

- pharmacotherapy to both prevent and treat
  variceal bleeding
- endoscopic options of injection therapy or
  variceal ligation
- radiologically placed transjugular intrahepatic
  porto-systemic shunts (TIPS)
- surgical options, which can be used to
  obliterate varices (devascularisation procedures)

or reduce portal pressure (surgical shunts and
liver replacement).

The selection of these options needs to be tailored
to the individual patient, taking into account the
general fitness of the patient, including severity of
any underlying liver disease, and the local medical
facilities and expertise available.

This chapter will outline briefly the causes, pathophysiology and natural history of portal hypertension, but will concentrate on the evaluation and
the management of both asymptomatic and acutely
bleeding patients with variceal bleeds together
with longer-term strategies. In addition, specific
recommendations will be made for the management
of ascites and for patients with hepatic venous outflow obstruction due to Budd–Chiari syndrome.

AETIOLOGY AND
PATHOPHYSIOLOGY OF
PORTAL HYPERTENSION

Traditionally, portal hypertension has been classified
as prehepatic, intrahepatic or posthepatic, with the
intrahepatic causes subdivided into presinusoidal,
sinusoidal or postsinusoidal (**Box 6.1**). Prehepatic
causes are usually due to portal vein thrombosis,
which is discussed later in this chapter. The main
cause of portal hypertension in the West is cirrhosis.

Box 6.1 • Causes of portal hypertension

PRESINUSOIDAL

Extrahepatic

Portal vein thrombosis

Splenic vein thrombosis

Increased splenic vein flow (tropical splenomegaly, myelofibrosis)

Intrahepatic

Schistosomiasis

Congential hepatic fibrosis

Sarcoidosis

SINUSOIDAL

Cirrhotic

Postviral (B,C,)

Alcoholic

Cryptogenic

Primary biliary cirrhosis

Primary sclerosing cholangitis

Chronic active hepatitis

Haemochromatosis

Wilson's disease

Non-cirrhotic

Acute alcoholic hepatitis

Cytotoxic drugs

POSTSINUSOIDAL

Budd–Chiari syndrome

Veno-occlusive disease

Caval web

Constrictive pericarditis

This is a sinusoidal obstruction to portal flow with varying causes. Viral hepatitis and alcoholic liver disease are the most common causes but others include primary biliary cirrhosis, primary sclerosing cholangitis, and haemochromatosis. Presinusoidal obstruction due to hepatic fibrosis occurs in schistosomiasis. Worldwide this is one of the commonest causes of portal hypertension, and as it is usually associated with normal liver function has a better prognosis. The main causes of postsinusoidal portal hypertension are hepatic venous thrombosis (Budd–Chiari syndrome) and veno-occlusive disease.

Experimental studies have demonstrated that the initial factor in the pathophysiology of portal hypertension is the increase in vascular resistance to portal blood flow. In cirrhosis, this increase in resistance occurs in the hepatic microcirculation (sinusoidal portal hypertension) and is a consequence of both a 'passive' and an 'active' component. The 'passive' component is the mechanical consequence of the hepatic architectural disorder resulting from histological cirrhosis and the 'active' component, the active contraction of portal/septal myofibroblasts, activated stellate cells and portal venules.[1-3] The increase in intrahepatic tone is probably a consequence of an imbalance between an increase in the endogenous vasoconstrictor substances such as endothelin, noradrenaline (norepinephrine), leukotrienes and angiotensin II, and a relative decrease in the endogenous vasodilator nitric oxide.[3-6] Vasodilatory drugs (e.g. calcium channel blockers) may restore the equilibrium in intrahepatic tone, although these are not used for this indication in clinical practice.

The other major pathophysiological factor contributing to portal hypertension is an increase in portal venous blood flow through the portal circulation resulting from splanchnic arteriolar vasodilatation caused by an excessive release of endogenous arteriolar vasodilators (endothelial, neural and humoral).[7-11] This can be corrected by means of splanchnic vasoconstrictors such as terlipressin and non-selective beta-blockers. Clearly, there is a crossover in the actions of many drugs that lower portal pressure; many of these drugs both reduce intrahepatic vascular resistance and decrease portal venous inflow.

An important but rare form, segmental or left upper quadrant portal hypertension, occurs in patients with splenic vein thrombosis. This should be suspected in patients with bleeding varices but normal liver function, particularly if there is a history of either acute or chronic pancreatitis.

NATURAL HISTORY OF PORTAL HYPERTENSION

The prevalence of oesophageal varices in patients with cirrhosis and portal hypertension is high.

When cirrhosis is diagnosed, varices are present in 40% of compensated and 60% of decompensated cirrhotics.[12] After the initial diagnosis of cirrhosis, varices develop with an incidence of 5% per year; subsequently, they may progress from small to large at an incidence of 10–15% per year.[13] Rapid progression of hepatic decompensation is associated with a rapid increase in size, whilst improvement in liver function, particularly when associated with removal of the injurious agent (e.g. abstinence from alcohol) may result in decrease in size or disappearance of the varices.[14,15]

The overall incidence of variceal bleeding following diagnosis is in the order of 25% in unselected patients.[16] The most important predictive factors of variceal bleeding are severity of liver dysfunction; size of varices; and intravariceal wall pressure (which although difficult to measure may correlate at endoscopy with the presence of red spots or red weals).[16,17] Traditionally liver dysfunction has been classified using the Child–Pugh score[18] (**Table 6.1**), but a more recent scoring system, the MELD (Model for End-stage Liver Disease) may be a better prognostic indicator.[19] Variceal size may be the best single predictor of variceal bleeding, and generally it is used to decide whether a patient should be given prophylactic therapy or not. Whether a patient dies from a variceal bleed depends on the severity of the accompanying liver failure; those with a high Child–Pugh or MELD score have been reported to have a risk of mortality as high as 30–50% within 6 weeks of the index bleed.[20] However, a more accurate figure may be a mortality of 20% at 6 weeks; immediate mortality from uncontrolled bleeding is as low as 5–8%. Indeed, in 40–50% of patients who bleed and develop hypotension, variceal bleeding stops spontaneously, probably as a result of reflex splanchnic vasoconstriction with associated reduction in portal pressure and blood flow; this beneficial response is nullified by overtransfusing the patient.[21]

The incidence of re-bleeding ranges between 30 and 40% within the first 6 weeks; this risk peaks in the first 5 days following the index bleed. Bleeding gastric varices, active bleeding at emergency endoscopy, low serum albumin levels, renal failure and a hepatic venous pressure gradient >20 mmHg have all been reported as significant indicators of an early risk of re-bleeding.[22–24] Patients surviving a first episode of variceal bleeding have a very high risk of re-bleeding (63%) and death (33%), and this is the basis for treating all patients to prevent further bleeding.[20]

PRESENTATION

Portal hypertension may present acutely with variceal bleeding or be discovered during the investigation of a patient with liver disease. Varices are usually diagnosed easily at endoscopy and patients will then be investigated systematically. A classification of the grading of varices is given in **Box 6.2**. Presentation in patients with liver disease is variable and ranges from non-specific tiredness to advanced encephalopthy with decompensation. External features of advanced liver disease such as spider naevi, palmar erythema and ascites are easy to detect, although these signs will be lacking in many patients. Splenomegaly is probably the most useful physical sign, though some patients will have the classic sign of dilated umbilical vein collaterals (caput medusae).

IMAGING

Doppler ultrasonography is a useful and easily obtained initial imaging modality for patients with suspected portal hypertension. Not only can portal and hepatic vein patency and direction of flow be obtained, but also the state of the liver parenchyma,

Table 6.1 • Child–Pugh classification: grade A, 5–6 points; grade B, 7–9 points; grade C, 10–15 points

	Number of points		
	1	2	3
Bilirubin (µmol/L)*	<34	34–51	>51
Albumin (g/L)	>35	28–35	<28
Prothrombin time prolonged by (s)	<3	3–10	>10
Ascites	None	Slight to moderate	Moderate to severe
Encephalopathy	None	Slight to moderate	Moderate to severe

*In primary biliary cirrhosis, the point scoring for bilirubin level is adjusted as follows: 1 = <68, 2 = 68–170, 3 = >170.

Box 6.2 • Classification of oesophageal and gastric varices

Oesophageal varices

Grade 0 (or absent)

Grade 1 (or small): Varices that collapse on insufflation of oesophagus with air.

Grade 2 (or medium): Varices that do not collapse on air insufflation.

Grade 3 (or large): Varices that are large enough to occlude the lumen.

Gastric varices

GOV 1: Gastro-oesophageal varices extending <5 cm from the oesophagus across the gastro-oesophageal junction.

GOV 2: Gastro-oesophageal varices extending into the fundus across the gastro-oesophageal junction.

IGV 1: Isolated gastric varices in the fundus.

IGV 2: Isolated non-fundic varices.

---

splenic size, and presence or absence of varices can usually be determined. Developments in computed tomography (CT) and magnetic resonance imaging (MRI) now allow detailed roadmaps of vascular anatomy to be obtained prior to any surgical intervention without the need for invasive angiography in most cases.

MANAGEMENT OF VARICES

The management of oesophageal varices will be considered in three sections: the prevention of bleeding in patients with varices that have never bled; the longer-term management of patients who have bled to prevent future bleeding episodes; and the emergency resuscitation and initial control of the acute bleeding episode. Though the emergency management of many patients will be in a district general hospital, patients may require referral to specialised centres with expertise in liver diseases and where recourse to specialised radiological intervention is available.

Because pharmacological therapy is employed in the majority of cases, the treatment aims of this require consideration. The hepatic venous pressure gradient (HVPG) reflects accurately portal pressure in sinusoidal portal hypertension and is measured readily. Varices do not develop until the HVPG increases to 10–12 mmHg, and the HVPG must be greater than 12 mmHg for the appearance of complications such as variceal bleeding and ascites.[25] Longitudinal studies of patients with complications of portal hypertension have demonstrated that when an HVPG decreases to less than 12 mmHg with pharmacological therapy, TIPS, or an improvement in liver function, variceal bleeding is prevented and varices may decrease in size or disappear altogether.[26] When this target is not reached, a substantial reduction in portal pressure by more than 20% still offers protection against variceal bleeding,[27] and thus these two parameters are regarded as the endpoints of therapeutic strategies to lower portal pressure. Recent evidence also suggests that these therapeutic endpoints may also reduce the risk of other complications of portal hypertension, including ascites; spontaneous bacterial peritonitis and hepatorenal syndrome.[27,28]

Oesophageal varices

PRIMARY PROPHYLAXIS FOR THE PREVENTION OF VARICEAL HAEMORRHAGE

All patients with cirrhosis should be screened for varices at the time of the first diagnosis of their cirrhosis. In patients with grade I varices at index endoscopy, a follow-up endoscopy should be performed after 12 months to detect the progression from grade II to III varices. Patients without varices should be re-evaluated in 2–3 years after their index endoscopy.

The mainstay of primary prophylactic therapy in the prevention of variceal haemorrhage is the non-selective beta-adrenergic receptor blocker (beta-blocker). Twelve trials using beta-blockers in this context have been reported. A meta-analysis has indicated that indefinite treatment with propranolol or nadolol reduces significantly the bleeding risk from 25% with non-active treatment or placebo to 15% with beta-blockers over a median follow-up period of 24 months; there was no significant reduction in mortality.[13] The benefit of therapy was only proven in those patients with grade II (or larger) varices; there was no evidence to support the use of primary prophylactic therapy in patients with grade I varices. Withdrawal of therapy was associated with a return to the same bleeding risk (25%) as the untreated subpopulation; indeed, there may be an increased risk of mortality over untreated patients in those individuals who stop therapy.[29,30]

Assessment of the success of primary prophylactic therapy is ideally undertaken by measurement of the HVPG before and after initiating therapy, with the aim being to reduce the HVPG to below 12 mmHg or to reduce it by >20% from its baseline value.[26] In practice, however, measurement of HVPG does require specific training and is probably not cost-effective for assessing primary prophylactic therapy. Thus, the clinician faces the question of how to adjust the dose of beta-blocker to maximise its beneficial effects. Traditional practice has recommended a stepwise increase in dose until the heart rate decreases by 25% or is <55 beats per minute or there is arterial hypotension or clinical intolerance. This means that the dose of the beta-blocker is titrated against its β_1 effects (cardiac) and clinical tolerance; however, a fall in portal pressure results from blockade of both β_1 and β_2 receptors, and the fall in portal pressure does not readily correlate with the fall in heart rate or blood pressure. Therefore, titration solely against clinical tolerance may be the most useful surrogate marker of the maximal dose of beta-blocker in the absence of HVPG measurement.

There appears to be no advantage of one non-selective beta-blocker over another. However, the newest approach to increase response to beta-blockers has been the use of carvedilol, a drug that combines a non-selective beta-blocker action with an α_1-adrenoceptor blocker action. This causes a marked decrease in portal pressure, but has the side effect of systemic hypotension. When compared with propranolol, carvedilol significantly increased the number of patients achieving a target reduction of HVPG (<12 mmHg or >20% reduction from baseline HVPG).[31] There is considerable controversy about how to give the carvedilol because of its hypotensive side effects; however, recent studies have demonstrated that lower doses (12.5 mg/day) or careful titration result in good tolerance.[31,32]

In patients who are unable to tolerate beta-blockers (15–20%) because of side effects or relative/absolute contraindications, treatment with nitrates is ineffective despite its portal pressure-lowering properties.[33] Therefore, variceal band ligation (VBL) therapy is the only option for patients with high-risk varices (grade II or above) and contraindications to beta-blockers. More controversially, a recent meta-analysis suggested that VBL is a more effective mode of treatment than beta-blockers for primary prophylaxis.[34] However, of the four trials included in this analysis, only two have been published in full; therefore, it seems reasonable to recommend that for the time being, beta-blockers remain the primary prophylactic therapy of choice in terms of cost and convenience. Of course, VBL does not reduce portal pressure (and therefore measurement of HVPG following endoscopic monotherapy is of no value) and this may leave the patient at risk of developing other complications of portal hypertension. An algorithm for the primary prevention of variceal bleeding is given in **Fig. 6.1**.

 Patients who have not bled from grade II varices or worse should receive beta-blocker therapy unless there are medical contraindications.

PREVENTION OF RE-BLEEDING FROM OESOPHAGEAL VARICES

Following a variceal bleed, patients with cirrhosis should be assessed in two ways; firstly, they should receive urgent and active treatment for the prevention of re-bleeding, and secondly, they should be examined for signs of physiological stress following their bleed, which might indicate a need for an elective liver transplant assessment (**Fig. 6.2**). Management of non-cirrhotic patients is discussed later in this chapter.

Endoscopic variceal band ligation (VBL) therapy or beta-blocker therapy are the treatments of choice for the prevention of re-bleeding from oesophageal varices. Meta-analyses of studies using β-blocker therapy to prevent re-bleeding have demonstrated both a significantly decreased mortality (27% in controls to 20% in beta-blocker-treated individuals) and a decreased incidence of re-bleeding (63% to 42%).[13] VBL also both improves survival and significantly decreases re-bleeding rates; it is superior to endoscopic sclerotherapy since it is associated with significantly fewer complications.[35,36] Currently, it is unclear whether pharmacological therapy is

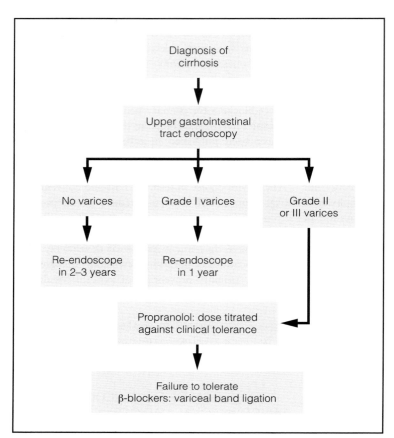

Figure 6.1 • Algorithm for primary prevention of variceal bleeding.

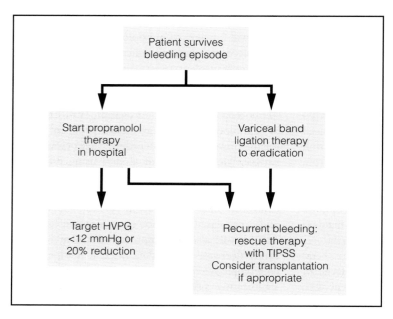

Figure 6.2 • Algorithm for secondary prevention of variceal bleeding.

better than VBL or vice versa; studies have demonstrated a variety of outcomes with reference to re-bleeding rates, but none has indicated any clear difference in survival.[27,37,38] A combination of pharmacological therapy and endoscopic therapy is commonly used, but evidence suggesting a better outcome with this combination compared with monotherapy is hard to find. Likewise, combination therapy of nitrates and beta-blockers has not been consistently shown to be more effective than beta-blockers alone or VBL.[27,39]

Re-bleeding is still common with pharmacological or endoscopic therapy (30–50% at 2 years), and in these cases, second-line therapies should be offered. This will depend on the underlying aetiology, and fitness and age of the patient, and may be TIPS, shunt surgery or liver transplantation.

There is strong evidence that beta-blocker therapy results in a decrease in incidence of re-bleeding and a significantly decreased mortality.

TREATMENT FOR BLEEDING OESOPHAGEAL VARICES

Variceal bleeding is a medical emergency and the first priority is to achieve adequate resuscitation of the patient in a safe environment, preferably a high-dependency or intensive care unit. On presentation, airway protection is essential, especially for intoxicated patients or those withdrawing from alcohol. Subsequent therapy is aimed at correcting hypovolaemic shock; blood volume replacement should maintain the haematocrit between 25 and 30% and preferably a pulmonary artery capillary wedge pressure of 10–15 mmHg. Overtransfusion should be avoided because of the risk of a rebound increase in portal pressure with continued bleeding or re-bleeding.[40] Antibiotics should be instituted from admission, since these increase the survival of bleeding patients; norfloxacin 400 mg/12 h or ciprofloxacin 250 mg/12 h are the antibiotics of choice.[41,42] Finally, early therapy should also involve starting a vasoactive drug from admission (usually terlipressin or octreotide); a number of randomised, controlled trials have demonstrated that early administration of vasoactive drugs facilitates endoscopy, improves control of bleeding, and reduces 5-day re-bleeding rate.[43–45] Initiation of these measures in association with endoscopic therapy

at the time of diagnostic endoscopy will control bleeding in about 75% of patients. However, as in most trials, in acute variceal bleeding, this combined approach failed to improve overall mortality compared with drug or endoscopic therapy alone. The optimal duration of vasoactive drug therapy is not well established and requires evaluation; current recommendations are to continue the drug for 5 days, since this covers the period of maximum risk of re-bleeding.

Endoscopic therapy should be performed at the time of diagnostic endoscopy, within 12 hours of admission in a resuscitated patient. However, if the patient is stable, endoscopic therapy can probably be postponed until normal working hours. There are multiple randomised controlled trials examining modes of endoscopic therapy in acute variceal bleeding. These have compared:

- endoscopic therapy with no therapy
- endoscopic therapy with vasoactive drug therapy
- endoscopic sclerotherapy with variceal band ligation therapy
- combined endoscopic therapy with variceal band ligation therapy
- endoscopic therapy with TIPS.

Endoscopic therapy is certainly superior to no therapy;[46] of the two endoscopic therapies, variceal band ligation therapy should be considered the treatment of choice since it is associated with significantly fewer complications (oesophageal stricturing or oesophageal ulcer formation) and significantly fewer sessions of therapy to eradicate the varices. However, there is probably no difference in re-bleeding or mortality rates between the two therapies. Likewise, there is little evidence to support combined endoscopic therapy for the treatment of bleeding varices,[47] although, in practice, it is sometimes beneficial for the endoscopist to use a small volume of sclerosant initially to improve vision in order to place some variceal bands to achieve eventual haemostasis. If endoscopic therapy fails to control bleeding, balloon tamponade should be used as a 'bridge' until definitive therapy can be offered. In practice, this usually means a further attempt at endoscopic band ligation therapy followed by second-line therapies. An algorithm for the management of variceal bleeding in cirrhotics is given in **Fig. 6.3**.

138

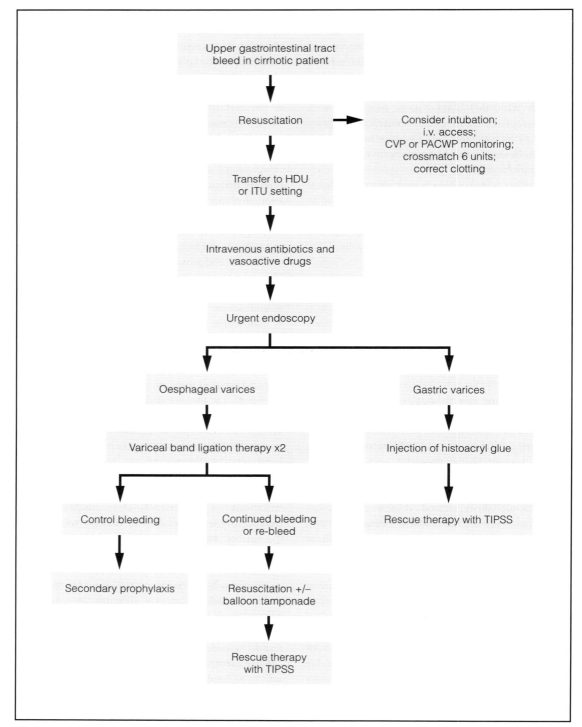

Figure 6.3 • Algorithm for the management of variceal bleeding.

The intravenous administration of antibiotics has been shown to increase survival in patients undergoing treatment for bleeding oesophageal varices.

Endoscopic band ligation is the initial treatment of choice for patients with bleeding oesophageal varices.

Gastric varices

Gastric varices are caused most commonly by cirrhosis complicated by portal hypertension and are the source of 5–10% of all upper gastrointestinal bleeding episodes. Patients with pancreatic disease, especially inflammatory pancreatic disease, can also develop splenic vein thromboses with subsequent formation of isolated gastric varices. There have been sporadic reports of gastric varices developing after endoscopic therapy for bleeding oesophageal varices, particularly after endoscopic sclerotherapy. The risk of bleeding from gastric varices is no greater than from oesophageal varices and it is probable that pharmacological therapy is equally as effective as primary prophylactic therapy in oesophageal varices, so patients with gastric varices should also receive non-selective beta-blockers as first-line therapy. There are no reports of primary attempts at prophylactic therapy using endoscopic-based therapy.

Treatment of acute gastric variceal bleeding is very challenging. Medical management is similar to the treatment of oesophageal varices. Terlipressin and octreotide are useful for control of acute bleeding, while beta-blockers may also be as effective as secondary prophylactic therapy. The Sengstaken–Blakemore tube may have some utility for controlling bleeding from junctional (GOV1 or GOV2) gastro-oesophageal varices but has little effect on controlling bleeding gastro-oesophageal varices in the fundus or further down the stomach. Some endoscopic therapies are promising, but quality data are scarce; sclerotherapy, glue injection, thrombin and variceal band ligation therapy have all been reported. Control of bleeding using sclerotherapy with cyanoacrylate has been reported as efficacious in 62–100% of cases, with successful obliteration of varices in 0–94%.[48,49] A recent randomised controlled trial confirmed that endoscopic sclerotherapy with cyanoacrylate was more effective and also safer than band ligation in the management of bleeding gastric varices.[50] Injection of human thrombin has also been successful in controlling gastric variceal bleeding in a few uncontrolled series; however, at present it is difficult to obtain authorisation for its use.[51] The major rescue therapy (indeed, some may consider it the primary therapy) for bleeding gastric varices used in the UK is TIPS, which has a >90% success rate for initial haemostasis and re-bleeding rates of 20–30%.

It is imperative that all patients treated with any of the above-mentioned interventions (for bleeding oesophageal and gastric varices) except medical management, also receive treatment with a proton pump inhibitor (PPI) to suppress acid secretion and to prevent complications related to acid interaction with bands, injection sites and treatment-related ulcers.

Endoscopic sclerotherapy with cyanoacrylate has been shown to be more effective and safer than band ligation in the management of bleeding oesophageal varices.

Portal hypertensive gastropathy

The presence of portal hypertensive gastropathy (PHG) is strongly correlated with the severity of cirrhosis; its overall prevalence in cirrhosis is about 80%.[52] However, the incidence of acute bleeding is low, occurring in about 2.5% of patients over an 18-month follow-up period, with an associated mortality of 12.5%; the incidence of chronic bleeding is significantly higher, at 12%. Propranolol, octreotide and terlipressin have all been proposed for the treatment of acute bleeding from PHG, based on their ability to decrease portal blood flow. In a randomised controlled trial, propranolol was found to reduce recurrent bleeding from PHG.[53] Once again, TIPS is considered as the rescue therapy of choice in patients who have repeated bleeding from PHG despite propranolol therapy.

Propranolol reduces significantly the risk of bleeding in patients with portal hypertensive gastropathy.

SECOND-LINE THERAPIES

Second-line therapies include the less invasive radiological techniques of TIPS, or open surgery, which can range from direct oversewing of bleeding veins to surgical shunts and ultimately liver replacement.

TIPS (TRANSJUGULAR INTRAHEPATIC PORTO-SYSTEMIC SHUNT)

TIPS is a non-surgical method of creating a porto-caval shunt. Its principal use is in treating variceal bleeding that is not controlled by medical and endoscopic means. It can therefore have a role in both elective and emergency situations. TIPS is also appropriate in selected cases of refractory ascites,[54] hepatic hydrothorax,[55] portal hypertensive gastropathy, Budd–Chiari syndrome and hepatorenal syndrome.[56] TIPS may also facilitate surgery in patients with portal hypertension requiring hepatic or other abdominal surgery, although it is not generally used prior to liver transplant without other specific indications.[57–59]

TIPS is created by needle puncture from a hepatic vein to a major intrahepatic portal vein branch. The track is dilated with a balloon catheter and lined by a metal stent. A variety of techniques have been described for performing the procedure to deal with anatomical difficulties. Most experience is with self-expanding (e.g. Wallstent, Memotherm) or balloon expandable types of stent (e.g. Palmaz), but recently covered or partly covered stent-grafts (e.g. Viatorr) have been introduced, which appear to have an improved patency rate.[60] The degree of shunting can be tailored to some extent by adjusting the diameter of the balloon-dilated shunt against the resulting pressure gradient, directly measured through the catheter.[61]

Occasionally there are severe and life-threatening complications but in the majority of cases few and only minor complications occur. The major disadvantage of TIPS is the relatively poor primary patency rate, but simpler radiological interventions can restore and maintain most narrowed or occluded TIPS. Patients require regular follow-up by Doppler ultrasound, and elective check venography may be performed at regular intervals (e.g. 6-monthly or yearly) to treat stenoses before clinically significant bleeding can recur. As with any shunt there is a risk of encephalopathy. This is greater in older patients,

wider diameter shunts and in those with prior encephalopathy or more advanced liver disease. Patients with precarious liver function may deteriorate into liver failure as a result of reduced portal perfusion.

TIPS has been compared unfavourably with surgery and other interventions because of cost due to the maintenance reinterventions needed.[62,63] However, the less invasive procedure is preferred in patients with worse liver function and long-term prognosis. TIPS is also preferred to surgery in those likely to need future transplantation. Patients with more severe liver disease may be candidates for liver transplantation, but TIPS can enable a patient to stabilise and survive long enough to receive a successful transplant. Child C patients have been shown to do worse in many studies of TIPS. Other methods used for evaluating likely survival and mortality following TIPS include MELD score,[64] BOTEM (Bonn TIPS early mortality score),[65] and hepatic perfusion studies.[66] Studies have shown renal function, intensive care, comorbidity and urgency of TIPS procedure to be important prognostic factors in addition to the standard liver function tests of prothrombin time, albumin and bilirubin, etc.[64,67,68]

TIPS FOR VARICEAL BLEEDING

Uncontrolled bleeding from oesophagogastric or ectopic varices in the presence of a patent portal vein can usually be controlled by TIPS. The procedure can be performed on patients requiring intensive care and in those considered too sick for surgery. The mortality of these patients is due more to their general condition rather than the TIPS procedure. The 30-day mortality after TIPS in the UK National Confidential Enquiry into Perioperative Death[69] study was 17%. In this study 80% of patients dying after TIPS had the procedure performed urgently or as an emergency for bleeding varices.

TIPS can be combined with embolisation of varices as there is direct access to the portal system. In selected cases the left gastric or short gastric veins can be catheterised for embolisation of the varices at the time of TIPS. This is done particularly in acute bleeding to further reduce the risk of haemorrhage. Reduction of extrahepatic porto-systemic shunting may also improve portal venous flow towards the liver and the TIPS. In some cases this may counter encephalopathy as well as helping to maintain flow in the TIPS.

Three meta-analyses of several trials[70–72] compare TIPS with endoscopic sclerotherapy and/or banding for prevention of recurrent variceal bleeding. Additional medical therapy was included in some. TIPS was generally more successful at preventing re-bleeding but with no overall improvement in mortality.[73–76] Encephalopathy was overall more frequent in the TIPS patients, but not in every trial. In some studies patients in the endoscopic groups were rescued by TIPS because of significant recurrent bleeding. The general consensus is that endoscopic and medical therapy should be the primary treatment and TIPS reserved for those cases where control is not achieved. TIPS may be combined effectively with medical treatment or endoscopic variceal eradication after bleeding has been controlled. Long-term TIPS surveillance and radiological reintervention may be less necessary in these circumstances.[77,78]

Other procedures have been used to control bleeding from varices when venous anatomy permits catheter access. Retrograde balloon occlusion gastric variceal embolisation has been mainly used in Asia as an alternative to TIPS when there is a patent gastro-splenic venous connection. This allows access for balloon catheters to enable embolisation of gastric varices via the left renal vein.[79] Experimental studies have also raised the possibility of radiological creation of a direct spleno-renal shunt.[80]

Endoscopic and medical therapy are considered as the optimal primary treatments in patients who have bled from varices, but TIPS should be considered in patients in whom endoscopic therapy is unsuccessful.

Surgical options

Until the application of endoscopic sclerotherapy in the early 1970s, the only practical options were surgical. These ranged from direct control of bleeding vessels by oversewing of varices to a variety of specific porto-systemic shunt procedures. More recently, liver transplantation has become the treatment of choice for patients with variceal bleeding who meet the acceptance criteria.

OESOPHAGEAL TRANSECTION AND DEVASCULARISATION PROCEDURES

These are mainly of historical interest and merit only brief mention. Early attempts at directly suturing the veins by transoesophageal ligation carried very high mortality rates. Oesophageal transection, which effectively interrupted the columns of veins in and around the lower oesophagus, became a relatively straightforward procedure with the advent of circular stapling gun devices. Control of acute bleeding was achieved in over 90% of patients but perioperative mortality rates were extremely high (over 70% as reported by Jenkins and Shield) with high later re-bleed rates in the survivors.[81]

A combination of oesophageal transection with devascularisation of the lower oesophagus and upper stomach is a much more extensive procedure, which was widely applied in Japan with low complication and re-bleeding rates. The Sugiura operation involved an additional vagotomy and pyloroplasty plus splenectomy.[82] However, these approaches have never had any significant application in the West and have been largely superseded by TIPS.

PORTO-SYSTEMIC SHUNTS

The variety of surgical shunts for portal hypertension is perhaps a testament to the ingenuity of surgeons (**Fig. 6.4**). With the passing of the 'shunt era' most surgical trainees will not have seen a shunt, which now has a limited application for a selected group of patients. Such patients are mainly those with non-cirrhotic portal hypertension and those living in areas where newer therapies are not available.

Shunt operations can be classified into selective or non-selective shunts. The latter carry lower rates of hepatic encephalopathy but are less successful in controlling acute bleeding situations. The two main procedures that have achieved popularity are the distal spleno-renal (Warren) shunt (DSRS)[83] and the interposition porto-caval or meso-caval shunt utilising a small-diameter polytetrafluoroethylene (PTFE) graft as described by Sarfeh et al.[84] A controlled crossover trial comparing DSRS with endoscopic sclerotherapy showed that shunting produced better control of bleeding but did not produce any survival advantage.[85] The Inokuchi left gastric–IVC (inferior vena cava) shunt (**Fig. 6.4**) has

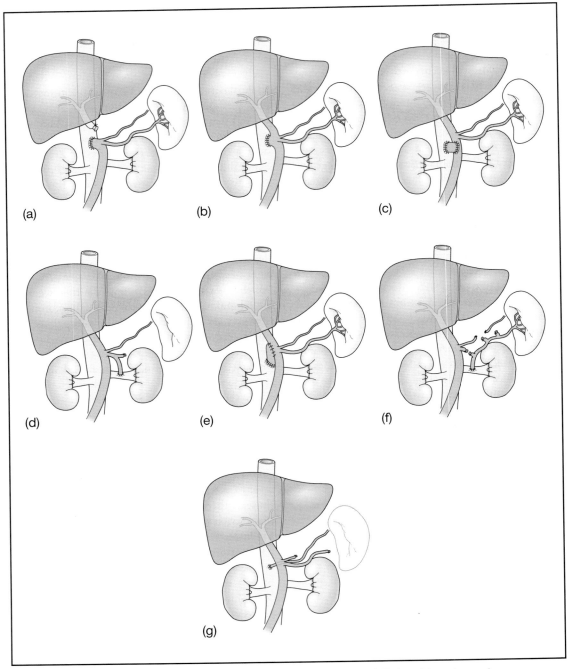

Figure 6.4 • Non-selective **(a–d)** and selective **(e–g)** porto-systemic shunts. **(a)** End-to-side porto-caval. **(b)** Side-to-side porto-caval. **(c)** Meso-caval (jugular vein graft or prosthesis). **(d)** Proximal spleno-renal. **(e)** Small-diameter PTFE H-graft porto-caval. **(f)** Distal spleno-renal. **(g)** Inokuchi left gastric-IVC.

not found favour outside of Japan perhaps because of the technical difficulty due to the fragility of the left gastric vein. Direct primary porto-caval anastomosis produces the most effective lowering of portal pressure but with the highest encephalopathy rates, and the advantage of the Sarfeh shunt is that it is selective and maintains some portal flow. This shunt has been compared to TIPS in a single-centre randomised trial, which reported a better control of bleeding in shunted patients than that seen in the TIPS patients.[60,86] The entry criterion was variceal bleeding in patients who had failed or 'were not amenable to' sclerotherapy or banding, which might suggest a low threshold to proceed with second-line therapies. The 30-day mortality rate was 20% for shunted patients and 15% for TIPS patients. It had already been established that shunt surgery for cirrhotics has significant postoperative mortality, being as high as 26.1% for Child C patients in specialised centres.[87] Furthermore, 5-year survival rates in patients with advanced liver disease are poor, and shunt surgery carries an additional burden due to the risks of hepatic encephalopathy. On the current evidence there is no role for routine shunting in cirrhotic patients, and the results of a larger multicentre trial comparing TIPS with DSRS in cirrhotic patients are awaited.[88]

Shunts are not usually appropriate for patients in whom transplantation is an option as they significantly increase the risk of surgery. If shunt surgery is deemed unavoidable due to failure of endoscopic and radiological approaches, surgery away from the liver hilum is recommended, either as a spleno-renal or interposition meso-caval shunt.

LIVER TRANSPLANTATION

With the improved results and wider application of liver transplantation, this has become the definitive treatment for many patients with variceal bleeding. However, results are inferior for patients transplanted around the time of an acute bleed. Furthermore, there are reports of oesophageal complications, including perforation, in grafted patients who have undergone recent endoscopic therapy. Thus the indications for liver replacement are more to do with the stage of the underlying liver disease although the priority for grafting will be influenced by a history of recent bleeding or a high risk for re-bleeding.

In 1997, minimal selection criteria were developed to aid such a process.[89] This was largely based on studies of the natural history of compensated chronic liver diseases.[90,91] The minimal listing criteria were: an estimated 1-year survival <90%; Child–Pugh score >7 (class B or C) or portal hypertensive bleeding or an episode of spontaneous bacterial peritonitis regardless of the Child–Pugh score. The basis of these criteria is that the expected outcome of the untreated patient would be significantly worse than that of the outcomes from liver transplantation. This recognises the significantly worse prognosis of decompensated cirrhosis, which in those with hepatitis C dramatically reduces from a 91% 5-year survival to 50%.[91] Spontaneous bacterial peritonitis carries an adverse outcome in these patients, with 1-year survival falling from 66% to 38% in one report,[92] and despite the many therapeutic modalities available for treatment, the only definitive therapy for recurrent variceal bleeding is liver transplantation.[93]

Broadly, liver transplantation should be considered in any patient who is able to cooperate with the treatment and in whom an anticipated survival rate of at least 50% at 5 years post grafting is likely to be achieved. The decision to proceed to liver replacement should be made by a multidisciplinary team including an experienced hepatologist.

SELECTION OF SECOND-LINE THERAPY

Non-cirrhotic

The easiest groups to consider are those without cirrhosis. If such patients fail with pharmacological or endoscopic therapy then a surgical shunt is the treatment of choice. For those with portal vein thrombosis a distal spleno-renal shunt is recommended and has the advantage of preserving the spleen. For non-cirrhotics with patent portal veins the choice rests between a porto-caval or distal spleno-renal depending on local expertise.

Cirrhotic

It is clear that patients who are potential transplant candidates should be assessed for this once the initial bleeding problem has been controlled. If the bleeding cannot be controlled they should be considered for urgent TIPS insertion and then consideration for liver replacement. Patients who are unsuitable for transplantation may be candiates for TIPS provided they do not have significant encephalopathy, as this may worsen following the procedure. Once the transplant candidates, patients who are high-risk because of comorbidity, and uncooperative patients who are actively drinking are identified as unsuitable for shunting, this leaves few potential candidates for this shunting procedure. Clearly in areas where transplantation is not available as an option, patients should be considered for shunting provided they are Child A or B.

MANAGEMENT OF ASCITES

Ascites is a common feature of portal hypertension, although the exact mechanisms remain under debate.[94] Ascites in chronic liver disease can be effectively treated by a number of medical, surgical or radiological techniques. A new occurrence of ascites should be investigated for the development of bacterial peritonitis, portal vein thrombosis or hepatic malignancy. Initial treatment involves dietary sodium restriction and diuretic therapy. Unresponsive patients may benefit from regular large-volume paracentesis with concurrent intravenous administration of 20% human albumin.[95] Though peritoneo-venous shunting is effective in controlling ascites, potential risks include disseminated intravascular coagulation, sepsis and cardiac failure. It has few advantages over large-volume paracentesis and is not recommended for patients who are transplant candidates.[96] Refractory ascites is an indication for transplant assessment. An alternative approach to the treatment of ascites is the construction of a sapheno-peritoneal shut.[97] A length of proximal saphenous vein is anastomosed to a small incision in the peritoneum in the groin. Early results are encouraging though there have been no comparative trials with other therapies.

TIPS can also be very effective in controlling ascites refractory to medical treatment, but many such patients have very advanced liver disease with poor prognosis. The immediate risk is worsening liver failure and hepatic encephalopathy, and advice from a skilled hepatologist should be sought before

a TIPS is placed. Older patients and those with renal dysfunction fare worse,[98] and if patients with severe ascites are liver transplant candidates this may be a better option than TIPS.[99] Some trials have shown TIPS to be more effective than medical treatment plus paracentesis, but patient selection is most important.[100–103] Patients with better liver function and disproportionate ascites, especially those with liver disease that can improve, for example by withdrawal from alcohol, can respond very well to TIPS. Some studies have shown an improved quality of life in patients having TIPS for ascites whereas others have not.[104] Surgical shunts are no longer recommended for resistant ascites due to high perioperative mortality and encephalopathy rates.

BUDD–CHIARI SYNDROME

Budd–Chiari syndrome is a rare condition resulting from the occlusion of the hepatic veins. It can present in various ways including acute abdominal pain, abdominal swelling due to ascites, acute fulminant liver failure or chronic liver failure, and can mimic many other conditions. CT scanning will often reveal abnormal perfusion, which can be difficult to interpret, and cases may be initially misdiagnosed as advanced hepatic malignancy. One specific feature is the compensatory hypertrophy of the caudate lobe of the liver. This occurs because it has venous drainage separate from the three main hepatic veins. This regenerated liver is clearly life preserving although pressure from the caudate may compound a tendency to caval thrombosis, which is seen in a proportion of patients. The majority of patients will have or will develop evidence of a thrombophilic state, and all should be assessed by an expert haematologist. Given the lifetime risks of further thromboses, all patients will require long-term anticoagulation.

Acute Budd–Chiari syndrome

In the acute presentation there will usually be abdominal pain and swelling, and the diagnosis is suggested by the failure at ultrasound to visualise normal venous phases flow in the hepatic veins. This finding should lead to referral to a specialised centre where hepatic venography and interventional radiological expertise is available. Depending on the pathological anatomy demonstrated by ultrasound and hepatic venography, a short stenosis or occlusion of the hepatic veins and/or IVC may be traversed and dilated with a balloon. The simplest and preferred method is catheter access via the transjugular or transfemoral route enabling safe balloon dilatation. In cases with good patent peripheral segments of hepatic vein not accessible from the cava a percutaneous transhepatic needle puncture into the patent vein will often permit the occlusion to be traversed. A guidewire passed through percutaneously is snared in the IVC or right atrium and balloon dilatation with a large balloon can proceed from the jugular access.[105,106] Occlusion or stenosis of the IVC (sometimes a web) may similarly respond to large balloon dilatation or double balloon inflation with one balloon inserted from the femoral vein and another from the jugular. If the dilated or recanalised segment of hepatic vein is not satisfactorily maintained after balloon inflation, a metal stent can be inserted with good effect to maintain the patent lumen.

These approaches have the benefit of restoring hepatic vein outflow in at least one of the main hepatic veins. Physiological hepatic venous drainage is theoretically preferred to decompression of the liver by a shunt. A non-randomised comparison of patients treated by angioplasty and shunt surgery showed better survival in the angioplasty patients.[107] However, the patients who had surgery probably had more extensive hepatic vein block, and indeed some of the surgical cases had previously tried and failed angioplasty.

Adjunctive pharmacological thrombolysis may assist in these procedures in selected cases, especially when acute thrombosis complicates an otherwise successful vein recanalisation. There are individual case reports of systemic thrombolysis producing improvement but these are rare. The status of thrombolysis for Budd–Chiari syndrome has recently been summarised.[108]

In Budd–Chiari patients with more extensive hepatic vein occlusion or no suitable patent vein segments to restore, TIPS may be performed as a less invasive equivalent to shunt surgery. TIPS can be used in both acute and chronic Budd–Chiari,[109,100] and would now be regarded as the treatment of choice for those not responding to medical therapy.[111] The advantage of TIPS is decompression of the portal vein above the compressed part of the IVC within the caudate lobe and avoidance of laparotomy. The disadvantage of TIPS, as ever, is the requirement for further procedures to maintain its patency. With their tendency to thrombosis, Budd–Chiari patients may have a greater need for reintervention than other TIPS patients.

TIPS can be successful treatment for Budd–Chiari syndrome complicated by portal and mesenteric vein thrombosis.[112,113] A few cases have been described in which TIPS was a successful stabilising factor before liver transplantation.[114] In our experience liver replacement is now rarely indicated as most Budd–Chiari patients with successful TIPS respond well and do not require surgical treatment. If TIPS cannot be achieved then surgical shunt can be performed, or liver transplant if there is significant liver failure. In summary there is a progressive hierarchy of radiological procedures that can manage a majority of Budd–Chiari patients according to their individual venous anatomy. These procedures are effective in combination with appropriate medical therapy.[115]

When the radiological approach has failed, the type of shunt possible will depend on the patency of the vena cava. If the cava is patent a meso-caval shunt using a length of autologous internal jugular vein between the superior mesenteric vein and the infrarenal vena cava is recommended. For cases with caval occlusion a meso-atrial shunt using a graft of reinforced PTFE between the superior mesenteric vein and the right atrium is required.[116] Selection of patients for shunting is not easy, and our experience suggests that patients with jaundice as an early symptom are at risk from liver decompensation and should be considered for liver grafting. If the patient develops fulminant hepatic failure then emergency liver transplantation is the only potential option. High success rates are reported but recurrence can occur and all patients will require long-term anticoagulation.

Chronic Budd–Chiari syndrome

Many patients present with significant ascites and marked changes on liver biopsy, which include significant fibrosis or even cirrhosis. It is likely that for some patients the hepatic venous obstruction is sequential and that the condition is asymptomatic until a second or final (third) hepatic vein is occluded. Despite worrying pathology, interventional radiology should still be considered, although again our local experience is that jaundice is an adverse prognostic sign and in these cases liver transplantation may be required. Either hepatic vein dilatation or TIPS should be performed, based on the presence of identifiable hepatic veins within the liver. Again, shunt procedures should be reserved for radiological approach failures. Our experience since developing an interventional radiological approach is that the vast majority of patients can be treated successfully in this way and that liver transplantation for Budd–Chiari syndrome is required rarely.[115]

Hepatic vein dilatation or stent insertion to restore venous outflow is the procedure of choice for Budd–Chiari syndrome when the venous anatomy permits. TIPS is the next procedure of choice in symptomatic acute and chronic Budd–Chiari syndrome in patients who do not respond to medical treatment.

NON-CIRRHOTIC PORTAL HYPERTENSION

Portal hypertension is uncommon in the absence of cirrhosis. The causes are mainly portal vein thrombosis, periportal fibrosis and segmental, usually left upper quadrant portal hypertension associated with splenic vein thrombosis.

Portal vein thrombosis

Portal vein thrombosis is rare in the West but seen more frequently in Third World countries, and is thought to be the result of umbilical sepsis in the neonatal period. Presentation can be in early childhood but is usually delayed to the early teenage years. The symptoms are usually that of a sudden variceal bleed, although some patients may be picked up by the presence of significant splenomegaly with or without haematological features of hypersplenism. The management of the acute bleed is similar to that in patients with cirrhosis. Re-

bleeding or the presence of large gastric varices should be considered as a clear indication for a surgical shunt. Given the risks of splenectomy in the young, a spleen-preserving procedure is recommended. In a small child spleno-renal shunts are less practical because of the small size of the vessels and interposition meso-caval shunts using autologous jugular vein have high success rates with good long-term patency.[117] In larger children the distal spleno-renal or Warren shunt is usually favoured, although side-to-side spleno-renal shunts have been reported in significant numbers from centres with a high prevalence of portal vein thrombosis.[118] The natural history of these patients is interesting in that as they grow the varices become less symptomatic, and certainly shunting is not indicated unless bleeding episodes have occurred.

Extensive mesenteric venous thrombosis is a potentially lethal complication seen in a few patients with portal vein thrombosis. Many patients present with gut infarction but those presenting late pose major management problems. Angiography may reveal particularly dilated mesenteric collaterals, which might allow ad hoc shunts to the cava, but currently only medical therapies to lower portal pressure can be recommended.

Segmental portal hypertension

Segmental portal hypertension should always be considered as the potential cause of bleeding in patients with pancreatic pathology as they have splenic vein thrombosis. Those with advanced pancreatic malignancy can usually be controlled with medical therapy or sclerotherapy. Patients with chronic pancreatitis who develop variceal bleeding secondary to splenic vein thrombosis should be considered for splenectomy, which will usually be curative.

TIPS and portal vein thrombosis

Experience with TIPS and interventional procedures in liver transplant patients have extended applications into the portal vein by both percutaneous transhepatic and transjugular routes.[119,120] This leads to the treatment of selected cases of acute portal vein thrombosis and even chronic portal vein obstruction by catheter and stent techniques. Provided access to the portal vein is achieved, limited portal vein thrombus is treated relatively easily by TIPS, which may be combined with mechanical thrombolysis such as clot disruption by balloon or other devices.[121,122] Patients with normal liver may only require transhepatic portal vein procedures for successful outcome, but those with hepatic portal hypertension in addition can benefit from TIPS combined with intraportal intervention.

Chronic portal vein thrombosis is usually associated with extensive portal collaterals forming a portal vein cavernoma. If there is only a limited underlying obstruction and an appropriate clinical need then some of these can be traversed and the main portal vein flow can be restored by balloon dilatation or stent insertion.[123] Cases with a more extensive occlusion involving the splenic and superior veins are less likely to be treated effectively,[124] and those with underlying liver disease fare worse than those with normal liver function.

Key points

Patients with grade II varices or worse who have not bled should be treated with beta-blockers unless there are medical contraindications.

Endoscopic band ligation is the initial treatment of choice for acute variceal bleeding.

After bleeding, patients should enter a programme of variceal ligation or beta-blockade to prevent recurrent bleeding.

TIPS should be considered in patients in whom endoscopic therapy is unsuccessful.

Liver transplantation should be considered in appropriate cases once variceal bleeding is problematic.

Shunt surgery should be considered for non-cirrhotic patients with recurrent variceal bleeding and for Child–Pugh stage A and B patients who live in areas where TIPS or transplantation is unavailable.

REFERENCES

1. Wiest R, Groszmann RJ. The paradox of nitric oxide in cirrhosis and portal hypertension: too much, not enough. Hepatology 2002; 35:478–91.

2. Pinzani M, Gentilini P. Biology of hepatic stellate cells and their possible relevance in the pathogenesis of portal hypertension in cirrhosis. Semin Liver Dis 1999; 19:397–410.

3. Rockey DC, Weisiger RA. Endothelin induced contractility of stellate cells from normal and cirrhotic rat liver: implications for regulation of portal pressure and resistance. Hepatology 1996; 24:233–240.

4. Ballet F, Chretien Y, Rey C et al. Differential response of normal and cirrhotic liver to vasoactive agents. A study in the isolated perfused rat liver. J Parmacol Exp Ther 1988; 244:233–5.

5. Graupera M, Garcia-Pagan JC, Gonzalez-Abraldes J et al. Cirrhotic livers exhibit a hyper-response to mehoxamine. Role of nitric oxide and eicosanoids. J Hepatol 2001; 34:66A.

6. Graupera M, Garcia-Pagan JC, Titos E et al. 5-lipoxygenase inhibition reduces intrahepatic vascular resistance of cirrhotic livers: a possible role of cysteinyl-leukotrienes. Gastroenterology 2002; 122:387–93.

7. Vorobioff J, Bredfelt J, Goszmann RJ. Hyperdynamic circulation in a portal hypertensive rat model: a primary factor for maintenance of chronic portal hypertension. Am J Physiol 1983; 244:G52–6.

8. Benoit JN, Barrowman JA, Harper SL et al. Role of humoral factors in the intestinal hyperaemia associated with chronic portal hypertension. Am J Physiol 1984; 247:G486–93.

9. Pizcueta MP, Pique JM, Bosch J et al. Effects of inhibiting nitric oxide biosynthesis on the systemic and splanchnic circulation of rats with portal hypertension. Br J Pharmacol 1992; 105:184–90.

10. Pizcueta MP, Pique JM, Fernandez M et al. Modulation of the hyperdynamic circulation of cirrhotic rats by nitric oxide inhibition. Gastroenterology 1992; 103:1909–15.

11. Wiest R, Goszmann RJ. Nitric oxide and portal hypertension: its role in the regulation of intrahepatic and splanchnic vascular resistance. Semin Liver Dis 1999; 19:411–26.

12. Schepis F, Camma C, Nicefero D et al. Which patients should undergo endoscopic screening for esophageal varices detection? Hepatology 2001; 33:333–8.

13. D'Amico G, Pagliaro L, Bosch J. Pharmacological treatment of portal hypertension: an evidence based approach. Semin Liver Dis 1999; 19:475–505.

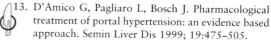
Meta-analysis illustrating the benefits of treating patients with beta-blockers after an episode of bleeding

oesophageal varices both in terms of decreasing risk of re-bleeding and decreasing mortality.

14. Zoli M, Merkel C, Magalotti D et al. Natural history of cirrhotic patients with small esophageal varices: a prospective study. Am J Gastroenterol 2000; 95:503–8.

15. Vorobioff J, Grozmann RJ, Picabea E et al. Prognostic value of hepatic venous pressure gradient measurements in alcoholic cirrhosis: a 10-year prospective study. Gastroenterology 1996; 111:701–9.

16. The North Italian Endoscopic Club for the Study and Treatment of Esophageal Varices. Prediction of the first variceal haemorrhage in patients with cirrhosis of the liver and esophageal varices: a prospective multicenter study. N Engl J Med 1988; 319:983–9.

17. Snady H, Feinman L. Prediction of variceal haemorrhage: a prospective study. Am J Gastroenterol 1988; 83:519–25.

18. Albers I, Hartmann H, Bircher J et al. Superiority of the Child–Pugh classification to quantitative liver function tests for assessing prognosis of liver cirrhosis. Scand J Gastroenterol 1989; 24:269–76.

19. Kamath PS, Wiesner RH, Malinchoc M et al. A model to predict survival in patients with end-stage liver disease. Hepatology 2001; 33:464–70.

20. D'Amico G, Luca A. Natural History. Clinical-haemodynamic correlations. Prediction of the risk of bleeding. Baillières Best Pract Res Clin Gastroenterol 1997; 11:243–56.

21. Polio J, Groszmann RJ, Picabea E et al. Hemodynamic factors involved in the development and rupture of esophageal varices: a pathophysiological approach to treatment. Semin Liver Dis 1986; 6:318–31.

22. Ben Ari Z, Cardin F, McCormik AP et al. A predictive model for failure to control bleeding during acute variceal haemorrhage. J Hepatol 1999; 31:443–50.

23. Goulis J, Armonis A, Patch D et al. Bacterial infection is independently associated with failure to control bleeding in cirrhotic patients with gastrointestinal haemorrhage. Hepatology 1998; 27:1207–12.

24. Moitinho E, Escorsell A, Bandi JC et al. Prognostic value of early measurements of portal pressure in acute variceal bleeding. Gastroenterology 1999; 117:626–31.

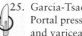
25. Garcia-Tsao G, Grozsmann RJ, Fisher RL et al. Portal pressure, presence of gastroesophageal varices and variceal bleeding. Hepatology 1985; 5:419–24.

26. Feu F, Garcia-Pagan JC, Bosch J et al. Relation between portal pressure response to pharmacotherapy and risk of recurrent variceal bleeding in patients with cirrhosis. Lancet 1995; 346:1056–9.

27. Villaneuva C, Minana J, Ortiz J et al. Endoscopic ligation compared with combined treatment with nadolol and isosorbide mononitrate to prevent variceal bleeding. N Engl J Med 2001; 345:647–55.

These references provide the rationale for the therapeutic aim of pharmacological therapy to decrease the HVPG to <12 mmHg or reduce it to 20% of its baseline value.

28. Tarantino I, Abraldes JG, Turnes J et al. The HVPG response to pharmacological treatment of portal hypertension predicts prognosis and the risk of developing complications of cirrhosis. J Hepatol 2002; 36(Suppl. 1):15A.

29. Bosch J, Abraldes JG, Groszmann R. Current management of portal hypertension. J Hepatol 2003; 38:S54–S68.

30. Abraczinskas DR, Ookubo R, Grace ND et al. Propranolol for the prevention of first esophageal haemorrhage: a lifetime commitment? Hepatology 2001; 34:1096–102.

31. Banares R, Moitinho E, Matilla A et al. Randomised comparison of long-term carvedilol and propranolol administration in the treatment of portal hypertension in cirrhosis. Hepatology 2002; 36: 1367–73.

32. Tripathi D, Therapondos G, Lui HF et al. Haemodynamic effects of acute and chronic administration of low dose carvedilol, a vasodilating beta-blocker, in patients with cirrhosis and portal hypertension. Aliment Pharmacol Ther 2002; 16:373–80.

33. Borroni G, Salerno F, Cazzaniga M et al. Nadolol is superior to isosorbide mononitrate for the prevention of the first variceal bleeding in cirrhotic patients with ascites. J Hepatol 2002; 37:315–21.

34. Imperiale TF, Chalasani N. A meta-analysis of endoscopic variceal ligation for primary prophylaxis of esophageal variceal bleeding. Hepatology 2001; 33:908–14.

35. De Franchis R, Primignami M. Endoscopic treatments for portal hypertension. Semin Liver Dis 1999; 19:439–55.

36. Laine L, El Newihi HM, Migikovsky et al. Endoscopic ligation compared with sclerotherapy for the treatment of bleeding esophageal varices. Ann Intern Med 1993; 119:1–7.

37. Patch D, Sabin CA, Goulis J et al. A randomised, controlled trial of medical therapy versus endoscopic ligation for the prevention of variceal rebleeding in patients with cirrhosis. Gastroenterology 2002; 123:1013–19.

38. Lo GH, Chen WC, Chen MH et al. Banding ligation versus nadolol and isosorbide mononitrate for the prevention of esophageal rebleeding. Gastroenterology 2002; 123:728–34.

39. Gournay J, Masliah C, Martin T et al. Isosorbide mononitrate and propranolol compared with

propranolol alone for the prevention of variceal re-bleeding. Hepatology 2000; 31:1239–1245.

40. Casteneda B, Debernadi-Vernon W, Bandi JC et al. The role of portal pressure in the severity of bleeding in portal hypertensive rats. Hepatology 2000; 31:581–6.

41. Bernard B, Grange JD, Khac EN et al. Antibiotic prophylaxis for the prevention of bacterial infections in cirrhotic patients with gastrointestinal bleeding: a meta-analysis. Hepatology 1999; 29:1655–61.

42. Rimola A, Garcia-Tsao G, Navasa M et al. Diagnosis, treatment and prophylaxis of spontaneous bacterial peritonitis: a consensus document. International Ascites Club. J Hepatol 2000; 32:142–53.

    Illustrations of the benefit to cirrhotic patients of prophylactic antibiotics following a variceal bleed by decreasing mortality.

43. Levacher S, Letoumelin P, Pateron D et al. Early administration of terlipressin plus glyceryl trinitrate to control active upper gastrointestinal bleeding in cirrhotic patients. Lancet 1995; 346:865–8.

44. Avgerinos A, Nevens F, Raptis S et al. Early administration of somatostatin and efficacy of sclerotherapy in acute variceal bleeds: the European acute bleeding oesophageal variceal episodes (ABOVE) randomised trial. Lancet 1997; 350:1495–9.

45. Cales P, Masliah C, Bernard B et al. Early administration of vapreotide for variceal bleeding in patients with cirrhosis. French club for the study of portal hypertension. N Engl J Med 2001; 344:23–8.

46. Infante-Rivard C, Esnaola S, Villeneuve JP. Role of endoscopic variceal sclerotherapy in the long-term management of variceal bleeding: a meta-analysis. Gastroenterology 1989; 96:1087–92.

47. Singh P, Pooran N, Indaram A et al. Combined ligation and sclerotherapy versus ligation alone for secondary prophylaxis of esophageal variceal bleeding: a meta-analysis. Am J Gastroenterol 2002; 97:623–9.

48. Huang YH, Yeh HZ, Chen GH et al. Endoscopic treatment of bleeding gastric varices by N-butyl-2-cyanoacrylate (Histoacryl) injection: long-term efficacy and safety. Gastrointest Endosc 2000; 52:512–9.

49. Kind R, Guglielmi A, Rodella L et al. Bucrylate treatment of bleeding gastric varices: 12 years' experience. Endoscopy 2000; 32:512–19.

50. Lo GH, Lai KH, Cheng JS et al. A prospective randomised trial of butyl cyanoacrylate injection versus band ligation in the management of bleeding gastric varices. Hepatology 2001; 33:1060–4.

    This was the first study to compare banding with the injection of 'glue' in the treatment of gastric varices as a prospective randomized trial.

51. Yang WL, Tripath D, Therapondos G et al. Endoscopic use of human thrombin in bleeding gastric varices. Am J Gastroenterol 2002; 97:1381–5.

52. Primignani M, Carpinelli L, Preatoni P et al. Natural history of portal hypertensive gastropathy in patients with liver cirrhosis. The new Italian endoscopic club for the study and treatment of esophageal varices (NIEC). Gastroenterology 2000; 119:181–7.

53. Perez-Ayuso RM, Pique JM, Bosch J et al. Propranolol in the prevention of recurrent bleeding from severe portal hypertensive gastropathy in cirrhosis. Lancet 1991; 337:1431–1434.

    Most helpful study demonstrating the use of pharmacological therapy in the prevention of recurrent bleeding from portal hypertensive gastropathy.

54. Rossle M, Ochs A, Gulberg V et al. A comparison of paracentesis and transjugular intrahepatic portosystemic shunting in patients with ascites. N Engl J Med 2000; 342:1701–7.

55. Siegersetter V, Deibert P, Ochs A et al. Treatment of refractory hepatic hydrothorax with transjugular intrahepatic portosystemic shunt: long-term results in 40 patients. Eur J Gastroenterol Hepatol 2001; 13:529–34.

56. Brensing KA, Textor J, Perz J et al. Long term outcome after transjugular intrahepatic portosystemic stent-shunt in non-transplant cirrhotics with hepatorenal syndrome: a phase II study. Gut 2000; 47:288–95.

57. Bilbao JI, Quiroga J, Herrero JI et al. Transjugular intrahepatic portosystemic shunt (TIPS): current status and future possibilities. Cardiovasc Intervent Radiol 2002; 25:251–69.

58. Rosado B, Kamath PS. Transjugular intrahepatic portosystemic shunts: an update. Liver Transplantation 2003; 9:207–17.

59. Tripathi D, Therapondos G, Redhead DN et al. Transjugular intrahepatic portosystemic stent-shunt and its effects on orthotopic liver transplantation. Eur J Gastroenterol Hepatol 2002;14:827–32.

60. Haskal ZJ, Weintraub JL, Susman J. Recurrent TIPS thrombosis after polyethylene stent-graft use and salvage with polytetrafluoroethylene stent-grafts. J Vasc Interv Radiol 2002; 13:1255–9.

    PTFE-covered stents may be the answer.

61. Rossle M, Siegerstetter V, Olchewski et al. How much reduction in portal pressure is necessary to prevent variceal rebleeding? A longitudinal study in 225 patients with transjugular intrahepatic portosystemic shunts. Am J Gastroenterol 2001; 96:3379–83.

    Observations on 225 patients having TIPS follow-up. Reduction of pressure gradient by 25–50% of original may be sufficient to prevent re-bleeding rather than the target of 12 mmHg.

62. Rosemurgy AS, Zervos EE, Blooston M et al. Post shunt resource consumption favors small-diameter prosthetic H-graft portocaval shunt over TIPS for patients with poor hepatic reserve. Ann Surg 2003; 237:820–5.

63. Helton WS, Maves R, Wicks K et al. Transjugular intrahepatic portosystemic shunt vs surgical shunt in good-risk cirrhotic patients: a case control comparison. Arch Surg 2001; 136:17–20.

64. Salerno F, Merli M, Cazzaniga M et al. MELD score is better than Child–Pugh score in predicting 3 month survival of patients undergoing transjugular intrahepatic portosystemic shunt. J Hepatol 2002; 36:494–500.

65. Brensing KA, Raab P, Textor J et al. Prospective evaluation of a clinical score for 60 day mortality after tranjugular intrahepetic portosystemic stent-shunt: Bonn TIPSS early mortality analysis. Eur J Gastroenterol Hepatol 2002; 14:723–31.

66. Walser E, Ozkan OS, Raza S et al. Hepatic perfusion as a predictor of mortality after transjugular intrahepatic portosystemic shunt creation in patients with refractory ascites. J Vasc Interv Radiol 2003; 14:1251–7.

67. Schepke M, Roth F, Fimmers R et al. Comparison of MELD, Child–Pugh and Emory model for the prediction of survival in patients undergoing trans-jugular intrahepatic portosystemic shunting. Am J Gastroenterol 2003; 98:1167–74.

68. Angermayr B, Cejna M, Karnel F et al. Child–Pugh versus MELD score in predicting survival in patients undergoing transjugular intrahepatic portosystemic shunt. Gut 2003; 52:879–85.

69. NCEPOD report on Vascular Interventional Radiology 2000. www.ncepod.org.uk.

70. Luca A, D'Amico G, La Galla R et al. TIPS for prevention of recurrent bleeding in patients with cirrhosis. Radiology 1999; 212:411–21.

71. Papatheodoridis GV, Goulis J, Leandro G et al. Transjugular intrahepatic portosystemic shunt compared with endoscopic treatment for prevention of variceal rebleeding. A meta-analysis. Hepatology 1999; 30:612–22.

72. Burroughs AK, Vangeli M. Transjugular intrahepatic portosystemic shunt versus endoscopic therapy: randomized trials for secondary prophylaxis of variceal bleeding: an updated meta-analysis. Scand J Gastroenterol 2002; 37:249–52.

73. Pomier-Layrargues G, Villeneuve JP, Deschenes M et al. Transjugular intrahepatic portosystemic shunt (TIPS) versus endoscopic variceal ligation in the prevention of variceal rebleeding in patients with cirrhosis: a randomised trial. Gut 2001; 48:390–6.

74. Escorell A, Banares R, Garcia-Pagan JC et al. TIPS versus drug therapy in preventing variceal rebleed-ing in advanced cirrhosis: a randomised controlled trial. Hepatology 2002; 35:385–92.

75. Gulberg V, Schepke M, Geigenberger G et al. Transjugular intrahepatic portosystemic shunting is not superior to endoscopic variceal ligation for prevention of variceal rebleeding in cirrhotic patients: a randomized controlled trial. Scand J Gastroenterol 2002; 37:338–43.

76. Sauer P, Hansmann J, Richter GM et al. Endoscopic variceal ligation plus propranolol vs. transjugular intrahepatic portosystemic stent shunt: a long term randomized trial. Endoscopy 2002; 34:690–7.

77. Brensing KA, Horsch M, Textor J et al. Hemodynamic effects of propranolol and nitrates in cirrhotic patients with transjugular intrahepatic portosystemic stent-shunt. Scand J Gastroenterol 2002; 37:1070–6.

78. Bellis L, Moitinho E, Abraldes JG et al. Acute propranolol administration effectively decreases portal pressure in patients with TIPS dysfunction. Transjugular intrahepatic portosystemic shunt. Gut 2003; 52:130–3.

79. Choi YH, Yoon CJ, Park JH et al. Balloon-occluded retrograde transvenous obliteration for gastric varices: Its feasibility compared with transjugular intrahepatic portosystemic shunt. Korean Journal of Radiology 2003; 4:109–16.

80. Kaminou T, Rosch J, Yamada R et al. Percutaneous retroperitoneal splenorenal shunt: an experimental study in swine. Radiology 1998; 206:799–802.

81. Jenkins SA, Shields R. Variceal haemorrhage after failed injection sclerotherapy: the role of emergency oesophageal transection. Br J Surg 1989; 76:49–51.

82. Sugiura M, Futagawa S. Esophageal transection with paraesophagogastric devascularizations (the Sugiura procedure) in the treatment of esophageal varices. World J Surg 1984; 8:673–9.

83. Warren WD, Zeppa R, Fomon JJ. Selective trans-splenic decompression of gastroesophageal varices by distal splenorenal shunt. Ann Surg 1967; 166:437–55.

84. Sarfeh IJ, Rypins EB, Conroy RM et al. Portocaval H-graft: relationships of shunt diameter, portal flow patterns and encephalopathy. Ann Surg 1983; 197:422–6.

85. Henderson JM, Kutner MH, Millikan WJ Jr et al. Endoscopic variceal sclerosis compared with distal splenorenal shunt to prevent recurrent variceal bleeding in cirrhosis. A prospective, randomized trial. Ann Intern Med 1990; 112:262–9.

Shunting produced better control of bleeding but did not produce any survival advantage.

86. Rosemurgy A, Serafini F, Zweibel B et al. Transjugular intrahepatic portosystemic shunt vs.

small-diameter prosthetic H-graft portacaval shunt: Extended follow-up of an expanded randomized prospective trial. J Gastroint Surg 2000; 4:589–97.

87. Rikkers LF. The changing spectrum of treatment for variceal bleeding. Ann Surg 1998; 228:536–46.

88. Henderson JM. Salvage therapies for refractory variceal haemorrhage. Clin Liver Dis 2001; 5:709–25.

89. Lucey MR, Brown KA, Everson GT et al. Minimal criteria for placement of adults on liver transplant waiting list: a report of a national conference organized by the American Association for the Study of Liver Diseases. Liver Transpl Surg 1997; 3:628–37.

90. Propst A, Propst T, Zangerl G et al. Prognosis and life expectancy in chronic liver disease. Dig Dis Sci 1995; 40:1805–15.

91. Fattovich G, Giustina G, Degos F et al. Morbidity and mortality in compensated cirrhosis type C: a retrospective follow up study of 384 patients. Gastroenterology 1997; 112:463–72.

92. Andreu M, Sola R, Sitges-Serra A et al. Risks for spontaneous bacterial peritonitis in cirrhotic patients with ascites. Gastroenterology 1993; 104:1133–8.

93. D'Amico G, Pagliaro L, Bosch J. The treatment of portal hypertension: a meta-analytic review. Hepatology 1995; 22:332–54.

94. Jalan R, Hayes PC. Hepatic encephalopathy and ascites. Lancet 1997; 350:1309–15.

95. Gines A, Fernandez-Esparrach G, Monescillo A et al. Randomized trial comparing albumin, dextran 70, and polygeline in cirrhotic patients with ascites treated by paracentesis. Gastroenterology 1996; 111:1002–10.

96. Gines P, Arroyo V, Vargas V et al. Paracentesis with intravenous infusion of albumin as compared with peritoneovenous shunting in cirrhosis with refractory ascites. N Engl J Med 1991; 325:829–35.

97. Vadeyar HJ, Doran JD, Charnley R et al. Saphenoperitoneal shunts for patients with intractable ascites associated with chronic liver disease. Br J Surg 1999; 86:882–5.

98. Deschenes M, Dufresne MP, Bui B et al. Predictors of clinical response to transjugular intrahepatic portosystemic shunt (TIPS) in cirrhotic patients with refractory ascites. Am J Gastroenterol 1999; 94:1361–5.

99. Thuluvath PJ, Bal JS, Mitchell S et al. TIPS for management of refractory ascites: response and survival are both unpredictable. Dig Dis Sci 2003; 48:542–50.

100. Lebrec D, Giuily N, Hadengue A et al. Transjugular intrahepatic portosystemic shunts: comparison with paracentesis in patients with cirrhosis and refractory ascites: a randomised trial. J Hepatol 1996; 25:135–44.

101. Rossle M, Ochs A, Gulberg V et al. A comparison of paracentesis and transjugular intrahepatic portosystemic shunting in patients with ascites. N Engl J Med 2000; 342:1701–7.

102. Gines P, Uriz J, Calahorra B et al. Transjugular intrahepatic portosystemic shunting versus paracentesis plus albumin for refractory ascites in cirrhosis. Gastroenterology 2002; 123:1839–47.

103. Sanyal AJ, Glenning C, Reddy KR et al. North American Study for Treatment of Refractory Ascites Group. Gastroenterology 2003; 124:634–41.

104. Gulberg V, Liss I, Bilzer M et al. Improved quality of life in patients with refractory ascites after insertion of transjugular intrahepatic portosystemic shunts. Digestion 2002; 66:127–30.

105. Cooper S, Olliff S, Elias E. Recanalisation of hepatic veins by a combined transhepatic, transjugular approach in three cases of Budd Chiari syndrome. J Intervent Radiol 1996;11:9–13.

106. Griffith JF, Mahmoud AE, Cooper S et al. Radiological intervention in Budd Chiari syndrome: techniques and outcome in 18 patients. Clin Radiol 1996; 51:775–84.

107. Fisher NC, McCafferty I, Dolapci M et al. Managing Budd Chiari syndrome: a retrospective review of percutaneous hepatic vein angioplasty and surgical shunting. Gut 1999; 44:568–74.

108. Sharma S, Texeira A, Texeira P et al. Pharmacological thrombolysis in Budd Chiari syndrome: a single centre experience and review of the literature. J Hepatol 2004; 40:172–80.

109. Gasparini D, Del Forno M, Sponza M et al. Transjugular intrahepatic portosystemic shunt by direct transcaval approach in patients with acute and hyperacute Budd–Chiari syndrome. Eur J Gastroenterol Hepatol 2002; 14:567–71.

110. Michl P, Bilzer M, Waggershauser T et al. Successful treatment of chronic Budd–Chiari syndrome with a transjugular intrahepatic portosystemic shunt. J Hepatol 2000 32:516–20.

111. Perello A, Garcia-Pagan JC, Gilabert R et al. TIPS is a useful long-term derivative therapy for patients with Budd Chiari syndrome uncontrolled by medical therapy. Hepatology 2002; 35:132–9.

Study showing that the majority of Budd–Chiari patients can be treated effectively by TIPS.

112. Mancuso A, Watkinson A, Tibballs J. Budd Chiari syndrome with portal, splenic and superior mesenteric vein thrombosis treated with TIPS: who dares wins. Gut 2003; 52:438.

113. Pfammatter T, Benoit C, Cathomas G et al. Budd–Chiari syndrome with spleno-mesenteric-portal

thrombosis: treatment with extended TIPS. J Vasc Intervent Radiol 2000; 11:781–4.

114. Ryu RK, Durham JD, Krysl J et al. Role of TIPS as a bridge to hepatic transplantation in Budd Chiari syndrome. J Vasc Intervent Radiology 1999; 10:799–805.

115. Olliff S. Radiological treatment of Budd Chiari syndrome. Imaging 1998; 10:81–8.

116. Stringer MD, Howard ER, Green DW et al. Meso-atrial shunt: a surgical option in the management of the Budd–Chiari syndrome. Br J Surg 1989; 76:474–8.

117. Gauthier F, De Dreuzy O, Valayer J et al. H-type shunt with an autologous venous graft for treatment of portal hypertension in children. J Pediatr Surg 1989; 24:1041–3.

118. Mitra SK, Rao KL, Narasimhan KL et al. Side-to-side lienorenal shunt without splenectomy in non-cirrhotic portal hypertension in children. J Pediatr Surg 1993; 28:398–401.

119. Ciccarelli O, Goffette P, Laterre PF et al. Trans-jugular intrahepatic portosystemic shunt approach and local thrombolysis for treatment of early post-transplant portal vein thrombosis. Transplantation 2001; 72:159–61.

120. Bhattacharjya T, Olliff SP, Bhattacharjya S et al. Percutaneous portal vein thrombolysis and endo-vascular stent for management of posttransplant portal venous conduit thrombosis. Transplantation 2000; 69:2195–8.

121. Granger DR, Klapman JB, McDonald V. Trans-jugular intrahepatic portosystemic shunt (TIPS) for Budd Chiari syndrome or portal vein thrombosis. Am J Gastroenterol 1999; 94:603–8.

122. Uflacker R. Applications of percutaneous mech-anical thrombectomy in transjugular intrahepatic portosystemic shunt and portal vein thrombosis. Tech Vasc Interv Radiol 2003; 6:59–69.

123. Cwikiel W, Solvig J, Schroder H. Stent recanalization of chronic portal vein occlusion in a child. Cardiovasc Intervent Radiol 2000; 23:309–11.

124. Stein M, Link DP. Symptomatic spleno-mesenteric-portal venous thrombosis: recanalization and reconstruction with endovascular stents. J Vasc Intervent Radiol 1999; 10:363–71.

Fenella K.S. Welsh and
John J. Casey

INTRODUCTION

The function and immunological importance of the spleen has only been fully appreciated in the last few decades. In reflection of this, the indications for splenectomy have evolved, and with the advent of minimal access technology, laparoscopic splenectomy is now a widely accepted technique. Furthermore, with advances in diagnostic imaging, surgical philosophy in splenic trauma has moved from nihilistic excision, to spleen-conserving surgery, through to non-operative management.

FUNCTIONAL ANATOMY AND PHYSIOLOGY OF THE SPLEEN

The known functions of the spleen are phagocytosis and the mounting of immune responses, haemopoiesis and erythrocyte storage. Splenic macrophages remove cell debris, microorganisms and old/deformed erythrocytes, leucocytes and platelets from the blood. They also capture, process and present foreign antigen. The spleen is a rich source of T- and B-lymphocytes, and as such is important in the mounting of humoral and cellular immune responses. There is proliferation of splenic macrophages and increased growth and differentiation of antibody-producing plasma cells in response to antigen stimulation. If the individual suffers repeated episodes of blood-borne infection such as malaria, the splenic tissues become permanently hypertrophied and the spleen enlarged. Physiologically, the spleen is an important haemopoietic organ only in the fetus. However, in some anaemias and myeloid leukaemia its haemopoietic function resumes.

SPLENECTOMY

Indications for splenectomy

Of the current indications for splenectomy (**Box 7.1**), the most common is for patients with idiopathic thrombocytopenic purpura (ITP). In patients with ITP, the spleen is the primary site of antiplatelet autoantibody synthesis and of antibody-sensitised platelet sequestration and destruction, and the severity of the disease is related to the magnitude of the thrombocytopenia. Of the other common haematological indications for splenectomy, it should be borne in mind that patients with hereditary spherocytosis should be screened for gallstones, so that cholecystectomy can be performed at the same time if appropriate.

The changing incidence and indications for splenectomy are illustrated in a study by Rose and

54

Box 7.1 • Indications for splenectomy

Elective

Haematological disorders (hereditary spherocytosis, immune thrombocytopenic purpura, autoimmune haemolytic anaemia)

In combination with distal pancreatectomy for pancreatic tumours/chronic pancreatitis

As part of extended resection of gastric tumours

Excision of splenic cysts/abscesses

Staging of haematological malignancies (e.g. Hodgkin's disease)

Treatment of splenic artery aneurysms

Resection of tumours of the spleen

Treatment of gastric varices

Emergency

Major trauma

Iatrogenic injury

Box 7.2 • Guidelines for the prevention and treatment of infection in patients with an absent or dysfunctional spleen

1. All splenectomised patients and those with functional hyposplenism should receive pneumococcal immunisation and undergo reimmunisation every five years. Patients not previously immunised should receive *Haemophilus influenzae* type B vaccine and meningococcal group C conjugate vaccine. Influenza immunisation should be given yearly. Life-long prophylactic antibiotics are recommended (oral phenoxymethyl-penicillin 250–500 mg 12-hourly or an alternative).

2. Some patients fail to mount an antibody response to the vaccine and remain unprotected. Patients taking prophylactic antibiotics remain vulnerable to infection by resistant organisms. Thus patients developing infection, despite measures, must be given systemic antibiotics and admitted urgently to hospital.

3. Patients should be given written information and carry a card to alert health professionals to the risk of overwhelming infection.

4. Patients should be educated as to the potential risks of overseas travel, particularly with regards to malaria and animal bites. Travellers abroad should receive a meningococcal vaccine that protects against group A infections.

5. Patient records should be clearly labelled. Vaccination and revaccination status should be clearly documented.

6. The vaccines should be given a minimum of 2 weeks before elective splenectomy in order to ensure an optimal antibody response. If this has not occurred, or the splenectomy was an emergency, the patient should be immunised as soon as possible.

Reproduced from Davies et al. Clin Med 2002; 2(5):440–3. With permission of the Royal College of Physicians of London.

colleagues, who reviewed all splenectomies performed at a single institution between 1986 and 1995.[1] In this period, 896 patients underwent splenectomy, with the principal indication being trauma (41.5%). The remaining cases included haematological malignancy (15.4%), cytopenia (15.6%), incidental (12.3%), iatrogenic (8.1%), portal hypertension (2.3%), diagnostic (2.0%), and a variety of infrequent pathologies (2.7%). Comparing the first and second 5-year time periods, they noted a 36.9% decrease in incidence of splenectomy for all indications. It is well established that there is an increased risk of overwhelming infection following splenectomy, and this was most marked for haematological malignancy (reduced by 51.4%).[1]

Current guidelines for postsplenectomy prophylaxis

The current guidelines for prevention of postsplenectomy infection were defined by a Working Party of the Clinical Haematology Task Force on behalf of the British Committee for Standards in Haematology in 1996[2] and further revised in 2002[3] (**Box 7.2**). In view of the uncertainty of the level of splenic function achieved by partial splenectomy or autotransplantation of splenic

tissue it is recommended that patients undergoing these procedures should be treated similarly to asplenic patients.

Open splenectomy: technical details

The incision is dependent on the indication for surgery; for example, midline for trauma, rooftop if combined with pancreatic resection. Of the two basic approaches to splenectomy, the medial approach involves early isolation of the splenic artery and vein and is recommended in cases of splenomegaly. The lateral approach involves division of the lienorenal ligament and mobilisation of the spleen into the wound prior to isolation of the vessels, and is favoured for trauma cases where spleen is normal in size.

Nasogastric decompression is not warranted in uncomplicated elective splenectomy although it may facilitate exposure. However, in complicated cases, particularly if there has been injury to the gastric fundus (haematoma or a serosal tear), a nasogastric tube should be placed at the time of surgery to prevent postoperative gastric distension until the gastric ileus resolves.

Meticulous haemostasis of the splenic bed should be a routine and essential part of splenectomy, and in an uncomplicated elective procedure abdominal drainage is unnecessary. Ugochukwu and Irving found an incidence of two subphrenic abscesses following 282 consecutive splenectomies (0.71%). This complication rate is low compared to published series, and they attribute this to the routine use of low-pressure closed suction drainage to the splenic bed and thus advocate this approach.[4] However, in a prospective randomised trial of closed suction drainage or no drainage following splenectomy, Patcher et al. found no difference in the incidence of subphrenic abscess between the two groups.[5]

Others argue that the routine use of open drainage systems increases the incidence of subphrenic abscess.[6,7] The authors would recommend selective drainage of the splenic bed following splenectomy in complicated elective cases or for trauma, although admit that the evidence for this is largely anecdotal and the literature outdated.

Complications of splenectomy

The complications of splenectomy are classified in **Table 7.1.** Their incidence ranges from 15 to 60%, with risk factors including the size of the spleen, the volume of blood lost intraoperatively, the indication for splenectomy, and the age of the patient. In a review of 2417 splenectomies performed in a single institution between 1949 and 1978, it was found that the majority of complications occurred in patients undergoing incidental splenectomy or splenectomy for trauma, not in patients with underlying haematological disease.[8] However, other authors have shown that splenectomy for myelofibrosis[9] or haematological malignancy[10] is associated with increased morbidity and mortality. The type of complication in collected series varies, but respiratory complications are most common (10–48%), followed by thromboembolic complications

Table 7.1 • Complications of splenectomy

	Immediate	Early	Late
Specific			
	Haemorrhage	Collection/abscess	Infection (encapsulated organisms, malaria parasites)
		Arteriovenous fistula	
		Thrombocytosis	Overwhelming postsplenectomy infection (OPSI)
		Splenic, portal, mesenteric vein thrombosis/ischaemic gut	Splenosis
		Pancreatic leak/fistula/pseudocyst	
		Gastric ileus/acute gastric dilatation	
		Gastric necrosis/perforation	
General			
	–	Basal atelectasis/pneumonia	Incisional hernia
		Deep vein thrombosis/pulmonary embolus	
		Wound infection	

(5–11%). Prophylactic aspirin is recommended to prevent this latter complication if the blood platelet count exceeds 10^6/mL. The incidence of subphrenic abscesses (4–8%), pancreatic injury (1–3%), and haemorrhage (1–2%) is much less common.[11]

Overwhelming postsplenectomy infection (OPSI) is rare, with an estimated incidence of 0.23–0.42% per year and a lifetime risk of 5%. Asplenic children under 5 and especially infants splenectomised for trauma have an infection rate of over 10%, much higher than in adults (<1%). The risk of dying of serious infection, although highest within 2 years after surgery, remains lifelong.[12] Early symptoms and signs of OPSI may be very non-specific, often resembling a flu-like illness, but there can be rapid progression to multiorgan failure and death. Hence, episodes of OPSI are emergencies, requiring immediate parenteral antibiotics and intensive care.[13,14] *Streptococcus pneumoniae* accounts for around 90% of cases of OPSI[15,16] and carries a mortality of up to 60%.[11,17] Infection with other encapsulated bacteria such as *Haemophilus influenzae* type b and *Neisseria meningitidis* (meningococcus)[18] can occur, as can infection with *Escherichia coli*,[19] malaria[20] and *Capnocytophaga canimorsus* (DF-2 bacillus associated with dog bites).[21]

OPSI can occur despite immunisation and/or prophylactic antibiotic administration,[22–24] often because of immunisation failure or the presence of resistant organisms. However, appropriate vaccination and antibiotic prophylaxis are not achieved in all asplenic patients. Kyaw et al. investigated the vaccine status and antibiotic prophylaxis in all patients who had undergone splenectomy in Scotland between 1988 and 1998. They found that the administration of pneumococcal vaccination (88%) was higher than that of *Haemophilus influenzae* type b (Hib) conjugate vaccine (70%) or meningococcal vaccine (51%). Only 47% of patients received all three vaccines. Coverage of influenza vaccine increased significantly from 76% in the 1997/1998 period to 96% in the 2000/2001 period. Antibiotic prophylaxis was received by 67% of all patients.[25] This evidence is supported by a retrospective review from Ejstrud et al., who showed that pneumococcal vaccination rates were inadequate (62%), particularly if patients underwent splenectomy during cancer surgery or because of inadvertent intraoperative trauma to the spleen. They also found that documentation of splenectomy and vaccine status was poor, as was communication to the primary care physician.[26] Moreover, education of asplenic patients as to their lifelong risk of infection and the action required should they become unwell is insufficient.[27] In a recent review of 77 reported cases of OPSI, it was found that only 31% of individuals had received pneumococcal vaccination before OPSI, and few patients had been advised adequately on antibiotic prophylaxis or other measures.[16] The overall mortality in this series was 50%.

Evolution of laparoscopic splenectomy

Laparoscopic splenectomy (LS) was first described by Delaitre and Maignien[28] in 1991, with a number of institutions reporting small series in 1992.[29–32] All were performed with the patient in the supine position, using a five-port technique, and the spleen was removed in a bag via the umbilical port after morcellation or finger-fracture. Since then the technique has become widely adopted as it illustrates many of the benefits of minimal-access surgery, although the procedure has evolved. The right lateral decubitus position with the left arm elevated was described by Delaitre[33] in 1995 and refined by Miles et al.[34] in 1996. This position allows the spleen to hang down from its diaphragmatic attachments, facilitating dissection, and allows a four-port rather than a five-port technique to be used. A case-controlled study comparing the results of LS using the anterior versus this lateral approach was performed by Trias et al.[35] The operation was completed laparoscopically in all of the patients who had a lateral approach, compared to 80% of the anterior approach group. The operative time, number of trocars used, transfusion requirements and hospital stay were significantly lower in the group with a lateral approach. Park and co-workers reported after their first 22 cases that the lateral approach afforded superior exposure, allowing easier dissection of splenic hilar structures, and concluded that it was the approach of choice for LS.[36] The same group have recently published their experience of 203 LSs: 3% underwent conversion to an open procedure, the mean operating time was 145 minutes, and 70% of patients were discharged before 48 hours. Their morbidity rate was 9.3%, with zero mortality. The proportion of

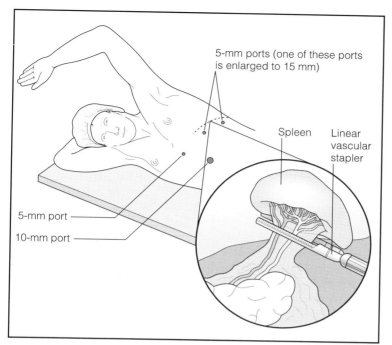

5-mm ports (one of these ports is enlarged to 15 mm)

Spleen

Linear vascular stapler

5-mm port

10-mm port

Figure 7.1 • Port sites for laparoscopic splenectomy. A linear vascular stapler is used to divide the splenic vessels.

of patients undergoing concomitant procedures, usually cholecystectomy for patients with hereditary spherocytosis,[37] was 8.4%. Two further large series report similar results. Corcione et al. describe 105 elective LSs and report a 1% conversion rate, a mean operating time of 95 minutes, and median hospital stay of 4.5 days.[38] Their morbidity rate was 8.6%, with 1% mortality. The second series of 103 consecutive LSs quotes a 4% conversion rate, 5.8% morbidity and zero mortality.[39]

 Laparoscopic splenectomy should be undertaken by the lateral approach with a 30° laparoscope, using the ultrasonic dissector and linear vascular stapler. The specimen is placed in a bag whence it is fragmented and then retrieved (**Fig. 7.1**).

Indications and contraindications to LS

The indications for LS are the same as for open splenectomy (OS). The only absolute contra-indications to laparoscopic splenectomy are severe cardiopulmonary disease or cirrhosis and portal hypertension, where the risk of bleeding from varices and coagulopathy is too great. The issues of

splenomegaly are discussed below. Obesity is not a contraindication; indeed, these patients are ideal for a laparoscopic approach.[40]

Specific complications of laparoscopic splenectomy

The sensitivity of laparoscopy in detecting accessory spleens remains unclear and there is concern that these may be missed due to a less thorough abdominal exploration. The estimated prevalence of accessory spleens ranges from 6 to 12% and thus necessitates a thorough search strategy. Complete exploration for accessory spleens should include the area around the splenic hilum, the greater omentum, close to the greater curvature of the stomach, and the gastrocolic, gastrosplenic and splenocolic ligaments. Meticulous technique to avoid tearing the splenic capsule and the use of a retrieval bag is advocated to prevent splenosis.

Some authors argue that pancreatic injury is more common in LS. Indeed, a retrospective review of 94 procedures by Chand et al. found that 15 patients (16%) had some evidence of pancreatic injury, including: asymptomatic hyperamylasaemia ($N = 6$); symptomatic hyperamylasaemia ($N = 2$); pancreatic

Table 7.2 • Comparison of open (OS) and laparoscopic (LS) splenectomy

Authors (year of publication)	Type of study (grade of recommendation*)	OS N	LS N	Conclusions LS vs. OS
Cordera et al. (2003)[43]	Retrospective, case control (C)	44	42	↑ operating time, ≡ cost ≡ morbidity, ≡ mortality, ↓ pain, ↓ hospital stay
Cogliandolo et al. (2001)[44]	Retrospective, case control (C)	24	20	≡ operating time, ↓ morbidity, ↓ hospital stay
Velanovich et al. (2001)[45]	Prospective, case control (C)	17	27	↓ pain
Park et al. (1999)[46]	Prospective, case control (C)	63	147	↑ operating time, ↓ cost, ↓ morbidity, ↓ hospital stay
Glasgow et al. (1997)[47]	Prospective, case control (C)	28	52	≡ operating time, ≡ morbidity, ↓ ileus, ↓ hospital stay, ↓ cost
Brunt ML et al. (1996)[48]	Retrospective, case control (C)	20	26	↑ operating time, ≡ morbidity, ↓ ileus, ↓ pain, ↓ hospital stay
Rhodes et al. (1995)[49]	Prospective, case control (C)	11	22	↑ operating time, ↓ hospital stay

*Grade C recommendation arises from Level III (non-randomised studies with contemporaneous controls) and Level IV (non-randomised studies with historical controls) evidence.

collections ($N = 6$) and pancreatic fistula ($N = 1$). They suggest that serum amylase should be measured routinely in the postoperative period to alert the surgeon early to a possible pancreatic injury and to thus alter postoperative management.[41] In contrast, other series report pancreatic injury rates of only 1–6%.[40]

Care should be taken to avoid injury to the tail of pancreas by keeping the plane of dissection close to the splenic hilum, and it is likely that increasing experience will minimise the operative morbidity. In a prospective review of 122 LSs, Targarona and colleagues found that the overall complication rate was 18%, the majority being either pulmonary (26%) or haemorrhagic (35%). A multivariate analysis revealed that the operator's learning curve, patient's age, spleen weight, and a diagnosis of malignancy were all independent predictors of complications.[42]

Evidence that laparoscopic splenectomy is preferable to the open approach

LS can be achieved safely and efficiently, but what is the evidence that the laparoscopic approach is better than open splenectomy (OS)? Indeed, minimal-access surgery has been criticised in the past by the medical community for being adopted rapidly and widely without sufficient evidence base. The authors believe that there is no published prospective randomised controlled trial of LS versus OS. **Table 7.2** details seven case–control studies that compare the two approaches.[43–49] These suggest that whilst LS may be associated with a longer operating time, it results in fewer complications, a shorter hospital stay and reduced cost compared to OS.

Laparoscopic removal of the enlarged spleen: is it feasible?

Splenomegaly was initially thought to be a relative contraindication to the laparoscopic approach, and it certainly increases the technical difficulty of the procedure. In assessing the evidence, it is apparent that there is no universally adopted definition of splenomegaly, particularly with regard to weight. Targarona et al. compared 105 prospective LSs to a retrospective cohort of 81 patients who underwent open splenectomy.[50] Patients were classified into three groups according to spleen weight: group A, <400 g; group B, 400–1000 g; and group C, >1000 g. Operative time was significantly longer for LS than for OS. However, LS morbidity, mortality and postoperative stay were all lower at similar spleen weights. Spleens weighing more than 3200 g required conversion to open surgery in all cases. When looking at the LS group only, the authors found that the operative time was significantly longer in patients with larger spleens, and an accessory incision was more frequently required. However, there were no significant differences in transfusion rate, length of stay, severe morbidity, or conversion rate between the three different weight groups.[51] Similar results were found by Heniford et al. in a prospective study of 142 patients undergoing LS, which compared the outcome of patients with normal-sized spleens (<150 g) and those with splenomegaly (>500 g). Whilst the mean operative times and estimated blood loss were lower for those patients with normal-sized spleens, there were no statistical differences between the two groups in terms of conversion rate, length of stay or complications.[52] It could be argued, however, that the definition of splenomegaly used in this latter study was somewhat conservative. Terrosu and colleagues performed a prospective analysis of 20 LSs for splenomegaly and 40 LSs for normal-sized spleens and found that for spleens weighing <2000 g, the outcome was comparable to that for normal spleens, whereas LS for spleens >2000 g was associated with a higher conversion rate, greater blood loss, a longer hospital stay, and increased morbidity.[53] This is supported by results from Patel and others in a series of 108 consecutive laparoscopic splenectomies.[54] They defined massive splenomegaly as a splenic weight of >1000 g, which represented 25% of their cases (median weight 2500 g). These patients had a significantly longer median operating time, conversion rate, postoperative morbidity and median postoperative stay compared to patients with spleens weighing <1000 g. Multivariate analysis found splenic weight to be the most powerful predictor of morbidity, and patients with splenomegaly (>1000 g) were 14 times more likely to have postoperative complications. Similar results were found by Mahon and Rhodes,[55] who also reported a zero conversion rate for LS in patients with a splenic weight of <1000 g (N = 29),

compared to a 60% conversion rate in patients with spleens >1000 g (N = 10). Thus whilst LS is feasible in patients with splenomegaly, for patients with massively enlarged spleens (>1000 g) the procedure seems to be associated with greater morbidity and the advantages of a laparoscopic approach are not so clear.

In the early experience of laparoscopic splenectomy for splenomegaly, preoperative selective embolisation of the splenic artery was used to facilitate the procedure.[56,57] However, with increased experience, adoption of the lateral approach and improved technology, any additional benefit of embolisation must be weighed against the potential complications of severe pain, migration of coils to the liver and splenic abscesses. This approach has, therefore, largely been abandoned. A more promising approach is the use of hand-assisted laparoscopy (HAL), which offers the same benefits of minimally invasive surgery while allowing safe manipulation and dissection of the enlarged spleen. Furthermore, when an abdominal incision for removal of an intact spleen is planned, the incision can be placed to facilitate surgery with HAL. Rosen and co-workers undertook a retrospective analysis of patients with splenomegaly undergoing conventional LS compared to hand-assisted LS (HALS).[58] They found that the HALS group had significantly larger spleens than the conventional LS group (mean weight 1516 g versus 1031 g) but that the mean operative time, estimated blood loss, length of hospital stay and complication rates were similar. Several authors are strong advocates of HALS in cases of splenomegaly, having found that it was associated with less morbidity, a shorter operative time, and a shorter hospital stay.[59,60]

 There is increasing evidence that either HALS or an open approach should be considered when performing splenectomy in patients with splenomegaly.

SPLENIC TRAUMA

Incidence

In the UK, fewer than 10% of severely injured patients require surgical intervention in the abdomen for blunt trauma.[61,62] However, the spleen remains the most commonly injured organ after blunt abdominal trauma despite its protected location inside the rib cage.

Aetiology

In addition to road traffic accidents (RTAs), causes of splenic trauma include falls, sporting injuries, and iatrogenic and spontaneous rupture. Rupture may result from minimal trauma in cases of spleno-megaly secondary to haematological disorders or infections such as malaria or Epstein–Barr virus. The extent of iatrogenic splenic injury is perhaps not appreciated. In a recent comprehensive literature review, Cassar and Munro found that up to 40% of all splenectomies performed during abdominal surgery are for iatrogenic injury.[63] They identified that the risk of splenic injury is highest during left hemicolectomy (1–8%), open antireflux procedures (3–20%), left nephrectomy (4–13%) and during exposure and reconstruction of the proximal abdominal aorta and its branches (21–60%). They showed that the consequences of such splenic injury included a prolonged operating time, increased blood loss, longer hospital stay, and a 2–10-fold increase in infection rate. The risk of injury to the spleen was higher in patients who had undergone previous abdominal surgery, in the elderly and in obese patients. Excessive traction or retraction and direct trauma are the commonest mechanisms of

injury. Iatrogenic splenic trauma can also occur less directly. It is a rare but recognised complication of colonoscopy[64] and has been reported as a consequence of cardiopulmonary resuscitation or following anticoagulation.

Classification of splenic injury

The classification of splenic injury described in 1989 by Moore and colleagues[65] and revised by them in 1994[66] has been adopted for general use by the American Association for the Surgery of Trauma (AAST) (**Table 7.3**). The injury grade is calculated from assessment of the splenic injury using information derived from radiological studies, operative findings or autopsy report; for multiple injuries to the spleen the grade is advanced by one stage. The organ injury score does not assign prognostic value to a specific injury, but rather provides a clearer description of the injury, to facilitate objective comparison of splenic trauma management.

Initial assessment

The initial assessment of a patient with suspected splenic injury is the same as for any trauma patient and should be according to the Advanced Trauma Life Support (ATLS) principles of primary survey and resuscitation, followed by secondary survey

Table 7.3 • Splenic Injury Scale used by the American Association for the Surgery of Trauma (AAST)

Grade		Injury description	
I	Haematoma	Subcapsular, <10% surface area	
	Laceration	Capsular tear, <1 cm parenchymal depth	
II	Haematoma	Subcapsular, 10–50% surface area	
		Intraparenchymal, <5 cm in diameter	
	Laceration	1–3 cm parenchymal depth, which does not involve a trabecular vessel	
III	Haematoma	Subcapsular, >50% surface area or expanding; ruptured subcapsular or parenchymal haematoma	
		Intraparenchymal haematoma >5 cm or expanding	
	Laceration	>3 cm parenchymal depth, or involving trabecular vessels	
IV	Laceration	Laceration involving segmental or hilar vessels producing major devascularisation (>25% of spleen)	
V	Laceration	Completely shattered spleen	
	Vascular	Hilar vascular injury that devascularises spleen	

Advance one grade for multiple injuries, up to grade III.

and definitive care. The concept of 'permissive hypotension', with which the vascular surgeon is familiar in the management of the leaking aortic aneurysm, is gaining support in trauma care.[67] It is now accepted that aggressive and multiple cycles of fluid resuscitation with the aim of elevating blood pressure to pre-injury levels and prior to operative control of the bleeding site may result in progressive and repeated re-bleeding ('popping the clot'), depletion of platelets and clotting factors, and hypothermia. Maintaining the systolic blood pressure just below 80 mmHg allows vital end-organ perfusion but limits haemorrhage, as the patient is being transferred to definitive care.

Management

The haemodynamically unstable patient with abdominal trauma requires a laparotomy. If haemodynamically stable, the patient should undergo contrast-enhanced computed tomography (CT), which is approximately 95% sensitive and specific for detection of splenic injury. A negative initial ultrasound in the stable patient should not be relied on, regardless of patient age. In cases of clinically suspected abdominal trauma, another assessment (e.g. CT) must be performed since, despite its high specificity, ultrasonography has an unexpectedly low sensitivity for the detection of both free fluid and organ lesions and tends to downgrade the severity of injury.[68,69]

> Haemodynamically stable patients with abdominal trauma should undergo contrast-enhanced CT scanning. Unless the CT shows a grade V splenic injury, or other injuries requiring laparotomy, the patient should be managed non-operatively in the first instance, within a high-dependency or intensive care unit. Evidence of ongoing haemorrhage or delayed recognition of other injuries necessitating laparotomy should be regarded as failure of non-operative management.

Increasing appreciation of the risk of OPSI has led to routine attempts at splenic conservation and non-operative management after trauma. This was initially adopted by paediatric surgeons in the 1970s, and by the late 1980s was coming into practice in adult trauma. This change in surgical philosophy

is illustrated by Pachter and colleagues, who compared management of splenic injury in a single trauma centre in two time-periods.[70] Before 1990, over an 11-year study period involving 193 patients, splenorrhaphy was the most common splenic salvage method noted (66% overall), with non-operative management employed in only 13% of blunt splenic injuries. Between 1990 and 1996, the authors found that in 190 consecutive patients with splenic injuries, 102/190 (54%) were managed non-operatively, including 96 (65%) of 147 patients with blunt trauma. Of the patients treated operatively, 56 (29%) patients underwent splenectomy and 32 splenorrhaphy (17%). Two patients failed non-operative therapy (2%) and underwent splenectomy, and one patient required splenectomy after partial splenic resection. There were no deaths among the patients treated non-operatively. Similar results were found in a retrospective review of 207 patients admitted with splenic trauma to a US hospital between 1965 and 1994. In this study, the number of patients treated by splenorrhaphy and observation markedly increased during the study period with no adverse outcome and achieving shorter hospital stays.[71]

Should splenic injury be managed differently in children or the elderly?

Non-operative management of splenic injury appears to be more successful in children and has been addressed in two recent large studies.[72,73] These confirm that the rate of spleen salvage and non-operative management is higher in children than in adults. The data suggest that this may be due to differing mechanisms of injury (more RTAs and motor cycle injuries in adults; more falls and sports injuries in children), which result in lower injury severity scores and splenic injury scores in children compared to adults.

Age greater than 55 years has been proposed as a predictor for failure of, and even a contraindication to, non-operative management of blunt splenic trauma. In a study of 251 consecutive patients admitted to a Level 1 Trauma Centre with blunt splenic trauma, Myers et al. performd a subgroup analysis of 23 patients aged 55 years. They found that 17/23 patients (74%) were treated successfully without operation.[74] In contrast, Tsugawa et al. suggest that the threshold for operative intervention in patients with splenic trauma should be lower in the elderly. In a retrospective review of 167 patients with blunt splenic trauma presenting between 1983 and 1997, they classified 116 patients as young (<60 years old) and 51 patients as elderly (>60 years old). They found higher injury severity scores, lower Glasgow Coma Scales and a higher mortality in the elderly. The younger patients had a higher rate of non-operative management compared to the elderly (63% versus 32%) and a lower incidence of splenectomy (29% versus 52%). Ten percent of elderly patients failed non-operative management, compared to 5% of young patients. They suggest that criteria for early operative intervention should be lowered in the elderly to include those with a grade IV splenic injury, because of the increased fragility of the spleen and decreased physiological reserve in this group.[75]

Improving non-operative management rates: the role of angiography

Davis et al. found that a contrast blush on CT was a predictor of failure of non-operative management and suggest that these patients should undergo aggressive surveillance for and embolisation of post-traumatic splenic artery pseudoaneurysms.[76] They found that this policy improved the rate of successful non-operative management of blunt splenic trauma to 61%, with a non-operative failure rate of only 6%.

It is not clear that all haemodynamically stable patients with blunt splenic injury should undergo mandatory angiography. In 1995, Sclafani et al. reported on the first series of splenic artery embolisation for treatment of patients with blunt splenic injury.[77] In that series, all patients with splenic injury underwent angiography, and the overall splenic salvage rate was 98.5%. In a Level 1 US Trauma Centre, it was found that the yield of angiography increased with the AAST grade of splenic injury and that less than 5% of angiograms in grade 1 injuries were positive.[78] The authors of this study advocate a selective policy, using angio-

graphy in stable patients with grade 3 or higher injuries and those with CT scan evidence of ongoing bleeding or the presence of pseudoaneurysm. This approach can achieve an overall non-operative management rate of 74%, with only 3% of patients failing non-operative management.

The criteria for angiography in haemodynamically stable patients with splenic trauma are patients with grade 3 or higher injuries and those with CT scan evidence of ongoing bleeding or the presence of pseudoaneurysm. A selective policy of angiography appears to be associated with an increased non-operative rate.

Time of discharge and follow-up after non-operative management

Most failures of non-operative management occur within 72 hours of admission.[78,79] After this length of time on a high-dependency unit, patients can be 'stepped-down' to the surgical ward and depending on their other injuries and home circumstances, discharge considered with strict limitation on activities.

A number of studies have addressed the issue of follow-up imaging studies (either CT or ultrasound) and all conclude that these are of little value since they only demonstrate progression of injury and do not change management in the stable, asymptomatic patient.[80–84]

Patients managed non-operatively should be in a high-dependency environment for the first three days.
Follow-up imaging studies, during non-operative management, should not be performed routinely.

Operative management of splenic injury

For splenic trauma, the incision should be in the upper midline, extending the wound below the umbilicus if other injuries are encountered in the infracolic compartment. The surgical principles for splenic trauma are control of haemorrhage, assessment of severity of splenic injury, and active exclusion of other injuries. If feasible the spleen should be conserved, otherwise splenectomy should be performed without causing further complications.

Once the abdomen is opened, all four quadrants are packed. With consideration to the anaesthetic team and the patient's condition, a full laparotomy is then performed in a systematic fashion. The extent of splenic injury is evaluated according to the AAST grade, which aids operative decision-making. Grade V splenic injuries will require splenectomy. Splenic conservation or preservation should be attempted in grade I–IV injuries, depending on individual circumstances (concomitant injuries, patient age and comorbidity). Available techniques to achieve this include fibrin glue,[85,86] an omental patch, use of an absorbable mesh bag,[87] or partial splenectomy. This approach is illustrated by the experience of Pickhardt's group, who reported their management of 170 adults with splenic injury identified at emergency laparotomy between 1982 and 1987.[88] Their rate of operative splenic salvage was 63% (107/170). Grade I splenic injuries were amenable to haemostatic agents alone, and suturing or mesh enclosure was necessary in 43% of grade II and in all grade III injuries. Grade IV disruption required anatomical splenic resection for haemorrhage control in 88% of cases. Of the 63 patients (37%) who underwent splenectomy, 76% had grade V injuries, and the remaining 24% were performed expeditiously in multisystem injured patients with concomitant life-threatening injuries.

Outcome of splenic trauma

The outcome of patients with splenic trauma depends on the extent of blood loss, their other injuries and underlying comorbidity. Carlin and colleagues reviewed the outcome of 546 consecutive patients with penetrating and blunt splenic trauma seen over a 17.5-year (1980–1997).[89] The most significant risk factors for death were all associated with major blood loss: transfusion requirements >6 units of blood, low initial blood pressure, associated abdominal vascular injuries and performance of a thoracotomy. The two most important organs injured in conjunction with the spleen that were significant predictors of postoperative infectious complications were the colon and the pancreas.

Key points

Laparoscopic splenectomy is safe and effective, even in splenomegaly. However, in massive splenomegaly (>1000 g), consider hand-assisted laparoscopic splenectomy or open splenectomy.

Overwhelming postsplenectomy infection (OPSI) is rare but associated with high mortality.

Postsplenectomy guidelines must be followed.

Stable splenic trauma must be assessed by CT, with the aim of managing grade I–IV injuries non-operatively in the first instance.

REFERENCES

1. Rose AT, Newman MI, Debelak J et al. The incidence of splenectomy is decreasing: lessons learned from trauma experience. Am Surg 2000; 66(5):481–6.

2. Working Party of the British Committee for Standards in Haematology Clinical Haematology Task Force. Guidelines for the prevention and treatment of infection in patients with an absent or dysfunctional spleen. Br Med J 1996; 312:430–4.

3. Davies JM, Barnes R, Milligan D. British Committee for Standards in Haematology. Working Party of the Haematology/Oncology Task Force. Update of guidelines for the prevention and treatment of infection in patients with an absent or dysfunctional spleen. Clin Med 2002; 2(5):440–3.

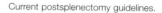
Current postsplenectomy guidelines.

4. Ugochukwu AI, Irving M. Intraperitoneal low-pressure suction drainage following splenectomy. Br J Surg 1985; 72(3):247–8.

5. Patcher HL, Hofstetter SR, Spencer FC. Evolving concepts of splenic surgery: splenorrhaphy versus splenectomy and postsplenectomy drainage. Experience in 105 patients. Ann Surg 1981, 194:262–9.

6. Olsen WR, Beaudois DS. Wound drainage after splenectomy. Am J Surg 1969, 117:615–20.

7. Cerise EJ, Pierce WA, Diamond DC. Abdominal drains: their role as a source of infection following splenectomy. Ann Surg 1970, 171:764–9.

8. Traetow WD, Fabri PJ, Carey LC. Changing indications for splenectomy. Arch Surg 1980; 115:447–51.

9. Arnoletti JP, Karam J, Brodsky J. Early postoperative complications of splenectomy for hematologic disease. Am J Clin Oncol 1999; 22(2):114–18.

10. Horowitz J, Smith JL, Weber TK et al. Postoperative complications after splenectomy for hematologic malignancies. Ann Surg 1996; 223(3):290–6.

11. Ellison E, Fabri PJ. Complications of splenectomy: etiology, prevention and management. Surg Clin North Am 1983; 63:1313–30.

Comprehensive review article.

12. Shaw JH, Print CG. Postsplenectomy sepsis. Br J Surg 1989; 76:1074–81.

13. Davidson RN, Wall RA. Prevention and management of infections in patients without a spleen. Clin Microbiol Infect 2001; 7(12):657–60.

14. Lynch AM, Kapila R. Overwhelming post-splenectomy infection. Infect Dis Clin North Am 1996; 10(4):693–707.

15. Styrt B. Infection associated with asplenia: risks, mechanisms, and prevention. Am J Med 1990; 88(5N): 33N–42N.

16. Waghorn DJ. Overwhelming infection in asplenic patients: current best practice preventive measures are not being followed. J Clin Pathol 2001; 54(3):214–18.

17. Holdsworth RJ, Irving AD, Cuschieri A. Post-splenectomy sepsis and its mortality rate: actual versus perceived risks. Br J Surg 1991; 78:1031–8.

18. Traub A, Giebink GS, Smith C et al. Splenic reticulo-endothelial function after splenectomy, spleen repair and spleen autotransplantation. N Engl J Med 1987; 317:1559–64.

19. Edwards LD, Digiola R. Infections in splenectomised patients. A study of 131 patients. Scand J Infect Dis 1976; 8:255–61.

20. Oster CN, Koontz LC, Wyler CJ. Malaria in asplenic mice: effects of splenectomy, congenital asplenia and splenic reconstitution on the course of infection. Am J Trop Med Hyg 1980; 29:1138–42.

21. McCarthy M, Zumla A. DF-2 infection. Br Med J 1988; 297:135–6.

22. Evans DI. Fatal post-splenectomy sepsis despite prophylaxis with penicillin and pneumococcal vaccine. Lancet 1984; 1:1124.

23. Ejstrud P, Kristensen B, Hansen JB et al. Risk and patterns of bacteraemia after splenectomy: a population-based study. Scand J Infect Dis 2000; 32:521–5.

24. Brivet F, Herer B, Frernaux A et al. Fatal post-splenectomy pneumococcal sepsis despite pneumococcal vaccine and penicillin prophylaxis. Lancet 1984; 2:356–7.

25. Kyaw MH, Holmes EM, Chalmers J et al. A survey of vaccine coverage and antibiotic prophylaxis in splenectomised patients in Scotland. J Clin Pathol 2002; 55(6):472–4.

26. Ejstrud P, Hansen JB, Andreasen DA. Prophylaxis against pneumococcal infection after splenectomy: a challenge for hospitals and primary care. Eur J Surg 1997; 163(10):733–8.

27. Brigden ML, Pattullo AL. Prevention and management of overwhelming postsplenectomy infection – an update. Crit Care Med 1999; 27(4):836–42.

28. Delaitre B, Maignien B. Splenectomy by the coelioscopic approach. Report of a case [Letter]. Presse Med 1991; 20:2263.

29. Thibault C, Mamazza J, Letourneau R et al. Laparoscopic splenectomy: operative technique and preliminary report. Surg Laparosc Endosc 1992; 2(3):248–53.

30. Delaitre B, Maignien B. Laparoscopic splenectomy – technical aspects. Surg Endosc 1992; 6(6):305–8.

31. Carroll BJ, Phillips EH, Semel CJ et al. Laparoscopic splenectomy. Surg Endosc 1992; 6(4):183–5.

32. Hashizume M, Sugimachi K, Ueno K. Laparoscopic splenectomy with an ultrasonic dissector. N Engl J Med 1992; 327(6):438.

33. Delaitre B. Laparoscopic splenectomy. The 'hanged spleen' technique. Surg Endosc 1995; 9(5):528–9.

34. Miles WF, Greig JD, Wilson RG et al. Technique of laparoscopic splenectomy with a powered vascular linear stapler. Br J Surg 1996; 83(9):1212–14.

35. Trias M, Targarona EM, Balague C. Laparoscopic splenectomy: an evolving technique. A comparison between anterior and lateral approaches. Surg Endosc 1996; 10(4):389–92.

36. Park A, Gagner M, Pomp A. The lateral approach to laparoscopic splenectomy. Am J Surg 1997; 173(2):126–30.

37. Park AE, Birgisson G, Mastrangelo MJ et al. Laparoscopic splenectomy: outcomes and lessons learned from over 200 cases. Surgery 2000, 128(4):660–7.

38. Corcione F, Esposito C, Cuccurullo D et al. Technical standardization of laparoscopic splenectomy: experience with 105 cases. Surg Endosc 2002; 16(6):972–4.

39. Katkhouda N, Hurwitz MB, Rivera RT et al. Laparoscopic splenectomy: outcome and efficacy in 103 consecutive patients. Ann Surg 1998; 228(4):568–78.

40. Katkhouda N, Mavor E. Laparoscopic splenectomy. Surg Clin North Am 2000; 80(4):1285–97.

Comprehensive review article, including details of operative technique.

41. Chand B, Walsh RM, Ponsky J et al. Pancreatic complications following laparoscopic splenectomy. Surg Endosc 2001; 15(11):1273–6.

42. Targarona EM, Espert JJ, Bombuy E et al. Complications of laparoscopic splenectomy. Arch Surg 2000; 135(10):1137–40.

43. Cordera F, Long KH, Nagorney DM et al. Open versus laparoscopic splenectomy for idiopathic

thrombocytopenic purpura: clinical and economic analysis. Surgery 2003; 134(1):45–52.

44. Cogliandolo A, Berland-Dai B, Pidoto RR et al. Results of laparoscopic and open splenectomy for nontraumatic diseases. Surg Laparosc Endosc Perc Tech 2001; 11(4):256–61.

45. Velanovich V, Shurafa MS. Clinical and quality of life outcomes of laparoscopic and open splenectomy for haematological diseases. Eur J Surg 2001; 167(1):23–8.

46. Park A, Marcaccio M, Sternbach M et al. Laparoscopic vs open splenectomy. Arch Surg 1999; 134(11):1263–9.

47. Glasgow RE, Yee LF, Mulvihill SJ. Laparoscopic splenectomy. The emerging standard. Surg Endosc 1997; 11(2):108–12.

48. Brunt ML, Langer JC, Quasebarth MA et al. Comparative analysis of laparoscopic versus open splenectomy. Am J Surg 1996; 172(5):596–601.

49. Rhodes M, Rudd M, O'Rourke N et al. Laparoscopic splenectomy and lymph node biopsy for hematologic disorders. Ann Surg 1995; 222(1):43–6.

50. Targarona EM, Espert JJ, Cerdan G et al. Effect of spleen size on splenectomy outcome. A comparison of open and laparoscopic surgery. Surg Endosc 1999; 13(6):559–62.

51. Targarona EM, Espert JJ, Balague C et al. Splenomegaly should not be considered a contraindication for laparoscopic splenectomy. Ann Surg 1998; 228(1):35–9.

52. Heniford BT, Park A, Walsh RM et al. Laparoscopic splenectomy in patients with normal-sized spleens versus splenomegaly: does size matter? Am Surg 2001; 67(9):854–7, discussion 857–8.

53. Terrosu G, Baccarani U, Bresadola V et al. The impact of splenic weight on laparoscopic splenectomy for splenomegaly. Surg Endosc 2002; 16(1):103–7.

54. Patel AG, Parker JE, Wallwork B et al. Massive splenomegaly is associated with significant morbidity after laparoscopic splenectomy. Ann Surg 2003, 238(2):235–40.

55. Mahon D, Rhodes M. Laparoscopic splenectomy: size matters. Ann R Coll Surg Engl 2003, 85:248–51.

56. Totte E, Van Hee R, Kloeck I et al. Laparoscopic splenectomy after arterial embolisation. Hepatogastroenterology 1998; 45(21):773–6.

57. Poulin EC, Mamazza J, Schlachta CM. Splenic artery embolisation before laparoscopic splenectomy. An update. Surg Endosc 1998; 12(6):870–5.

58. Rosen M, Brody F, Walsh RM et al. Hand-assisted laparoscopic splenectomy vs conventional laparoscopic splenectomy in cases of splenomegaly. Arch Surg 2002; 137(12):1348–52.

59. Ailawadi G, Yahanda A, Dimick JB et al. Hand-assisted laparoscopic splenectomy in patients with splenomegaly or prior upper abdominal operation. Surgery 2002; 132(4):689–94.

60. Targarona EM, Balague C, Cerdan G et al. Hand-assisted laparoscopic splenectomy (HALS) in cases of splenomegaly: a comparison analysis with conventional laparoscopic splenectomy. Surg Endosc 2002; 16(3):426–30.

61. Templeton J, Bickley S. The organisation of trauma care in the UK. J Royal Soc Med 1998; 91:23–5.

62. Bain IH, Kirby RM, Cook AL et al. Role of general surgeons in a British trauma centre. Br J Surg 1996; 83:1248–51.

63. Cassar K, Munro A. Iatrogenic splenic injury. J R Coll Surg Edin 2002; 47(6):731–41.

64. Moses RE, Leskowitz SC. Splenic rupture after colonoscopy. J Clin Gastrol 1997; 4(4):257–8.

65. Moore EE, Shackford SR, Patcher HL et al. Organ injury scaling system: spleen, liver and kidney. J Trauma 1989; 29:1664–6.

66. Moore EE, Cogbill TH, Jurkovich GJ et al. Organ injury scaling system: spleen and liver (1994 revision). J Trauma 1995; 38:323–4.

67. Mattox KM. Permissive hypotension [Editorial]. Available online: http://www.trauma.org 8:1, Jan 2003.

Succinct and elegant argument for permissive hypotension in trauma care.

68. Stengel D, Bauwens K, Sehouli J et al. Systematic review and meta-analysis of emergency ultrasonography for blunt abdominal trauma. Br J Surg 2001; 88(7):901–12.

69. Krupnick AS, Teitelbaum DH, Geiger JD et al. Use of abdominal ultrasonography to assess paediatric splenic trauma. Potential pitfalls in the diagnosis. Ann Surg 1997; 225(4):408–14.

Two studies illustrating the problems with ultrasound assessment in splenic trauma.

70. Pachter HL, Guth AA, Hofstetter SR et al. Changing patterns in the management of splenic trauma: the impact of nonoperative management. Ann Surg 1998; 227(5):708–17, discussion 717–19.

71. Morrell DG, Chang FC, Helmer SD. Changing trends in the management of splenic injury. Am J Surg 1995; 170(6):686–9, discussion 690.

72. Powell M, Courcoulas A, Gardner M et al. Management of blunt splenic trauma: significant differences between adults and children. Surgery 1997; 122(4):654–60.

73. Konstantakos AK, Barnoski AL, Plaisier BR et al. Optimizing the management of blunt splenic injury in adults and children. Surgery 1999; 26(4):805–12, discussion 812–13.

74. Myers JG, Dent DL, Stewart RM et al. Blunt splenic injuries: dedicated trauma surgeons can achieve a high rate of non-operative success in patients of all ages. J Trauma 2000; 48(5):801–5, discussion 805–6.

75. Tsugawa K, Koyanagi N, Hashizume M et al. New insight for management of blunt splenic trauma: significant differences between young and elderly. Hepatogastroenterology 2002; 49(46):1144–9.

76. Davis KA, Fabian TC, Croce MA et al. Improved success in nonoperative management of blunt splenic injuries: embolisation of splenic artery pseudoaneurysms. J Trauma 1998; 44(6):1008–13; discussion 1013–5.

77. Sclafani SJ, Shaftan GW, Scalea TM et al. Non-operative salvage of computed tomography-diagnosed splenic injuries: utilization of angiography for triage and embolisation for haemostasis. J Trauma 1995; 39:818–27.

78. Haan J, Ilahi ON, Kramer M et al. Protocol-driven non-operative management in patients with blunt splenic trauma and minimal associated injury decreases length of stay. J Trauma 2003; 55(2):317–21, discussion 321–2.

79. Meguid AA, Bair HA, Howells GA et al. Prospective evaluation of criteria for the nonoperative management of blunt splenic trauma. Am Surg 2003; 69(3):238–42, discussion 242–3.

80. Allins A, Ho T, Nguyen TH et al. Limited value of routine follow-up CT scans in non-operative management of blunt liver and splenic injuries. Am Surg 1996; 62(11):883–6.

81. Thaemert BC, Cogbill TH, Lambert PJ. Non-operative management of splenic injury: are follow-up computed tomographic scans of any value? J Trauma 1997; 43(5):748–51.

82. Lawson DE, Jacobson JA, Spizarny DL et al. Splenic trauma: value of follow-up CT. Radiology 1995; 194(1):97–100.

83. Lyass S, Sela T, Lebensart PD et al. Follow-up imaging studies of blunt splenic injury: do they influence management? Israel Med Assoc J 2001; 3(10):731–3.

84. Rovin JD, Alford BA, McIlhenny TJ et al. Follow-up abdominal computed tomography after splenic trauma in children may not be necessary. Am Surg 2001; 67(2):127–30.

85. Ochsner MG, Maniscalco-Theberge ME, Champion HR. Fibrin glue as a haemostatic agent in hepatic and splenic trauma. J Trauma 1990; 30(7):884–7.

86. Kram HB, del Junco T, Clark SR et al. Techniques of splenic preservation using fibrin glue. J Trauma 1990; 30(1):97–101.

87. Fingerhut A, Oberlin P, Cotte JL et al. Splenic salvage using an absorbable mesh: feasibility, reliability and safety. Br J Surg 1992; 79(4):325–7.

88. Pickhardt B, Moore EE, Moore FA et al. Operative splenic salvage in adults: a decade perspective. J Trauma 1989; 29(10):1386–91.

89. Carlin AM, Tyburski JG, Wilson RF et al. Factors affecting the outcome of patients with splenic trauma. Am Surg 2002; 68(3):232–9.

Eight

Gallstones

Leslie K. Nathanson and
Ian M. Shaw

INTRODUCTION

Gallstones remain one of the commonest surgical problems in the developed world, and despite major therapeutic advances in recent years, there has been no progress in the prevention of gallstone development. In the UK it has been estimated from autopsy studies that approximately 12% of men and 24% of women of all ages have gallstones present.[1] The prevalence in North America is comparable to that in the UK, and it is believed that 10–30% of gallstones become symptomatic. There is a high prevalence in American Indians, who have an incidence of 50% in men and 75% in women in the age group 25–44 years, and this points to the importance of genetic factors in the aetiology of gallstones. In the UK more than 40 000 cholecystectomies are performed each year,[2] whereas in the USA approximately 500 000 operations are performed annually.[3] The incidence of common bile duct stones found before or during cholecystectomy is approximately 12%,[4] indicating that in the UK alone more than 4000 common bile ducts require stone clearance annually.

Composition, formation and risk factors

Gallstones are usually designated as cholesterol stones, mixed stones or pigment stones.[5] Pure cholesterol and pure pigment stones account for only 20% of gallstones, and mixed stones are considered as variants of cholesterol stones as they usually contain over 50% cholesterol and account for about 80% of gallstones in Western countries. Chemical analysis shows a continuous spectrum of stone composition rather than three mutually exclusive stone types, and 10–20% contain enough calcium to be rendered radio-opaque.

The two most important determinants of gallstone frequency in any population are age and gender; gallstones become more common with increasing age and are at least twice as common in women.[6] The increased frequency in women becomes manifest at puberty, and an increased risk of gallstones is conferred by parity and by the ingestion of oral contraceptives.[7] Other factors related to the development of cholesterol gallstones include obesity, ileal disease or resection, cirrhosis, cystic fibrosis, diabetes mellitus, long-term parenteral nutrition, impaired gallbladder emptying, ingestion of clofibrate,[8] heart transplant,[9] and periods of dieting on a very low fat diet.[10] A positive family history of previous cholecystectomy also increases the risk of developing symptomatic gallstone disease.[11] Increasing evidence is emerging that impaired colonic motility contributes to stone formation, and speculation arises for this as a means of prevention.[12]

Little is known of the epidemiology and cause of bilirubin stones. They are especially common in the Far East and become more frequent with increasing age, although occurring with equal frequency in men and women. They may be associated with haemolytic anaemia, cirrhosis and infection of bile with β-glucuronidase-producing bacteria such as *Escherichia coli* and *Bacteroides* species, and occur in diseases affecting the ileum due to increased enterohepatic cycling of bilirubin.[13] The metabolic mechanisms responsible for the formation of cholesterol gallstones centre on the solubility of the main constituents of bile.[14] The bile acid conjugates have detergent-like properties and form micelles in aqueous solution. Lecithin is incorporated with bile acids into micelles, and these also incorporate cholesterol, thereby promoting its solubility in the aqueous environment of bile. The capacity of this solubilising system may, under certain circumstances, be exceeded and bile is then converted into a state of cholesterol supersaturate, thereby favouring the nidation of cholesterol microcrystals. There is evidence to suggest that factors responsible for cholesterol microcrystal nucleation and for its inhibition are present in bile.[15,16] Excessive secretion of cholesterol in the bile may account for the increased predisposition to gallstones in obese patients, those ingesting oestrogens, and during pregnancy.

Biliary stasis, diminished gallbladder function, and diet have similarly been implicated. Suture material has been identified in almost one-third of patients with ductal stones following cholecystectomy and may be an important nidus for stone formation.[17]

PRESENTATION

Gallstones present with symptoms related to the site of the gallstones and are therefore considered according to site.

Cholecystolithiasis

Gallstones confined to the gallbladder may present with an acute episode of pain from acute cholecystitis, biliary colic, chronic recurrent abdominal discomfort from repeated episodes of mild biliary colic, or from a vague collection of symptoms usually referred to as flatulent dyspepsia.

PATHOPHYSIOLOGY

Impaction of a stone in the neck of the gallbladder is thought to result in gallbladder spasm, which produces biliary colic. As the stone falls back, the gallbladder empties and the pain stops, whereas continuing impaction of the stone in the gallbladder neck produces continuing pain. The trapped bile alters in composition producing local inflammation, which creates a more constant pain that may take several days to resolve. The gallbladder contents may become infected in approximately 30% of patients with gallstones.[18] This will add to the patient's toxaemia, and may lead to the development of empyema or possible gangrene and perforation. An empyema will produce pain, right upper quadrant tenderness and a swinging pyrexia. Urgent intervention is required since conservative measures rarely succeed in resolution. Increasing oedema and intramural vascular compromise may result in infarction of the gallbladder wall with consequent perforation of the organ.

The pathophysiology behind 'flatulent dyspepsia' is not understood. The gallbladder may be shrunken and contracted from episodes of subclinical inflammation but it is not unusual to find a normal looking gallbladder at cholecystectomy in patients with gallstones causing 'flatulent dyspepsia'. Contraction of the gallbladder against stones is the traditional explanation for postprandial discomfort, but there is a poor correlation between such symptoms and the presence of gallstones in a general population. A mucocoele may develop when a gallstone impacts in Hartmann's pouch in an empty gallbladder. The gallbladder secretes mucus behind the obstructing stone producing a steady increase in the size of the gallbladder, which may be easily palpable.

CLINICAL FEATURES

There is a poor correlation between pathological findings in the gallbladder wall and the presenting clinical features. Typically, acute cholecystitis presents with sharp, constant, right upper quadrant pain, which frequently is of sudden onset but may have been preceded by years of postprandial epigastric discomfort. It will be worse on inspiration or movement and frequently radiates to the back or to the tip of the right shoulder blade. It may be associated with nausea, vomiting or loss of appetite, and may persist for several days. Examination may reveal signs of toxaemia; the abdomen is tender in the right upper quadrant and classically a positive Murphy's sign is elicited. In more advanced cases, there may be a palpable inflammatory mass, which is usually due to an enlarged oedematous gallbladder surrounded by adherent omentum. Clinical signs of swinging pyrexia, tachycardia and impaired cardio-respiratory function should raise clinical suspicion of an empyema. The development of diffuse upper abdominal peritonism is a sign of perforation of the gallbladder. The presence of jaundice suggests choledocholithiasis although the possibility of common bile duct compression from an inflamed and oedematous gallbladder may need to be considered (Mirizzi's syndrome).

Biliary colic presents in a similar fashion to acute cholecystitis but is usually not affected by movement and lasts only for several hours. It is often precipitated by ingestion of fatty foods but resolution is spontaneous. Chronic pain due to gall-stones is attributed to the occurrence of 'flatulent dyspepsia' characterised by bouts of postprandial fullness, belching, nausea and a sensation of regurgitation of food. A family history of gallstone disease is not unusual, and factors predisposing to the development of gallstones may be present. Patients presenting with flatulent dyspepsia or recurrent episodes of biliary colic have little to find on examination.

Choledocholithiasis

PATHOPHYSIOLOGY

It is uncertain whether all common bile duct (CBD) stones produce symptoms. It is traditionally held that the CBD cannot produce colicky pain as it does not contain smooth muscle, but pain in the right upper quadrant following cholecystectomy may be a sign of retained bile duct stones. A stone impacted in the lower end of the CBD may also be associated with nausea and vomiting, and undoubtedly the muscular spasms of the sphincter of Oddi or duodenum could account for the pain that is often felt radiating through to the back. Obstructive jaundice results when a stone becomes impacted within the CBD, usually in the ampulla. A stone may pass spontaneously or fall back into the CBD ('ball-valving') with spontaneous regression of the jaundice, or it may remain impacted until it is

removed. A stone at the lower end of the CBD may also cause pancreatitis by temporary obstruction of the pancreatic duct, and this may be associated with transient jaundice (see Chapter 11). Ascending cholangitis results from infection within an obstructed or poorly draining biliary system. In patients with CBD stones, coliforms are identified within the bile in around 80% of cases.[18] The classic Charcot's triad of symptoms produced by bile duct stones with cholangitis consists of pain, obstructive jaundice and fever (with or without rigors). Acute cholangitis may progress to acute obstructive suppurative cholangitis with pain, obstructive jaundice, fever, hypotension and mental obtundation (Reynolds' pentad) requiring early recognition and prompt drainage to save life.[19]

CLINICAL FEATURES

Presentation of a patient with right upper quadrant pain some time after cholecystectomy may indicate choledocholithiasis. However, CBD stones are more likely to be either silent and found at the time of cholecystectomy or present due to one of the complications of obstructive jaundice, pancreatitis or ascending cholangitis. Pain is associated more frequently with obstructive jaundice due to gall-stones as opposed to an underlying malignancy. In addition to the presence of bilirubin in the urine and pale stool, obstructive jaundice may be associated with pruritus and steatorrhoea. Examination will not normally reveal a palpable gallbladder, and features of pancreatitis should be sought. Ascending cholangitis should be suspected in the presence of rigors and swinging pyrexia associated with jaundice. The patient may demonstrate signs of bacteraemia or septicaemia with a flushed appearance, tachycardia and hypotension.

INVESTIGATION

The diagnosis of gallstone disease is suspected on clinical grounds but relies on the relevant laboratory or radiological investigations for confirmation. The differentiation between gallstone causes for pain and other intra-abdominal disease should include an erect chest radiograph, and may require a plain radiograph of the abdomen. Less than 10% of gallstones are radio-opaque and therefore the yield from abdominal radiographs is low. Occasionally, in cases of intestinal obstruction, air is seen in the biliary tree, suggesting a cholecyst-enteric fistula and gallstone ileus.

Blood tests

Liver function tests (LFTs) should be performed routinely in patients with suspected gallstones. Although these may not be affected by the presence of cholecystolithiasis, they may be abnormal in the presence of choledocholithiasis. An isolated increase of unconjugated bilirubin is present in prehepatic jaundice such as is seen with excessive haemolysis. The biochemical picture of hepatic jaundice, as seen with hepatitis, is one of raised conjugated and unconjugated bilirubin, high aspartate (AST) and alanine (ALT) transaminase levels, but associated with a relatively normal or slightly raised alkaline phosphatase (ALP). Posthepatic (obstructive) jaundice is associated with a raised conjugated bilirubin only, high ALP and normal AST and ALT. In late cases of obstructive jaundice or in acute cholangitis, the transaminase levels will rise as hepatocellular damage proceeds. Minor abnormalities in the LFTs occur with non-obstructing stones in the CBD. These minor abnormalities may prompt the undertaking of an operative cholangiogram at the time of surgery if a selective operative cholangiogram policy is being pursued.[20,21]

Approximately 60% of patients with CBD stones (including asymptomatic stones) will have one or more abnormal liver function tests,[22] although a substantial number of patients with an abnormal liver function test will not have CBD stones. Bilirubin, ALP and gamma glutamyl transpeptidase (GGT) are the most sensitive tests routinely used.[23,24] In the acute situation, a serum amylase or lipase level should also be ascertained to exclude a diagnosis of pancreatitis, and a raised white blood cell count may support a clinical diagnosis of acute cholecystitis.

Ultrasonography

Ultrasound is the investigation used most widely to confirm the diagnosis of cholelithiasis. It is easy to perform, causes little discomfort to the patient, avoids irradiation and potentially toxic contrast media, and may be useful in demonstrating and assessing other structures in the upper abdomen. The gallbladder wall, as well as its contents, can be assessed and this may give additional information useful for planning management. Gallstones are seen as bright echoes within the gallbladder, and large stones cast an acoustic shadow behind them. Their size and number can be assessed. CBD stones may be harder to identify, although the presence of a dilated CBD and small stones within the gallbladder give clues as to their presence. The reliability of ultrasound in diagnosing gallbladder stones is very high. If the gallbladder cannot be identified, the presence of an echogenic focus in the gallbladder area is nearly as specific a finding as that of calculi in a distended gallbladder. With high-quality ultrasound scanning, gallstones should be detected in at least 95% of patients with stones. Its reliability in detecting CBD stones varies between 23 and 80% depending on body habitus and experience of the ultrasonographer.[25,26]

Endoscopic ultrasound (EUS)

Prat and colleagues have reported EUS with a sensitivity of 93% and specificity of 97% in detecting CBD stones, showing some promise of approaching values achieved by endoscopic retrograde cholangiopancreatography (ERCP) (89% and 100%).[27] In a more recent series, EUS was used as the gold standard in detecting CBD stones. This was performed under general anaesthetic and followed by ERCP and sphincterotomy if stones were observed.[24] Endoscopic ultrasound has also been reported as more sensitive than the transabdominal approach. Norton and Alderson reported confirmation of gallstone disease in 15 of 44 patients with 'idiopathic' pancreatitis who underwent EUS.[28]

Oral cholecystography

The use of oral cholecystography in the detection of gallstones has diminished dramatically with the increasing use of ultrasonography. The examination relies on a functioning gallbladder for concentration of the contrast media. False-negative rates for small gallstones of 6–8% are reported.[29] Non-functioning gallbladders are common with cholelithiasis, and although absence of function may imply the presence of gallbladder stones, it is by no means definitive.

Oral cholecystography may have a role in the identification of patients with biliary dyskinesia, but has no part to play in the identification of CBD stones.

CT scanning

Computed tomography (CT) may be more accurate than ultrasound in identifying CBD stones, with a sensitivity of 75% for CBD stones causing obstructive jaundice.[30] However, the relatively low rate of gallbladder stone detection may be due, in part, to cholesterol stones being isodense with bile on CT scanning. The newer generation spiral CT and magnetic resonance imaging (MRI) may be better but their potential advantage over abdominal ultrasound scanning is not readily apparent. Spiral CT following intravenous infusion cholangiography has been shown to allow accurate reconstruction of cystic duct/CBD anatomy.[31]

Radioisotope scanning

Technetium-labelled hydroxy-imino-diacetic acid (HIDA) is excreted in the bile after intravenous injection. It may be useful for demonstrating the patency of the biliary tree or of biliary-enteric anastomoses but its use with gallstones is limited. Failure to demonstrate a gallbladder due to blocked cystic duct may assist in the diagnosis of acute cholecystitis but images are too poor to reveal CBD stones. HIDA scanning may be helpful in patients with right upper quarter pain, fever, gallstones and right lower lobe pneumonia. Referred pain and tenderness can give confusing clinical signs, and the presence of a functional gallbladder makes the diagnosis of cholecystitis much less likely. HIDA scanning is of no value in cases of severe jaundice, since the isotope is not excreted into an obstructed system.

Intravenous cholangiography

The advent of laparoscopic cholecystectomy has ensured a revival in the use of intravenous cholangiography (IVC) as a means of identifying suspected CBD stones. Failure to opacify the biliary tree, however, arises in 3–10% of cases.[32,33] Although improvements in intravenous cholangi-

ography make it a useful occasional alternative to ultrasonographic assessment of the bile duct, factors such as time, cost and occasional failure, together with a low risk of allergic reaction, make it less attractive. The adoption of infusional cholangiography improves the safety of the investigation, and tomography improves imaging of the bile duct, though anatomical delineation is not as clear as preoperative cholangiography.[34] The use of IVC is therefore limited in that it cannot be employed in patients who are allergic to iodine or in those patients with biliary obstruction, as secretion of the contrast into the biliary tree does not occur.

Magnetic resonance cholangiography (MRCP)

Emerging developments of fast image acquisition in a few seconds and improving software have allowed imaging of the biliary and pancreatic tree in enough detail to approach the resolution of ERCP.[35] The technique relies on the principle of imaging fluid columns that are static and so give detail of bile and static fluid in the duodenum and stomach. Better images are obtained with dilated ducts, and bile flow can be a source of error in false-positive stone detection. The presence of CBD calculi can be detected with a sensitivity of 95%, specificity of 89% and accuracy of 92%. The ability to detect anatomical variation of the extrahepatic bile ducts is less established.[36] Following standard non-invasive tests, Liu et al. stratified suspicion of CBD stones into four categories. Patients at extremely high risk of CBD stone underwent ERCP. Patients at high risk underwent magnetic resonance cholangiopancreatography (MRCP) followed by ERCP if stones were seen. With diagnostic accuracies greater than 90% many patients were spared unnecessary ERCP.[37] The strength of this system lies in accurate triage and experience in interpreting MRCP. However, the capital expense and running costs of MRI still limit widespread availability in all but the most affluent of medical environments.

Percutaneous transhepatic cholangiography

Percutaneous transhepatic cholangiography (PTC) is best performed in patients who have a dilated biliary tree, but is not employed routinely in patients with suspected gallstone biliary obstruction. Despite the use of a fine-gauge needle, there is a risk of bile leakage and haemorrhage in patients with abnormal clotting.

Endoscopic retrograde cholangiopancreatography (ERCP)

ERCP is considered the gold standard in pre-operative CBD imaging. With direct visualisation of the papilla using a side-viewing duodenoscope, the papilla can be selectively cannulated to provide images of both the pancreatic and common bile ducts. Water-soluble contrast medium is injected to outline the biliary tree, and offers the advantage over other biliary tree imaging techniques of thera-peutic intervention with sphincterotomy and stone extraction at the time of examination (**Fig. 8.1**). The role of ERCP in the management of CBD stones is discussed later in this chapter.

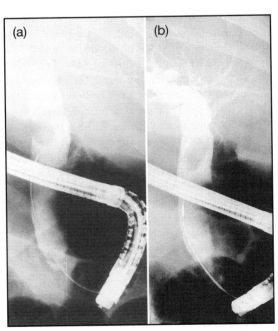

Figure 8.1 • **(a)** A large stone has been demonstrated by endoscopic retrograde cholangiography within the common bile duct. **(b)** The common bile duct stone has been snared by a Dormia basket ready for extraction.

MANAGEMENT OF GALLBLADDER STONES

Asymptomatic stones

There has been much debate regarding the need for surgical intervention in patients with asymptomatic gallstones. In one American study, which assessed the natural history of subjects with asymptomatic stones, individuals with gallstones were diagnosed by ultrasound scan on entry to a large university health care plan.[38] Only 2% of patients with inci-dentally diagnosed gallstones became symptomatic each year and presented with biliary colic or chole-cystitis rather than the more serious complications of jaundice, empyema or cholangitis.[38] Only 10% of the asymptomatic patients, followed for a mean of almost 5 years by McSherry and colleagues, developed symptoms, and only 7% required operation.[39] Although stones are undoubtedly associated with an increased risk of gallbladder cancer, only one of the 691 gallstone patients followed in this study[39] was found eventually to have an incidental carcinoma at operation, and further data are required to clarify this issue.

 There is no evidence to support interventional treatment of patients with asymptomatic gallstones since natural history studies have shown that symptoms develop at a rate of less than 2% per year.

Non-operative treatments for gallstones

DISSOLUTION

In the early 1970s there was great interest in the use of dissolution agents, principally chenodeoxycholic acid (CDCA), in the treatment of gallstones.[40] Pre-requisites for attempting dissolution therapy were a functioning gallbladder, multiple small stones (which have a greater total surface area for contact with the dissolution agent rather than a smaller number of larger stones) and radiolucency (indi-cative of pure cholesterol stones without a calcium or pigment matrix to impede dissolution). Success was slow to be achieved in most subjects, usually taking 6–12 months as judged by the disappear-ance of stones on ultrasound. Side effects of treatment included abdominal cramps, diarrhoea and occasional liver function test abnormalities. Despite the early encouraging results, gallstones often recurred when dissolution therapy was stopped. Ursodeoxycholate (UDCA) has been shown to be equally effective as CDCA in dissolving gallstones. Cohort studies followed for up to 18 years have also shown a significant reduction in biliary symptoms in patients taking UDCA.[41] UDCA is associated with fewer side effects but still requires years of compliance. Costs of development, rates of recurrence of stones and non-compliance have prevented its popular use.[42]

In patients administered dissolution agents, O'Donnell and Heaton[43] found that recurrence rates increased rapidly in the first few years, with rates of 13% at 1 year, 31% at 3 years, 43% at 4 years and 49% at 11 years. Although recurrent stones were readily redissolved, they generally recurred when therapy ceased.

LITHOTRIPSY

Success with lithotripsy for renal stones led to the use of the same techniques for gallbladder stones. Early lithotripters, with immersion in large water baths, were soon succeeded by smaller devices with a limited area of contact via a water-filled cushion. The biliary anatomy, however, did not lend itself to a repeat of the success observed with renal stones. The tidal flow of bile into and out of the gallbladder, along with the presence of multiple gallstones, were factors that contributed to the failure of the technique. Ahmed et al. reported 45% of patients undergoing lithotripsy required subsequent cholecystectomy.[44] Lithotripsy has therefore been retained only for the management of ductal stones resistant to endoscopic removal.[45]

 The potential role of oral dissolution therapy and lithotripsy has been superseded by the advent of laparoscopic cholecystectomy.

Operative treatment of gallbladder stones

OPEN CHOLECYSTECTOMY

In the decade before the establishment of laparoscopic cholecystectomy, it did appear that the traditional practice of many surgeons was being eroded by alternative treatment for gallstones, including dissolution therapy and extracorporeal shockwave lithotripsy.

The operative mortality of open cholecystectomy for cholelithiasis had fallen in the years before the introduction of laparoscopic surgery, with many series reporting operative mortality rates of less than 1%.[46,47] Common duct exploration was regarded as increasing the risk of open cholecystectomy by 4–8-fold.[48] In a comparative study between a North American and a European centre, 12–14% of patients developed complications, and the bile duct was explored in 8.6% of the patients in Toronto as opposed to 17.9% in Geneva, the incidences of positive exploration being 61% and 73% respectively.[47] Factors increasing the risk of postoperative mortality were advancing age, acute admission, admission to hospital within 3 months of the index admission, and the number of discharge diagnoses.[48] Only 18% of postoperative deaths in this study were related to the gallstone disease or the surgery, with underlying cardiovascular or respiratory disease contributing to 48% of deaths.

There has been considerable uncertainty regarding the true incidence of bile duct injury at open cholecystectomy, and the surveys available cite figures of one injury per 300–1000 operations.[49,50] At cholecystectomy, injury results from imprecise dissection and inadequate demonstration of the anatomical structures.[51] Although some patients do have anatomical anomalies or pathological changes that increase the risk of duct injury, it is noteworthy that in the extensive Swedish review, the patients most at risk appear to be young, slim females who have not undergone previous surgery.[49]

In a detailed analysis of a consecutive group of patients undergoing cholecystectomy for presumed biliary pain in a District General Hospital between 1980 and 1985, Bates and his colleagues compared the outcome of an age- and sex-matched control group of surgical patients without gallstone disease.[52] Flatulent dyspepsia was more frequent in gallstone patients but operation markedly reduced these symptoms to an incidence almost identical to that of the control group.

However, within 1 year of cholecystectomy, no less than 34% of patients still suffered some abdominal pain and none of the 35 patients referred back to hospital for investigation had evidence of retained ductal stones. Multivariant analysis showed that preoperative flatulence and long durations of attacks of pain were risk factors for postoperative dissatisfaction.

Given that the basis for symptoms before chole-cystectomy often remains uncertain, it is evident that a substantial number of patients continue to experience problems after operation.

MINILAPAROTOMY CHOLECYSTECTOMY

In the few years before the advent of laparoscopic cholecystectomy, there had been a resurgence of interest in open cholecystectomy through a small incision, the so-called minilaparotomy cholecyst-ectomy, in an effort to reduce the trauma of open surgery.

There have been few controlled trials; of those that have been performed, one showed laparoscopic cholecystectomy to be superior and the other showed mini-laparotomy cholecystectomy as superior.[53,54] The most recent randomised trial has again con-firmed a smoother convalescence for laparoscopic cholecystectomy although operating times remained longer.[55]

The technique relies on retractors to provide exposure for a fundus-first cholecystectomy carried out without the surgeon's hands entering the abdominal cavity. Cholangiography is possible but not performed in most reports of the technique. The authors' limited first-hand experience of the technique has not persuaded them that the view of the cystic duct/CBD junction is comparable to that achieved by laparoscopic cholecystectomy. The true incidence of bile duct injury with this technique is unknown and cannot be equated to the open era of large incisions.

There is no evidence to support the routine use of minicholecystectomy in the treatment of symptomatic gallstone disease.

LAPAROSCOPIC CHOLECYSTECTOMY

Despite the paucity of randomised controlled trials, enthusiasm for the technique of laparoscopic chole-cystectomy continues unabated, driven predomi-nantly by patient satisfaction, with less pain and an earlier return to normal activities. Surgeons are attracted by the excellent view of the gallbladder and biliary tree afforded by the laparoscope, and health providers and purchasers are attracted by the short hospital stay, which offers significant cost savings.

Symptomatic gallstones

The laparoscopic procedure can be offered to all patients with symptomatic gallstones, providing their cardiorespiratory status did not preclude lapar-oscopy. Of all patients presenting for operation, 95% can be completed successfully by laparoscopic means. Obesity, acute inflammation, adhesions and previous abdominal surgery do not usually prevent a laparoscopic cholecystectomy, but may require some adaptations of technique to complete the procedure.[56–64] Techniques of laparoscopic chole-cystectomy have been previously well described,[56,57] including cases performed under regional anaes-thesia in patients with chronic pulmonary disease.[58] Laparoscopic cholecystectomy has been widely reported in pregnancy,[59] and in patients with cirrhosis.[60] In a substantial audit of seven European centres,[61] 96% of procedures were completed successfully in the 1236 patients and only four bile duct injuries were reported. There were no post-operative deaths and a median hospital stay of 3 days with a median return to normal activities of only 11 days was observed.

Acute cholecystitis

Fears that laparoscopic cholecystectomy in the management of acute cholecystitis could carry an unacceptable risk of disseminating infection or of perpetrating an injury to the bile duct appear unfounded.[64] Several large series report success and safety with this procedure although the incidence of bile duct injury and conversion to open oper-ation remain slightly higher.[65,66] In difficult cases, improvement in the exposure of Calot's triangle may require additional or different positioning of the laparoscopic cannulas, the use of oblique viewing telescopes and placement of endoscopic retractors. Decompression of a distended or inflamed gallbladder may also improve access.

Complications

The mortality rate in a good-risk patient undergoing elective operation is less than 1%, and operative risks usually arise from comorbid conditions. The laparoscopic technique is associated with lower wound infection rates than open surgery.[67]

Furthermore, a recent meta-analysis has shown that antibiotic prophylaxis is not warranted in low-risk patients undergoing laparoscopic cholecystectomy.[68]

Day-case laparoscopic cholecystectomy

Worldwide, laparoscopic cholecystectomy is being performed in the day-case setting with good pre-operative patient selection, improved techniques, and improved postoperative control of pain, nausea and vomiting.[69]

Needlescopic cholecystectomy

This technique has been described using 2-mm and 3-mm instruments and a 3-mm laparoscope. A randomised trial has shown less pain and smaller scars when this technique was used in patients with chronic cholecystitis.[70]

Bile duct injury

Anxieties regarding an increased incidence of bile duct injury with the introduction of laparoscopic cholecystectomy have not been substantiated by multicentre studies from Europe[61] and the USA,[62] with a reported incidence of injury to the CBD of 1 in 200–300 cases. In a study in the West of Scotland, a prospective audit of laparoscopic cholecystectomy was undertaken.[71] A total of 5913 laparoscopic cholecystectomies were undertaken by 48 surgeons, and 37 laparoscopic bile duct injuries were reported. Major bile duct injuries were defined as those where laceration to more than 25% of the bile duct diameter occurred, where the common hepatic duct or CBD was transected, or in those instances when a bile duct stricture developed in the postoperative period. Of the 37 injuries, 20 were classified in this way, giving an incidence of 0.3%. Delayed identification of bile duct injury occurred in 19 patients and, although it was noted by the authors that cholangiography did not play a part in the identification of bile duct injuries, it was note-worthy that imaging was used in only 8.8% of all laparoscopic procedures. During the course of this 5-year study, the annual incidence of bile duct injury peaked at 0.8% in the third year but had fallen to 0.4% in the final year of audit. A meta-analysis of more than 100 000 cases reported an injury rate of 0.5%.[72] Archer et al. emphasised the importance of supervised surgical training to allow attenuation of the trainee surgeon's learning curve by the experience of his/her proctoring surgeon.

The importance of cholangiography in the early detection of bile duct injury was also emphasised.[73] Way et al. analysed bile duct injuries from a cognitive psychological perspective and concluded that errors that led to bile duct injury stemmed from anatomical misperceptions as opposed to errors of skill or judgement (**Fig. 8.2**). This analysis concluded with a list of rules to help prevent injuries.[74]

CHOLECYSTOSTOMY

For patients whose symptoms of acute cholecystitis do not settle, cholecystostomy was often undertaken in those cases where open cholecystectomy was thought to carry an unacceptable risk of injury to the biliary tree. The procedure could be undertaken under local anaesthesia and following decompression of the gallbladder and stone removal, a drain could be left in situ. With the demonstration that acute cholecystectomy could be undertaken safely,[64] cholecystostomy has become an infrequent surgical procedure. The technique can also be undertaken percutaneously under ultrasound or CT guidance and is currently most used in the frail patient with cardiorespiratory instability requiring time to control. It may rarely be of value during a difficult laparoscopic cholecystectomy when the risk of conversion to an open procedure may be considered unacceptable in the frail patient. In such instances, a drain can be inserted through one of the 5-mm cannulas, which can be introduced directly into the gallbladder by reinsertion of a trocar.

SUBTOTAL CHOLECYSTECTOMY

This is another strategy to consider if dense fibrosis or large vessels are present in the area of Calot's triangle and the cystic duct is clearly identified and confirmed by cholecystogram. The cystic duct is ligated and excision of the gallbladder is undertaken leaving its posterior wall intact on the liver. This situation probably arises most in those patients with cirrhosis and portal hypertension.

Laparoscopic cholecystectomy is associated with less pain, shorter hospital stay, faster return to normal activity and less abdominal scarring than open surgery and is therefore preferred to open surgery in the management of symptomatic gallstone disease.

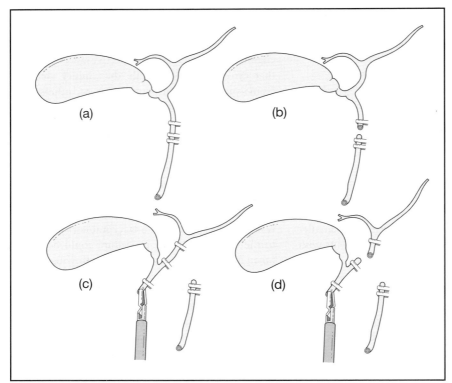

Figure 8.2 • The 'classical' laparoscopic bile duct injury. **(a)** The common duct is misidentified as the cystic duct and is doubly clipped. **(b)** The common duct is then divided. **(c)** The gallbladder is retracted to the right, stretching the common hepatic duct and placing it in contact with the gallbladder. This is identified as an accessory duct, and double clipped. **(d)** A high transection of the common hepatic duct results in the excision of most of the extrahepatic biliary tree.

INTRAOPERATIVE CHOLANGIOGRAPHY (IOC)

The debate over the potential benefit of operative cholangiography has spanned the open and laparoscopic eras.

Routine IOC

Many surgeons who had previously performed the technique routinely at the time of open cholecystectomy abandoned cholangiography during laparoscopic cholecystectomy, since it was thought to be too difficult to undertake. In a large population-based study in Western Australia, Fletcher et al. concluded that operative cholangiography had a protective effect for complications of cholecystectomy.[75] In a large study of over 1.5 million Medicare patients undergoing cholecystectomy, Flum and his colleagues demonstrated

that surgeons performing operative cholangiography routinely had a lower rate of bile duct injuries than those who did not, and this difference disappeared when IOC was not used.[76] The authors believe that operative cholangiography has an important role in laparoscopic cholecystectomy, not only to detect CBD stones but also to confirm, beyond doubt, the anatomy of the biliary tree, since the severity of bile duct injury appears far greater in laparoscopic surgery. The addition of cholangiography to the total dissection time of laparoscopic cholecystectomy is relatively short. On the basis that the time to learn operative cholangiography is not during the management of a difficult case, we recommend that it should be performed as a routine but should not be seen as a substitute for careful dissection of the infundibulum of the gallbladder and the cystic duct close to the gallbladder.[51] By dissecting these structures both anteriorly and posteriorly, the gall-bladder is displaced (sometimes called the 'flag' technique) to enable the surgeon to see behind the gallbladder and thus minimise the risk of injury to the portal structures. Routine IOC also improves the surgeon's skills to enable successful transcystic exploration of the CBD.

Selective IOC

There are data supporting a selective approach to intraoperative cholangiography at open[21] and laparoscopic cholecystectomy.[77] Unsuspected stones on routine cholangiography at laparoscopic chole-cystectomy occurred in only 2.9%, and residual CBD stones causing symptoms in patients not undergoing routine cholangiography were found in only 0.30%. The strength of any selective policy for IOC will depend on the predictive values of preoperative investigations. Numerous studies have examined risk factors for choledocholithiasis but, from multivariate analysis, it would appear that an increased diameter of the CBD and the presence of multiple (>10) gallstones are the only significant independent indicators.[20] During laparoscopic cholecystectomy, the surgeon may have difficulty in assessing CBD diameter, and palpation of the extrahepatic biliary tree, which some surgeons consider a useful adjunct in detecting CBD stones, cannot be undertaken.[78]

BILE DUCT INJURY

The principal cause of damage is due to mis-identification of the CBD as the cystic duct. As dissection proceeds an 'accessory duct' (in reality the common hepatic duct) is visualised, clipped and divided, resulting in resection of most of the extra-hepatic biliary tree (**Fig. 8.2**). Operative cholangi-ography adds to the certainty that the cannula is in the cystic duct. If only the distal biliary tree is filled, the surgeon is alerted to the error before any duct is completely divided. Although critics of operative cholangiography will argue that the CBD has been injured by the incision through which the chol-angiogram catheter is introduced, the injury at this point is recoverable, either by direct suture or insertion of a T-tube (**Fig. 8.3**). In the rarer situation when the cystic duct arises from the right hepatic duct, and dissection has not progressed correctly, cholangiography identifies such anomalies and helps to avert more major injury (**Fig. 8.4**).

(a)

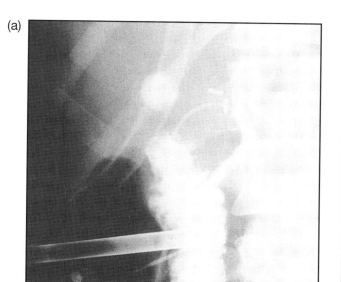

(b)

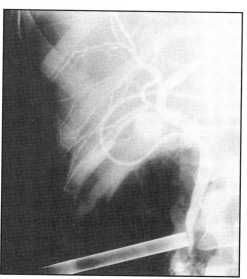

Figure 8.3 • **(a)** The small diameter common bile duct has been mistaken for the cystic duct. Only the distal common bile duct and duodenum are shown, with no proximal filling of the ducts. Recognition of the error at this stage averts a major injury to the common duct. **(b)** After further dissection, the cystic duct was identified and a T-tube placed in the incision in the common duct. A subsequent T-tube cholangiogram confirms the normal anatomy and laparoscopic cholecystectomy was completed successfully.

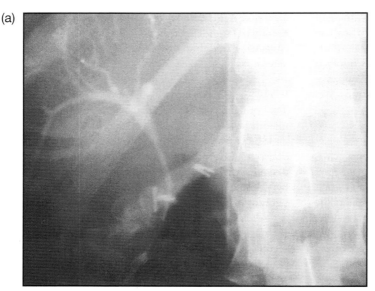

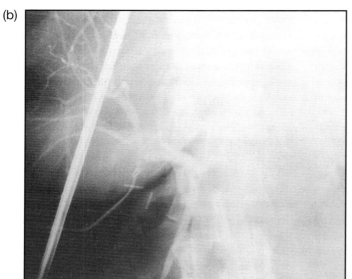

Figure 8.4 • **(a)** During what appeared to be a very straightforward laparoscopic cholecystectomy, the routine operative cholangiogram showed only the right hepatic duct and right hepatic biliary tree. **(b)** Repositioning of the catheter and the LigaClip showed the remainder of the biliary tree and made clear that the structure initially thought to be the cystic duct was the distal right hepatic duct below an anomalous origin of the cystic duct.

LAPAROSCOPIC ULTRASOUND (LUS)

The emergence of ultrasound probes that can be passed down the laparoscopic ports has further improved the accurate measurement of CBD diameter, as well as the stone load within the gallbladder. Both mechanical sectoral and linear array laparoscopic ultrasound probes have been shown to be as useful as cholangiography in the detection of CBD stones.[79–81] LUS is less invasive, less time consuming, allows less radiation exposure and has similar failure rates to IOC when performed in well-trained hands. In a large series the common hepatic duct and the CBD were identified in 93% and 99% of cases, respectively. Sensitivity and specificity for identifying bile duct stones was 92% and 100%, respectively. A normal CBD diameter at LUS was also an excellent negative predictor of CBD stones.[82] The same authors later concluded that LUS could replace IOC.[83] Others feel IOC and LUS should be seen as complementary tests rather than competitive.[84] Laparoscopic ultrasonography may facilitate a policy of selective cholangiography. Despite reports of accurate identification of anatomy it remains to be seen whether this will translate to prevention of bile duct injury. A cost benefit also remains to be demonstrated given the capital outlay for the equipment.

The use of intraoperative cholangiography allows detection of CBD stones during cholecystectomy and when interpreted appropriately is associated with a lower risk of CBD injury.

MANAGEMENT OF COMMON BILE DUCT STONES

The natural history of a given common bile duct (CBD) stone remains difficult to predict. In a prospective study of 1000 cases of symptomatic gallstones it was found that 73% of cases that presented with features suggestive of CBD stones had no CBD stone at the time of operation and were therefore considered to have passed the stone spontaneously. Cases of cholangitis or jaundice were less likely to pass stones spontaneously.[85]

Primary bile duct stones form within the CBD usually due to ampullary stenosis, diverticula or impaired bile duct motility. Management of these stones will often require choledochojejunostomy depending on the circumstances and patient age.[86,87] Treatment of primary duct stones with choledochotomy and T-tube drainage alone is associated with recurrence rates up to 41%.[88] Laparoscopic choledochoduodenostomy remains an option for the advanced laparoscopic surgeon,[89,90] although there may be concerns regarding the longer-term consequences of bilioenteric reflux.

Secondary bile duct stones are stones that originate within the gallbladder and are found in the CBD prior to, at the time of, or within 2 years of cholecystectomy. Approximately 12% of patients undergoing surgery for symptomatic gallbladder stones will also have stones in the CBD. More than 90% of these patients will have preoperative indications such as a history of jaundice or pancreatitis or abnormal liver function tests, but 5–10% have no indication of stones in the bile duct other than a positive finding (filling defect, absence of filling of the terminal segment of the common duct, delay

or absence of flow into the duodenum) on the peroperative cholangiogram.

The best management of CBD stones is still a matter of debate. Discussion of different practices is presented here in the order the authors consider most practical, and a suggested algorithm is presented.

Laparoscopic transcystic common bile duct exploration

Laparoscopic common bile duct (CBD) exploration has been described through the cystic duct or common duct using either fibreoptic instruments or radiologically guided wire baskets or balloons.[91–94] The laparoscopic approach to the common duct was developed initially by the transcystic route because of the ease of closure without the need for a suture technique. The authors stress the importance of differentiating between laparoscopic transcystic exploration of the CBD and laparoscopic choledochotomy. Careful evaluation of the CBD diameter and stone load is required to determine the best approach.

The authors' preferred method of laparoscopic exploration is by fluoroscopic means using a C-arm image intensifier, which is mobile and provides dynamic images with angulation. We employ a 5.5-Fr 70-cm radio-opaque nylon catheter with soft tip and end hole along with a side arm that connects to a catheter for injection of contrast (**Fig. 8.5**) (also in colour, see Plate 5, facing p. 20). Once the cystic duct is opened distal to a previously applied clip, the ducts are milked to push stones through the cystic duct incision and a cholangiogram is performed (**Fig. 8.6a**). Once the cystic and CBD diameters have been assessed, the transcystic exploration proceeds by passing a feed wire, 75-cm-long stone extractor (Cook®, Wilson-Cook Medical GI Endoscopy Inc., North Carolina). The basket tip should be positioned well back from the cannula tip to avoid perforation of the duct. Once the cannula tip is advanced, under image intensification, the basket is advanced within the cannula to allow engagement of the stone, which is withdrawn into the basket before being extracted via the cystic duct (**Fig. 8.6b**). It is useful to remove the proximal stones first, and vital to avoid opening the basket within the duodenum or drawing the ampulla with the

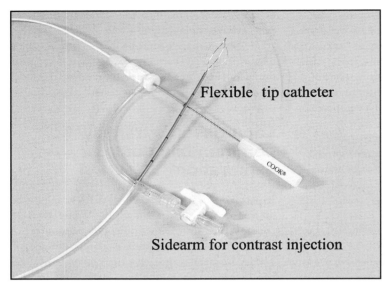

Flexible tip catheter

Sidearm for contrast injection

Figure 8.5 • Composite cholangiogram catheter and stone extraction basket used for laparoscopic transcystic exploration of the common bile duct. See also Plate 5, facing p. 20. Reproduced with permission of Cook Australia.

basket wires open. Any impacted stones can be dislodged by passing a 4-Fr Fogarty catheter beyond the stone and withdrawing the catheter with the balloon inflated. Failed disimpaction may require choledochoscopy and lithotripsy (**Box 8.1**).

Traditionally at open surgery, the common duct was decompressed postoperatively with a T-tube until it was known that the bile was draining satisfactorily through the ampulla and there was no bile leak. Most series of laparoscopic transcystic common duct explorations do not report the routine use of drainage of the common duct. A subhepatic drain is routine.

There is accumulating evidence, including two randomised trials,[95–97] that 60–70% of patients are able to have their calculi cleared via the cystic duct.[98,99]

Laparoscopic choledochotomy

In up to 35% of patients laparoscopic transcystic exploration of the CBD will fail to clear the CBD.[95,96] Choledochotomy then needs to be considered. The only absolute contraindication to choledochotomy is a CBD diameter of less than 8 mm (**Box 8.2**). It should also be borne in mind that approximately one-third of stones detected at cholangiography may be passed spontaneously, and that exploration

Box 8.1 • Techniques for improving transcystic clearance

- Careful dissection of cystic duct/CBD junction
- Avoidance of the spiral valves when incising cystic duct
- Careful examination of cholangiogram ('did that stone pass through the cystic duct?')
- Approach cystic duct from different or extra ports
- Dilatation of cystic duct with balloon
- Choledochoscopy via cystic duct
- Vary retraction on fundus

Box 8.2 • Indications for choledochotomy

- Unsuccessful transcystic exploration
- Cystic duct diameter smaller than size of stones
- CBD diameter >8 mm
- Multiple large stones
- Impacted stones with clinical features of cholangitis
- Ampullary diverticulum on IOC
- Previous Billroth II gastrectomy
- Previous failed ERCP
- Contraindication to postoperative ERCP
- ERCP unavailable

(a)

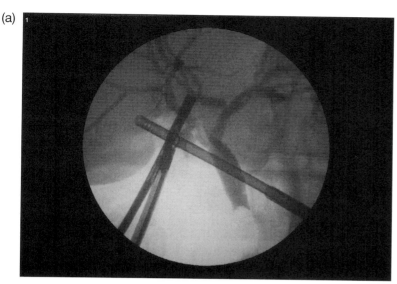

(b)

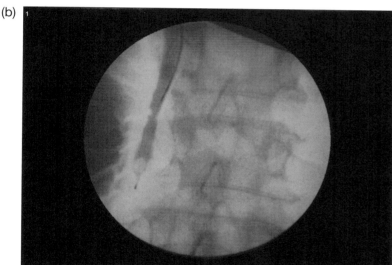

Figure 8.6 • **(a)** Composite cholangiogram demonstrating a filling defect at lower end of common bile duct. **(b)** Fluoroscopic view of bile duct showing a four-wire basket retrieving a lower common bile duct stone.

of a small duct may result in increased morbidity for the patient.[100] Therefore, laparoscopic choledochotomy is only an option for appropriately trained surgeons (**Box 8.3**).

Once clearance of the duct has been confirmed by choledochoscopy, a T-tube is inserted or primary closure can be considered with the insertion of an antegrade stent across the ampulla.[95] Antegrade stenting, placement of a T-tube or cystic duct tube decompression of the CBD is wise where doubt

Box 8.3 • Useful tips in performing laparoscopic choledochotomy

- Deflate duodenum with nasogastric tube (NGT)
- Extra port to retract duodenum
- Leave cholangiocatheter in to prevent deflation
- Laparoscopic knife for choledochotomy
- Intraoperative lithotripsy preferably by lithoclast

exists about free postoperative bile drainage through the ampulla. This is most likely where a stone was impacted, ampullary manipulation has been extensive or with established cholangitis. Placement of a subhepatic drain is essential

Open choledochotomy

Successful exploration of the CBD can only be achieved through an adequately sized choledochotomy to facilitate both removal of any obvious stones and choledochoscopy. The gradual adoption of operative choledochoscopy during the 1970s and 1980s saw a decline in the incidence of retained CBD stones following surgery, from about 10% to 1.2%, with a number of surgeons reporting large series of patients with no retained stones.[22,101–103] On initial examination of the proximal ducts, it is normally possible to visualise several generations of ducts when these are dilated. Once it has been ascertained that the upper ducts are clear, the distal biliary tree can be examined. It is mandatory to clearly visualise the rather ragged appearance of the ampulla of Vater and then withdraw the choledochoscope. If a stone is visualised it can be retrieved with a stone basket and the procedure repeated until the duct is clear. The common duct is closed with or without a T-tube.[104–106] The latter is probably unnecessary for an experienced choledochoscopist but, for the less experienced surgeon, it allows access to the biliary tree for postoperative cholangiography to confirm ductal clearance and to allow re-exploration of the duct without the need for re-operation.

With the advent of laparoscopic cholecystectomy, ERCP and endoscopic sphincterotomy (ES) have become the usual procedure for treating common duct stones, since laparoscopic common duct exploration is not yet a widely practised technique (**Box 8.4**). Moreover, cholecystectomy without cholangiography is commonly performed in the expectation that ERCP and ES will be effective in dealing with unrecognised retained common duct stones at a later date. Such a policy, however, does expose the patient to an additional and often unnecessary procedure. Laparoscopic common duct exploration by whatever route has the advantage for the patient of being able to deal with both gallbladder and CBD stones at the same time.[107,108]

Box 8.4 • Reasons to consider converting to open choledochotomy

- Unsuccessful transcystic CBD exploration
- Unsuccessful laparoscopic choledochotomy
- Multiple (>10) CBD stones
- Large CBD stones
- Intrahepatic or proximal ductal stones
- Impacted stones
- Failed or unavailable ERCP

Endoscopic retrograde cholangiopancreatography (ERCP)

There is general agreement that endoscopic removal of bile duct stones is preferable to surgery in post-cholecystectomy patients, and in high-risk surgical patients when the gallbladder is still present, that is, patients with severe acute cholangitis and selected patients with acute biliary pancreatitis.[109–112] The authors believe ERCP becomes an option when transcystic CBD exploration has failed, but should not be considered the first-line management of all CBD stones.

Duct clearance can be expected in 90–95% of patients undergoing successful sphincterotomy, and this results in an overall success rate for endoscopic stone clearance of 80–95%, the highest success rates being recorded as experience increases.[109,111,113] Major complications occur in up to 10% of patients, and include haemorrhage, acute pancreatitis, cholangitis and retroduodenal perforation, but the overall procedure-related mortality is less than 1%.[109] However, the 30-day mortality can reach 15%, reflecting the severity of the underlying disease. In selected patients with calculi less than 15 mm in diameter, morbidity may be reduced by papillary dilatation rather than sphincterotomy.[110] Difficulties in removing CBD stones endoscopically may be due to unfavourable or abnormal anatomy, such as periampullary diverticulum or previous surgery. Stones larger than 15 mm and those situated intrahepatically or proximal to a biliary stricture may be difficult to remove (**Box 8.5**). Adjuvant techniques include mechanical lithotripsy,

Box 8.5 • Difficult bile duct stones at ERCP

- Stones greater than 15 mm
- Intrahepatic stones
- Multiple stones
- Impacted stones
- Stone proximal to a biliary stricture
- Tortuous bile duct
- Disproportionate size of the bile duct stone
- Duodenal diverticulum
- Billroth II reconstruction
- Surgical duodenotomy

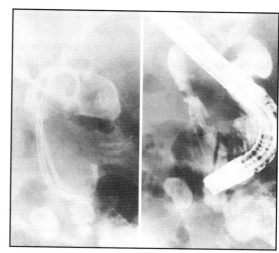

Figure 8.7 • Multiple common bile duct stones lying above a mid-common bile duct stricture and not amenable to endoscopic extraction. Biliary drainage is maintained with two endoscopically placed stents.

extracorporeal shockwave lithotripsy and chemical dissolution.[111–116] Although successful stone fragmentation has been reported in up to 80% of patients, the major drawback is the need for multiple treatment sessions and at least one subsequent ERCP to extract stone fragments.

The establishment of ERCP in the prelaparoscopic era was based on the avoidance of an open exploration of the CBD, a procedure that was believed to have significant morbidity.[117] ERCP was, therefore, generally reserved for the high-risk surgical patients but open cholecystectomy and exploration of the CBD was reserved for the younger patient. In the laparoscopic era, management strategies vary considerably and are based on local endoscopic and laparoscopic resources and expertise.

ERCP STENT INSERTION

In the 5% or less of situations where extraction of CBD stones is incomplete or impossible, a nasobiliary tube or stent should be inserted to provide biliary decompression and prevent stone impaction of the distal CBD (**Fig. 8.7**).[118] Such manoeuvres may allow improvement of the patient's clinical condition until complete stone clearance can be achieved by further endoscopic manoeuvres or subsequent surgery. Temporary biliary endoprosthesis placement avoids accidental or intentional dislodgement of the nasobiliary catheter by a confused or uncooperative patient. The stent may become blocked after a few months, but bile drainage often continues around the stent, and the presence of the stent alone may be sufficient to prevent stones from becoming impacted at the lower end of the CBD. In the surgically unfit patient, a change of stent may be required if jaundice recurs. Recurrent episodes of cholangitis may result in secondary biliary cirrhosis in the long term, and careful consideration of the patient's level of fitness must be made before surgery is totally discounted.

PREOPERATIVE ERCP

For some, ERCP is the chosen method of preoperative CBD stone detection for any patient with suspected CBD stones. The advantage of this strategy is that duct clearance preoperatively removes the dilemma as to how to manage CBD stones found at operation. This management policy, however, will expose a substantial number of patients to an unnecessary endoscopic intervention. Since approximately 12% of patients undergoing elective cholecystectomy have CBD stones, it is therefore likely that more than 25% of cholecystectomies would require ERCP preoperatively with this strategy. In the UK, this would entail an additional 10 000 ERCPs per annum, and if it were assumed that all these examinations were purely diagnostic, there would be approximately 100 major complications per year from this investigation.

A randomised study has shown no significant advantage for patients treated by preoperative sphincterotomy as opposed to open cholecystectomy and exploration of CBD alone.[119] Despite this, ERCP and ES has become popular practice in the management of CBD stones, with an increased reliance on ERCP and a reluctance among surgeons to perform surgical exploration of the CBD.[120]

Cholecystectomy should routinely follow clearance of the CBD except in those considered too frail or unfit for general anaesthetic. It can be expected that if the gallbladder is left intact following ERCP and ES, up to 47% of patients will develop at least one recurrent biliary event, with many requiring cholecystectomy.[99]

INTRAOPERATIVE ERCP

There have been several reports over the years describing this technique with success but few centres consider this the most appropriate use of resource.[121]

POSTOPERATIVE ERCP

If ductal stones are not suspected preoperatively, their presence can be determined at laparoscopic cholecystectomy by intraoperative cholangiography (IOC). CBD stones identified in this way could be referred for postoperative endoscopic clearance if the surgeon was unable to explore the duct. Such a policy would reduce dramatically the number of ERCPs undertaken by a policy of routine or selective preoperative ERCP. This would leave only a small proportion of patients, in whom stones could not be cleared by ERCP, requiring a second operation.[122] If the surgeon is trained in laparoscopic exploration of the CBD, ERCP should be reserved for the few patients in whom laparoscopic ductal clearance fails. Unpublished randomised trial data have shown that this approach is safe and represents an effective management plan (L. K. Nathanson, personal data).

At the present time, the precise role of ERCP remains to be defined but is likely to be dictated by local expertise and practice (see 'Laparoscopic choledochotomy' above). A number of acceptable algorithms have been proposed to manage the laparoscopic cholecystectomy patients suspected of harbouring CBD stones.[123]

There is argument for leaving small stones (<5 mm) found intraoperatively. On follow-up for up to 33 months in a small group of patients, 29% in this category developed symptoms, but were safely managed with ERCP.[124]

TRANSCYSTIC EXPLORATION OF THE CBD VERSUS PREOPERATIVE OR POSTOPERATIVE ERCP

At present, the array of management strategies for common duct stones requires data to guide us, with the techniques employed depending on local circumstances. In hospitals with ready access to ERCP, a surgeon may see little need for ascending the learning curve of laparoscopic CBD exploration, whereas those units with less ready access to ERCP see many attractions in dealing with common duct stones by laparoscopic means.

Preoperative ERCP and laparoscopic clearance of the CBD have been shown to be equivalent in overall outcomes.[96] However, those patients whose ductal stones were cleared transcystically experienced a far shorter hospital stay.

Postoperative ERCP clearance in a small single-surgeon study showed equivalent overall outcome to laparoscopic CBD clearance.[97] However, the number of choledochotomies was small, and the retained stone rate high. Placement of biliary stents at the time of operation may improve the success of postoperative ERCP and stone clearance.

With experience, the majority of CBD stones can be treated at the time of surgery provided a flexible approach is employed. No single technique will be applicable to the management of all stones. In general, if the stones are few in number, small (<1 cm) in size, situated in the common duct, or distal to cystic duct entry then transcystic exploration has a high chance of success. If the stone, or stones are large and numerous, or if the stones are situated in the common hepatic duct or intrahepatic biliary tree, a choledochotomy and exploration with the larger 5 mm choledochoscope is the preferred option. For those embarking on laparoscopic exploration careful consideration of the strategies to be employed, equipment required and adequacy of assistance will go a long way to simplifying what can be a complex procedure. When laparoscopic transcystic exploration fails, the surgeon has three options:

- to ligate the cystic duct, complete the cholecystectomy and rely on postoperative ERCP

- to perform a laparoscopic choledochotomy
- to perform a laparotomy and open exploration of the CBD.

If laparoscopic choledochotomy fails, the options include insertion of a T-tube and subsequent extraction of the retained stones via the T-tube track after 6 weeks; postoperative ERCP and sphincterotomy; or conversion to open exploration CBD. Individual circumstances will dictate which option is the most suitable although this should be discussed carefully with the patient before a management strategy is implemented.

It has been suggested that preoperative ERCP is the most cost-effective management of patients at high risk for CBD stone.[125] There is evidence accumulating, however, that where transcystic clearance is successful this leads to less morbidity and more rapid recovery.[95,96] Intraoperative stone fragmentation remains an option for stones found at operation that are unable to be dislodged at laparoscopic or open surgery. The authors believe the most cost-effective approach is laparoscopic cholecystectomy, intraoperative cholangiography (IOC) and transcystic clearance of CBD stones, preserving ERCP for retained stones. Learning the techniques to achieve this seems worthwhile.

In a recent extensive review of the literature, it was concluded that laparoscopic CBD exploration is safe and effective for all patients presenting with gallstones and may be a better way of removing CBD stones than ERCP.[126,127]

Recurrent or retained CBD stones

Recurrent CBD stones occur in up to 10% of cases. In a retrospective series of 169 patients followed for up to 19 years, recurrences were more common in patients with primary duct stones, large CBD diameters (around 16 mm), and periampullary diverticula. Lowest recurrence rates were found in those patients undergoing choledochoduodenostomy.[88]

Retained CBD stones found at postoperative T-tube cholangiography are best dealt with by ERCP. If ERCP is unsuccessful or not available, exploration of the CBD via the T-tube tract is indicated. It usually takes approximately 6 weeks for the T-tube track to mature, at which time percutaneous radiologically guided stone extraction or

percutaneous choledochoscopy can be performed. A cholangiogram is obtained immediately prior to the procedure as a proportion of stones will have passed spontaneously.

The T-tube is removed, a guidewire is left in situ, and either a steerable catheter or choledochoscope is advanced down the track and into the CBD. With choledochoscopy, the remainder of the technique is identical to that carried out at open operation.[128] With the steerable catheter technique, fluoroscopy and further cholangiograms are taken as the stones are retrieved with a stone basket.[129,130]

If there is uncertainty as to the completeness of clearance, a straight tube may be inserted to keep the track open for a further attempt a few days later. Both techniques are successful in more than 95% of cases and carry less risk of complications such as pancreatitis or haemorrhage than ERCP. Providing there are no time constraints and the patient is happy to be managed as an outpatient with a T-tube, the technique is effective.

TRANSHEPATIC STONE RETRIEVAL

In a few patients, particularly those who have previously undergone a Pólya gastrectomy, the ampulla will not be readily accessible for ERCP. Access to the common duct can be achieved using a percutaneous transhepatic technique. Over a percutaneously inserted guidewire, a series of dilators are advanced into the biliary tree, so as to develop a transhepatic tract. Following insertion of a sheath, a choledochoscope or steerable catheter can be inserted and stones retrieved.[131]

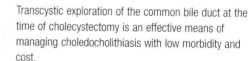

Transcystic exploration of the common bile duct at the time of cholecystectomy is an effective means of managing choledocholithiasis with low morbidity and cost.

ERCP is effective in managing the remaining patients in whom this is not achievable and is the accepted means of managing the patient presenting with acute cholangitis.

ACALCULOUS BILIARY PAIN

Given the poor understanding of the mechanisms of pain production in patients with acalculous biliary disease, the outcome for patients following cholecystectomy is uncertain. There is gathering evidence that some patients have abnormal motility of the sphincter of Oddi, in addition to the gallbladder. Some authors have reported improvement in symptoms in as many as 85–95% of patients with acalculous biliary pain after cholecystectomy,[132] but it is conceivable that surgery confers a placebo effect. Controversy exists over the use of cholecystokinin (CCK) provocation tests as a means of reproducing symptoms and predicting which patients might benefit from cholecystectomy. In one study, all 26 patients with positive CCK tests showed improvement after removal of the gallbladder,[133] whereas 10 of the 16 patients with negative tests were found to have other pathology accounting for their pain. Despite these encouraging results, other investigators have failed to demonstrate differences in outcome in patients with positive CCK tests when compared to those with negative tests.[134] Objective criteria on which to base the decision to recommend cholecystectomy in such patients are difficult to define. It is clear, however, that, despite the minimally invasive nature of laparoscopic cholecystectomy, there should be no relaxation in the indications for cholecystectomy with patients with acalculous biliary pain.

Key points

Asymptomatic gallstones do not require surgical intervention.

The standard treatment for symptomatic gallstones is now laparoscopic, and there are few exceptions to a trial of a laparoscopic approach in all comers.

All surgeons undertaking cholecystectomy, by whatever technique, should be capable of performing operative cholangiography.

The use of operative cholangiography appears to be associated with a lower incidence of bile duct injury.

Experience is accumulating that transcystic clearance of the CBD at the time of cholecystectomy is effective, with low morbidity and cost. In the one-third of patients where this is not achievable, ERCP is probably the best means of clearance.

An algorithm for the management of common bile duct stones is shown in **Fig. 8.8**. The management strategy chosen will depend on personal experience, equipment availability, time, and the availability of other departmental expertise. There is no consensus as to the ideal approach.

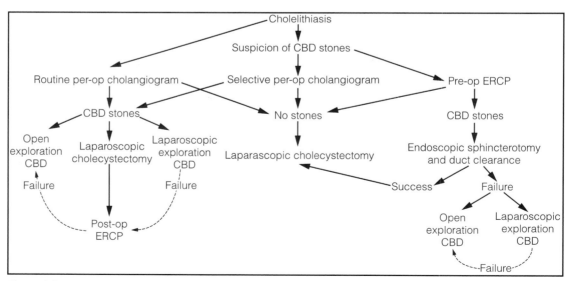

Figure 8.8 • Algorithm showing the available strategies for management of common bile duct stones.

REFERENCES

1. Godfrey PJ, Bates T, Harrison M et al. Gallstones and mortality: a study of all gallstone related deaths in a single health district. Gut 1984; 25:1029–33.

2. Hospital In-patient Inquiry, 1980: Main tables. Department of Health and Social Security/Office of Population Census and Surveys. London: HMSO, 1989, Chicago.

3. Socio-economic fact book for surgery. Socio-economic Affairs Department, American College of Surgeons, 1988, Chicago.

4. Motson RW. Operative cholangiography. In: Motson RW (ed.) Retained common duct stones. Prevention and treatment. London: Grune and Stratton, 1985; pp. 8–9.

5. Neoptolemos JP, Hofmann AF, Moossa AR. Chemical treatment of stones in the biliary tree. Br J Surg 1986; 73:515–24.

6. Bennion LJ, Grundy SM. Risk factors for the development of cholelithiasis in man. N Engl J Med 1978; 299:1161–221.

7. Scragg RKR, McMichael AJ, Seamark RF. Oral contraceptives, pregnancy and endogenous oestrogen in gallstone disease – a case controlled study. Br Med J 1984; 288:1795–9.

8. Scragg RKR, McMichael AJ, Paghurst PA. Diet, alcohol and relative weight in gallstone disease: a case controlled study. Br Med J 1984; 288:1113–18.

9. Richardson WS, Surowiec WJ, Carter KM et al. Gallstone disease in heart transplant recipients. Ann Surg 2003 237:273–6.

10. Festi D, Colecchia A, Orsini M et al. Gallbladder motility and gallstone formation in obese patients following very low calorie diets. Int J Obes Relat Metab Disord 1998; 22(6):592–600.

11. Nakeeb A, Comuzzie AG, Martin L et al. Gallstones: genetics versus environment. Ann Surg 2002; 235(6):842–9.

12. Dowling RH, Veysey MJ, Pereira SP et al. Role of intestinal transit in the pathogenesis of gallbladder stones. Can J Gastroenterol 1997; 11(1):57–64.

   Recent case-controlled study implicating impaired colonic motility as a cause of gallstone formation.

13. Brink MA, Slors JF, Keuleman YC et al. Entero-hepatic cycling of bilirubin: a putatative mechanism for pigment gallstone formation in ileal Crohn's disease. Gastroenterology 1999; 116(6):1420–7.

14. Smith BF, LaMont JT. The central issue of cholesterol gallstones. Hepatology 1986; 6:529–31.

15. Burnstein MJ, Ilson RG, Petrunka CN et al. Evidence for important nucleating factor in the gall bladder bile of patients with cholesterol gallstones. Gastroenterology 1983; 85:801–7.

16. Dowling RH. Review: pathogenesis of gallstones. Aliment Pharmacol Ther 2000; May 14 Suppl 2:39–47

17. Wosiewitz U, Schenk J, Sabinski F et al. Investigations on common bile duct stones. Digestion 1983; 26:43–52.

18. Keighley MRB. Micro-organisms in the bile. A preventable cause of sepsis after biliary surgery. Ann R Coll Surg Eng 1977; 59:328–34.

19. Glenn F, Moody FG. Acute obstructive suppurative cholangitis. Surg Gynecol Obstet 1961; 113:265–73.

20. Taylor TV, Torrance B, Rimmer S et al. Operative cholangiography: is there a statistical alternative? Am J Surg 1983; 145:640–3.

21. Wilson TG, Hall JC, Watts JM. Is operative cholangiography always necessary? Br J Surg 1986; 73:637–40.

   Two studies that have sought to identify which patients undergoing open cholecystectomy might benefit from a policy of selective cholangiography.

22. Menzies D, Motson RW. Operative common bile duct imaging by operative cholangiography and flexible choledochoscopy. Br J Surg 1992; 79:815–17.

23. Trondsen E, Edwin B, Reiertsen O et al. Prediction of common bile duct stones prior to cholecystectomy: A prospective validation of a discriminant analysis function. Arch Surg 1998; 133:162.

24. Prat F, Meduri B, Ducot B et al. Prediction of common bile duct stones by noninvasive tests. Ann Surg 1999; 229(3):362–8.

25. Pasen P, Partanen K, Pikkarainen P et al. Ultra-sonography, CT, and ERCP in the diagnosis of choledochal stones. Acta Radiol 1992; 33:53–6.

26. Lindsel DRM. Ultrasound imaging of pancreas and biliary tract. Lancet 1990; 335:390–3.

27. Prat F, Amouyal G, Amouyal P et al. Prospective controlled study of endoscopic ultrasonography and endoscopic retrograde cholangiography in patients with suspected common bile duct lithiasis. Lancet 1996; 347(8994):75–9.

   A study making the case for endoscopic ultrasonography as an alternative to ERCP for the detection of common bile duct stones.

28. Norton SA, Alderson D. Endoscopic ultrasonography in the evaluation of idiopathic acute pancreatitis. Br J Surg 2000; 87:1650–5.

29. Berk RN, Cooperberg PL, Gold RP et al. Radiography of the bile ducts. A symposium on the use of new modalities for diagnosis and treatment. Radiology 1982; 145:1–9.

30. Baroll RL. Common bile duct stones. Reassessment of criteria for CT diagnosis. Radiology 1987; 162:419–24.

31. Ichii H, Takada M, Kashiwagi R et al. Three-dimensional reconstruction of biliary tract using spiral computed tomography for laparoscopic cholecystectomy. World J Surg 2002; 26:608–11.

32. Hammerstrom L-E, Holmin T, Stridbeck H et al. Routine preoperative infusion cholangiography at elective cholecystectomy: a prospective study in 694 patients. Br J Surg 1996; 83:750–4.

33. Bloom ITM, Gibbs SL, Keeling-Roberts CS et al. Intravenous infusion cholangiography for investigation of the bile duct – a direct comparison with ERCP. Br J Surg 1996; 83:755–7.

34. Joyce WP, Keane R, Burke GJ et al. Identification of bile duct stones in patients undergoing laparoscopic cholecystectomy. Br J Surg 1991; 78:1174–6.

35. Hochwalk SN, Dobransky MBA, Rofsky NM et al. J Gastrointest Surg 1998; 2(6):573–9.

36. Masui T, Takehara Y, Fujiwara T et al. MR and CT cholangiography in evaluation of the biliary tract. Acta Radiol 1998; 39(5):557–63.

37. Liu TH, Consorti ET, Kawashima A et al. Patient evaluation and management with selective use of magnetic resonance cholangiography and endoscopic retrograde cholangiopancreatography before laparoscopic cholecystectomy. Ann Surg 2001; 234(1):33–40.

This article outlines a simple system to allow stratification of the risk of CBD stones based on routine blood tests. With selective use and accurate reporting of MRCP many patients are saved unnecessary ERCP.

38. Gracie WA, Ransahoff DF. The natural history of silent gallstones: the innocent gallstone is not a myth. N Engl J Med 1982; 307:798–800.

39. McSherry CK, Glenn F. The incidence and causes of death following surgery for non-malignant biliary tract disease. Ann Surg 1980; 191:271–5.

Two important studies that have documented the natural history of asymptomatic gallstones.

40. Iser JH, Dowling RH, Mok HYI et al. Chenodeoxycholic acid treatment of gallstones. N Engl J Med 1975; 293:333–78.

41. Tomida S, Abel M, Yamaguchi Y et al. Long term ursodeoxycholic acid therapy is associated with reduced risk of biliary pain and acute cholecystitis in patients with gallbladder stones; a cohort analysis. Hepatology 1999; 30(1):6–12.

42. Kelly E, Williams JD, Organ CH. A history of the dissolution of retained choledocholithiasis. Am J Surg 2000; 180:86–98.

43. O'Donnell LDJ, Heaton KW. Recurrence and re-recurrence of gallstones after medical dissolution: a long-term follow-up. Gut 1988; 29:655–8.

A study highlighting the limitation of oral dissolution therapy of gallstones.

44. Ahmed R, Freeman JV, Ross B et al. Long term response to gallstone treatment – problems and surprises. Eur J Surg 2000; 166:447–54.

45. Sauerbruch T, Stern M. Fragmentation of bile duct stones by extracorporeal shockwaves. A new approach to biliary calculi after failure of routine endoscopic measures. Gastroenterology 1989; 96:146–52.

46. Herzog U, Messmer P, Sutter M et al. Surgical treatment for cholelithiasis. Surg Gynecol Obstet 1992; 175:238–42.

47. Clavien PA, Sanabria JR, Mentha G et al. Recent results of elective open cholecystectomy in a North American and a European centre – comparison of complications and risk factors. Ann Surg 1992; 216:618–26.

48. Bredesen J, Jorgensen T, Andersen TF et al. Early postoperative mortality following cholecystectomy in the entire female population of Denmark – 1977–1991. World J Surg 1992; 16:530–5.

Both these papers document the results of open cholecystectomy prior to the advent of laparoscopic cholecystectomy.

49. Andren-Sandberg A, Alinder A, Bengmark S. Accidental lesions of the common bile duct at cholecystectomy: pre- and peroperative factors of importance. Ann Surg 1985; 201:328–33.

Frequently cited study that documents risk factors implicated in injury to the common bile duct during open cholecystectomy.

50. Banting S, Carter DC. Expectations of cholecystectomy. In: Paterson-Brown S, Garden J (eds) Principles and practice of surgical laparoscopy. London: WB Saunders, 1994; pp. 53–66.

51. Garden OJ. Iatrogenic injury to the bile duct. Br J Surg 1991; 78:1412–13.

52. Bates T, Ebbs SR, Harrison M et al. Influence of cholecystectomy on symptoms. Br J Surg 1991; 78:964–7.

Important study comparing outcome (and expectations) of open cholecystectomy compared to an age- and sex-matched control group of patients without gallstone disease.

53. MacMahon AJ, Russell IT, Baxter JN et al. Laparoscopic versus minilaparotomy cholecystectomy: a randomised trial. Lancet 1994; 343:135–8.

54. Majeed AW, Troy G, Nicholl JP et al. Randomised, prospective, single-blind comparison of laparoscopic versus small-incision cholecystectomy. Lancet 1996; 347:989–94.

55. Ros A, Gustafsson L, Krook H et al. Laparoscopic cholecystectomy versus mini-laparotomy cholecystectomy: a prospective, randomised, single-blind study. Ann Surg 2001; 234(6):741–9.

Three randomized controlled trials of laparoscopic versus mini-cholecystectomy arriving at different conclusions.

56. Dubois F, Icard P, Berthelot G et al. Coelioscopic cholecystectomy. Ann Surg 1990; 211:60–2.

57. Nathanson LK, Shimi S, Cuschieri A. Laparoscopic cholecystectomy: the Dundee technique. Br J Surg 1991; 78:155–9.

58. Gramatica L, Brasesco OE, Mercado LA et al. Laparoscopic cholecystectomy performed under regional anaesthesia in patients with chronic obstructive pulmonary disease. Surg Endosc 2002; 16:472–5.

59. Ghumman E, Barry M, Grace PA. Management of gallstones in pregnancy. Br J Surg 1997; 84:1646–50.

60. Yeh CN, Chen MF, Jan YY. Laparoscopic cholecystectomy in 226 cirrhotic patients. Experience of a single centre in Taiwan. Surg Endosc 2002; 16:1583–7.

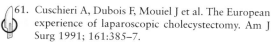
61. Cuschieri A, Dubois F, Mouiel J et al. The European experience of laparoscopic cholecystectomy. Am J Surg 1991; 161:385–7.

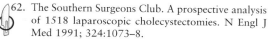
62. The Southern Surgeons Club. A prospective analysis of 1518 laparoscopic cholecystectomies. N Engl J Med 1991; 324:1073–8.

Two important early audits of laparoscopic cholecystectomy in Europe and the USA.

63. Wilson P, Leese T, Morgan WP et al. Elective laparoscopic cholecystectomy for 'all comers'. Lancet 1991; 338:795–7.

64. Unger SW, Rosenbaum G, Unger HM et al. A comparison of laparoscopic and open treatment of acute cholecystitis. Surg Endosc 1993; 7:408–11.

65. Navez B, Mutter D, Russier Y et al. Safety of laparoscopic approach for acute cholecystitis: retrospective study of 609 cases. World J Surg 2001; 25(10):1352–6.

66. Schwesinger WH, Sirinek KR, Strodel WE. Laparoscopic cholecystectomy for biliary tract emergencies: state of the art. World J Surg 1999; 23:334–42.

67. Richards C, Edwards J, Culver D et al. Does using a laparoscopic approach to cholecystectomy decrease the risk of surgical site infection? Ann Surg 2003; 3:358–62.

68. Al-Ghnaniem R, Benjamin IS, Patel AG. Meta-analysis suggests antibiotic prophylaxis is not warranted in low-risk patients undergoing laparoscopic cholecystectomy. Br J Surg 2003; 90:365–6.

69. Lau H, Brooks DC. Contemporary outcomes of ambulatory laparoscopic cholecystectomy in a major teaching hospital. World J Surg 2002; 26:1117–21.

70. Cheah WK, Lenzi JE, So BY et al. Randomised trial of needlescopic versus laparoscopic cholecystectomy. Br J Surg 2001; 88:45–7.

71. Richardson MC, Bell G, Fullarton GM and The West of Scotland Laparoscopic Cholecystectomy Audit Group. Incidence and nature of bile duct injuries following laparoscopic cholecystectomy: an audit of 5913 cases. Br J Surg 1996; 83:1356–60.

Large audit of UK practice of laparoscopic cholecystectomy attempting to assess the causation and incidence of common bile duct injuries during laparoscopic cholecystectomy.

72. MacFadyen BV, Vecchio R, Ricardo AE et al. Bile duct injury after laparoscopic cholecystectomy. Surg Endosc 1998; 12:315–21.

73. Archer SB, Brown DW, Hunter JG et al. Bile duct injury during laparoscopic cholecystectomy: results of a national survey. Ann Surg 2001; 234(4):549–59.

74. Way LW, Stewart L, Hunter JG et al. Causes and prevention of laparoscopic bile duct injuries. Analysis of 252 cases from a human factors and cognitive psychology perspective. Ann Surg 2003; 4:460–9.

75. Fletcher DR, Hobbs M, Tan P et al. Complications of cholecystectomy. Risks of the laparoscopic approach and protective effects of operative cholangiography: a population-based study. Ann Surg 1999; 229(4):449–57.

76. Flum DR, Dellinger EP, Cheadle A et al. Intraoperative cholangiography and risk of common bile duct injury during cholecystectomy. JAMA 2003; 289:1639–44.

Large study on 1.5 million patients demonstrating an increased risk of common bile duct injury when intraoperative cholangiography was not used during laparoscopic cholecystectomy.

77. Snow LL. Evaluation of operative cholangiography in 2043 patients undergoing laparoscopic cholecystectomy. A case for the selective operative cholangiogram. Surg Endosc 2001; 15:14–20.

78. Cassey GP, Kapadia CR. Operative cholangiography or extraductal palpation: an analysis of 418 cholecystectomies. Br J Surg 1981; 68:516–17.

79. Windsor JA, Garden OJ. Laparoscopic ultrasonography. Aust NZ J Surg 1993; 63:1–2.

80. John TG, Banting SW, Pye S et al. Preliminary experience with intracorporeal laparoscopic ultrasonography using a sector scanning probe. A prospective comparison with intraoperative cholangiography in the detection of choledocholithiasis. Surg Endosc 1994; 8:1176–81.

81. Greig JD, John TG, Mahadaven M et al. Laparoscopic ultrasonography in the evaluation of the biliary tree during laparoscopic cholecystectomy. Br J Surg 1994; 84:1202–6.

82. Tranter SE, Thompson MH. Potential of laparoscopic ultrasonography as an alternative to operative cholangiography in the detection of bile duct stones. Br J Surg 2001; 88:65–9.

83. Tranter SE, Thompson MH. A prospective single-blinded controlled study comparing laparoscopic ultrasound of the common bile duct with operative cholangiography. Surg Endosc 2003; 17:216–19.

84. Catheline JM, Turner R, Paries J. Laparoscopic ultrasonography is a complement to cholangiography for the detection of choledocholithiasis at laparoscopic cholecystectomy. Br J Surg 2002; 89:1235–9.

85. Tranter SE, Thompson MH. Spontaneous passage of bile duct stones: frequency of occurrence and relation to clinical presentation. Ann R Coll Surg Engl 2003; 85:174–7.

86. Lygidakis NJ. A prospective randomised study of recurrent choledocholithiasis. Surg Gynecol Obstet 1982; 155(5):679–84.

87. Panis Y, Fagniez PL, Brisset D et al. Long-term results of choledochoduodenostomy versus choledochojejunostomy for choledocholithiasis. Surg Gynecol Obstet 1993; 177(1):33–7.

Two studies stressing the need to consider a surgical drainage procedure if ductal stones are thought to represent primary calculi.

88. Uchiyama K, Onishi H, Tani M et al. Long-term prognosis after treatment of patients with choledocholithiasis. Ann Surg 2003; 238(1):97–102.

89. Jeyapalan M, Almeida JA, Michaelson RL et al. Laparoscopic choledochoduodenostomy: review of a 4-year experience with an uncommon problem. Surg Laparosc Endosc 2002; 12(3):148–53.

90. Rhodes M, Nathanson L. Laparoscopic choledochoduodenostomy. Surg Laparosc Endosc 1996; 6(4):318–21.

91. Khoo D, Walsh CJ, Murphy C et al. Laparoscopic common bile duct exploration: evolution of a new technique. Br J Surg 1996; 83:341–6.

92. Rhodes M, Nathanson L, O'Rourke N et al. Laparoscopic exploration of the common bile duct: lessons learned from 129 consecutive cases. Br J Surg 1995; 82:666–8.

93. Petelin JB. Clinical results of common bile duct exploration. Endosc Surg Allied Technol 1993; 1(3):125–9.

94. Berci G, Morgenstern L. Laparoscopic management of common bile duct stones. A multi-institutional SAGES study. Society of American Gastrointestinal Endoscopic Surgeons. Surg Endosc 1994; 8:1168–74.

95. Martin IJ, Bailey IS, Rhodes M et al. Towards T-tube free laparoscopic bile duct exploration: a methodologic evolution during 300 consecutive procedures. Ann Surg 1998; 228(1):29–34.

96. Cuschieri A, Lezoche E, Morino M et al. E.A.E.S. multicentre prospective randomised trial comparing two-stage vs. single-stage management of patients with gallstone disease and ductal calculi. Surg Endoscopy 1999; 13(10):952–7.

97. Rhodes M, Sussman L, Cohen L et al. Randomised trial of laparoscopic exploration of common bile duct versus postoperative endoscopic retrograde cholangiography for common bile duct stones. Lancet 1998; 351:159–61.

Two important randomized studies and the author's (Nathanson) own experience indicating success of laparoscopic bile duct exploration.

98. Riciardi R, Islam S, Canete JJ et al. Effectiveness and long-term results of laparoscopic common bile duct exploration. Surg Endosc 2003; 17:19–22.

99. Boerma D, Rauws EAJ, Keulemans YCA et al. Wait-and-see policy of laparoscopic cholecystectomy after endoscopic sphincterotomy for bile-duct stones: a randomised trial. Lancet 2002; 360:761–5.

100. Collins C, Maguire D, Ireland A et al. A prospective study of common bile duct calculi in patients undergoing laparoscopic cholecystectomy: natural history of choledocholithiasis revisited. Ann Surg 2004; 239(1):28–33.

A small study showing that a third of incidental common bile duct stones pass spontaneously following laparoscopic cholecystectomy.

101. Finnis D, Rowntree T. Choledochoscopy in exploration of the common bile duct. Br J Surg 1977; 64:661–4.

102. Grange D, Maillard J-N. La choledochoscopie peroperatoire. Gastroenterol Clin Biol 1981; 5:857–65.

103. Griffin WT. Choledochoscopy. Am J Surg 1976; 132:697–8.

104. Lygidakis NJ. Choledochotomy for biliary lithiasis: T-tube drainage or primary closure. Effects on postoperative bacteremia and T-tube bile infection. Am J Surg 1983; 146(2):254–6.

105. Payne RA, Woods WG. Primary closure or T-tube drainage after choledochotomy. Ann R Coll Surg Engl 1986; 68(4):196–8.

106. Williams JA, Treacy PJ, Sidey P et al. Primary duct closure versus T-tube drainage following exploration of the common bile duct. Aust NZ J Surg 1994; 64(12):823–6.

107. Fielding GA. The case for laparoscopic common bile duct exploration J Hepatobil Pancreat Surg 2002; 9:723–8.

108. Tanaka M. Bile duct clearance, endoscopic or laparoscopic? J Hepatobil Pancreat Surg 2002; 9:729–32.

109. Leese T, Neoptolemos JP, Carr-Locke DL. Successes, failures, early complications and their management: results of 394 consecutive patients from a single centre. Br J Surg 1985; 72:215–19.

110. Ochi Y, Mukawa K, Kiyosawa K et al. Comparing the treatment outcomes of endoscopic papillary dilation and endoscopic sphincterotomy for removal of bile duct stones. J Gastroenterol Hepatol 1999; 14(1):90–6.

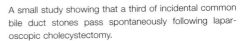

111. Vaira D, Ainley C, Williams S et al. Endoscopic sphincterotomy in 1000 consecutive patients. Lancet 1989; ii:431–4.

Three reports supporting use of endoscopic removal of common bile duct stones in high-risk surgical patients.

112. Rosso PG, Kortan P, Haber G. Selective common bile duct cannulation can be simplified by the use of a standard papillotome. Gastrointest Endosc 1993; 39:67–9.

113. Lambert ME, Betts CD, Hill J et al. Endoscopic sphincterotomy – the whole truth. Br J Surg 1991; 78:473–6.

114. Birkett DH. Biliary laser lithotripsy. Surg Clin North Am 1992; 72:641–52.

115. Webber J, Ademak HE, Riemann JF. Extracorporeal piezo-electric lithotripsy for retained bile duct stones. Endoscopy 1992; 24:239–43.

116. Shaw MJ, Mackie RD, Moore JP et al. Results of a multi-centre trial using a mechanical lithotriptor for the treatment of large bile duct stones. Am J Gastroenterol 1993; 88:730–3.

117. Leese T, Neoptolemos JP, Baker AR et al. Management of acute cholangitis and the impact of endoscopic sphincterotomy Br J Surg 1986; 73:988–92.

118. Leung JWC, Cotton PB. Endoscopic nasobiliary catheter drainage in biliary and pancreatic disease. Am J Gastroenterol 1991; 86:389–94.

119. Neoptolemos JP, Carr-Locke DL, Fossard NP. A prospective randomised study of pre-operative endoscopic sphincterotomy versus surgery alone for common bile duct stones. Br Med J 1987; 294:470–4.

120. Barwood NT, Valinsky LJ, Hobbs M et al. Changing methods of imaging the common bile duct in the laparoscopic cholecystectomy era in Western Australia. Implications for surgical practice. Ann Surg 2002; 235(1):41–50.

121. Tatulli F, Cuttitta A. Laparoendoscopic approach to treatment of common bile duct stones. J Laparoendosc Adv Surg Tech 2000; 10(6):315–17.

122. Ng T, Amaral J. Timing of endoscopic retrograde cholangio-pancreatography and laparoscopic cholecystectomy in the treatment of choledocholithiasis. J Laparoendosc Adv Surg Tech 1999; Part A 9(1):31–7.

123. Lichtenstein D, Carr-Locke D. Closed treatment of choledocholithiasis. In: Paterson-Brown S, Garden J (eds) Principles and practice of surgical laparoscopy. London: WB Saunders, 1994; pp. 105–40.

124. Ammori BJ, Birbas K, Davides D et al. Routine vs 'on demand' postoperative ERCP for small bile duct calculi detected at intraoperative cholangiography. Surg Endosc 2000; 14:1123–6.

125. Urbach DR, Khanjanchee YS, Jobe BA et al. Cost-effective management of common bile duct stones. Surg Endosc 2001; 15:4–13.

126. Tranter SE, Thompson MH. Comparison of endoscopic sphincterotomy and laparoscopic exploration of the common bile duct. Br J Surg 2002; 89:1495–1504.

127. Tranter Thompson. All-comers policy for laparoscopic exploration of the common bile duct. Br J Surg 2002; 89:1608–12.

128. Menzies D, Motson RW. Percutaneous flexible choledochoscopy: a simple method for retained common bile duct stone removal. Br J Surg 1991; 78(8):959–60.

129. Burhenne HJ. The technique of biliary duct stone extraction. Radiology 1974; 113:567–72.

130. Mason R. Percutaneous extraction of retained gallstones via the T-tube track – British experience of 131 cases. Clin Radiol 1980; 31:587–97.

131. Nussinson E, Cairns SR, Vaira D et al. A 10-year single centre experience of percutaneous and endoscopic extraction of bile duct stones with T-tube in situ. Gut 1991; 32:1040–3.

132. Nathan MH, Newman MA, Murray DJ et al. Cholecystokinin cholecystography. Four years evaluation. Am J Roentgenol 1970; 110:240–51.

133. Lennard TWJ, Farndon JR, Taylor RMR. Acalculous biliary pain: diagnosis and selection for cholecystectomy using the cholecystokinin test for pain reproduction. Br J Surg 1984; 71:368–70.

134. Sunderland GT, Carter DC. Clinical application of the cholecystokinin provocation test. Br J Surg 1988; 75:444–9.

Nine

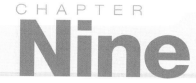

Benign biliary tract diseases

Benjamin N.J. Thomson and
O. James Garden

INTRODUCTION

Apart from those disorders related to chole-docholithiasis, benign diseases of the biliary tree are relatively uncommon (**Box 9.1**). The most challenging issues are in patients who present with symptoms associated with biliary strictures, which more commonly arise following iatrogenic injury during cholecystectomy. Congenital abnormalities such as choledochal cysts and biliary atresia are usually in the domain of the paediatric surgeon although later presentation of cysts may occur after missed diagnosis or when revisional surgery is required. Most of the published literature regarding benign non-gallstone biliary disease is retrospective or at best prospectively gathered, non-randomised data, but clear guidelines can be followed based upon observation.

CONGENITAL ANOMALIES

Biliary atresia

Biliary atresia is thought to be an inflammatory process that occurs before birth leading to the failure of development of the biliary lumen in all or part of the extrahepatic biliary tree. This occurs in approximately 1 per 10 000 live births but its aetiology remains unclear.

Box 9.1 • Benign causes of biliary strictures

Strictures of the extrahepatic biliary tree
Iatrogenic biliary injury
Post-cholecystectomy
Trauma
Other
Gallstone related
Mirizzi's syndrome
Inflammatory
Recurrent pyogenic cholangitis
Parasitic infestation
Clonorchis sinensis
Opisthorchis viverrini
Echinococcus
Ascaris
Primary sclerosing cholangitis
Benign strictures imitating malignancy
Pancreatitis
Lymphoplasmacytic pancreatitis
Inflammatory pseudotumour
HIV cholangiopathy

Presentation is usually in the early neonatal period with prolongation of neonatal jaundice. Most patients are treated in specialist neonatal surgical units; however, occasionally patients may be referred to adult units for assessment for liver transplantation. Treatment in the neonate is by portoenterostomy (Kasai's operation), which involves anastomosis of a Roux limb of jejunum to the tissue of the hilum. Restoration of bile flow has been reported in 86% of infants treated before 8 weeks of age, but only 36% in older children, with a probability of survival without liver transplantation of 60% at 5 years.[1]

Choledochal cysts

The earliest description of a choledochal cyst was by Douglas in 1952,[2] who described a 17-year-old girl with jaundice, fever and a painful mass in the right hypochondrium. However, presentation is usually in childhood and around 25% are diagnosed in the first year, although prenatal diagnosis is now possible with improvements in antenatal ultrasonography.[3] Adult centres treat a small proportion of those with delayed diagnosis as well as complications from previous cyst surgery.

The incidence of choledochal cysts in Western countries is around 1 in 200 000 live births but it is much higher in Asia. There is a frequent association with other hepatobiliary disease such as hepatic fibrosis as well as an aberrant pancreatico-biliary duct junction.[4]

Traditionally diagnosis has included abdominal ultrasonography, computed tomography (CT) scanning and endoscopic retrograde cholangio-pancreatography (ERCP). However, magnetic resonance cholangiopancreatography (MRCP) now allows images that are superior to traditional cholangiography (**Fig. 9.1**), and it should be recommended due to its non-invasive nature.[5]

CLASSIFICATION

The modified Todani classification can be employed to describe the various forms of choledochal cyst[6] (**Fig. 9.2**). Type I is the most common and represents a solitary cyst characterised by fusiform dilatation of the common bile duct. Type II comprises a diverticulum of the common bile duct, whilst type III cysts are choledochoceles. Type IV is the second

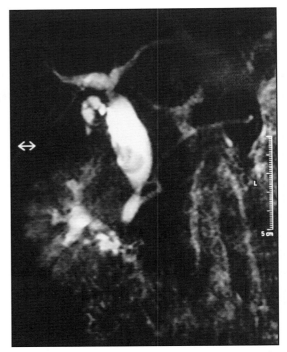

Figure 9.1 • MRCP demonstrating a type I choledochal cyst.

most common, with extension of cysts into the intrahepatic ducts. Lastly, type V involves intrahepatic cystic disease with no choledochal cyst, which merges into the syndrome of Caroli's disease.

RISK OF MALIGNANCY

In the Western literature the incidence of cholangiocarcinoma is considered to be lower (0–14%)[7–9] than that reported in Japanese series (17.5%).[10] The association with biliary malignancy is poorly understood but may be related to the reflux of pancreatic fluid into the biliary system leading to biliary epithelial damage. Recently, mutations of the tumour suppressor genes *p53* and *Smad-4* as well as the oncogene K-*ras* have been identified in resected specimens of choledochal cysts and aberrant pancreatico-biliary duct junctions.[11,12] Cyst drainage without cyst excision does not prevent later malignant change, and there is continuing debate regarding the precise on-going risk following cyst resection. The overall risk increases with time, with an age-related incidence of 0.7% in the first decade rising to 14% after 20 years of age.[13]

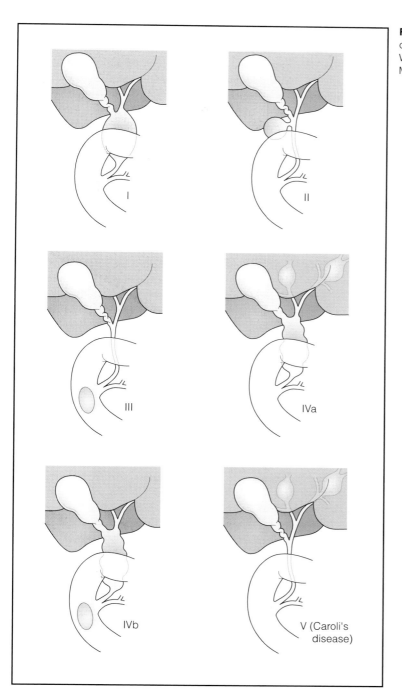

Figure 9.2 • Modified Todani classification for choledochal cysts.[7] With permission from Excerpta Medica Inc.

MANAGEMENT

Surgical resection is required to prevent recurrent episodes of sepsis and pain, to prevent the risk of pancreatitis from passage of debris and calculi, and because of the association with cholangiocarcinoma. Complete cyst excision with preservation of the pancreatic duct is required, with hepaticojejunostomy for reconstruction. Some authors advocate liver resection for type IV cysts with intrahepatic extension for complete removal of the cyst, although the advantage is debatable.[10,14]

Cyst-enterostomy, or drainage of the cyst into the duodenum, should no longer be performed as the cyst epithelium remains unstable and malignant potential remains. If previous drainage has been performed, symptoms of cholangitis generally persist and conversion to a Roux-en-Y hepaticojejunostomy is advisable.

SPECIAL OPERATIVE TECHNIQUES

During operative exposure intraoperative ultrasound is very useful to identify the biliary confluence, the intrahepatic extension of the cyst and the relationship with the right hepatic artery above and to the pancreatic duct below (**Fig. 9.3a,b**). Small aberrant hepatic ducts may enter the cyst below the biliary confluence and these are frequently missed on preoperative imaging.[15] Such aberrant ducts are usually identified once the cyst has been opened, although intraoperative ultrasound may occasionally detect these. The cyst is normally best excised in its entirety and this is facilitated by opening it along its anterior length. This aids identification of the vessels from which the cyst is freed. Early identification of the biliary confluence aids the surgeon in planning the incorporation of any segmental duct into the eventual hepatico-jejunal Roux-en-Y anastomosis. Dissection into the head of the pancreas is made easier by use of bipolar scissors and the CUSA™ (ultrasonic surgical aspiration system, ValleyLab, Boulder, CO) if the plane of dissection is obscured by fibrosis or inflammation. It may be necessary to leave a small oversewn lower common bile duct stump to avoid compromise to the pancreatic duct lumen.

(a)
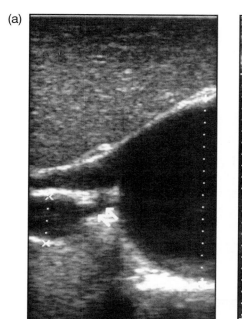

(b)
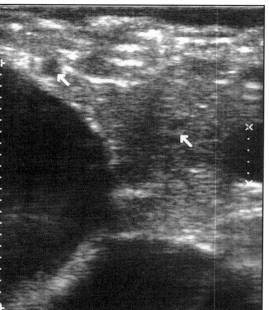

Figure 9.3 • **(a)** Operative ultrasound scan of a type I choledochal cyst. The junction of the undilated proximal biliary tree with the cyst (long dotted line) is demonstrated. The right hepatic artery is posterior (two arrows) as is the right branch of the portal vein (short dotted line). **(b)** Operative ultrasound scan of a type I choledochal cyst. This scan is of the pancreatic head with a choledochal cyst (long dotted line). The gastroduodenal artery (left arrow), pancreatic duct (right arrow) and splenoportal junction are demonstrated (short dotted line).

There is an accepted association between choledochal cyst and cholangiocarcinoma. The cyst should be excised and the biliary tree reconstructed by means of a hepatico-jejunostomy Roux-en-Y.

IATROGENIC BILIARY INJURY

The commonest cause of an injury to the extra-hepatic biliary tree is as a result of an iatrogenic injury at the time of cholecystectomy. Although it is recognised that injury may also occur during other gastric or pancreatic procedures, this is much less common with the reduction in ulcer surgery and increasing specialisation in pancreatico-biliary surgery. Rarely the injury may be related to abdominal trauma, injection of scolicidal agents in the management of hydatid cyst, or radiotherapy.

The true incidence of biliary injury following laparoscopic cholecystectomy remains obscure. It has been suggested that there was a slight decrease in the incidence of injuries following initial intro-duction of the laparoscopic technique,[16] with a reported incidence of 0.3–0.7%.[17–19] Nevertheless, an anonymous survey performed in British Columbia identified that surgeons performing laparoscopic cholecystectomy had a 1 in 2 chance of causing a biliary injury in their working lifetime.[20]

Open cholecystectomy is said to have a lower incidence of biliary injury, with a rate of 0.13%.[21,22] In our own unit's series of 114 bile duct injuries, 35% occurred during laparoscopic cholecystectomy, 33% in patients converted to open cholecystectomy, and 26% during open cholecystectomy. A further 6% occurred during upper gastrointestinal surgery,[23] a figure not dissimilar to that reported in the North American literature.[24]

Aetiology

Previous reports of injury during laparoscopic chole-cystectomy suggested that injury was more likely to occur when performed for pancreatitis, cholangitis or acute cholecystitis.[25] However, the majority of cholecystectomies are performed for biliary colic. In a recent prospective analysis of patients referred following biliary injury, 71% occurred in patients in whom the indication for cholecystectomy was biliary colic alone,[26] and thus surgeons should always be vigilant regardless of the indication.

In the majority of patients the problem is misinterpretation of the biliary anatomy, with the common bile duct confused with the cystic duct. Injury to the right hepatic artery often occurs in association as it is mistaken for the cystic artery. Partial injury may occur to the common bile duct after a diathermy burn or due to rigorous traction on the cystic duct, leading to its avulsion from the bile duct. Occasionally perforation of the bile duct may occur secondary to the passage of a cholangiogram catheter.[26]

Techniques to avoid injury

Many techniques have been described to decrease the risk of injury to the common bile duct during cholecystectomy. The main risk factors are thought to be inexperience, aberrant anatomy and inflammation.[27] However, in a recent analysis of 252 laparoscopic bile duct injuries, the primary cause of error was a visual perceptual illusion in 97% of cases, whilst faults in technical skill were present in only 3% of injuries.[28]

Identification of the biliary anatomy is essential in avoiding injury to the extrahepatic bile duct. Dissection of Hartmann's pouch should start at the junction of the gallbladder and cystic duct and con-tinue lateral to the cystic lymph node thus staying as close as possible to the gallbladder. The biliary tree and hepatic arterial anatomy is highly variable and therefore great care must be taken in identify-ing all structures within Calot's triangle before ligation. In Couinaud's published study of biliary anatomy, 25% had drainage of a right sectoral duct directly into the common hepatic duct.[29] Sometimes this structure may follow a prolonged extrahepatic course where it can be at greater risk from chole-cystectomy. The right hepatic artery may also course through this area. All structures should be traced into the gallbladder to minimise the risk of injury.

Extensive diathermy dissection should be avoided in Calot's triangle as diathermy injury may occur to the lateral wall of the common hepatic duct. Furthermore, arterial bleeding in this area should not be cauterised blindly. Most bleeding can be controlled with several minutes of direct pressure with a laparoscopic forceps compressing Hartmann's pouch onto the bleed point.

During the era of open cholecystectomy many advocated complete excision of the cystic duct to its insertion into the common bile duct to avoid a cystic duct stump syndrome. However, extensive dissection around the common bile duct with diathermy may cause an ischaemic stricture due to the intricate blood supply of the common hepatic duct, and the cystic duct is known often to pursue a long course into the pancreatic region whilst being densely adherent to the common hepatic duct.

Many authors argue that operative cholangiography is essential to avoid biliary injury.[15,18,25,30] Fletcher et al. reported an overall twofold reduction in biliary injuries with the use of operative cholangiography, with an eightfold decrease in complex cases.[25] Flum and colleagues analysed retrospectively the Medicare database in the USA and identified 7911 common bile duct injuries following cholecystectomy. After adjusting for patient-level factors and surgeon-level factors the adjusted relative risk when intraoperative cholangiography was not used was 1.49 (95% confidence interval 1.38–2.28).[18] When the use of intraoperative cholangiography has undergone cost analysis, routine cholangiography has been found to be the most cost effective during high-risk operations when employed by less experienced surgeons.[31]

Unfortunately, many operative cholangiograms are interpreted incorrectly and injuries are missed.[32] In reported series of biliary injuries only 6–33% of operative cholangiograms were interpreted correctly.[26,32–34] For correct anatomical interpretation of the proximal biliary tree, both right sectoral/sectional ducts and the left hepatic duct should be visualised. In the presence of an endoscopic sphincterotomy contrast will preferentially flow into the duodenum and the patient may need to be placed in a head-down position to fill the intrahepatic ducts. When operative cholangiography is used and the anatomy is unclear, no proximal clip should be placed on what is presumed to be the cystic duct, to avoid a crush injury to what may be the common hepatic duct.

Retrograde cholecystectomy has previously been described as a safe technique when inflammation around Calot's triangle makes identification of the anatomy difficult. Nonetheless, care still needs to be exercised during dissection to avoid injury to the right hepatic artery and common hepatic duct, which may be adherent to an inflamed gallbladder. If identification remains impossible then the gallbladder can be opened to facilitate identification of the cystic duct. A subtotal cholecystectomy should be considered if a safe plane of dissection cannot be established, thus avoiding injury to the common hepatic or left hepatic ducts. Originally described for open cholecystectomy, these techniques have now also been performed laparoscopically.[35]

Bile duct injury can be avoided by careful identification of the biliary anatomy, dissection close to the gallbladder and avoidance of diathermy in Calot's triangle. The use of operative cholangiography and its correct interpretation is associated with a reduced incidence of bile duct injury.

Classification

Injury to the distal biliary tree is less technically demanding to repair than involvement of the biliary confluence. The success of reconstruction depends on the type of injury and the anatomical location.[36] Bismuth first described a classification system for biliary strictures reflecting the relationship of the injury to the biliary confluence (**Table 9.1**).[37] Strasberg and colleagues further proposed a broader classification to include a number of biliary complications including cystic stump leaks, biliary leaks and partial injuries to the biliary tree (**Fig. 9.4**).[22]

Table 9.1 • Bismuth classification of biliary strictures

Bismuth classification	Definition
Bismuth 1	Low common hepatic duct stricture – hepatic duct stump >2 cm
Bismuth 2	Proximal common hepatic duct stricture – hepatic duct stump <2 cm
Bismuth 3	Hilar stricture with no residual common hepatic duct – hepatic duct confluence intact
Bismuth 4	Destruction of hepatic duct confluence – right and left hepatic ducts separated
Bismuth 5	Involvement of aberrant right sectoral hepatic duct alone or with concomitant stricture of the common hepatic duct

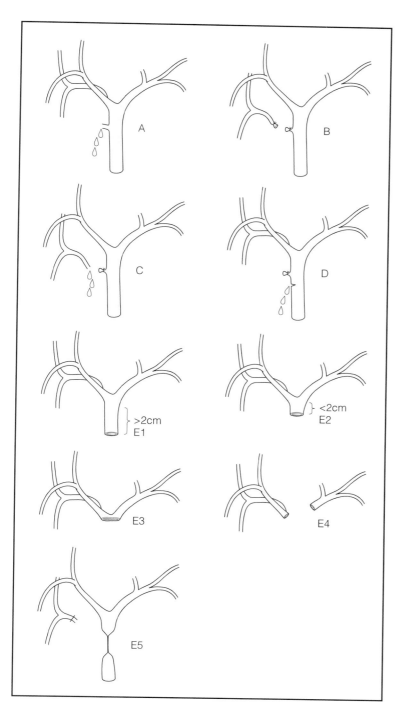

Figure 9.4 • Strasberg classification. Injuries E1–E5 include the Bismuth classification (**Table 9.1**).[22] From Strasberg SM et al. J Am Coll Surg 1995; 180:102–25, with permission.

Type A injuries include leakage from the cystic duct or subvesical ducts. Type B involves occlusion of part of the biliary tree, most usually an aberrant right hepatic duct. If the former injury involves transection without ligation this is termed a type C injury. A lateral injury to the biliary tree is a type D injury. Type E injuries are those described by Bismuth and subdivided into his classification (**Table 9.1**). Unfortunately neither system allows perfect description of all injuries that may arise following surgery, but the type E, or Bismuth, classification of injuries are those that arise most frequently at laparoscopic cholecystectomy.

Presentation

It is preferable that injuries are recognised at the time of surgery to allow the best chance of repair. However, this occurs in less than a third of patients. An unrecognised injury may present early with a postoperative biliary fistula, symptoms of biliary peritonitis or jaundice. Early symptoms or signs may be lacking but ductal injury should be suspected in the patient whose recovery is not immediate or is complicated by symptoms of peritoneal or diaphragmatic irritation and/or associated with deranged liver function tests. Signs may range from localised abdominal tenderness through to generalised peritonitis with overwhelming sepsis. Ligation of the bile duct will present early with jaundice; however, later presentation may occur as a result of stricture formation from a partial injury, localised inflammation or ischaemic insult.

Ligation of sectoral ducts may cause subsequent or late atrophy of the drained liver segments, which may become infected secondarily. Occasionally injuries may present late with secondary biliary cirrhosis, which may require liver transplantation when liver failure results.

In many patients there is a delay until referral, despite evidence of a biliary injury. In a report by Mirza et al. the median interval until referral was 26 days.[38] This delay is not inconsequential as the opportunity for an early repair is lost and results in the liver sustaining further damage. Johnson et al. demonstrated an association between hepatic fibrosis and early cirrhosis on liver biopsy if there had been a significant delay in referral.[39]

Management

INTRAOPERATIVE RECOGNITION

In a review by Carroll et al., only 27% of patients underwent a successful repair by the primary surgeon responsible for the injury whilst 79% of repairs performed following referral had a successful outcome.[40] If experienced help is not at hand, no attempt should be made to remedy the situation since this may compromise subsequent successful management. A T-tube or similar drain should be placed to the biliary injury and drains left in the subhepatic space followed by referral to a specialist centre. No attempt should be made to repair a transection or excision of the bile duct. A partial injury to the bile duct may sometimes be managed with direct closure with placement of a T-tube through a separate choledochotomy. Primary repair with or without a T-tube for complete transection of the common bile duct is nearly always unsuccessful. This may result from unappreciated loss of common duct or arterial injury, or result from local diathermy injury or devascularisation of the duct from overzealous dissection of the common bile duct[41] (**Fig. 9.5a,b**).

If an injury to the biliary tree is suspected during cholecystectomy then help must be sought from an experienced hepatobiliary surgeon. A successful repair by the surgeon who has caused the injury is far less likely than one performed by a surgeon experienced in performing a hepatico-jejunostomy.

POSTOPERATIVE RECOGNITION: BILIARY FISTULA

Any patient who is not fit for discharge at 24 hours due to ongoing abdominal pain, vomiting, fever or bile in an abdominal drain should be considered to have a biliary leak. The lack of bile in an abdominal drain does not exclude the possibility of a biliary leak, particularly if there is liver function test derangement. Symptoms and signs vary widely, and widespread soiling of the abdominal cavity may be present with few signs.

Initial investigation should include full blood examination and determination of serum levels of urea, electrolytes, creatinine and liver function tests. Ultrasound is usually the initial investigation. However, it cannot readily differentiate bile and blood from a residual fluid collection following uneventful cholecystectomy. It does, however, provide important information about the presence of intra-abdominal or pelvic fluid, biliary dilatation or retained stones within the bile duct.

If there is evidence of significant peritoneal irritation from widespread biliary peritonitis,

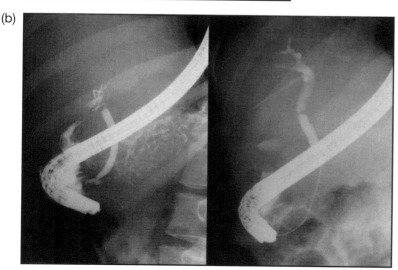

laparoscopy allows confirmation of this and provides an opportunity for abdominal lavage. The porta hepatis can be inspected to determine the cause of the bile leak. Whilst dislodged clips from the cystic duct can be managed by application of further clips or suture, any other form of bile leak should lead to specialist referral. Drains can be placed to the subhepatic space as well as the sub-diaphragmatic space and pelvis if required. No attempt should be made to repair an injury laparoscopically. If laparotomy is required, this should be considered in conjunction with specialist assistance if bile duct injury is suspected.

Further assessment depends on the clinical situation. The majority of biliary fistulas are due to leaks from the cystic duct stump or subvesicle ducts, and ERCP allows anatomical definition as well as endoscopic sphincterotomy or stent placement. Almost all simple cystic duct stump leaks can be resolved by endoscopic stenting if cannulation is possible at ERCP.[42,43] Occasionally side injury to the biliary tree may also be controlled with endoscopic stent placement.[42,44]

If ERCP is unsuccessful or the bile duct ligated or occluded by clips, percutaneous transhepatic cholangiography allows diagnosis, delineates the biliary anatomy and may facilitate biliary decompression if necessary. Occasionally both sides of the liver may need to be externally drained to gain control of a biliary fistula, especially with E4 injuries

Figure 9.5 • **(a)** Failure of primary repair with T-tube. Primary repair was performed for an injury to the common bile duct presenting with biliary peritonitis. A T-tube was inserted through the anastomosis and this was removed at 4 weeks. An anastomotic stricture developed and the patient required a hepatico-jejunostomy 2 months later. **(b)** Failure of primary repair for ligation of the common bile duct. A complete transection of the common bile duct identified at postoperative endoscopic retrograde cholangiopancreatography (ERCP). Immediate repair was performed with a direct duct-to-duct repair. A tight anastomotic stricture is demonstrated at a later ERCP.

to the biliary confluence. However, injury to the biliary tree detected in this way may allow surgical repair to be considered within the first week of injury in the stable non-septic patient, and again such further investigation or management decisions should only be considered following specialist referral.

Where the diagnosis of bile duct injury has been delayed, the aim should be to control the biliary fistula with external drainage using surgical or radiologically placed drains. Further control may be required with endoscopic stenting or external biliary drainage. Delayed repair can be considered subsequently once sepsis and intra-abdominal soiling has resolved, as a planned elective procedure in a specialist unit usually 2–3 months following injury. Such an initial conservative approach renders a potentially difficult operation into a repair, which will be considerably easier.

Diagnosis of a bile duct injury in the postoperative period should lead to immediate referral to a specialist centre since inappropriate attempts to manage this outwith a specialist centre will compromise the outcome.

POSTOPERATIVE RECOGNITION: BILIARY OBSTRUCTION

Ligation or inadvertent clipping of the biliary tree presents early in the postoperative period with jaundice. Later, stricture formation may occur as a result of direct trauma during dissection, clips placed inadvertently on the cystic duct but compromising the bile duct, or from damage to the intricate vascular supply of the bile duct by extensive mobilisation or diathermy.

Initial investigation should include haematology, assessment of coagulation by estimation of prothrombin time, and by liver function tests. Ultrasound may indicate the level of obstruction or exclude the presence of a correctable cause of obstructive jaundice, such as a retained stone in the common bile duct.

ERCP will identify a stricture or complete transection of the bile duct. Overzealous instillation of contrast should be avoided, and placement of an endoscopic stent should only be considered after consultation with a specialist unit since this may introduce sepsis into the biliary tree and compromise

further management. Furthermore, an undrained biliary tree may allow proximal biliary dilatation thereby facilitating later reconstruction. Although some units have reported satisfactory resolution of biliary strictures with endoscopic stenting alone,[44,45] the reported follow-up has usually been short and in our experience almost all patients require later surgery. Partial occlusion of the duct by a clip may be remedied by balloon dilatation with or without placement of a stent; however, delay in diagnosis may result in subsequent recurrent stricture formation. In a report by Familiari and colleagues, biliary strictures were managed with progressive insertion of 10 French plastic stents up to a maximum of four endoprostheses, which were left in situ for a mean of 20 months until disappearance of the stenosis. Of the 17 strictures so treated, 11 resolved completely, 3 were still being treated, 2 required surgery and 1 refused further endoscopic surgery (median follow-up 40 months).[44] It may be that such an approach is appropriate for a frail elderly patient although repeated interventions over a prolonged period of time put the patient at risk of recurrent cholangitis.

If the diagnosis of ductal obstruction is made early within the first week post-surgery, if the bilirubin level is only moderately elevated and there is no coexisting coagulopathy or sepsis, then immediate repair will offer the best chance of a successful outcome.

If repair needs to be delayed, stent placement may still be avoidable and a decision will generally be made based on the individual patient circumstances. Suspicion or evidence of arterial injury may influence the management decision.

For strictures that declare late, appropriate indications for stent placement are the presence of sepsis, severe itch resistant to medical therapy, or significant hepatic dysfunction.

THE TIMING OF REPAIR

Early repair

When an injury is recognised in the early postoperative period and there is minimal peritoneal contamination or sepsis, a definitive repair by an experienced surgeon can be successful (**Fig. 9.6**) (also in colour, see Plate 6, facing p. 20). In our series of 114 patients with biliary injury, none of the 21 patients who had definitive repair in our unit

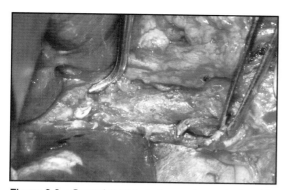

Figure 9.6 • Operative picture of an early repair of an E4 injury. A right-angle forceps is placed in the opening of the left hepatic duct whilst the open right hepatic duct is visible below. The portal vein is skeletonised with ligation and excision of both the extrahepatic biliary tree and right hepatic artery (held by forceps). See also Plate 6, facing p. 20.

within the first postoperative week have required revisional surgery to date. Of the 83 delayed repairs or revisions, 13 (16%) have required further surgery.[46] The most important factor for revisional surgery was a repair performed before referral. Forty-one of 52 (79%) patients in whom repair was attempted before referral required further surgery whilst only 3 of 52 (6%) patients repaired after referral required further revisional surgery.

Delayed repair

Many injuries continue to be unrecognised or referral delayed. In a recent prospective audit of major bile duct injuries from Australia, the median delay before referral was 9 days (2–28 days), and this included five patients with generalised peritonitis.[26]

The first treatment aim is to control the biliary injury and associated sepsis. This may require endoscopic or percutaneous biliary decompression of the bile duct, allowing jaundice to settle or biliary sepsis to be drained. Intra-abdominal collections may be drained percutaneously, or in the early postoperative period this may be better achieved by laparoscopic means. It is accepted, however, that bile collections are frequently loculated and difficult to eradicate in patients with intra-abdominal sepsis or widespread biliary contamination or peritonitis. The most effective treatment may be laparotomy with extensive lavage and the placement of large intra-abdominal drains. Definitive repair should not be contemplated if there is severe peritoneal soiling since injudicious attempts to repair the injury may aggravate the injury and result in a poor outcome.

Once these objectives have been met, the patient should be allowed to recover from the combined insult of surgery and sepsis. A period of rehabilitation at home is generally required before repair is contemplated in these compromised patients. Abdominal and biliary drainage can be managed on an outpatient basis with community nursing support. Nutritional supplementation may be required, particularly in those who have required a prolonged admission to the intensive care unit and hospital. Attention should be paid to the consequences of prolonged external biliary drainage and consideration given to recycling of bile.

Associated vascular injury

Abdominal CT scanning is required to ensure resolution of intra-abdominal collections and before repair to exclude the presence of liver atrophy. Atrophy can occur from prolonged obstruction to the segmental, sectional or hepatic ducts but is generally associated with the presence of a vascular injury, most usually of the right hepatic artery. Liver resection may occasionally be needed at the time of definitive repair to remove a source of ongoing sepsis or if satisfactory and secure reconstruction to the left or right duct is not possible.

Buell and colleagues identified associated vascular injury as an independent predictor of mortality, with 38% of patients dying compared to 3% ($P < 0.001$) where no arterial injury was present.[47] Some authors advocate arteriography before repair to identify such associated vascular injury as a repair is less likely to be successful.[48] However, in a recent paper by Alves and colleagues,[49] 55 patients with postcholecystectomy strictures who underwent surgical reconstruction with a left duct approach had preoperative coeliac axis and superior mesenteric artery angiography. Twenty-six patients (47%) had an associated vascular injury, of which 20 (36%) were of the right hepatic artery. In this series only one patient in each group (vascular injury vs. no injury) developed a recurrent stricture after repair.[49] A proximal anastomosis may offer a better blood supply, minimising the risk of anastomotic stricturing. In support of this theory Mercado and colleagues demonstrated that patients with an anastomosis fashioned below the biliary confluence were more likely to require revisional surgery (16%) compared to an anastomosis performed at the biliary confluence (0%; $P < 0.05$).[50] Recent improvements in magnetic resonance imaging (MRI) and spiral CT are producing impressive arterial and venous anatomical reconstructions, which may negate the need for invasive arteriography (**Fig. 9.7**).

Injury to the hepatic arterial supply may present with haemobilia or intra-abdominal haemorrhage from a false aneurysm, usually associated with on-going subhepatic sepsis and most frequently of the right hepatic arteries. If suspected, urgent angiography is required (**Fig. 9.8**). Haemorrhage may be controlled by embolisation of the feeding vessel although re-bleeding can occur and necessitate further embolisation. However, in our experience,

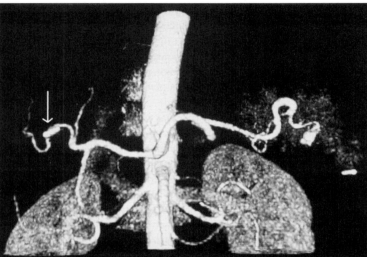

Figure 9.7 • Spiral CT arterial reconstruction. A clip is visible on the right posterior sectoral artery (arrow).

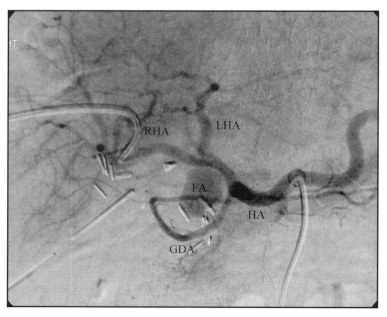

Figure 9.8 • Digital subtraction angiogram demonstrating a false aneurysm of the common hepatic artery. Embolisation was required for control. The patient has undergone a primary repair for a complete transection of the common bile duct. FA, false aneurysm; HA, common hepatic artery; GDA, gastroduodenal artery; RHA, right hepatic artery; LHA, left hepatic artery.

further bleeding in the presence of ongoing sepsis usually requires laparotomy for control of bleeding and drainage of any subhepatic collection.

Further imaging

For patients with injury to the biliary confluence (E3 and E4), preoperative imaging will help in the planning of future repair. In the presence of a biliary stricture, invasive cholangiography by ERCP or percutaneous transhepatic cholangiogram (PTC) risks introducing sepsis. However, if PTC is required for external biliary drainage, an adequate cholangiogram may be obtained at this time. The quality of MRCP continues to improve, and detailed biliary anatomical reconstructions can be produced, thereby negating the need for more invasive imaging.

OPERATIVE TECHNIQUES

Biliary reconstruction should be performed under optimal circumstances at the time of injury or soon thereafter. Once this opportunity has been lost, repair should only be considered when the patient has been optimised, in the absence of intra-abdominal sepsis and when sufficient time has elapsed to allow for maturation of adhesions and the tissues at the porta hepatis.

We use a right subcostal incision for access, which can be extended across the midline if required. Retraction is provided with Doyen's blades and the Omni-tract® (Omni-tract surgical, St Paul MN) mechanical retractor. Laparotomy is undertaken to assess the liver and to allow adhesiolysis thereby freeing the small bowel for reconstruction. Frequently the omentum, hepatic flexure, duodenum and hepatoduodenal ligament are involved in a dense inflammatory mass, and occasionally an unsuspected fistula between bile duct and duodenum or colon is identified. Dissection is often easier if commenced laterally and then directed towards the biliary structures. The common bile duct can be difficult to identify, particularly in the presence of extensive fibrosis, and intraoperative ultrasound is a useful tool in allowing its location and relationship to vessels to be determined (**Fig. 9.9**).

For injuries that involve the biliary confluence, lowering of the hilar plate allows easier identification of the left and right hepatic ducts. This may be aided by the use of an ultrasonic dissector (CUSA), which is also employed to break down the

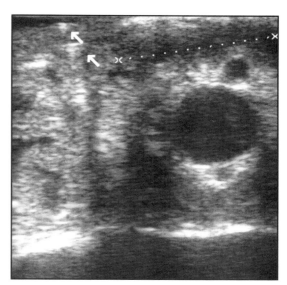

Figure 9.9 • Operative ultrasound scan to identify the biliary tree. The dotted line identifies the biliary tree above the ligation with clips (arrows). The right hepatic artery and portal vein are seen posteriorly.

contracted fibrotic tissue in the gallbladder bed and facilitate the division of any bridge of liver tissue between segments 3 and 4. Opening these two planes on the right and left sides facilitates identification of and access to the biliary confluence.

Since the blood supply to the bile duct is often damaged at the time of injury, the common hepatic duct should be opened as proximally as possible, although frequently there has been retraction of the fibrotic remnant superiorly. Extension of the incision into the left hepatic duct allows a wide anastomosis to be fashioned with adequate views of the left- and right-sided ducts. Care should be taken since there may be a small superficial arterial branch crossing the left duct anteriorly and running above to segment 4. For injuries with separation of the confluence, the right and left hepatic ducts can be anastomosed together before formation of a hepatico-jejunostomy, allowing a single biliary anastomosis. Injuries to an isolated right sectoral duct are best repaired or drained into a Roux limb of bowel. Simple ligation will lead to atrophy of the drained segments, which may become a nidus for sepsis.

Repair should be effected by a hepatico-jejunostomy with a 70-cm Roux limb of jejunum thereby minimising the risk of enteric reflux and chronic damage to the biliary tree. Moraca and colleagues advocate hepatico-duodenostomy for biliary injury on the basis that it is more physiological, quicker to perform and allows later ERCP for imaging and intervention.[51] They found no difference in outcome following hepatico-duodenostomy when compared with hepatico-jejunostomy, although median follow-up was only 54 months. Hepatico-duodenostomy has largely been abandoned in the treatment of other benign biliary disease due to ongoing enteric reflux. There have been anecdotal reports of the late development of cholangiocarcinoma,[52,53] as well as the need to undertake liver transplantation in patients so managed when secondary biliary cirrhosis due to enteric reflux has resulted.

Fine absorbable interrupted sutures of 4/0 or 5/0 polydioxanone sulphate (PDS II) should be used to fashion an end-to-side hepatico-jejunostomy, with care being taken to produce good mucosal apposition. Some authors advocate the use of an access limb, particularly for E3 and E4 injuries[54] to allow subsequent radiological intervention for dilatation of recurrent strictures.[55] However, others believe that advances in percutaneous transhepatic techniques have made this unnecessary and have achieved satisfactory results without using this surgical approach.

Partial injury to the biliary tree can be repaired with fine interrupted sutures, although when resulting from diathermy dissection, formal hepatico-jejunostomy may be necessary as conduction of the thermal injury may cause later stricture formation. If a T-tube is placed to protect a primary duct repair, this should be placed through a separate choledochotomy.

MANAGEMENT OF COMPLICATIONS RELATED TO REPAIR

Revisional surgery

Many patients with biliary injury continue to suffer from complications despite reconstruction. Factors such as the experience of the initial surgeon, the level of injury, the associated sepsis and liver atrophy all increase the chance of an unsuccessful repair. Following primary repair of a ductal tear or laceration, further stricture formation may result if there has been extensive dissection around the common hepatic duct. In such instances, surgical revision with the formation of a Roux-en-Y hepatico-jejunostomy is indicated.

The majority of patients requiring revisional surgery will have undergone a previous biliary enteric drainage procedure. Anastomotic stricturing will require revision of the anastomosis, with extension of the choledochotomy into the left hepatic duct. Choledocho-duodenotomy will require conversion to a Roux-en-Y hepatico-jejunostomy to avoid on-going problems with biliary enteric reflux.

Liver resection and transplantation

In the acute setting of bile duct injury, long-term damage to the hepatic parenchyma is difficult to predict. Major vascular injury or unrecognised segmental biliary obstruction may lead to atrophy of the liver, chronic intrahepatic infection, abscess formation or secondary biliary cirrhosis. In such patients, careful operative assessment is required; CT scanning should be performed to identify areas of associated liver atrophy and to exclude portal vein thrombosis.

In our experience, the majority of patients requiring liver resection are those with ongoing sepsis in an obstructed segment or those where drainage of the extrahepatic biliary tree is not possible due to sectoral duct damage or fibrosis. Very rarely, resection may be needed to gain access to the biliary tree, especially when the injury involves the biliary confluence (E4). The right lobe is most commonly affected by sepsis and atrophy as the right-sided sectoral ducts and arterial supply are more likely to be damaged during cholecystectomy, although both left- and right-sided hepatic resections have been reported in patients with severe biliary injury. Resection of the right liver can be performed, for example, at the time of delayed reconstruction if there is any doubt regarding the integrity of the anastomosis to the right sectoral or hepatic duct and when a satisfactory anastomosis can be achieved to the long extrahepatic left duct.

Failed reconstruction and persistent cholangitis may lead to end-stage liver failure within a few years,[56] and this may require liver transplantation[57] (**Fig. 9.10**). A long interval between injury and referral is known to be associated with end-stage liver disease.[57] Rarely, liver transplantation may be needed when the combined biliary and vascular injury is so severe as to preclude attempted reconstruction.[58]

PROGNOSIS

Success of repair

Successful repair has been well described and can be achieved in 90% of patients in a specialised unit.[34] However, anastomotic strictures, liver atrophy and cirrhosis may occur many years following repair. Predictors of a poor outcome include involvement of the biliary confluence,[36,54] repair by the injuring surgeon,[40,59,60] three or more previous attempted repairs,[36] and recent active inflammation.[60]

Survival

Mortality following injury to the biliary tree is significant. Death may follow the acute injury itself, following the biliary repair, or occur later as a result of biliary sepsis or cirrhosis. In a recent report of a nationwide analysis of survival following biliary injury after cholecystectomy, Flum and colleagues identified 7911 (0.5%) injuries from 1 570 361 cholecystectomies.[59] Within the first year after

cholecystectomy the mortality rate was 6.6% in the uninjured group and 26.1% in those with injury to the common bile duct. The adjusted hazard ratio for death during follow-up was higher for those with an injury (2.79; 95% CI 2.71–2.88). The risk of death increased significantly with advancing age and comorbidities. If the initial repair was performed by the injuring surgeon then the adjusted hazard of death increased by 11%.

Quality of life

Boerma and colleagues first undertook an assessment of quality of life in patients who had sustained biliary injury or leak that required additional intervention.[61] Five years after injury, quality of life in the physical and mental domains was significantly worse than controls, despite a successful outcome in 84% of treated patients and regardless of the type of treatment or severity of injury. However, the length of treatment was an independent predictor of a poor mental quality of life. In another study of the quality of life in 89 patients who had undergone biliary repair following laparoscopic cholecystectomy, it was interesting to note that there was no difference in the physical or social domains when compared to controls.[62] However, in the pyschological domain, patients were significantly worse, particularly in the 31% of patients who sought legal recourse for their injury.

Associated malignancy

A small number of reports exist about the development of cholangiocarcinoma at the site of anastomosis 20–30 years following repair.[52] It is possible that enteric reflux into the biliary tree with sepsis and the production of mutagenic secondary bile salts may be responsible.[53] Furthermore, hepatocellular carcinoma may develop due to secondary biliary cirrhosis (**Fig. 9.11**) (**Fig. 9.11b** also in colour, see Plate 7, facing p. 20).

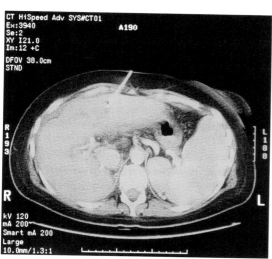

Figure 9.10 • Contrast-enhanced CT scan of the liver after unsuccessful revisional hepatico-jejunostomy. The surgeon who performed the laparoscopic cholecystectomy performed the hepatico-jejunostomy for an E4 injury. A revisional hepatico-jejunostomy was performed before referral, which was complicated by an anastomotic stricture and portal vein thrombosis. The CT shows evidence of right lobe atrophy and splenomegaly as well as a percutaneous biliary drain.

BENIGN BILIARY STRICTURES

Mirizzi's syndrome

Mirizzi first described the syndrome of extrahepatic biliary stricture in association with cholelithiasis

(a)

(b)

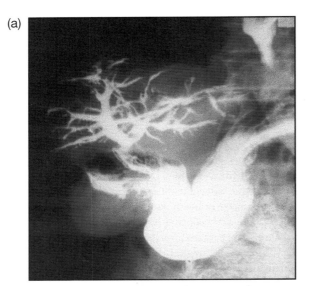

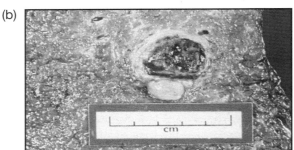

Figure 9.11 • Hepatocellular carcinoma as a consequence of biliary injury. This patient required a liver transplant for secondary biliary cirrhosis, which developed following hepato-duodenostomy for a biliary injury **(a)**. At pathological examination a hepatocellular carcinoma was detected in the explanted liver **(b)** (see also Plate 7, facing p. 20).

in 1948,[63] a condition that occurs in fewer than 0.5% of cholecystectomies.[64] Obstruction of the common hepatic duct may occur for two reasons: (i) a stone impacted in the cystic duct may cause direct pressure or oedema (Mirizzi type 1), or (ii) occasionally the stone may erode through the wall of the cystic duct and into the common hepatic duct (Mirizzi type 2).

PRESENTATION

Diagnosis can be difficult as symptoms may be the same as for acute cholecystitis, but all patients with the disease process will have abnormal liver function tests and some may present with jaundice.

Occasionally the diagnosis is made at the time of laparoscopic cholecystectomy.

MANAGEMENT

The investigations may be aimed at excluding a diagnosis of bile duct or gallbladder cancer. Ultrasound assessment will identify dilatation of the biliary tree proximal to the stricture and may even have features suggestive of a Mirizzi's syndrome. An ultrasound finding of a decompressed gallbladder with stones involving the common hepatic duct would be more suggestive of a Mirizzi syndrome. An associated mass or lymphadenopathy would be more in keeping with biliary malignancy, but associated sepsis or an empyema of the gallbladder may lead the operator to diagnose Mirizzi's syndrome as cancer. Both conditions may coexist. ERCP allows endoscopic stent placement to relieve jaundice and may demonstrate a fistula between the gallbladder and common hepatic duct (type 2). A smooth, tapered stricture is more typical of a benign rather than malignant cause of jaundice. Endoscopic stenting provides resolution of jaundice, an anatomical roadmap and also may help with identification of the common hepatic duct at operation.

When Mirizzi's syndrome is difficult to distinguish from a malignant stricture, CT scanning may aid in the diagnosis.[65,66] Occasionally laparoscopic ultrasound may be necessary to further delineate the stricture and exclude tumour dissemination. Although the two conditions may appear similar, vascular invasion may be seen and targeted biopsy may confirm a malignant diagnosis.[67]

Successful completion of cholecystectomy by laparoscopic means has been reported for apparent type 1 Mirizzi's syndrome,[68] although this would be inappropriate where there was a clear fistulous communication between gallbladder and common hepatic duct. One of these reported patients has subsequently developed a biliary stricture (O.J. Garden, personal communication). The conventional approach for type 1 strictures is to perform an open cholecystectomy or to convert from a laparoscopic procedure to allow adequate assessment of the associated biliary stricture. Operative cholangiography should be performed, and in those with persistent strictures a hepaticojejunostomy should be performed. For type II, where a defect results from the removal of the gallbladder and stent, the common bile duct should be explored. The majority of patients will require a hepatico-jejunostomy although apparently successful reconstructions using grafts of Hartmann's pouch have been described.[69] Long-term results of this innovative approach are awaited.

In a recent report, Schafer and colleagues identified Mirizzi's syndrome in 39 (0.3%) of 13 023 patients undergoing a laparoscopic cholecystectomy.[70] Thirty-four (87%) patients had a type I Mirizzi's syndrome. Of these, 23 patients underwent cholecystectomy alone, 10 patients required bile duct exploration and T-tube insertion, and 1 patient had a Roux-en-Y reconstruction. Twenty-four (74%) of the 34 patients had required open conversion. Of the remaining five patients with a type II Mirizzi's syndrome, three underwent a hepatico-jejunostomy and two had simple closure with a T-tube drainage. All had required open conversion and, interestingly, four (10%) patients were found to have a gallbladder carcinoma on histopathology.

Mirizzi's syndrome is an uncommon cause of obstructive jaundice secondary to gallstone disease. This condition will normally necessitate conversion to open surgery if a laparoscopic cholecystectomy is attempted, and a hepatico-jejunostomy will normally be required for a type II lesion.

Recurrent pyogenic cholangitis (Oriental cholangiohepatitis)

Oriental cholangiohepatitis is most common in South-East Asia and Hong Kong and is characterised by recurrent attacks of primary bacterial cholangitis with fever, rigors, abdominal pain and jaundice.[71] Recently there has been a decline in incidence, possibly related to improved economic conditions and changes in diet.[72] The cause is unknown although *Clonorchis sinensis*, ascariasis and nutritional insufficiency have been suggested as associated factors in its causation.

Pathologically there is gross irregular dilatation and intrahepatic stricture formation of the biliary tree, which frequently contains stones, debris and pus.[73] Bile duct proliferation, and portal and periportal inflammation and fibrosis are seen, and occasionally there is liver abscess formation. The bile is infected in 96% of patients with hepatolithiasis, most usually with *E. coli*.[74]

Diagnosis is based on history and demographic features, and investigation includes liver biochemistry and abdominal ultrasonography. Ultrasound is usually diagnostic although abdominal CT scan may add further information regarding associated liver atrophy or abscess formation. ERCP will provide important anatomical detail and will allow endoscopic stenting if required. If stricture formation or stones prevent filling of the intrahepatic ducts MRCP should provide further information, avoiding the risk of PTC.

MANAGEMENT

In an acute attack, treatment of cholangitis is initiated with broad-spectrum antibiotics. A third-generation cephalosporin and metronidazole with the addition of ampicillin for resistant enterococci will provide broad cover for most biliary pathogens. Intravenous fluid resuscitation and analgesia are required. Conservative treatment fails in around 30% of cases, and is more likely in those with obstruction of the extrahepatic biliary tree rather than an isolated segment.[75] When conservative treatment fails, biliary decompression is required by either an endoscopic, radiological or surgical approach.

Following resolution of an acute attack definitive surgery is required. A full spectrum of interventions from simple exploration and stone removal, hepatico-jejunostomy or liver resection through to liver transplantation may be required. A multidisciplinary approach to management will require involvement of radiologists, surgeons and gastroenterologists.

Parasitic infestation

LIVER FLUKES (TREMATODES)

Infestation with liver flukes is caused through consuming inadequately cooked, pickled or salted infected fish. The immature fluke passes into the biliary tree, where it grows to maturity. Ova are passed into the gastrointestinal tract and subsequently to water supplies infecting molluscs and fish. Infection with *Clonorchis sinensis* occurs in China, Japan and South-East Asia, whilst *Opisthorchis viverrini* is found in parts of eastern Europe and Siberia. Infection may be asymptomatic or the patient may present with an acute febrile illness or chronic symptoms. Chronic infestation results in periductal fibrosis, obstruction and calculi formation, and secondary bacterial infection may lead to pyogenic cholangitis. Later in the disease, biliary cirrhosis and liver failure may develop. Cholangiocarcinoma is a recognised complication and this continues to be a problem in developing countries.[76]

Diagnosis is possible by the detection of ova within the stool or in duodenal aspirates, and an eosinophilia may also be present on blood film. ERCP may demonstrate slender filling defects within the bile duct as well as associated changes of fibrosis and calculus formation. Medical therapy with praziquantel is effective, and the chronic damage to the biliary tree should be managed as for Oriental cholangiohepatitis (see above).

ECHINOCOCCUS

Hydatid cysts involving the liver remain endemic in parts of the Mediterranean and Far East as well as sheep farming areas of Australia, New Zealand, South America and South Africa. Infection is from *Echinococcus granulosus*, and less commonly *Echinococcus multilocularis* in central Europe. The intermediate host is usually cattle or sheep; however, humans are infected following the ingestion of eggs after faecal contamination from the definitive hosts – canines (*E. granulosus*) or rodents and wolves (*E. multilocularis*). The ingested parasites enter the portal circulation and implant in the liver to form cysts.

Biliary obstruction can occur due to local compression of the common hepatic duct by the expanding cyst, or when daughter cysts pass down the common hepatic duct following rupture of the cyst into intrahepatic radicles. Secondary sclerosing cholangitis has been described following inappropriate injection of scolicidal agents into the hepatic cyst when there is communication with the biliary tree.[77]

Diagnosis

A diagnosis is based often on the presentation, demography and the history of contact with animals. There may be calcification of the cyst wall on plain radiography. Abdominal ultrasonography and CT may provide the diagnosis if hydatid sand or daughter cysts are seen within the main hepatic lesion. Sometimes the cyst may still be indistinguishable from a simple hepatic cyst or cystic liver tumour.

Diagnostic aspiration is dangerous due to the potential to leak cyst fluid and disseminate infection. Immunoelectrophoresis to detect the specific antigen 'Arc 5' is diagnostic of active infection,[78] as is the detection of three of Arc antigens 1–4.

Treatment

Preoperative endoscopic cholangiography may identify debris within the biliary tree, and endoscopic sphincterotomy may prevent further episodes of biliary obstruction. Endoscopic stenting may also allow resolution of obstruction secondary to a large intrahepatic cyst.

A discussion about the treatment of intrahepatic cysts is outside the scope of this chapter; however, cysts should be excised if possible. Cyst deroofing with aspiration of the contents and daughter cysts should be reserved for those unable to be resected by formal hepatectomy or pericystectomy. Medical treatment with albendazole has been found to be equivalent to surgical therapy in uncomplicated disease.[79] The use of pre- and postoperative albendazole may sterilise the cyst before surgery and reduce the risk of disseminating infection.

The secondary sclerosing cholangitis produced by inappropriate instillation of a scolicidal agent into the biliary tree will often only be amenable to hepatic replacement. Surgical bypass may be possible for localised strictures.

ASCARIS LUMBRICOIDES

The roundworm *Ascaris lumbricoides* is the commonest worm to infect humans. The adult worm resides within the small bowel, and ova are passed into the gut lumen. Infection occurs after contact with contaminated food or water, when the ingested larvae pass into the duodenum and then burrow through the bowel wall to enter the portal circulation. They pass to the liver before migrating through to the lungs, where they are coughed up and reingested to mature in the small bowel.

Rarely, an infected patient can present with obstructive jaundice due to migration of the worm into the biliary tree and this is difficult to distinguish from stone disease. The more frequent presentation is from cholangitis due to the worm traversing the ampulla. *Ascaris* has also been associated with recurrent pyogenic cholangitis.[80]

Ultrasound sometimes identifies a long, linear filling defect within the biliary tree. Identification may occur at the time of ERCP where endoscopic extraction may be possible. Medical treatment exists with the anthelmintics mebendazole or albendazole, which are often curative. The late complication of papillary stenosis can be treated with endoscopic sphincterotomy.

Primary sclerosing cholangitis

AETIOLOGY

Primary sclerosing cholangitis is a rare condition, and although the precise cause has yet to be determined there is increasing evidence of an immunological basis. Around 70% of patients will have ulcerative colitis, or more rarely Crohn's disease. There are other reports of association with Riedel's thryoiditis, retroperitoneal fibrosis and lymphoplasmacytic sclerosing pancreatitis.[81] Two reports have demonstrated a strong association with HLA-B8 and HLA A1 B8 DR3.[82,83]

PRESENTATION

Primary sclerosing cholangitis is a progressive obliterative fibrosis of the intrahepatic and extrahepatic biliary tree with a wide clinical spectrum and frequent remissions and relapses. In the early stages of disease most patients are asymptomatic but later in the disease process patients may have pruritus, ill-defined pain, fever, jaundice and weight loss. Many asymptomatic patients are diagnosed by detection of abnormal liver function tests during the investigation of inflammatory bowel disease. Although some patients may present at an advanced stage, signs of liver failure develop over a period of time. Sudden deterioration may suggest the development of cholangiocarcinoma, with which there is a strong association.

INVESTIGATION

Liver biochemistry demonstrates a cholestatic picture. Although antineutrophil cytoplasmic antibodies are present in the serum of around 80% of patients,[84] testing for autoantibodies is usually performed to exclude primary biliary cirrhosis, a condition with which it can be difficult to differentiate.

The mainstay of investigation is cholangiography, which usually demonstrates a diffuse picture of stricturing and attenuated intrahepatic bile ducts. As well as providing anatomical details of the biliary tree, ERCP enables endoscopic therapy and the opportunity for brush cytology if malignancy is suspected. MRCP is highly sensitive, with a diagnostic accuracy comparable to ERCP,[85] and is now preferred as a means of both diagnosing and assessing the extent of disease to avoid the introduction of bacteria, possibly causing severe biliary sepsis.

MANAGEMENT

The prognosis of primary sclerosing cholangitis is poor, with only 75% of patients alive at 9 years post-diagnosis.[86] Survival may improve with earlier diagnosis and liver transplantation. The use of ursodeoxycholic acid in the treatment of pruritus has been associated with improvements in biochemical function and histological appearance.[87] Episodes of cholangitis can be treated with antibiotics covering biliary pathogens. There is no evidence that colectomy for inflammatory bowel disease alters disease progression.

Endoscopic or transhepatic dilatation of short dominant strictures has been described as effective, safe and well tolerated.[88] The addition of endoscopic or percutaneous stents following biliary dilatation is more likely to cause procedure-related complications,[89] and there is a considerable risk that endoscopic treatment may introduce infection leading to cholangitis, liver abscess formation or precipitation of liver failure. In those patients without cirrhosis but with jaundice secondary to a dominant stricture, surgical drainage with an access limb has been described. However, adhesions and cholangitis following surgery may compromise later liver transplantation.[90] Furthermore, liver disease may progress following an apparently successful drainage procedure.[91]

Liver transplantation is necessary to treat end-stage liver disease. However, it is now more usual for patients to be considered if there is persistent jaundice, intractable pruritus, recurrent cholangitis, malnutrition or fatigue. Many patients are now transplanted before liver failure, with survival rates of 86% at 5 years.[92]

EXCLUSION OF ASSOCIATED MALIGNANT STRICTURE

Cholangiocarcinoma and gallbladder cancer complicates 10–36% of patients with primary sclerosing cholangitis,[93] and needs to be excluded before liver transplantation. The majority of patients have recurrence of cholangiocarcinoma following transplantation,[94] with only a 30% survival at 1 year and no 6-year survivors.[93]

In the majority of patients, concern regarding occult cholangiocarcinoma is small, and liver transplantation is undertaken in the absence of a dominant stricture. Serum carbohydrate antigen (CA) 19-9 has been used in an attempt to identify cases with an occult biliary malignancy. In patients with a level >100 U/mL, the test had a 75% sensitivity and an 80% specificity in identifying cholangiocarcinoma.[95]

Patients with a sudden rapid deterioration in their clinical state or with a dominant stricture must be considered to have a cholangiocarcinoma and be investigated extensively. Brush cytology at ERCP may provide the diagnosis if a malignant smear is obtained. In a recent prospective study of biliary brush cytology at ERCP the sensitivity for diagnosing cholangiocarcinoma was found to be 80%.[96] CT scanning or MRI may demonstrate a mass lesion in association with the biliary tree, although the usual appearance is of a stricture indistinguishable from a benign disease. Positron emission tomography (PET) scanning may be of value in differentiating between primary sclerosing cholangitis and cholangiocarcinoma but further studies are awaited.[97]

Laparoscopy identifies the majority of patients with unresectable biliary tract cancer,[98] and may be of use in assessing those considered for transplantation in whom a cholangiocarcinoma is suspected since tumour dissemination often occurs early. Laparoscopic ultrasound may further aid assessment, and occasionally laparotomy may be required if there is diagnostic doubt regarding cholangiocarcinoma.

Biliary strictures imitating malignancy

It is not unusual for benign biliary pathology to be found in resected specimens of the pancreatic head that had been thought to be malignant. Around 10% of Whipple resections for malignancy will be found to have benign pathology.[99,100] Most commonly the pathology is chronic pancreatitis related to alcohol or gallstone disease. However, other confounding pathologies include lymphoplasmacytic sclerosing pancreatitis, primary sclerosing cholangitis, choledocholithiasis and inflammatory pseudotumours.

LYMPHOPLASMACYTIC SCLEROSING PANCREATITIS

Lymphoplasmacytic sclerosing pancreatitis is also known as autoimmune pancreatitis, sclerosing pancreatitis or primary inflammatory pancreatitis. The disease is associated with other autoimmune diseases such as Sjögren's syndrome, Riedel's thyroiditis, retroperitoneal fibrosis, ulcerative colitis and primary sclerosing cholangitis.[81,101] Although only accounting for about 2.4% of pancreatic resections,[101] the condition is important since a proportion of patients will develop either biliary anastomotic strictures or intrahepatic strictures following resection. In a series of 31 patients, 8 (28%) went on to develop recurrent jaundice after resection.[101]

Recently, increased levels of IgG4 have been described in association with the disease,[102] and successful treatment with steroids has been described.[103] As yet the value of steroid treatment in the prevention and treatment of recurrent strictures is not well described.

INFLAMMATORY PSEUDOTUMOUR

Inflammatory pseudotumours can mimic malignant lesions of the bile duct. Although rare they have been reported in up to 8% of patients undergoing surgery for presumed malignant hilar obstruction.[104] It is usually impossible to differentiate them from malignancy preoperatively and thus resection is often attempted if feasible. Successful treatment has been described with the use of steroids.[105]

HIV cholangiopathy (AIDS cholangiopathy)

HIV (human immunodeficiency virus)-related infections may affect the biliary tree causing acalculous cholecystitis,[106] a condition that needs prompt recognition and drainage.[107] HIV cholangiopathy is a secondary sclerosing cholangitis caused by opportunistic infections that can affect the entire biliary tree. It incorporates the pathologies of sclerosing cholangitis, papillary stenosis, and extrahepatic biliary strictures.[108-110] Causative organisms include cytomegalovirus, *Cryptosporidium*, *Mycobacterium avium* complex, microsporidia, herpes simplex virus[111] and giardiasis.[112] Up to 50% of patients will not have a causative organism isolated.[111]

Most patients with HIV will have abnormal liver function tests during the course of their disease, most commonly as a result of drug interactions or viral hepatitis. For those with obstructive or mixed liver function tests, initial investigation should include abdominal ultrasonography to identify areas of biliary dilatation.

ERCP allows identification of biliary strictures and has the ability to facilitate biliary biopsies and sample bile for culture. Endoscopic sphincterotomy is effective in relieving pain in the first 12 months although the abnormal liver function tests generally do not improve.[113] Treatment directed at the pathogen is rarely successful.[111]

Biliary strictures may respond to endoscopic stenting, and surgical treatment is rarely warranted as the 1-year survival for HIV cholangiopathy is only 41%.[110]

FUNCTIONAL BILIARY DISORDERS

Most patients who present for investigation of sphincter of Oddi have already undergone cholecystectomy for presumed gallbladder pain. However, up to 39–90% of patients with idiopathic recurrent pancreatitis may also have sphincter of Oddi dysfunction.[114] In those patients with postcholecystectomy pain, the presentation and investigation identifies three types.[115]

- Type 1 – Abdominal pain, obstructive liver function tests, biliary dilatation and delayed emptying of contrast at ERCP.
- Type 2 – Pain with only one or two of the above-mentioned criteria.
- Type 3 – Recurrent biliary pain only.

Between 65 and 95% of group 1 patients will be found on biliary manometry to have sphincter of Oddi dysfunction compared to only 12–28% of type 3.[114] Diagnosis is usually by exclusion of other causes of abdominal pain. Liver function tests, abdominal ultrasonography, CT scanning, endoscopy and MRCP have often been already performed.

At ERCP, biliary manometry is not required if there is delayed drainage of contrast in type 1 or 2 patients. This investigation should be reserved for those patients in whom the diagnosis remains unclear.

Medical therapy with calcium channel blockers, nitrates and botulinum toxin is available but long-term results are unknown. Endoscopic sphincterotomy is the usual treatment; however, 5–16% of patients will develop postprocedural pancreatitis.[116,117] Surgical sphincterotomy is now indicated rarely due to the lower cost and lower morbidity of endoscopic sphincterotomy but it may be required if the endoscopic approach has been unsuccessful.

Key points

Choledochal cysts should be treated with complete cyst excision and hepatico-jejunostomy due to the risk of malignancy in the remaining biliary epithelium.

Identification of the biliary anatomy and minimisation of diathermy near the common bile duct are essential during laparoscopic cholecystectomy to avoid biliary injury.

Operative cholangiography is a useful tool for delineating the biliary anatomy during cholecystectomy; however, many cholangiograms are not interpreted correctly at the time of biliary injury.

Any patient who is not fit for discharge at 24 hours due to ongoing abdominal pain, vomiting, fever or bile in an abdominal drain should be considered to have a biliary leak.

Diagnosis of a bile duct injury in the postoperative period should lead to immediate referral to a specialist centre since inappropriate attempts to manage this outwith a specialist centre will compromise the outcome.

In the absence of sepsis, repair of injuries to the biliary tree can be performed successfully within the first week.

REFERENCES

1. Mieli-Vergani G, Howard ER, Portmann B et al. Late referral for biliary atresia: missed opportunities for effective surgery. Lancet 1989; i:421–3.

   A review of the management of 147 cases of biliary atresia that demonstrated a better outcome with early repair.

2. Douglas AH. Case of dilatation of the common bile duct. Monthly J M Sci 1852; 14:97–101.

3. Mackenzie TC, Howell LJ, Flake AW et al. The management of prenatally diagnosed choledochal cysts. J Pediatr Surg 2001; 36:1241–3.

4. Suda K, Miyano T, Suzuki F et al. Clinicopathologic and experimental studies on cases of abnormal pancreatico-choledocho-ductal junction. Acta Pathol Jpn 1987; 37:1549–62.

5. Kim SH, Lim JH, Yoon HK et al. Choledochal cyst: comparison of MR and conventional cholangiography. Clin Radiol 2000; 55:378–83.

6. Todani T, Watanabe Y, Narusue M et al. Congenital bile duct cysts: classification, operative procedures, and review of thirty-seven cases including cancer arising from choledochal cyst. Am J Surg 1977; 134:263–9.

7. Atkinson HDE, Fischer CP, de Jong CHC et al. Choledochal cysts in adults and their complications. HPB 2003; 5:105–10.

8. Hewitt PM, Krige JE, Bornmann PC et al. Choledochal cysts in adults. Br J Surg 1995; 82:382–5.

9. Lenriot JP, Gigot JF, Segol P et al. Bile duct cysts in adults: a multi-institutional retrospective study. French Associations for Surgical Research. Ann Surg 1998; 228:159–66.

10. Todani T, Watanabe Y, Toki A et al. Carcinoma related choledochal cysts with internal drainage operations. Surg Gynecol Obstet 1987; 164:61–4.

11. Shimotake T, Aoi S, Tomiyama H et al. DPC-4 (Smad-4) and K-ras gene mutations in biliary tract epithelium in children with anomalous pancreaticobiliary ductal union. J Pediatr Surg 2003; 38:694–7.

12. Matsumoto Y, Fujii H, Itakura J et al. Pancreatico-biliary maljunction: pathophysiological and clinical aspects and the impact on biliary carcinogenesis. Langenbecks Arch Surg 2003; 388:122–31.

13. Voyles CR, Smadja C, Shands WC et al. Carcinoma in choledochal cysts. Age-related incidence. Arch Surg 1983; 118:986–8.

14. Nakayama H, Masuda H, Ugajin W et al. Left hepatic lobectomy for type IV-A choledochal cyst. Am Surg 2000; 66:1020–2.

15. Narasimhan KL, Chowdhary SK, Rao KL. Management of accessory hepatic ducts in choledochal cysts. J Pediatr Surg 2001; 36:1092–3.

16. Morgenstern L, McGrath MF, Carroll BJ et al. Continuing hazards of the learning curve in laparoscopic cholecystectomy. Am Surg 1995; 61:914–18.

17. Ludwig K, Bernhardt J, Steffen H et al. Contribution of intra-operative cholangiography to incidence and outcome of common bile duct injuries during laparoscopic cholecystectomy. Surg Endosc 2002; 16:1098–104.

18. Flum DR, Dellinger EP, Cheadle A et al. Intra-operative cholangiography and risk of common bile duct injury during cholecystectomy. JAMA 2003; 289;1691–2.

    A retrospective analysis of more than 1.5 million chole-cystectomies detailing the risk of injury and the decreased risk if operative cholangiography is used.

19. Richardson MC, Bell G, Fullarton GM and the West of Scotland Laparoscopic Cholecystectomy Audit Group. Incidence and nature of bile duct injuries following laparoscopic cholecystectomy: An audit of 5913 cases. Br J Surg 1996; 83:1356–60.

    A prospective audit of biliary injury following chole-cystectomy in Scotland. One of the first studies to record the rate of biliary injury and the more severe nature of the injuries at laparoscopic surgery.

20. Francoeur JR, Wiseman K, Buczkowski AK et al. Surgeons' anonymous response after bile duct injury during cholecystectomy. Am J Surg 2003; 185:468–75.

21. Moore MJ, Bennett CL. The learning curve for laparoscopic cholecystectomy. The Southern Surgeon's Club. Am J Surg 1995; 170:55–9.

    A paper that demonstrated early in the life of laparoscopic cholecystectomy that surgeon inexperience was an important factor in the occurrence of bile duct injuries.

22. Strasberg SM, Hertl M, Soper NJ. An analysis of the problem of biliary injury during laparoscopic chole-cystectomy. J Am Coll Surg 1995; 180:102–25.

    This paper describes a very useful classification system for biliary injury that includes the Bismuth classification as well as other less major injuries.

23. Thomson BNJ, Madhavan KK, Parks RW et al. Early repair of biliary injury – successful in selected patients. BJS 2005, in press.

24. Lillemoe KD, Melton GB, Cameron JL et al. Post-operative bile duct strictures: management and out-come in the 1990s. Ann Surg 2000; 232:430–41.

25. Fletcher DR, Hobbs MS, Tan P et al. Complications of cholecystectomy: risks of the laparoscopic approach and protective effects of operative chol-angiography: a population-based study. Ann Surg 1999; 229:449–57.

    A retrospective audit of biliary injury in Western Australia that identified the increased risk of biliary injury after laparoscopic cholecystectomy compared to open cholecystectomy. This study also identified a significantly reduced risk of injury if operative cholangiography was performed.

26. Thomson BNJ, Cullinan MJ, Banting SW et al. Recognition and management of biliary complications after laparoscopic cholecystectomy. Austr NZ J Surg. 2003; 73:183–8.

27. Strasberg SM. Avoidance of biliary injury during laparoscopic cholecystectomy. J Hepatobiliary Pancreat Surg 2002; 9:543–7.

28. Way LW, Stewart L, Gantert W et al. Causes and prevention of laparoscopic bile duct injuries: analysis of 252 cases from a human factors and cognitive psychology perspective. Ann Surg 2003; 237:460–9.

Analysis of 252 bile duct injuries according to the principles of the cognitive science of visual perception, judgement and human error showing that the majority of errors result from misperception, not errors of skill, knowledge or judgement.

29. Couinaud C. Le Foi. Etudes anatomogiques et chirurgicales. Paris: Masson, 1957.

30. Woods MS, Traverso LW, Kozarek RA et al. Biliary tract complications of laparoscopic cholecystectomy are detected more frequently with routine intra-operative cholangiography. Surg Endosc 1995; 9(10):1076–80.

31. Flum DR, Flowers C, Veenstra DL. A cost-effectiveness analysis of intra-operative cholangiography in the prevention of bile duct injury during laparoscopic cholecystectomy. J Am Coll Surg 2003; 196:385–93.

32. Andren-Sandberg A, Alinder G, Bengmark S. Accidental lesions of the common bile duct at cholecystectomy. Pre- and perioperative factors of importance. Ann Surg 1985; 201:328–32.

33. Olsen D. Bile duct injuries during laparoscopic cholecystectomy. Surg Endosc 1997; 11:133–8.

34. Slater K, Strong RW, Wall DR et al. Iatrogenic bile duct injury: the scourge of laparoscopic cholecystectomy. Aust NZ J Surg 2002; 72:83–8.

35. Mahmud S, Masuad M, Canna K et al. Fundus-first laparoscopic cholecystectomy. Surg Endosc 2002; 16:581–4.

36. Chapman WC, Halevy A, Blumgart LH et al. Postcholecystectomy bile duct strictures. Arch Surg 1995; 130:597–604.

37. Bismuth H. Postoperative strictures of the bile duct. In: Blumgart LH (ed.) The biliary tract. Clinical surgery international. Edinburgh: Churchill Livingstone, 1982; pp. 209–18.

Description of the Bismuth classification of biliary injury, now often incorporated into the Strasberg classification.

38. Mirza DF, Narsimhan KL, Ferras Neto BH et al. Bile duct injury following laparoscopic cholecyst-ectomy: referral pattern and management. Br J Surg 1997; 84:786–90.

39. Johnson SR, Koehler A, Pennington LK et al. Long-term results of surgical repair of bile duct injuries following laparoscopic cholecystectomy. Surgery 2000; 128:668–77.

40. Carroll BJ, Birth M, Phillips EH. Common bile duct injuries during laparoscopic cholecystectomy that result in litigation. Surg Endosc 1998; 12(4):310–13.

A retrospective review that demonstrated a poor chance of successful repair of biliary injury if performed by the surgeon that caused the injury.

41. Stewart L, Way LW. Bile duct injuries during laparoscopic cholecystectomy: factors that influence the results of treatment. Arch Surg 1995; 130:1123–9.

42. Woods MS, Traverso LW, Kozarek RA et al. Characteristics of biliary tract complications during laparoscopic cholecystectomy: a multi-institutional study. Am J Surg 1994; 167:27–33.

43. Adams DB, Borowicz MR, Wootton FT 3rd et al. Bile duct complications after laparoscopic cholecystectomy. Surg Endosc 1993; 7:79–83.

44. Familiari L, Scaffidi M, Familiari P et al. An endo-scopic approach to the management of surgical bile duct injuries: nine years' experience. Dig Liver Dis 2003; 35:493–7.

45. al-Karawi MA, Sanai FM. Endoscopic management of bile duct injuries in 107 patients: experience of a Saudi referral center. Hepatogastroenterology 2002; 49:1201–7.

46. Thomson BNJ, Wakefield CH, Madhavan KK et al. Early repair for bile duct injuries – satisfactory in selected patients. Br J Surg 2003; 90:3–4.

47. Buell JF, Cronin DC, Funaki B et al. Devastating and fatal complications associated with combined vascular and bile duct injuries during cholecyst-ectomy. Arch Surg 2002; 137:703–8.

48. Gupta N, Solomon H, Fairchild R et al. Management and outcome of patients with combined bile duct and hepatic artery injuries. Arch Surg 1998; 133:176–81.

49. Alves A, Farges O, Nicolet J et al. Incidence and consequence of an hepatic artery injury in patients with postcholecystectomy bile duct strictures. Ann Surg 2003; 238:93–6.

An analysis of arterial injury during cholecystectomy and its impact on the success of hepaticojejunostomy in patients with bile duct injury. All patients had a left duct approach for repair and there was no difference in out-come between those with and without arterial injury.

50. Mercado MA, Chan C, Orozco H et al. Acute bile duct injury. The need for a high repair. Surg Endosc 2003; 17:1351–5.

51. Moraca RJ, Lee FT, Ryan JA et al. Long-term biliary function after reconstruction of major bile

duct injuries with hepaticoduodenostomy or hepaticojejunostomy. Arch Surg 2002; 137:889–93.

52. Strong RW. Late bile duct cancer complicating biliary enteric anastomosis. Am J Surg 1999; 177:472–4.

53. Bettschart V, Clayton RA, Parks RW et al. Cholangiocarcinoma arising after biliary-enteric drainage procedures for benign disease. Gut 2002; 51:128–9.

54. Al-Ghnaniem R, Benjamin IS. Long-term outcome of hepaticojejunostomy with routine access loop formation following iatrogenic bile duct injury. Br J Surg 2002; 89:1118–24.

55. Hutson DG, Russell E, Yrizarry J et al. Percutaneous dilatation of biliary strictures through the afferent limb of a modified Roux-en-Y choledochojejunostomy or hepaticojejunostomy. Am J Surg 1998; 175:108–13.

56. Kozicki I, Bielecki K. Hepaticojejunostomy in benign biliary stricture – influence of careful postoperative observations on long term results. Dig Surg 1997; 14:527–33.

57. Nordin A, Halme L, Makisalo H et al. Management and outcome of major bile duct injuries after laparoscopic cholecystectomy: from therapeutic endoscopy to liver transplantation. Liver Transplantation 2002; 8:1036–43.

58. Robertson AJ, Rela M, Karani J et al. Laparoscopic cholecystectomy: an unusual indication for liver transplantation. Transpl Int 1998; 11:449–51.

59. Flum DR, Cheadle A, Prela C et al. Bile duct injury during cholecystectomy and survival in medicare beneficiaries. JAMA 2003; 290:2168–74.

A retrospective analysis of survival following bile duct injury among Medicare beneficiaries in the USA. This study demonstrates the increased hazard ratio of death following injury in comparison to a control group of routine cholecystectomy patients.

60. Huang CS, Lein HH, Tai FC et al. Long-term results of major bile duct injury associated with laparoscopic cholecystectomy. Surg Endosc 2003; 17:1362–7.

61. Boerma D, Rauws EA, Keulemans YC et al. Impaired quality of life 5 years after bile duct injury during laparoscopic cholecystectomy: A propsective analysis. Ann Surg 2001; 234:750–7.

A prospective analysis of quality of life that demonstrated a poor outcome at 5 years, despite successful repair.

62. Melton GB, Lillemoe KD, Cameron JL et al. Major bile duct injuries associated with laparoscopic cholecystectomy: effect of surgical repair on quality of life. Ann Surg 2002; 235:888–95.

A study of the impact of biliary injury on quality of life that demonstrated a significantly worse psychological domain, especially in those pursuing legal action.

63. Mirizzi PL. Sindrome del conducto hepatico. J Int Chir 1948; 8:731–77.

64. Johnson LW, Sehon JK, Lee WC et al. Mirizzi's syndrome: experience from a multi-institutional review. Am Surg 2001; 67:11–14.

65. Callery MP, Strasberg SM, Doherty GM et al. Staging laparoscopy with laparoscopic ultrasonography: optimizing resectability in hepatobiliary and pancreatic malignancy. J Am Coll Surg 1997; 185:33–9.

66. Baer HU, Matthews JB, Schweizer WP et al. Management of the Mirizzi syndrome and the surgical implications of cholecystocholedochal fistula. Br J Surg 1990; 77:743–5.

67. Garden OJ, Paterson-Brown S. The gallbladder and bile ducts. In: Garden OJ (ed.) Intraoperative and laparoscopic ultrasonography. Oxford: Blackwell Science, 1995; pp. 17–43.

68. Binnie NR, Nixon SJ, Palmer KR. Mirizzi syndrome managed by endoscopic stenting and laparoscopic cholecystectomy. Br J Surg 1992; 79:647.

69. Shah OJ, Dar MA, Wani MA et al. Management of Mirizzi syndrome: a new surgical approach. Aust NZ J Surg 2001; 71:423–7.

70. Schafer M, Schneiter R, Krahenbuhl L. Incidence and management of Mirizzi syndrome during laparoscopic cholecystectomy. Surg Endosc 2003; 17:1186–90.

A large review of 39 patients with surgical management of Mirizzi syndrome.

71. Lam SK, Wong KP, Chan PKW et al. Recurrent pyogenic cholangitis as studied by endoscopic retrograde cholangiography. Gastroenterology 1978; 74:1196–203.

72. Lo CM, Fan ST, Wong J. The changing epidemiology of recurrent pyogenic cholangitis. Hong Kong Med J 1997; 3:302–4.

73. Choi TK, Wong J, Ong GB. The surgical management of primary intrahepatic stones. Br J Surg 1982; 69:86–90.

74. Tabata M, Nakayama F. Bacteriology of hepatolithiasis. Prog Clin Biol Res 1984; 152:163–74.

75. Fan ST, Lai ECS, Mok FPT et al. Acute cholangitis secondary to hepatolithiasis. Arch Surg 1991; 126:1027–31.

76. Watanapa P, Watanapa WB. Liver fluke-associated cholangiocarcinoma. Br J Surg 2002; 89:962–70.

77. Belghiti J, Benhamou JP, Houry S et al. Caustic sclerosing cholangitis. A complication of the surgical treatment of hydatid disease of the liver. Arch Surg 1986; 121:1162–5.

78. Hira PR, Bahr GM, Shweiki HM et al. An enzyme-linked immunosorbent assay using arc 5 antigen for the diagnosis of cystic hydatid disease. Ann Trop Med Parasitol 1990; 84:157–62.

79. Gil-Grande LA, Rodriguez-Caabeiro F, Prieto JG et al. Randomised controlled trial of efficacy of albendazole in intra-abdominal hydatid disease. Lancet 1993; 342:1269–72.

80. Khuroo MS, Sarjar SA, Mahajan R. Hepatobiliary and pancreatic ascariasis in India. Lancet 1990; 335:1503–6.

81. Montefusco PP, Geiss AC, Bronzo RL et al. Sclerosing cholangitis, chronic pancreatitis, and Sjögren's syndrome: A syndrome complex. Am J Surg 1984; 147:822–6.

82. Chapman RW, Kelly PM, Heryet A et al. Expression of HLA-DR antigens on bile duct epithelium in primary sclerosing cholangitis. Gut 1988; 29:422–7.

83. Donaldson PT, Farrant JM, Wilkinson ML et al. Dual association of HLA DR2 and DR3 with sclerosing cholangitis. Hepatology 1991; 13:129–33.

Both articles support an autoimmune aetiology for primary sclerosing cholangitis.

84. Duerr RH, Targan SR, Labders CJ et al. Neutrophil cytoplasmic antibodies: A link between primary sclerosing cholangitis and ulcerative colitis. Gastroenterology 1991; 100:1385–91.

85. Textor HJ, Flacke S, Pauleit D et al. Three-dimensional magnetic resonance cholangio-pancreatography with respiratory triggering in the diagnosis of primary sclerosing cholangitis: comparison with endoscopic retrograde cholangiography. Endoscopy 2002; 34:984–90.

86. Helseberg JH, Petersen JM, Boyer JL. Improved survival with primary sclerosing cholangitis. A review of clinicopathologic features and comparison of symptomatic and asymptomatic patients. Gastroenterology 1987; 92:1869–75.

87. Beuers U, Spengler U, Kruis W et al. Ursodeoxycholic acid for treatment of primary sclerosing cholangitis: a placebo-controlled trial. Hepatology 1992: 16:707–14.

A prospective randomized double-blind trial that demonstrated the efficacy of ursodeoxycholic acid in the treatment of primary sclerosing cholangitis.

88. Wagner S, Gebel M, Meier P et al. Endoscopic management of biliary tract strictures in primary sclerosing cholangitis. Endoscopy 1996; 28:576–7.

89. Kaya M, Petersen BT, Angulo P et al. Balloon dilation compared to stenting of dominant strictures in primary sclerosing cholangitis. Am J Gastroenterol 2001; 96:1059–66.

90. Ismail T, Angrisani L, Powell JE et al. Primary sclerosing cholangitis: surgical options, prognostic variables and outcome. Br J Surg 1991; 78:564–7.

91. Lemmer ER, Borman PC, Krige JE et al. Primary sclerosing cholangitis. Requiem for biliary drainage operations? Arch Surg 1994; 129:723–8.

92. Graziadei IW, Wiesner RH, Marotta PJ et al. Long-term results of patients undergoing liver transplantation for primary sclerosing cholangitis. Hepatology 1999: 30:1121–7.

93. Nashan B, Schlitt HJ, Tusch G et al. Biliary malignancies in primary sclerosing cholangitis: Timing for liver transplantation. Hepatology 1996; 23:1105–11.

94. Rosen CB, Nagorney DM, Wiesner RH et al. Cholangiocarcinoma complicating primary sclerosing cholangitis. Ann Surg 1991; 213:21–5.

95. Chalasani N, Baluyut A, Ismail A et al. Cholangiocarcinoma in patients with primary sclerosing cholangitis: a multicenter case-control study. Hepatology 2000; 31:247–8.

96. Glassbrenner B, Ardan M, Boeck W et al. Prospective evaluation of brush cytology of biliary strictures during endoscopic retrograde cholangio-pancreatography. Endoscopy 1999; 31:758–60.

97. Keiding S, Hansen SB, Rasmussen HH et al. Detection of cholangiocarcinoma in primary sclerosing cholangitis by positron emission tomography. Hepatology 1998; 29:700–6.

98. Weber SM, DeMatteo RP, Fong Y et al. Staging laparoscopy in patients with extrahepatic biliary carcinoma. Analysis of 100 patients. Ann Surg 2002; 235:392–9.

99. Powell JJ, Parks RW, Pleass H et al. Whipple's resection of non-neoplastic pathology in patients with presumed malignancy. Br J Surg 2003; 90:49.

100. Abraham SC, Wilentz RE, Yeo CJ et al. Pancreatico-duodenectomy (Whipple resections) in patients without malignancy: are they all 'chronic pancreatitis'? Am J Surg Pathol 2003; 27:110–20.

101. Weber SM, Cubukcu-Dimopulo O, Palesty JA et al. Lymphoplasmacytic sclerosing pancreatitis: Inflammatory mimic of pancreatic carcinoma. J Gastrointest Surg 2003; 7:129–37.

102. Hamano H, Kawa S, Horiuchi A et al. High serum IgG4 concentrations in patients with sclerosing pancreatitis. N Engl J Med 2001; 344:732–8.

103. Ito T, Nakano I, Koyanagi S et al. Autoimmune pancreatitis as a new clinical entity. Three cases of autoimmune pancreatitis with effective steroid therapy. Dig Dis Sci 1997; 42:1458–68.

104. Hadjis NS, Collier NA, Blumgart LH. Malignant masquerade at the hilum of the liver. Br J Surg 1985; 72:659–61.

105. Saint-Paul MC, Hastier P, Baldini E et al. Inflammatory pseudotumor of the intrahepatic biliary tract. Gastroenterol Clin Biol 1999; 23:581–4.

106. French AL, Beaudet LM, Benator DA et al. Cholecystectomy in patients with AIDS: clinicopathologic correlations in 107 cases. Clin Infect Dis 1995; 21:852–8.

107. Keaveny AP, Karasik MS. Hepatobiliary and pancreatic infections in AIDS: Part one. AIDS Patient Care STDs 1998; 12:347–57.

108. Cello J. Acquired immunodeficiency syndrome cholangiopathy: spectrum of disease. Am J Med 1989: 86:539–46.

109. Bonacini M. Hepatobiliary complications in patients with human immunodeficiency virus infection. Am J Med 1992; 92:404–10.

110. Ducreux M, Buffet C, Lamy P et al. Diagnosis and prognosis of AIDS-related cholangitis. AIDS 1995; 9:875–80.

111. Keaveny AP, Karasik MS. Hepatobiliary and pancreatic infections in AIDS: Part II. AIDS Patient Care STDs 1998; 12:451–6.

112. Aronson NE, Cheney C, Rholl V et al. Biliary giardiasis in a patient with human immunodeficiency virus. J Clin Gastroenterol 2001; 33:167–70.

113. Cello JP, Chan MF. Long-term follow-up of endoscopic retrograde cholangiopancreatography sphincterotomy for patients with acquired immune deficiency syndrome papillary stenosis. Am J Med 1995; 99:600–3.

114. Corazziari E. Sphincter of Oddi dysfunction. Dig Liver Dis 2003; 35:S26–S29.

115. Geenen JE, Hogan WJ, Dodds WJ et al. The efficacy of endoscopic sphincterotomy after cholecystectomy in patients with sphincter of Oddi dysfunction. N Engl J Med 1989; 320:82–7.

116. Lehman GY, Sherman S. Sphincter of Oddi dysfunction. Int J Pancreatol 1996; 20:11–25.

117. Sherman S, Hawes RH, Troiano FP et al. Sphincter of Oddi manometry decreased risk of clinical pancreatitis with the use of a modified aspirating catheter. Gastrointest Endosc 1990; 36:462–6.

Ten

Malignant lesions of the biliary tract

Cynthia-Michelle Borg and
Irving S. Benjamin

Cancer of the bile ducts can be divided into intra-hepatic (arising in a segmental or a more peripheral duct), hilar (arising in common hepatic, first- or second-order ducts) and distal extrahepatic tumours. Hilar and distal extrahepatic cholangiocarcinoma, gallbladder carcinoma and carcinoma of the ampulla of Vater will be discussed in this chapter. Intra-hepatic cholangiocarcinoma has been discussed in Chapter 4.

CHOLANGIOCARCINOMA

Incidence

Biliary tract cancer is rare in Western countries, accounting for less than 2% of all human malignancies.[1] The reported autopsy incidence is 0.01–0.5%.[2] This varies widely in different parts of the world. The age-standardised annual incidence in France was 1.7 and 0.5 per 100 000 for males and females respectively,[3] whereas in northeast Thailand the rates were 135.4 and 43.0 per 100 000 (see below).[4]

The frequency of all types of bile duct cancer increases with age. Up to two-thirds of patients with cholangiocarcinoma are more than 65 years old, with a peak incidence in the eighth decade of life.[5]

Several studies have shown a worldwide increase in the mortality from intrahepatic cholangio-carcinoma over the last three decades.[6–10] In contrast, the mortality rates for extrahepatic cholangiocarcinoma and gallbladder carcinoma have shown a decreasing trend in most countries over the same period of time.[7,8,10] The reasons for these epidemiological changes are unknown.

Location

Cholangiocarcinoma arises from the biliary epithelium anywhere from the ampulla of Vater to the small intrahepatic biliary radicles. The hilar confluence is the site of predilection: attention was first drawn to this in 1965 in a report of 13 patients by Klatskin,[11] and cholangiocarcinoma at the hilum continues to bear his name.

In a retrospective analysis of 294 cases of cholangiocarcinoma,[12] 67% of tumours were found in the hilar region. Intrahepatic tumours accounted for 6%, while 27% affected the distal extrahepatic biliary tree. Up to 5% of the tumours may be multi-centric or diffuse.[13]

Risk factors

The majority of cases of cholangiocarcinoma are spontaneous. A number of factors have, however, been implicated in its aetiology. Most of these are associated with long-standing chronic inflammation to the bile duct mucosa.

There is a strong association between **primary sclerosing cholangitis** (PSC) and cholangiocarcinoma. Occult cholangiocarcinoma has been found in up to 40% of autopsy specimens and in up to 36% of liver explants from patients with PSC.[14] Some authors believe that pericholangitis, PSC and cholangiocarcinoma are parts of the spectrum of the same disease. Cholangiocarcinoma in PSC patients tends to be diffuse or multicentric.

Up to 70% of patients with PSC also suffer from ulcerative colitis but only a minority of patients with ulcerative colitis develop PSC. Patients with ulcerative colitis in the absence of symptomatic PSC also have an increased risk of cholangio-carcinoma. Surgical or medical treatment of ulcer-ative colitis does not decrease the risk of developing cholangiocarcinoma.

Patients with **congenital biliary cystic disease** also have an increased risk of developing cholangio-carcinoma. The incidence of malignant trans-formation in choledochal cysts ranges between 10 and 30%.[15] The risk is highest in patients who were not treated before the age of 20 years and in those treated with cyst drainage only rather than excision.[16] It seems that malignant change occurs more frequently in choledochal cysts associated with an anomalous pancreatico-biliary ductal junction (APBDJ).[15] Suda et al.[17] found an APBDJ in 14% of cases of biliary tract carcinoma, in all four cases of congenital biliary dilatation but in none of 200 control patients with no biliary tract disease. Ohta et al.[18] showed epithelial mucosal atypia with papillary proliferation and epithelial hyperplasia in patients with APBDJ. Bile from patients with congenital choledochal cysts was found to promote proliferation of human cholangiocarcinoma cells compared to normal bile in vitro.[19]

Parasitic infestation by the **biliary parasites**, *Opisthorchis viverrini* and *Clonorchis sinensis*, may be responsible for the higher incidence of these malignancies in South-East Asia.[20,21] These parasites are endemic to the area and may be transmitted in inadequately cooked fish. Several potential carcinogenic mechanisms have been described, including hyperplasia and dysplasia caused by chronic inflammation, nitric oxide formation,

intrinsic nitrosation and activation of cytochrome P450 isoenzymes.

Tocchi et al.[22] reviewed retrospectively 1003 patients who previously had had **biliary-enteric drainage** for benign disease. The incidence of cholangiocarcinoma was 5.8% in patients who had undergone transduodenal sphincteroplasty, 7.6% in choledocho-duodenostomy patients, and 1.9% in patients who had undergone hepatico-jejunostomy. The effect of endoscopic sphincterotomy is not known.

Bile duct **adenomas** and multiple biliary papilloma-tosis may also carry a malignant transformation potential.[23,24]

Thorotrast, a contrast medium used between 1930 and 1960, has been associated with numerous tumours including primary liver tumours (intra-hepatic cholangiocarcinomas, hepatocellular carcin-oma and angiosarcoma), gallbladder carcinoma and tumours of the extrahepatic bile ducts.[25,26] In the German Thorotrast Study, 45.6% of the patients who were exposed to Thorotrast had developed liver cancer by the 15th year of exposure compared to 0.3% of controls.[27]

Hepatolithiasis (recurrent pyogenic cholangio-hepatitis or Oriental cholangiohepatitis) is thought to result from chronic portal bacteraemia and gives rise to intrahepatic duct stones. This leads to recurrent episodes of cholangitis and ductal strictures and carries a 10% risk of developing cholangiocarcinoma.[28]

Carcinogens, including aflatoxins,[29] methylene chloride,[30] vinyl chloride monomer,[31] and nitrosamines,[32,33] have also been implicated. Less well-documented risk factors include smoking and chronic typhoid carriage. Intrahepatic cholangio-carcinoma was also reported to be associated with cirrhosis due to hepatitis C infection.[34]

Oncogenes

A number of mutations in oncogenes and in tumour suppressor genes have been found in biliary tract tumours. Mutations in K-*ras*, c-*myc*, c-*neu*, c-*erb*-b2 and c-*met* oncogenes have been described. Muta-tions have also been found in tumour suppressor genes p53, APC and *Bcl*-2.[35–38] These mutations can lead to detectable phenotypic changes. However, these changes can also be seen in non-malignant pathology and thus their use in clinical practice is questionable.

Pathology

Up to 90% of extrahepatic bile duct tumours are adenocarcinomas.[5] The WHO classification for carcinomas of the extrahepatic bile duct is shown in **Box 10.1**.

In a review of 3468 histologically proven bile duct cancers, Carriaga and Henson found that 71.9% of tumours were adenocarcinomas while the second commonest were papillary adenocarcinomas (9.3%). Carcinoma in situ was only found in about 0.5% of cases.[5]

Carcinoid tumours also rarely involve the extrahepatic bile duct. They are difficult to diagnose preoperatively and account for 0.2–2% of all gastrointestinal carcinoids. Unlike cholangiocarcinoma, the majority involve the common bile duct, and are commoner in young women. Aggressive local invasion by the tumour is rare, while distant metastasis occurs in about a third of cases.[39]

Cases of Kaposi's sarcoma and lymphoma of the biliary tract have also been described in patients with acquired immunodeficiency syndrome (AIDS).

Prognosis in bile duct cancer has been linked to its histological type. Papillary carcinomas are associated with the best outcome while the poorest outcome is associated with mucinous adenocarcinoma.

MACROSCOPIC APPEARANCE

Three gross appearances of cholangiocarcinoma have been described[40] (**Fig. 10.1**) (also in colour, see Plate 8, facing p. 20). The sclerosing variant accounts for 70% of tumours and is commoner in the hilar area than in the distal common bile duct. The duct wall appears thickened (>1 cm) and the tumour often extends into but remains demarcated from the surrounding liver tissue. These changes may be difficult to distinguish from changes in benign conditions such as PSC.

Nodular tumours usually affect the upper and mid bile duct. The duct wall is thickened and the luminal surface of the tumour appears irregular.

Papillary tumours are usually found in the mid to distal part of the common bile duct and account for about 10% of cholangiocarcinomas. They usually

Box 10.1 • WHO classification of carcinomas of the extrahepatic bile duct

Carcinoma in situ

Invasive adenocarcinomas:

  Adenocarcinoma

  Papillary adenocarcinoma

  Adenocarcinoma, intestinal-type

  Mucinous adenocarcinoma

  Clear-cell carcinoma

  Signet-ring-cell carcinoma

  Adenosquamous carcinoma

Squamous cell carcinoma

Small-cell carcinoma

Undifferentiated carcinoma

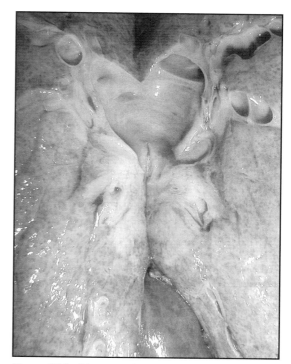

Figure 10.1 • Macroscopic appearance of hilar cholangiocarcinoma. The resected specimen is opened and shows stenosis of the hepatic duct at the hilus, and local invasion of the adjacent hepatic parenchyma. See also Plate 8, facing p. 20.

appear as an intraluminal soft, pink or grey-white growth.

MICROSCOPIC APPEARANCE

Adenocarcinomas show acinar and solid structures on microscopy. The tumour cells are larger than normal cells and are usually associated with varying amounts of desmoplastic (fibrous) stroma. This can be so extensive that biopsy specimens may consist mainly of fibrous tissue with only few sporadic malignant cells, making it difficult to distinguish this from inflammatory bile duct disease, especially on frozen section. Many express carcinoembryonic antigen (CEA) on histochemical staining, and this may help to identify foci of malignancy in small biopsy specimens.[41] Mucin production is common in cholangiocarcinoma, and there is a tendency to spread between hepatocyte plates, along duct walls and in relation to nerves. Dysplastic changes in adjacent bile duct epithelium may be present.[41] The tumours also show a strong tendency to longitudinal subepithelial growth. This may extend 5–50 mm proximally (towards the liver) and 5–30 mm distally (towards the duodenum), depending on the type of tumour.[42]

Multicentricity is frequently described but may be due to retrograde seeding. These factors make it difficult to ascertain the limits of tumour invasion on gross inspection.

The tumours may cause changes proximally due to obstruction. Such associated changes may include intracanalicular cholestasis, portal tract inflammation, oedema and ductal proliferation. Atrophy of the draining liver segment/lobe may also occur.

GRADING

Adenocarcinomas can be graded from 1 to 4 depending on the percentage of tumour that is composed of glandular tissue, and this is related to outcome. Some types of adenocarcinoma, including papillary adenocarcinoma, clear-cell carcinoma and carcinoma in situ, are not graded. Squamous cell carcinoma is graded according to the least differentiated area.

SPREAD

In general, haematogenous spread of hilar cholangiocarcinoma is rare, while nodal metastases are present in up to 50% of cases at initial presentation.[13]

Lymphatic spread is via the pericholedochal nodes to the coeliac nodes. In a review of 110 patients who underwent surgical resection and lymph node dissection for cholangiocarcinoma, 47% of patients did not have lymph node metastasis, 36% had regional lymph node metastasis, and 17% had both regional and para-aortic lymph node spread. The commonest nodes involved were the pericholedochal nodes, followed by the periportal, common hepatic and posterior pancreatico-duodenal nodes.[43]

In a study by Bhuiya et al.,[44] the overall incidence of perineural invasion in 70 resected specimens of cholangiocarcinoma was 81%. This study found a significant correlation between perineural invasion and the macroscopic appearance (commoner in nodular infiltrating/infiltrating subtypes). Perineural invasion was commoner in less-differentiated tumours and more frequent when the tumours invaded the subserosal layer and beyond. Perineural invasion was associated with a lower 5-year survival rate (32% compared with 67% when perineural invasion was not present) in this study.

Tumour spread can also occur along the intrahepatic bile ducts. The peribiliary capillary plexus is thought to play an important role in intrahepatic extension of hilar tumours. The tumour invades both adjacent liver tissue and vessels (portal vein and hepatic artery). Ampullary tumours are not usually accompanied by evidence of venous invasion while more proximal, sclerosing and nodular tumours may show venous involvement in up to 20%.

STAGING OF CHOLANGIOCARCINOMA

There is no universally accepted clinical staging system for hilar cholangiocarcinoma but any such staging system must take account of both biliary and vascular involvement.

Bismuth et al.[45] described a classification of perihilar bile duct tumours based on the degree of bile duct involvement by the tumour (**Box 10.2**). This classification does not take into account radial tumour growth, vascular involvement and lobar atrophy, and so is not indicative of resectability or survival. Many tumours originate eccentrically in the right or left duct and subsequently involve the confluence, so that some lesions require major hepatic resection for their eradication.[46] Such resections must take account of a possible atrophy/hyperplasia complex and must leave adequately

Box 10.2 • Bismuth–Corlette classification for hilar tumours

- Type I tumours – entirely below the confluence
- Type II tumours – affecting the confluence
- Type III tumours – occluding the confluence and extending to the first-order right (IIIa) or left (IIIb) intrahepatic ducts
- Type IV – involving both hepatic ducts or are multicentric

Box 10.3 • TNM classification for extrahepatic bile duct cancer

Primary tumour (T)

TX: Primary tumour cannot be assessed

T0: No evidence of primary tumour

Tis: Carcinoma in situ

T1: Tumour confined to the ductal wall

1a: Mucosa

1b: Muscle

T2: Tumour invades perimuscular connective tissue

T3: Tumour invades adjacent structures: liver, pancreas, duodenum, gallbladder, colon, stomach

Regional lymph nodes (N)

NX: Regional lymph nodes cannot be assessed

N0: No regional lymph node metastasis

N1: Metastasis in cystic duct, pericholedochal and/or hilar lymph nodes (i.e. in the hepatoduodenal ligament)

N2: Metastasis in peripancreatic (head only), periduodenal, periportal, coeliac and/or superior mesenteric lymph nodes

Distant metastasis (M)

MX: Presence of distant metastasis cannot be assessed

M0: No distant metastasis

M1: Distant metastasis

Stage grouping

Stage 0	Tis, N0, M0
Stage I	T1, N0, M0
Stage II	T2, N0, M0
Stage III	T1, N1, M0
	T1, N2, M0
	T2, N1, M0
	T2, N2, M0
Stage IVA	T3, any N, M0
Stage IVB	Any T, any N, M1

functioning liver tissue, and not an atrophic and possibly infected lobe.[47]

Formal pathological staging is by the TNM system (**Box 10.3**), but such complete staging can only be made after surgery and pathological examination of the resected specimen.

A modified preoperative T staging was proposed by Jarnagin et al. in 2001.[48] Stage T1 includes tumours that involve the biliary confluence with or without unilateral extension to second-order biliary radicles. Tumours involving the biliary confluence with or without unilateral extension to second-order biliary radicles and ipsilateral portal vein involvement with or without ipsilateral hepatic lobar atrophy are classified as T2 tumours. T3 tumours involve the biliary confluence with bilateral extension to second-order biliary radicles; or unilateral extension to second-order biliary radicles with contralateral portal vein involvement; or unilateral extension to second-order biliary radicles with contralateral hepatic lobar atrophy; or main or bilateral portal venous involvement. This staging system does not take into account nodal metastasis and distant spread but the incidence of these was found to increase with the T-stage. This system was used to analyse resectability in 219 patients with hilar cholangiocarcinoma. Resectability was 59% in group T1, progressively decreasing to 0% in stage T3. In the same study, a negative resection margin, concomitant hepatic resection and well-differentiated tumour histology were found to be independent predictors of long-term survival.

Presentation

Obstructive jaundice is the presenting feature in 90–98% of patients.[14] Jaundice tends to occur early in cases of common bile duct, common hepatic and ampullary cancer but may be absent in the cases of intrahepatic cholangiocarcinoma and in tumours that only involve the left or the right hepatic duct. The disease may be extensive even before jaundice develops. Lymph node metastases are present in up to 50% of patients at diagnosis, and up to 20% of cases have peritoneal metastatic disease on presentation.[13] Jaundice may be intermittent in cases of papillary tumours.

Itching may precede the onset of jaundice, and non-specific symptoms include weight loss and abdominal pain. Of 94 patients with biliary cancer seen at the Hammersmith Hospital, 40% had episodes of ill-defined pain for some time before diagnosis, and 37% had cholelithiasis.[49] Cholangitis is a rare initial presenting feature unless endoscopic or percutaneous instrumentation of the biliary tree has been performed.

Some cases may be diagnosed incidentally as a result of investigation of deranged liver function tests or abdominal ultrasound for other indications.

Investigative techniques

Hilar cholangiocarcinoma was first described clinically by Altemeier et al. in 1957,[50] but for almost two decades the diagnosis was rarely made during life, and often missed at laparotomy. Improvements in diagnostic techniques have changed this situation, and most of these tumours are now recognised preoperatively.

LABORATORY

Liver function tests are useful only in defining the degree of obstructive jaundice. Raised alkaline phosphatase may be an early isolated abnormality in a symptomatic but anicteric patient.

Tumour markers are of limited value: CEA is expressed in the cells of bile duct cancer,[51] and may be raised in the serum. Cancer antigens CA19-9 and CA50 are frequently raised, but these are not specific.[52] CA19-9 has been found to be useful in detecting cholangiocarcinoma in patients with PSC awaiting liver transplant. Recently, the muci Muc5AC was found in significant concentrations in patients with cholangiocarcinoma. Its sensitivity was 62.6% and it had a high specificity.[53] Serum Muc5AC levels are also associated with larger tumour volume and a poorer prognosis.[54] Other tumour markers

associated with cholangiocarcinoma include biliary fibronectin[55] and serum interleukin 6.[56]

Haematological tests should include measurement of coagulation status. Many patients are chronically anaemic on presentation, and leucocytosis may be a significant adverse prognostic factor in obstructive jaundice.

Nutritional status has a major impact on surgical risk. Low haemoglobin may be regarded as a nutritional index, but the most significant parameters are low serum albumin and history of recent weight loss.[57]

There are no tumour markers specific for cholangiocarcinoma but patients with suspected cholangiocarcinoma should have a combination of serum tumour markers measured.

RADIOLOGICAL

Ultrasound (US) can identify the level of obstruction in practically all cases although it may not be able to identify small tumours.[58] The presence of gallbladder stones should be readily identified, and abnormalities of the gallbladder wall may raise suspicion of gallbladder cancer. Duplex scanning may show invasion or encasements of the portal vein or hepatic artery. Masses within the liver may indicate secondaries, or microabscesses secondary to biliary obstruction. A skilled operator can identify the site of biliary obstruction as well as the presence or absence of portal vein involvement with 93% sensitivity and 99% specificity using duplex ultrasonography.[14]

Endoscopic ultrasound has been shown to be valuable in the assessment of cholangiocarcinoma, especially of the middle and distal thirds of the bile duct, and in determining the presence of lymphadenopathy. Ultrasound, however, cannot distinguish benign from malignant nodes.[59] Endosonography-guided fine-needle aspiration may help to determine the nature of the lymphadenopathy.[60]

Computed tomography (CT) may have some advantages over ultrasound in the diagnosis of malignant biliary tumours, especially in detecting intrahepatic spread of tumour or local lymphadenopathy. Engels et al.[61] detected lymphadenopathy in three-quarters of patients with gallbladder or bile duct cancer at presentation. CT is of specific value in defining lobar or segmental hepatic atrophy. Lobar atrophy appears as a small, often hypoperfused lobe with crowded and dilated intrahepatic bile ducts.

Magnetic resonance imaging (MRI) permits the visualisation of the hepatic parenchyma as well as the intrahepatic and extrahepatic biliary tree and vascular structures. Being non-invasive, MRI avoids bile duct intubation and its subsequent risk of cholangitis.[62,63] Combined with MRC and MRA (see below), it is possible to achieve full diagnostic imaging with a single investigation.

Cholangiography (Fig. 10.2) helps to delineate the full extent of tumour involvement of the biliary system, including definition of all hepatic segmental ducts; examinations carried out before referral to a specialist centre are often incomplete. Endoscopic retrograde cholangiopancreatography (ERCP) and percutaneous transhepatic cholangiography (PTC) remain the most common modalities, and local availability and expertise may dictate the choice between these. Arguably ERCP is the procedure of

first choice for distally placed tumours whereas for suspected upper biliary tract lesions, PTC is preferable, because the proximal extent of disease is important in staging and planning of treatment. Both procedures may be required for complete diagnosis.[64] PTC and ERCP are associated with a considerable complication rate (up to 9%). Complications include pancreatitis, sepsis, haemobilia and bowel perforation.[65] Diffuse abnormalities of the biliary tree as in PSC may make it impossible to delineate a tumour exactly.[66]

Nimura et al.[67] have extended the use of complete cholangiography to map all segmental ducts prior to surgery by PTC with drainage and percutaneous **cholangioscopy**, with a 96% positive rate on cholangioscopic biopsy. By contrast, some surgeons regard complete cholangiography before operation

(a)

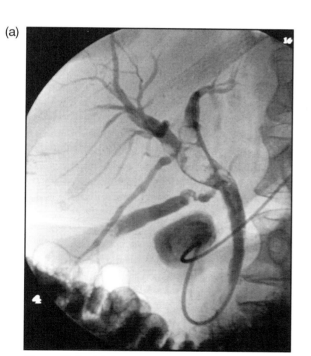

(b)

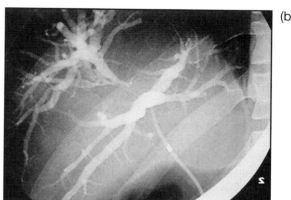

(c)

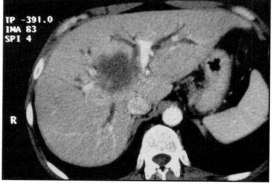

Figure 10.2 • **(a)** Endoscopic retrograde cholangiopancreatography (ERCP) and nasobiliary tube in a case of bulky intraductal papillary tumour expanding the hilar ducts. **(b)** Hilar cholangiocarcinoma involving mainly the right intrahepatic ducts. The anterior and posterior sectoral ducts are separated by the tumour, and a guidewire has been placed through the stricture as a first step in placement of a metallic stent. **(c)** CT scan in the same patient as (b). The tumour mass can be seen involving the right intrahepatic ducts and displacing and invading the contrast-filled portal venous branches.

as undesirable because of the risks of introducing infection, and rely on intraoperative cholangiography and/or ultrasound. This is a minority view, and most prefer to enter operative management with maximum anatomical information. Broadspectrum antibiotic prophylaxis and careful, low-pressure cholangiography should minimise the risks of infection. The possibility of interventional procedures should be considered before the diagnostic manoeuvre is undertaken; there should be close consultation between radiologist and endoscopist and the surgeon at the time of the procedure.

Magnetic resonance cholangiopancreatography (MRCP) was introduced in 1991 by Wallner et al.[68] It allows non-invasive visualisation of the biliary tree and has reported sensitivities approaching 90–95% in cases of biliary and pancreatic ductal dilatation and strictures. It also helps to identify obstructed and isolated ducts that may not be identified by PTC or ERCP. In a study by Yeh et al. comparing ERCP and MRCP,[65] ERCP was not possible in 5% of cases. Both tests detected the presence of obstruction in cases of cholangioarcinoma, but MRCP was found to be better in identifying the cause of the obstruction and the anatomical extent of the disease.

Cytology of bile samples taken from percutaneous stents may yield malignant cells in 40% of cases of cholangiocarcinoma. The use of brush biopsies can increase this to up to 70%. However, due to the desmoplastic nature of these tumours, biopsies may yield non-diagnostic tissue. In our study of over 200 aspiration biopsies or cytological brushings at ERCP or PTC,[69] we found predictive values of positive and negative results of 98% and 53%, respectively. Thus negative results should not be treated as implying no malignancy.

Histological diagnosis is not mandatory prior to exploration.

Angiography is used selectively. Arterial encasement is virtually diagnostic of malignant tumour. Information about the portal vein can often be satisfactorily obtained at ultrasound, especially with the use of duplex scanning. However, when there remains doubt with potentially operable lesions then visceral angiography remains the gold standard. MRI is gradually replacing invasive angiography.

Laparoscopy can detect small peritoneal nodules or liver secondaries missed on ultrasound and CT, and may eliminate an unnecessary laparotomy.

Laparoscopy is, however, less accurate in assessing vascular invasion, lymph node metastasis and the extent of biliary involvement.[70] Weber et al.[71] studied 100 patients with hilar or gallbladder carcinoma that were deemed resectable radiologically and found that the accuracy of laparoscopic staging (laparoscopy ± laparoscopic ultrasound) for hilar and gallbladder carcinoma was 67% for gallbladder carcinoma and 48% for hilar carcinoma. In this study, laparoscopy prevented unnecessary laparotomy in a third of the patients and no mortality was reported as a result of the procedure.

Positron emission tomography (PET) scanning, using the glucose analogue [18F]fluoro-2-deoxy-D-glucose (FDG), can be of value in diagnosing cholangiocarcinoma, especially in differentiating between benign PSC-related strictures and malignant change.[72] Cholangiocarcinoma cells accumulate FDG (due to relatively low levels of glucose-6-phosphatase) causing hot spots to appear on scanning (increased uptake values, lesion to normal liver background ratio >2 and standard uptake value >3.5).[73] Several small studies have shown that PET scanning may detect cholangiocarcinoma as small as 1 cm in diameter. In a study by Kluge et al.,[74] PET was found to have a sensitivity of 92.3% and specificity of 92.9% in diagnosing cholangiocarcinoma. However, the detection of regional lymph node metastasis was poor (sensitivity of 13%).

Other less frequently used, experimental imaging modalities include intraductal ultrasound,[75,76] endoscopic and percutaneous flexible cholangiography and radiolabelled antibody[77] and ligand imaging.[78,79]

Patients should have initial US screening and a combined MRI and MRCP. If MRI or MRCP is not available, a contrast-enhanced spiral CT should be undertaken.

Invasive cholangiography should be reserved for tissue diagnosis or therapeutic decompression where there is cholangitis, a need for stent insertion and in irresectable cases.

These investigations may be complementary and all investigations may be necessary as part of a surgical assessment.

The role of newer imaging techniques such as endoscopic ultrasound and PET have yet to be determined.

Management of cholangiocarcinoma

At present, only surgical excision of all detectable tumour is associated with an improvement in 5-year survival for patients with cholangiocarcinoma.[66] However, surgery is only able to cure a minority of patients, with a 20–30% 5-year survival for distal lesions and a 9–18% 5-year survival for more proximal lesions.[13] Relief of biliary obstruction is therefore a mandatory aim in management, and long-term prevention of cholangitis will ensure the best quality of life. On these principles, a judgement must be made between the complementary forms of therapy – endoscopic, radiological or operative. Because of the infrequency of these tumours they should be discussed in a multidisciplinary team setting, and most referred to specialist centres.

SURGICAL MANAGEMENT OF HILAR CHOLANGIOCARCINOMA

The patient's general fitness must be assessed before any procedure. Poor performance status and major cardiopulmonary disease are the most common patient-related factors that preclude surgical exploration. Patients with Child B or C cirrhosis are not candidates for curative resection if this will involve a liver resection. Poor nutritional status, sepsis and severe cholestasis also predict a poor outcome but can be corrected preoperatively to some extent.

Assessment of resectability

Preoperative staging should have been carried out before operation is undertaken. Having excluded distant metastases (e.g. lung), the extent of ductal and vascular involvement will determine local resectability, or the need for hepatic resection.

The following criteria would suggest an irresectable tumour:[80]

- involvement of bilateral second-order intrahepatic ducts, or multifocal tumour on cholangiography
- extensive involvement of the main stem of the portal vein
- involvement of major vessels or ducts on opposite sides of the liver
- liver atrophy or infection inconsistent with a viable liver remnant after resection

- nodal metastasis to N2 lymph nodes (peripancreatic, periduodenal, coeliac, superior mesenteric or posterior pancreatico-duodenal lymph nodes).

Lymph node involvement and intraperitoneal spread may be difficult to determine preoperatively: laparoscopy may help in this situation.

Potentially curative surgery – resection of hilar cholangiocarcinoma

Worldwide experience of resection for hilar cholangiocarcinoma has remained relatively small. Resectability rates reported from specialist units vary widely. The majority of Western series report a resectability rate of 15–33%.[49,66,81–83] Adoption of a more aggressive policy leads to higher resectability rates of 35–66%.[66,84–86] The resectability rate described in Japanese series (52–92%),[87–90] some with large numbers of patients, has been consistently higher than in Western reports. It is not absolutely clear why this should be so, but it reflects in part an increased readiness to undertake extensive resections in these patients, including resections of the portal vein, radical lymphadenectomy, and major hepatic resection.

The importance of negative resection margins for long-term survival has been shown in several studies, and the willingness of surgeons to use liver resection routinely to obtain clear margins has increased significantly. In a review article by Chamberlain and Blumgart,[14] this approach was found to produce negative resection margins (R0 resection) in more than 50% of cases, and has been associated with a significant trend towards prolonged survival, with 40–60% 3-year survival rates in most series. The mean operative mortality of such surgery was found to be 6% (range 0–14%).

Some surgeons feel that the caudate lobe (segment 1) should be removed routinely when resecting hilar cholangiocarcinomas, especially if the tumour involves the left duct, because of the risk of leaving residual tumour.[88,91,92] In a histological review of 45 consecutive cases of hilar cholangiocarcinoma, the caudate lobe was found to be involved in 44 cases (98%). The 3-year survival rate for patients surviving the curative excision was 55.1%, and the 5-year survival rate was 40.5%.[88] Resection of the nodes and lymphatics along the hepatoduodenal ligament may also be important for survival, but the value of more radical lymphatic clearance including the coeliac nodes is uncertain. Relatively few authors recommend major excision and reconstruction of the hilar vessels since there is no evidence that more extended resections and vascular reconstruction confer any survival benefit.[92] However, if a short segment of the portal vein is involved by tumour it is perfectly feasible to resect and reanastomose it end-to-end.[93]

> En bloc resection of the supraduodenal common bile duct, gallbladder, cystic duct and extrahepatic hepatic ducts together with regional lymphadenectomy and Roux-en-Y hepatico-jejunostomy is recommended for Bismuth type I and II tumours without major vessel involvement. A tumour-free proximal margin of at least 5 mm is required.
>
> Type III tumours require additional hepatic resection.
>
> Type IV tumours may require an extended right or left hepatectomy in addition to local resection and regional lymphadenectomy.
>
> Resection of segment I (caudate lobe) is recommended for type II, III and IV tumours as these often involve the ducts of this lobe.
>
> Distal cholangiocarcinoma is managed by pancreatico-duodenectomy.
>
> Intrahepatic cholangiocarcinoma is treated by resection of the involved liver.

SURGICAL RESECTION FOR DISTAL EXTRAHEPATIC TUMOURS

Pancreato-duodenectomy is the operation of choice in cases of resectable cholangiocarcinoma of the distal bile duct. Commonly, a pylorus-preserving Whipple procedure is performed. This is dealt with in Chapter 13.

ADJUVANT THERAPY

The use of radiotherapy in the management of cholangiocarcinoma was first advocated by Fletcher et al. in 1981.[94]

Intraoperative radiotherapy has been reported from a few specialised centres. Busse et al.[95] treated 15 patients with advanced bile duct cancer over a 5-year period, using 5–20 Gy, with postoperative radiotherapy administered also in 13 of these. There was little morbidity and a low mortality, though the effects on survival are undefined. One study of nine patients[96] found no significant difference in mean survival or 1-year survival between those patients treated with intraoperative radiotherapy (16.8 months, 56%) and those treated by external beam irradiation with or without iridium-192 (11 months, 46%).

In a small study, nine patients with extrahepatic cholangiocarcinoma were given **neoadjuvant chemoradiation** consisting of continuous infusion of 5-fluorouracil and external beam radiotherapy. Three of these patients had a pathological complete response while the rest all had negative resection margins.[97]

Pitt et al.[98] found that in patients who had undergone resection for localised perihilar tumours, **postoperative radiotherapy** did not improve survival. Kamada et al.,[99] however, suggested that radiotherapy may increase survival in patients with positive hepatic duct resection margins. If radiotherapy is to be used postoperatively, metal clips may be placed to mark the area of the anastomosis after resection, or areas of known or suspected residual tumour.

None of these studies were randomised and, while larger randomised and controlled studies would be desirable before routine use of adjuvant or neoadjuvant therapy, such studies are difficult to organise, so such data may not readily become available.

PALLIATIVE MEASURES

Most patients with hilar cholangiocarcinoma are not suitable for surgical resection. If a patient is deemed irresectable, histological or cytological confirmation should be obtained. Biliary decompression should be performed in order to relieve intractable pruritus and prevent or relieve cholangitis. This can be achieved by surgical, endoscopic or percutaneous techniques.

Surgical bypass

Biliary-enteric bypass for proximal biliary cancer is more difficult than for distally placed tumours, but it is often possible to carry out a hepatico-jejunostomy to the left duct. If the confluence has not been disconnected by the tumour, the right liver will also be drained by this procedure. Even in the absence of such a communication, effective palliation will still be obtained, provided there is no sepsis within the right liver. When the left duct is involved by tumour it is possible to gain access to an intrahepatic duct within the left liver.

In the Longmire procedure, part of the left lobe is resected to locate an intrahepatic duct.[100] This procedure has now been superseded by a bypass to the duct of segment 3, accessed by splitting the liver just to the left of the umbilical fissure, popularised by Bismuth et al. Operative morbidity and mortality for these procedures are low[101,102] and the palliation is excellent.[101] Jarnagin et al.[103] showed that the long-term patency rate for segment 3 bypass in patients with cholangiocarcinoma is high (up to 80% at 1 year). However, patients with gallbladder carcinoma who underwent the same procedure still had poor survival (due to the aggressive and advanced nature of the disease) and thus segment 3 bypass may not be a suitable alternative for such patients. Bypass to the right sectoral ducts was associated with greater morbidity and mortality and 60% patency rate at 1 year.[103]

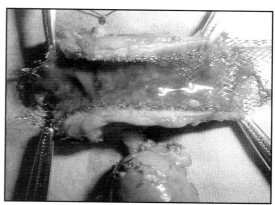

Figure 10.3 • Local excision of a short localised cholangiocarcinoma of the common hepatic duct. A metallic stent had been previously placed, and was excised in situ within the duct. The mesh has already become firmly embedded in the duct lining. The gallbladder is attached at the bottom of the picture. See also Plate 9, facing p. 20.

Surgical bypass should be considered in patients with good estimated life expectancy.

Operative intubation

The transhepatic U-tube first described by Praderi was popularised by Terblanche and his colleagues.[104] Although the technique found favour with other groups, it has been supplanted by the use of endoscopic or radiological methods.

Stenting

Ideally, routine biliary drainage should be avoided before assessing resectability or preoperatively, except in certain clinical situations such as acute suppurative cholangitis or patients who have severe renal dysfunction or are severely malnourished.

For pancreatic cancer, several trials have now demonstrated that stenting and surgical bypass are equally effective in the relief of obstructive jaundice,[105] and stenting is attended by a lower hospital mortality rate and a shorter stay. However, for patients with the relatively favourable tumours of the bile duct and anticipated longer survival, the rate of recurrent jaundice and cholangitis may be greater for those with an endoprosthesis than for those treated by surgical bypass. The development of large-calibre (up to 1 cm) self-expanding metallic stents may confer a significant improvement in long-term patency (**Fig. 10.3**) (also in colour, see Plate 9, facing p. 20). Initial concerns about the cost of metal stents were not borne out in ran-

domised clinical trials, as they were associated with longer complication-free survival, shorter hospital stay and lower overall cost, especially in those patients surviving longer than 6 months.[106–108]

Percutaneous stenting

For patients who are unsuitable for resection, permanent percutaneous stenting may follow diagnostic and staging PTC.[109–111] Insertion of percutaneous stents in hilar cholangiocarcinoma is usually technically more difficult than in patients with distal tumours. This is because more than one stent may be necessary if there is disruption of the confluence. The patency rate for metallic stents at the hilar region is also less than for those placed in the distal bile duct. Becker et al.[112] reported 1-year patency rates of 46% and 89% for Wallstents® (Boston Scientific, Natick, MN) inserted in the hilum and in the distal common bile duct, respectively. In most series, there is a restenting rate of 25% with Wallstents inserted in the hilar area. Percutaneous placement of conventional plastic stents may require a period of external drainage and dilatation of the track, but self-expanding metal stents can be placed in a single stage. Tumour ingrowth may be less of a problem with cholangiocarcinoma than with pancreatic or ampullary tumours because of their relatively low cellularity and dense stroma. Tumour 'overgrowth' above or below the stent may be more of a problem, but this can be overcome by placing the longest stent available. Occluded stents can often be cleared by further percutaneous interventions.[113,114] The use of cyclical antibiotics and ursodeoxycholic acid (UDCA) did not improve the patency rate of plastic stents.[115] In our own early experience of 202 patients with malignant biliary strictures over 7 years, 41 were treated with Wallstent endoprosthesis with a reintervention rate of 12%, compared with 22% in 100 patients treated with plastic stents.[110] The recently developed semicovered stents should reduce tumour ingrowth but are as yet unproved to have superior long-term patency.[13]

Endoscopic stenting
Metallic stents can also be placed endoscopically, combining the advantages of both techniques.[116] The techniques must not be looked upon as competitive, but complementary, and when intubation from below proves difficult or impossible, a combined procedure may be considered, using a percutaneous wire passed through the tumour from above. When endoscopic stenting is possible, it is usually regarded as a less invasive procedure, and is the first choice for a route of access over percutaneous methods.

In a study by Cheng et al.,[117] endoscopic Wallstent insertion was found to achieve successful palliation without the need for further biliary reintervention in the majority (69%) of patients with irresectable hilar cholangiocarcinoma. The 30-day mortality rate in this group was 6%, and 31% of patients required further stenting.

Stenting and complications
High rates of biliary bacterial contamination are found in patients with complete and incomplete biliary obstruction by tumour. The rate of cholangitis and bacterobilia increases with instrumentation of the biliary tree. The rate of occurrence of infective complications is highest if biliary stents are left in situ, and patients with stents are more likely to have polymicrobial infections.[118] In a study by Hochwald et al.,[119] patients who were stented preoperatively had a two-fold increase in postoperative infective complications after surgery for hilar cholangiocarcinoma. In the same study, preoperative biliary stenting was not found to improve the outcome or decrease morbidity but was associated with a higher intraoperative blood loss and increased difficulty in operative dissection. Increased compli-

cations were also described with preoperative biliary stenting and pancreato-duodenectomy.[120]

 Routine biliary drainage before assessing resectability or preoperatively should be avoided.

Palliative use of radiotherapy
The beneficial effects of radiotherapy in the adjuvant and in the palliative settings remain to be demonstrated in prospective randomised studies.

External beam radiotherapy (total doses used varying between 20 and 60 Gy) may cause radiation duodenitis and intractable gastrointestinal bleeding. To circumvent this problem, brachytherapy has been given, using iridium-192, a beta emitter with only a few millimetres depth of penetration, which might slow local progression and delay the onset of biliary obstruction or stent overgrowth. The local dose of 30–50 Gy can be supplemented by another 30–45 Gy external beam irradiation. Delivery has mostly been transhepatic,[121,122] but can be achieved endoscopically via nasobiliary tubes.[123,124]

A small study in our patients with locally advanced cholangiocarcinoma treated with combinations of external beam and iridium-192 therapy showed that although treatment was generally well tolerated, no additional benefit could be demonstrated.[125] Similar results were obtained by other groups.[126]

A retrospective comparison of stenting alone versus stenting with radiotherapy (internal and external) in non-resectable cholangiocarcinomas did not show significant survival benefit in the radiotherapy group. Patients in this group also had longer hospital stays and higher incidence of stent changes.[127]

Chemotherapy
Bile duct cancer has conventionally been regarded as chemoresistant. Oberfield and Rossi[128] reported a significant local response rate in 29% of 97 patients treated with 5-fluorouracil (5-FU) and mitomycin C, alone or in combination with Adriamycin (doxorubicin) (FAM). A report from UCLA[129] described significant response rates and possible survival improvement in seven patients receiving continuous 5-FU, with intermittent folinic acid (leucovorin), mitomycin C and dipyridamole. Our patients in King's College Hospital, London, have also shown promising responses to continuous infusional 5-FU with intermittent epirubicin and

cisplatin.[130] Sanz-Altamira et al., using a platinum salt (carboplatin), 5-FU and folinic acid, showed a total response rate of 21.4%, which is comparable to other single agents and combinations.[131]

Intra-arterial therapy produced a partial response rate of more than 50%, and a complete response in one of 11 patients in one series including both bile duct and gallbladder cancers, and suggested improved survival for both groups.[132] There remains, however, little evidence from controlled studies for the value of chemotherapy for tumours of the bile duct.

Photodynamic therapy

Photodynamic therapy (PDT) involves administration of a photosensitising drug that accumulates in tumour cells, followed by exposure of the tumour to laser light of the appropriate wavelength. The photosensitiser becomes activated and forms cytotoxic reaction products, including oxygen radicals, thereby destroying the photosensitised cells.[133] In a prospective, single-arm phase-II trial,[134] 23 patients were treated with PDT and endoprosthesis. Ninety-one percent survived for up to 6 months post-diagnosis compared with less than 50% of historical controls. The median survival time for patients with Bismuth III and IV tumours treated with PDT in this study was 11 months.

Complications associated with PDT include epigastric pain, acute-phase reactions, acute and chronic cholangitis, haemobilia and skin phototoxic changes. As with chemotherapy and radiotherapy, randomised trials are awaited.

All patients who have inoperable tumours or who have had a non-curative resection should be encouraged to participate in chemotherapy or similar trials.

Liver transplantation

The literature is confused by the reporting of intrahepatic and extrahepatic cholangiocarcinomas as one group. Provided regional nodal metastases and other sites of extrahepatic tumour can be excluded, then total hepatectomy with orthotopic liver transplantation (OLT) may be possible for patients with cholangiocarcinoma. Pichlmayr et al.[135] found no significant difference in 1- and 5-year survival in patients with proximal bile duct carcinoma undergoing surgical resection or liver transplantation especially in early tumour stages.

However, in a study of 207 patients who underwent liver transplantation for perihilar and intrahepatic cholangiocarcinoma or cholangiohepatoma, at least 51% of patients had recurrence of their tumour. Most of the recurrences occurred in the allograft, while the lungs were the second commonest site of metastatic spread. Most of the recurrences occurred within 2 years of the transplantation, and the survival after recurrence was rarely more than 1 year. Patients with hilar lymph node involvement had a higher recurrence rate and thus a worse prognosis after transplantation.[136]

In pilot studies, liver transplantation following preoperative chemoradiation for irresectable cholangiocarcinoma has resulted in long-term survival in carefully selected patients.[137] Those with incidental cholangiocarcinoma (found on explant histopathological evaluation) but without lymphatic involvement, may also result in acceptable patient survival.[138]

The dilemma, therefore, remains that patients with well-localised tumours are likely to survive transplantation and immunosuppression, but these are also the patients likely to be amenable to conventional local resection.

OLT should not be considered as standard therapy for hilar cholangiocarcinoma.

RESULTS

There remains no clear consensus as to the optimum methods of evaluation or treatment of these difficult cases. On the one hand, several authors are reporting higher resectability rates and more complex forms of resection, whereas on the other hand, radiologists and endoscopists have made technical advances resulting in more expeditious treatment of patients and shorter hospital stay. Although philosophically it is reasonable to accept that the only prospects of cure are afforded by complete resection of the cancer, it is by no means certain that this is so, nor indeed that complete as opposed to almost complete resection followed by adjuvant therapy confers a significant survival advantage in the majority of cases.[139] Little[140] has reviewed this dichotomy of views. The consistent view that stands out through all these reports is the need for a unified approach to assessment of quality of survival and palliation. Bismuth et al.[45] defined the 'Comfort Index' – the proportion of a patient's actual survival that is spent in good condition, effectively palliated – and demonstrated excellent results from a left-sided biliary-enteric anastomosis.

In looking at outcome, it is important to take account of the mortality of surgical treatment. Mortality is low for those not requiring hepatectomy and is becoming increasingly safe for those in whom liver resection is required (Table 10.1). One recent series[48] reported eight deaths from post-operative complications (median time from operation 1.1 months) in 80 patients undergoing resection for hilar cholangiocarcinoma. This group also reported a 35-month median survival and a 30% 5-year survival in the resected group.

The reported 5-year survival following resection for cholangiocarcinoma varies. Among the best results are those from Nimura,[88] detailed below. Our own early experience[139] in almost 200 patients treated from 1978 to 1988 was that only 44 cases (22%) underwent resection, of whom 40 patients had elective resection alone and were available for follow-up. The overall median survival of those who left hospital was 25 months. All those with involved margins died within 5 years, whereas the actuarial 5-year survival for those with clear margins approached 25%.

Our more recent experience at King's College Hospital reflects a continuing determination to resect the tumours whenever possible. Of 155 patients referred during 1991–2000, 76 (49%) had no operative procedure, 12 (15%) had a surgical bypass, and 50 (32% of all cases and 63% of those explored) underwent resection, including 17 hepatic resections and 6 pancreato-duodenectomies. There was one perioperative death. Excluding patients with follow-up of under 1 year, the median survival in 9 patients who had 'curative' resection was 26 months, compared with 11 months in 15 who had 'palliative' resection.[141] Nimura et al.[92] described the management of 127 cases of hilar cholangio-carcinoma over 16 years; 110 were operated upon with 100 resections. All but nine patients had combined hepatic and hilar ductal resection, including the caudate lobe, with an overall hospital mortality following resection of 10%. Resection was thought to be 'curative' in 82/100, and in this group there was a 33-month median survival and a 31% 5-year actuarial survival. In the 'palliative'

Table 10.1 • Four retrospective studies comparing outcome of resection for proximal bile duct carcinoma

Author	Nimura et al.[88]	Nakeeb et al.[12]	Pichlmayr et al.[135]	Jarnagin et al.[48]
Year	1990	1996	1996	2001
Number of patients evaluated	66	196	249	225
Number of patients who underwent resection (%)	55	109 (56%)	125 (50.2%)	80
% of resected patients with negative margins	83.6	26	72.8	78
% of resected patients who had liver resection	81.8	14	76	78
Operative/early postoperative mortality	6.4%	4%	8.8%	10%
Median survival in patients who underwent resection			19 months	35 months
5-year survival in resected group	40.5% (excluding patients who died in perop. period)	11%	25%	30%

group the comparable figures were 18 month median and 14% 3-year survival, and no patient survived 4 years. The 'curative' group included 27 patients with portal vein resection and 12 with synchronous pancreato-duodenectomy en bloc (5 with both), a formidable procedure; the 5-year survival for those with portal vein resection was only 5%, and for those without this manoeuvre it was 43%.

Accurate diagnosis of cholangiocarcinoma, including a full anatomical assessment of the tumour, is necessary. Preoperative diagnosis may be aided by cytological examination.

Surgical resection for cure is only achieved in a minority of cases. Long-term palliation depends on draining the maximum volume of functioning hepatic tissue possible, and this may involve palliative tumour clearance only when final histology is available. Stenting, especially with metallic stents, provides reliable palliation in most irresectable patients, and operative bypass is mostly now confined to patients who are explored but found to be irresectable, or in whom stenting has failed or been attended by severe recurrent cholangitis.

Radiotherapy has no clear role in the management of cholangiocarcinoma. The results of current trials of photodynamic therapy and chemotherapy are awaited.

 Episodes of recurrent cholangitis must be treated vigorously. Stenting is worthwhile for local recurrence and can give a useful period of prolonged palliation.

CARCINOMA OF THE GALLBLADDER

The gallbladder is the commonest site of cancer in the biliary tract; however, gallbladder neoplasia represents only 2% of all cancers. It is characterised by rapid progression and a poor 5-year survival (less than 10% in most series).[142] Only about a quarter of the cases are resectable for cure.

Risk factors

Gallbladder carcinoma is three times more common in females than males.[143,144] Incidence increases with age, and the tumour is commonest in the seventh decade.[5]

It is thought that longstanding inflammation of the gallbladder may predispose to cancer but the exact method of pathogenesis is not known. Up to 90% of patients with gallbladder cancer have gallstones, in contrast to about 13% for other biliary cancers.[3] The risk increases if the gallstones are large and symptomatic.[142,145]

Bacterial infection of bile may be found in up to 80% of patients with gallbladder cancer. Chronic inflammation due to typhoid, in association with cholelithiasis, appears to carry an increased risk.[146–148]

'Porcelain' gallbladder (**Fig. 10.4**) (**Fig. 10.4b** also in colour, see Plate 10, facing p. 20), with intramural calcification, is a premalignant condition.[142]

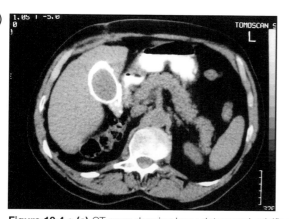

(a)

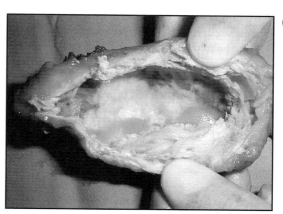

(b)

Figure 10.4 • **(a)** CT scan showing heavy intramural calcification in a 'porcelain' gallbladder. **(b)** Excised gallbladder from the case shown in (a). The wall is extensively replaced by calcium salt deposits and there is destruction of the epithelium. In this case there was no gallbladder cancer (see also Plate 10, facing p. 20).

The majority of gallbladder polyps are cholesterol polyps, but while true adenomatous polyps also occur,[149] there is little convincing evidence that benign polyps undergo malignant change. Malignant gallbladder polyps tend to be single, larger than 10 mm and occur in patients over 50 years of age.[150,151]

The incidence of gallbladder cancer is increased 14.7-fold 20 years after surgery for gastric ulcer, but there is no increase in the incidence of tumours in the rest of the biliary tract.[152]

There are high-risk ethnic groups, most notably South-West American Indians, and there are other, unexplained, areas of high incidence, including Poland, Czech Republic, Chile and northwest India.[144,153] Familial clustering of gallbladder cancer has also been described.[154]

Gallbladder carcinoma has also been associated with a high body mass index,[148] high total energy intake, high carbohydrate intake, chronic diarrhoea[155] and anomalous pancreato-biliary duct junction (APBDJ).[156] The incidence may be increased when APBDJ is not associated with choledochal cyst.[157,158] Other rare associations include inflammatory bowel disease and polyposis coli.[159]

Pathology

Most gallbladder tumours are adenocarcinomas (80–95%), though a small percentage are squamous or adenosquamous (2–10%). Other rarer types including undifferentiated, mesenchymal and carcinoid tumours have been described. Most of these tumours (60%) begin in the fundus, 30% commence in the body and 10% in the neck.

Three macroscopic appearances have been described: infiltrative, nodular or papillary. The commonest type is the infiltrative type, while papillary tumours carry the best prognosis.[5] Gallbladder carcinoma spreads early with lymphatic and haematogenous spread as well as direct extension to the liver. Spread can also occur along needle biopsy tracks, in surgical incisions and along laparoscopic port sites. Peritoneal seeding is also common.

STAGING

Several staging systems have been described. The most commonly used are the TNM (**Box 10.4**) and

Box 10.4 • TNM classification for gallbladder cancer

Primary tumour (T)

TX: Primary tumour cannot be assessed

T0:   No evidence of primary tumour

Tis: Carcinoma in situ

T1:   Tumour invades lamina propria or muscle layer

T1a: Tumour invades lamina propria

T1b: Tumour invades muscle layer

T2:   Tumour invades perimuscular connective tissue: no extension beyond serosa or into liver

T3:   Tumour perforates serosa (visceral peritoneum) or directly invades the liver and/or one other adjacent organ or structure, e.g. stomach, duodenum, colon, pancreas, omentum, extrahepatic bile ducts

T4:   Tumour invades main portal vein or hepatic artery, or invades two or more extrahepatic organs or structures

Regional lymph nodes (N)

NX: Regional lymph nodes cannot be assessed

N0:   No regional lymph node metastasis

N1:   Regional lymph node metastasis

Distant metastasis (M)

MX: Presence of distant metastasis cannot be assessed

M0:   No distant metastasis

M1:   Distant metastasis

Stage grouping

Stage 0	Tis, N0, M0
Stage IA	T1, N0, M0
Stage IB	T2, N0, M0
Stage IIA	T3, N0, M0
Stage IIB	T1, N1, M0
	T2, N1, M0
	T3, N1, M0
Stage III	T4, any N, M0
Stage IV	Any T, any N, M1

From Sobin LH, Wittekind C (eds) TNM classification of malignant tumours, 6th edn. Wiley-Liss, 2002. Reprinted with permission of John Wiley & Sons, Inc.

the modified Nevin staging systems, the latter of which assesses grade and stage of disease.

In the Nevin system,[160] the grade is divided into groups I–III, corresponding to well, moderately or poorly differentiated. Stage I tumours are confined to the mucosa; stage II tumours breach the muscularis mucosae; stage III tumours extend through the muscularis propria; stage IV additionally involves the cystic node; and stage V involves the liver or other organs, usually segments 4 and 5 in the gallbladder bed. Nevin's score, a sum of stage and grade, directly affects survival: no patients in his series with a score of more than 6 survived 1 year.

Presentation

The peak age of incidence is 70–75 years. Gallbladder cancer may be silent for a long time, and the diagnosis is commonly made postoperatively in gallbladders removed for stone disease. Incidental cancer is found approximately in 1 in every 100 cholecystectomies performed.[161] This may be a particular problem in laparoscopic cholecystectomy, because of the risk of tumour implantation at the extraction port and intraoperative bile spillage.

Presentation may be indistinguishable from that of gallbladder stones and chronic cholecystitis. Some patients with gallbladder cancer present with acute cholecystitis or with empyema of the gallbladder; in order not to miss such a diagnosis, biopsy of the gallbladder is mandatory in patients treated by cholecystostomy. Symptomatic cancers may present with biliary obstruction, and at this stage the tumours are usually bulky and inoperable.

Investigation

Laboratory tests are non-specific. The tumour markers CEA and CA19-9 may be raised, and can be helpful when the imaging is equivocal.

A **plain abdominal radiograph** is of limited value, but may show calcification suggestive of gallstones or gallbladder wall calcification ('porcelain gallbladder').

The preoperative diagnosis may be suggested by a mass on **ultrasound**. Other features suggestive of carcinoma include a discontinuous gallbladder mucosa, echogenic mucosa, submucosal echolucency and a polypoid lesion. Ultrasonography is less

sensitive to identify the full extent of the disease especially in the detection of peritoneal and lymph node metastasis.[162]

These findings may be confirmed by **CT scanning**. Diffuse gallbladder wall thickening secondary to tumour infiltration and inflammatory change is a common manifestation of advanced carcinoma. Associated changes that suggest malignancy include biliary dilatation, invasion of adjacent structures, and liver and nodal deposits.[163]

MRI in cases of gallbladder carcinoma will usually demonstrate the tumour as focal gallbladder thickening with an eccentric mass. Direct liver involvement as well as lymphadenopathy and biliary and vascular invasion may also be demonstrated.

Direct cholangiography may be required. A long stricture of the hepatic duct/common bile duct may be found in cases of gallbladder carcinoma. Involvement of the duct of segment 5 by a gallbladder mass is highly suggestive of cancer. **Arteriography** may show vascular involvement in advanced disease. This may also be shown on duplex ultrasound.

PET with FDG may also have a role in the evaluation of gallbladder masses. In a small study by Koh et al., this imaging modality was found to have sensitivity of 75% and specificity of 87.5%.[164] More recently developed methods include **endoscopic ultrasound** and percutaneous or endoscopic cholangiography.[165]

Management

PROPHYLACTIC CHOLECYSTECTOMY

Prophylactic cholecystectomy for patients with asymptomatic cholelithiasis and no other risk factors is not recommended.[66] Porcelain gallbladder is an indication for cholecystectomy even in asymptomatic patients as up to 25% of cases are associated with gallbladder cancer.

INCIDENTAL TUMOUR

Frozen-section histology should be performed if the retrieved gallbladder is suspected to harbour tumour during routine open or laparoscopic cholecystectomy.

When cancer of the gallbladder is discovered incidentally at open cholecystectomy, the surgeon should if possible make a full assessment at the time of operation and decide whether a curative excision is reasonable. If a well-localised tumour is found, a wedge resection of the gallbladder bed or a formal excision of segments 4b and 5 may be considered.[166] Incidental tumours found after laparoscopic cholecystectomy and not localised to the mucosa (i.e. T2 and above), warrant re-exploration and more radical resection.[161]

Simple open and laparoscopic cholecystectomy utilises the subserosal plane and may thus leave a positive margin. This may also lead to dissemination of the tumour within the peritoneal cavity.[161] Thus during re-exploration, an accurate laparotomy should exclude peritoneal secondaries. The incidence of port-site metastasis is reported to range between 14 and 20% and this incidence is not affected by the tumour stage. Damage to the gallbladder wall and excessive use of electrocautery may increase the incidence of port-site metastasis. Consideration should be given to excision of the port sites as part of the definitive resection for these tumours.

SUSPECTED/KNOWN CANCER

Patients suspected or known to have gallbladder cancer should undergo open exploration. Treatment of the established tumour depends on staging, and on the mode of presentation.[166] The T stage of the tumour is directly proportional to the likelihood of lymph node disease and of peritoneal dissemination.

T1 tumours

Tumours confined to the mucosa can be safely treated by simple open cholecystectomy alone. If this lesion is identified intraoperatively, the cystic duct node and pericholedochal nodes may be sampled to exclude metastatic disease. Tsukada et al. did not demonstrate any lymph node metastasis in 15 patients with T1 lesions.[167] Such tumours, though rare, are associated with an excellent prognosis.

If the cystic duct stump is involved, re-resection of the duct or common duct with Roux-en-Y reconstruction is necessary.

T2–4 tumours

These tumours should be treated by extended cholecystectomy and liver resection to obtain negative resection margins, as well as en-bloc lymphadenectomy of the porta hepatis and superior pancreatic nodes.

Excision of segments 4 and 5 (gallbladder bed) is usually sufficient for adequate clearance. Right hepatectomy may be necessary to obtain negative resection margins and when the tumour involves the right portal triad.

It is important to mobilise the duodenum and remove the retroduodenal nodes as the lymphatic drainage of the gallbladder is mainly in the caudal direction. In tumours involving or close to the cystic duct, excision of the extrahepatic bile duct and Roux-en-Y reconstruction is usually necessary.

Presence of N2 or M1 disease on preoperative imaging precludes curative resection.

ADJUVANT THERAPY

Some authors have reported useful responses and some long-term survival after external beam radiotherapy, but there are no controlled data.[168] Conventionally regarded as chemoresistant, gallbladder tumours have sometimes shown significant responses to combination chemotherapy, similar to that used in cholangiocarcinoma.[169]

PALLIATIVE THERAPY

The median survival for patients with irresectable disease is 2–4 months with a 1-year survival of less than 5%. Once cancer of the gallbladder has invaded the hilar ducts and caused obstructive jaundice, it is rarely resectable. These patients are best palliated by stenting or by internal bypass. The round ligament or left duct approach may be valuable, because the anastomosis is at a safe distance from the tumour.

RESULTS OF RESECTIONS

Fong et al.,[161] in the Memorial Sloan-Kettering Cancer Center, found 102 of 410 patients with gallbladder cancer whose tumours were potentially resectable. Their operative mortality was 3.9%, and the median survival in resected patients was 26 months with a 5-year survival of 38%. The median survival was 5.4 months in patients who were not resectable. There was no statistical difference in mortality, complications and long-term survival when comparing patients who had an incomplete prior resection and patients who had a definitive procedure at the first laparotomy.

In a series of 72 patients who underwent radical resection for stage IV gallbladder cancer, there were 14 postoperative deaths (19%). The 3-year survival in this series was 15%.[170] Local invasion remains the overwhelming determinant of survival even after radical excision.

AMPULLARY TUMOURS

Ampullary tumours are relatively uncommon and account for about 6% of all periampullary tumours. The prognosis of ampullary carcinoma is better than that for pancreatic adenocarcinoma, and the 5-year survival is between 20% and 60%.[171]

The first documented resection of an ampullary tumour was performed by Halstead in 1898. Unfortunately the patient died after 7 months from tumour recurrence.[172]

Predisposing factors

Adenomas, especially villous adenomas, are known to be premalignant. Familial adenomatous polyposis is associated with an increased risk for developing periampullary adenomas and carcinomas.[173] This usually happens one to two decades after the associated colon cancers. Other possible but not well-established risk factors include cholecystectomy, sphincterotomy and tobacco.

Pathology

Many of these tumours have in the past been wrongly classified along with cancer of the head of the pancreas, leading to the erroneous identification of 5-year survivors following bypass for 'pancreatic cancer'.[174] Most are adenocarcinomas though a number of other tumours, such as carcinoids, other neuroendocrine tumours and sarcomas, may arise from the ampulla. An important variant is benign villous adenoma, which may be part of an adenomatous syndrome such as Gardner's syndrome. There may be a true adenoma–carcinoma sequence.

Bad prognostic factors after resection for ampullary cancer include:

- lymph node involvement[175]
- poorly differentiated tumours
- tumours larger than 2 cm
- presence of tumour at the resection margins
- perineural invasion
- extension of the tumour into the pancreas.[171,176]

Spread of the tumours is by local extension to involve the pancreas and duodenum, and metastasis to regional lymph nodes. The commonest site for lymph node metastasis is the inferior pancreatico-duodenal nodes.[175] Ampullary carcinoma is staged using the TNM staging system (**Box 10.5**).

Box 10.5 • TNM classification for tumours of ampulla of Vater

Primary tumour (T)	
TX:	Primary tumour cannot be assessed
T0:	No evidence of primary tumour
Tis:	Carcinoma in situ
T1:	Tumour limited to ampulla of Vater or sphincter of Oddi
T2:	Tumour invades duodenal wall
T3:	Tumour invades 2 cm or less into pancreas
T4:	Tumour invades more than 2 cm into pancreas and/or into other adjacent organs

Regional lymph nodes (N)	
NX:	Regional lymph nodes cannot be assessed
N0:	No regional lymph node metastasis
N1:	Regional lymph node metastasis*

Distant metastasis (M)	
MX:	Presence of distant metastasis cannot be assessed
M0:	No distant metastasis
M1:	Distant metastasis

Stage grouping	
Stage 0	Tis, N0, M0
Stage I	T1, N0, M0
Stage II	T2, N0, M0
	T3, N0, M0
Stage III	T1, N1, M0
	T2, N1, M0
	T3, N1, M0
Stage IV	T4, any N, M0
	Any T, any N, M1

*Regional lymph nodes are: Superior: superior to head and body of pancreas. Inferior: inferior to head and body of pancreas. Anterior: anterior pancreatico-duodenal, pyloric, and proximal mesenteric. Posterior: posterior pancreatico-duodenal, common bile duct and proximal mesenteric. From Sobin LH, Wittekind C (eds) TNM classification of malignant tumours, 5th edn. Wiley-Liss, 1997. Reprinted with permission of John Wiley & Sons, Inc.

Presentation

Most patients present with biliary obstruction in the sixth or seventh decades. Jaundice may be intermittent due to repeated necrosis and sloughing, and associated with anaemia due to chronic gastrointestinal bleeding. A classic but rare occurrence is of grey or silvery stools as a result of biliary obstruction combined with melaena.

Investigation

Laboratory tests showing intermittent biliary obstruction and a microcytic hypochromic anaemia are characteristic. As with most other tumours of the biliary tract **tumour markers** are variable, with CEA and CA19-9 often raised.

Imaging is important, and simultaneous bile duct and pancreatic duct dilatation on **ultrasound** (the 'double-duct' sign) suggests a possible periampullary cancer. **Endoscopy** will make the diagnosis and allow biopsy in the majority of cases, missing only small intra-ampullary tumours. **Endoscopic ultrasound** is valuable in assessing the depth of invasion and resectability.[177,178] **Biopsies** should be obtained in every case, but false negatives may occur because of difficulty in accurate placement of the biopsy. **Helical CT scanning** produces information complementary to ultrasound and endoscopic ultrasound.[178] The classic appearance of the 'inverted 3' sign in the duodenum used to be reported in **barium meals**, but this investigation is now rarely used. **Cholangiography** is usually obtained by ERCP unless there is an impassable tumour at the ampulla. In this case PTC may show the ductal anatomy and demonstrate the extent of duct involvement.

Management

SURGERY

Management depends on the stage of the tumour and the condition of the patient. Very elderly and frail patients who are not considered suitable for surgical exploration are often well palliated by endoscopic stenting, or even simply by sphincterotomy, which may have to be repeated. For patients fit for surgery, resection offers a significantly higher cure rate than that for cancer of the head of pancreas and also excellent palliation. The choice lies between local excision and pancreato-duodenectomy.

In patients with very small tumours, local excision may be curative, but pancreato-duodenectomy is the procedure of choice. Transduodenal radical excision of a bulky ampullary cancer may, in fact, be more hazardous than resection of the head of pancreas because of the risks of pancreatitis and duodenal or pancreatic fistula formation. Pylorus preserving pancreato-duodenectomy[179] may be particularly applicable to these tumours. Fear that this procedure would compromise radicality has not been borne out by experience.[180,181]

Patients unsuitable for resection can be treated by palliative bypass (hepatico-jejunostomy) though this leaves the potential problems of future bleeding or gastric outlet obstruction. In a randomised trial, Lillemoe and colleagues found that performing a prophylactic gastro-jejunostomy prevented the development of gastric outlet obstruction, which subsequently occurred in 19% of the control group. There was no difference in morbidity between the two groups.[182]

ADJUVANT THERAPY

There is no good evidence regarding the role of chemotherapy or radiotherapy in surgically resected ampullary cancers. However, some authors believe that chemoradiation may be beneficial in patients with bad prognostic signs.[183] Studies of unresected tumours generally include both ampullary and pancreatic cancers, so conclusions are impossible for this tumour type.

Results

The overall 5-year survival rates reported for radical resection and for local excision are rather similar, ranging from 25 to 55%. In a series of 123 patients with ampullary carcinoma, the median survival in resected patients was 58.8 months (46% 5-year survival) versus 9.7 months in unresected patients (0% 5-year survival). The operative mortality rate was 5%.[184]

OPERATIVE APPROACHES

Preoperative preparation

Attention to nutrition is of great importance, because of the general effects of the tumour and of obstructive jaundice and malabsorption. Renal function and preoperative hydration are extremely important because of the increased tendency to acute renal failure in obstructive jaundice.

A controlled trial of percutaneous transhepatic biliary drainage showed that rehydration alone produced as great an improvement in renal function as rehydration combined with biliary drainage.[185] Preoperative biliary drainage remains controversial. Nakayama et al.[186] claimed a significant reduction in mortality by using external biliary drainage. However, several controlled trials have failed to show such improvement.[119,187–189] Internal drainage by means of endoscopic stenting may still be indicated for patients who are severely jaundiced, and particularly those suffering from acute cholangitis.[190]

Biliary resection and reconstruction for hilar cancer: a general operative approach

INCISIONS AND EXPLORATION

The bilateral subcostal ('rooftop') incision and a fixed retractor system (Omni-tract®) provide wide access to the upper abdomen, and allow mobilisation of the liver. The use of a fixed retractor system (such as the Omnitract) allows constant wide exposure.

After a thorough laparotomy, the umbilical ligament is divided between ligatures, the falciform ligament is divided using diathermy, and the liver is gently mobilised upwards.

DISSECTION OF THE HILAR PLATE

The left hepatic duct is an extrahepatic structure and can be accessed below segment 4 (Sg4). A broad-bladed retractor is placed beneath Sg4 and gently lifted, and the hilar plate is identified. The bridge connecting Sg3 and 4 at the umbilical fissure is of variable thickness and is divided to lower the hilar plate. If there is tumour involvement of the left duct and bypass alone is to be performed, this approach can be abandoned in favour of accessing the Sg3 duct to the left of the umbilical ligament.

MOBILISATION AND RESECTION OF THE BILIARY TREE

Resectability should be ascertained initially by dissection of the hilar plate as described and by

intraoperative ultrasound. The bile duct can be divided distally as low as possible, and is mobilised with the associated tumour from the underlying vessels. It is important to be aware of the common variant of a replaced right hepatic artery arising from the superior mesenteric artery. The thickened lymphatic, other periductal tissues and the peritoneum should be elevated en bloc, and the lymphatics surrounding the hepatic artery dissected forwards with the specimen. If invasion of the anterior surface of the portal vein is present, a palliative resection may still be performed, leaving if necessary a small rim of tumour on the portal vein, or by resection of part of the vein. The vein can often be re-anastomosed end-to-end after Kocherisation of the duodenum to remove tension from the vein, or a short length of graft of jugular vein or artificial material can be inserted (**Fig. 10.5**) (also in colour, see Plate 11, facing p. 20).

Once the tumour can be lifted as far as the confluence, the dissection can be continued from below to above, or the left hepatic duct divided and the tumour removed from left to right. Frozen section of the resection margins at this stage can be attempted though its value is limited because of difficulties in identifying tumour, unless an

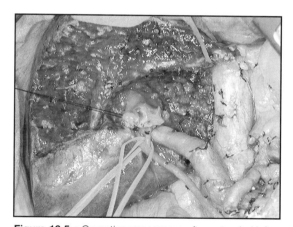

Figure 10.5 • Operative appearance after extended left hepatectomy (Sg1–5 + 8) for a hilar cholangiocarcinoma. On the right the vena cava is exposed. A blue sling is placed around the right hepatic vein. Red slings mark the residual right hepatic artery, and above this the opened ducts of Sg6 and 7 are seen. The portal vein was involved by the tumour at the bifurcation, and has been resected and reconstructed end to end: the anastomosis is clearly shown. Resection margins were all clear. See also Plate 11, facing p. 20.

experienced specialist pathologist is available. The techniques for combining resection of hilar tumours with major liver resection have been described in detail elsewhere, and will not be elaborated upon in this chapter.[191]

If postoperative radiotherapy is to be contemplated, metal clips may be used to mark areas of residual tumour or the area of the anastomosis. The use of an access loop may be helpful for bile duct cancers, since local recurrence may require treatment by stenting.

PREPARATION OF ROUX LIMB

It is our practice to use a 70 cm length, brought up in a retrocolic position to the right of the middle colic vessels since reflux has been demonstrated along the full length of a 40 cm limb. If an access loop is to be used, a side-to-side anastomosis should be performed a few centimetres from the apex to allow tension-free apposition of the free end to the peritoneum of the abdominal wall.

TECHNIQUE OF HEPATICO-JEJUNOSTOMY

Fine interrupted absorbable sutures are used, such as 4/0 PDS or Vicryl, to produce an inverting mucosa-to-mucosa anastomosis.[192] The anterior row of sutures is placed and held in order with the needles attached. The posterior row of the hepatico-jejunal anastomosis sutures is placed and the jejunum can be 'railroaded' down into position and all the stitches tied. The held anterior row of sutures is used to pick up the anterior wall of the jejunum and tied, achieving a good mucosal apposition with a small amount of inversion.

ACCESS LOOP

The ability of the radiologist to puncture an access loop successfully is entirely dependent on the positioning and quality of the marking of the loop.[193,194] A 2/0 stainless-steel braided suture is placed around the end of the Roux loop using shallow seromuscular bites, encircling the point of exit of the transanastomotic tube as a loose 'purse-string'. The tube is then brought out through the abdominal wall, and the end of the loop tacked to the peritoneum using four quadrant sutures of Vicryl. The loop should lie away from the midline to avoid difficulties for the radiologist, and should

be neither redundant nor under tension. This position must be carefully assessed before choosing the site in the Roux limb for the hepatico-jejunal anastomosis. This technique has proved useful for benign stricture reconstruction, where future intervention is likely, such as strictures of Bismuth type III and IV,[195] but may also be used selectively after reconstruction for malignant disease.

PALLIATIVE LEFT OR RIGHT DUCT BYPASS

The left hepatic duct can be identified if necessary by aspiration with a fine needle after lowering the hilar plate. Stay sutures are placed in the duct, the duct is opened using a knife, and the opening extended with fine-angled scissors. A length of 2–3 cm may be obtained by extending the opening in the left duct as far as the base of the umbilical fissure. In some difficult circumstances, the duct of Sg5 may be accessed at the base of the gallbladder bed and used for anastomosis.

THE ROUND LIGAMENT APPROACH

This technique is useful when tumour obliterates the left hepatic duct. The duct of Sg3 runs in a relatively constant position to the left of the umbilical fissure, and can be accessed by dividing the liver anteriorly just to the left of the falciform ligament, where no significant portal vein branches should be encountered in front of the duct. Intraoperative ultrasound may be useful in locating the duct in difficult cases. The use of the Cavitron ultrasonic surgical aspirator (CUSA) to divide the liver to the left of the falciform ligament may help to keep the field bloodless, which is important for identifying the duct. Once the duct is found an opening is made that can be extended proximally and distally, and often an anastomosis of 1 cm or longer can be achieved. The technique of anastomosis is as described above.

Postoperative management

The general management of the patient will not be detailed here, except to note that continued attention must be paid to fluid and electrolyte balance, to renal function and to the coagulation status. It is the author's practice to place a closed tube drain close to the anastomosis in every case. This drain can often be removed after 48 hours, but if there is any bile leakage it should be left in place longer. If a transanastomotic tube has been placed then a cholangiogram can be performed at 1 week, and the anastomosis checked for any small residual leaks.

This cholangiogram allows identification of all anastomosed ducts, which may be important for the future if problems of cholangitis should arise. The tube can usually be removed at 7 days. The marked site of the access loop remains visible for future radiological access (**Fig. 10.6**).

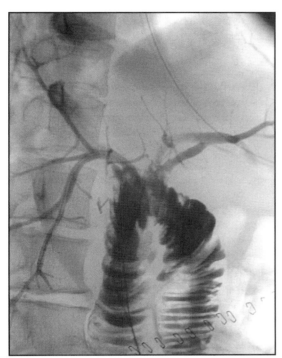

Figure 10.6 • Postoperative tubogram on day 7 after local excision cholangiocarcinoma of the hilar ducts with bilateral hepatico-jejunostomy Roux-en-Y. The fine tube enters through the blind end of the Roux loop, which is fixed to the abdominal wall as an access loop. The tube is removed after the cholangiogram, which gives a 'baseline' study, and marking of the loop allows radiological puncture and intubation in the event of future problems.

Key points

Tumours of the gallbladder and proximal biliary tree share much in common in relation to pathology, presentation and management, while tumours of the ampullary region are often confused with cancer of the head of the pancreas.

Precise anatomical diagnosis for biliary tumours is now possible in the majority of cases, often by non-invasive imaging, and provides the key to the planning of management.

Resection is the ideal, and although increasingly used it is still achieved in only a minority of cases.

Tumour clearance often demands complex surgery, including extended hepatic resections, regional lymphadenectomy and biliary recon-struction, and such cases should only be treated in specialist units.

Long-term survival remains poor, and has not been shown to be improved by radiotherapy. Combination chemotherapy may have an increasing role.

The technical advances in stenting have resulted in better palliation for irresectable cases, but patients should be fully assessed by multi-disciplinary teams before undergoing such treatments: preoperative biliary decompression is only indicated in selected cases.

REFERENCES

1. Parker SL. Cancer statistics. CA Cancer J Clin 1996; 46:5–27.

2. Zimmermann A. Tumors of the bile ducts – pathological aspects. In: Blumgart LH (ed.) Surgery of the liver and biliary tract, 3rd edn. W. B. Saunders: London, 2000; pp. 953–75.

3. Renard P, Boutron MC, Faivre J et al. Biliary tract cancers in Côte d'Or (France): incidence and natural history. J Epidemiol Community Health 1987; 41:344–8.

4. Green A, Uttaravichien T, Bhudhisawasdi V et al. Cholangiocarcinoma in North East Thailand. A hospital-based study. Trop Geogr Med 1991; 43:193–8.

5. Carriaga MT, Henson DE. Liver, gallbladder, extrahepatic bile ducts, and pancreas. Cancer 1995; 75(Suppl. 1):171–90.

6. Patel T. Increasing incidence and mortality of primary intrahepatic cholangiocarcinoma in the United States. Hepatology 2001; 33(6):1353–7.

7. Patel T. Worldwide trends in mortality from biliary tract malignancies. BMC Cancer 2002; 2:10. Epub 2002 May 03.

8. Taylor-Robinson SD, Toledano MB, Arora S et al. Increase in mortality rates from intrahepatic cholangiocarcinoma in England and Wales 1968–1998. Gut 2001; 48:816–20. Erratum in Gut 2001; 49(2):315.

9. Khan SA, Taylor-Robinson SD, Toledano MB et al. Changing international trends in mortality rates for liver, biliary and pancreatic tumours. J Hepatol 2002; 37(6):806–13.

10. Kocher HM, Patel AG, Benjamin IS. World-wide trends in biliary tract carcinoma [abstract]. Gastroenterology 2002; 122:A-569.

11. Klatskin G. Adenocarcinoma of the hepatic duct at its bifurcation within the porta hepatis: an unusual tumor with distinctive clinical and pathological features. Am J Med 1965; 38:241–56.

12. Nakeeb A, Pitt HA, Sohn TA et al. Cholangiocarcinoma. A spectrum of intrahepatic, perihilar and distal tumors. Ann Surg 1996; 224:463–75.

13. Khan SA, Davidson BR, Goldin R et al. Guidelines for the diagnosis and treatment of cholangiocarcinoma: consensus document. Gut 2002; 51(Suppl. VI):vi1–vi9.

Current UK guidelines for the investigation and management of cholangiocarcinoma from the British Society of Gastroenterology.

14. Chamberlain RS, Blumgart LH. Hilar cholangiocarcinoma: a review and commentary. Ann Surg Oncol 2000; 7:55–66.

15. Metcalfe MS, Wemyss-Holden SA, Maddern GJ. Management dilemmas with choledochal cyst. Arch Surg 2003; 138:333–9.

16. de Vries JS, de Vries S, Aronson DC et al. Choledochal cysts: age of presentation, symptoms, and late complications related to Todani's classification. J Paediatr Surg 2002; 37:1568–73.

17. Suda K, Miyano T, Suzuki F et al. Clinicopathologic and experimental studies on cases of abnormal pancreato-choledocho-ductal junction. Acta Pathol Jpn 1987; 37:1549–62.

18. Ohta T, Nagakawa T, Ueno K et al. Clinical experience of biliary tract carcinoma associated with anomalous union of the pancreatic ductal system. Jpn J Surg 1990; 20:36–43.

19. Wu GS, Zou SQ, Luo XW et al. Proliferative activity of bile from congenital choledochal cyst patients. World J Gastroenterol 2003; 9:184–7.

20. Nakanuma Y, Hoso M, Terada T. Clinical and pathological features of cholangiocarcinoma. In: Okuda K, Tabor E (eds) Liver cancer. New York: Churchill Livingstone, 1997; pp. 279–90.

21. Watanapa P, Watanapa WB. Liver-fluke associated cholangiocarcinoma. Br J Surg 2002; 89:962–70.

22. Tocchi A, Mazzoni G, Liotta G et al. Late development of bile duct cancer in patients who had biliary-enteric drainage for benign disease: a follow-up study of more than 1,000 patients. Ann Surg 2001; 234:210–14.

23. Callea F, Sergi C, Fabbretti G et al. Precancerous lesions of the biliary tree. J Surg Oncol Suppl 1993; 3:131–3.

24. O'Shea M, Fletcher HS, Lara JF. Villous adenoma of the extrahepatic biliary tract: a rare entity. Am Surg 2002; 68:889–91.

25. Lipshutz GS, Brennan TV, Warren RS. Thorotrast-induced liver neoplasia: a collective review. J Am Coll Surg 2002; 195:713–18.

26. Ishikawa Y, Wada I, Fukumoto M. Alpha-particle carcinogenesis in Thorotrast patients: epidemiology, dosimetry, pathology and molecular analysis. J Environ Pathol Toxicol Oncol 2001; 20:311–15.

27. van Kaick G, Wesch H, Luhrs H et al. Neoplastic diseases induced by chronic alpha-irradiation – epidemiological, biophysical and clinical results of the German Thorotrast Study. J Radiat Res (Tokyo) 1991; 32(Suppl. 2):20–33.

28. Lee CC, Wu CY, Chen GH. What is the impact of co-existence of hepatolithiasis on cholangiocarcinoma? J Gastroenterol Hepatol 2002; 17;1015–20.

29. Olsen JH, Dragsted L, Autrup H. Cancer risk and occupational exposure to aflatoxins in Denmark. Br J Cancer 1988; 58:392–6.

30. Lanes SF, Cohen A, Rothman KJ. Mortality of cellulose fibre production workers. Scand J Work Environ Health 1990; 16:247–51.

31. Bond GG, McLaren EA, Sabel FL et al. Liver and biliary tract cancer among chemical workers. Am J Ind Med 1990; 8:19–24.

32. Mitacek EJ, Brunnemann KD, Suttajit M et al. Exposure to N-nitroso compounds in a population of high liver cancer regions in Thailand: volatile nitrosamine (VNA) levels in Thai food. Food Chem Toxicol 1999; 37:297–305.

33. Mitacek EJ, Brunnemann KD, Hoffmann D et al. Volatile nitrosamines and tobacco-specific nitrosamines in the smoke of Thai cigarettes: a risk factor for lung cancer and a suspected risk factor for liver cancer in Thailand. Carcinogenesis 1999; 20:133–7.

34. Kobayashi M, Ikeda K, Saitoh S et al. Incidence of primary cholangiocellular carcinoma of the liver in Japanese patients with hepatitis C virus-related cirrhosis. Cancer 2000; 188:2471–7.

35. Holzinger F, Z'graggen K, Buchler MW. Mechanisms of biliary carcinogenesis: a pathogenetic multistage cascade towards cholangiocarcinoma. Ann Oncol 1999; 10(Suppl. 4):122–6.

36. Sturm PD, Baas IO, Clement MJ et al. Alterations of the p53 tumor-suppressor gene and K-ras oncogene in perihilar cholangiocarcinomas from a high-incidence area. Int J Cancer 1998; 78:695–8.

37. Petmitr S. Cancer genes and cholangiocarcinoma. Southeast Asian J Trop Med Public Health 1997; 28(Suppl. 1):80–4.

38. Okuda K, Nakanuma Y, Miyazaki M. Cholangiocarcinoma: Recent progress. Part 2: Molecular pathology and treatment. J Gastroenterol Hepatol 2002; 17:1056–63.

39. Chamberlain RS, Blumgart LH. Carcinoid tumors of the extrahepatic bile duct. A rare cause of malignant biliary obstruction. Cancer 1999; 86:1959–65.

40. Weinbren K, Mutum SS. Pathological aspects of cholangiocarcinoma. J Pathol 1983; 139:217–38.

41. Davis RI, Sloan JM, Hood JM et al. Carcinoma of the extrahepatic biliary tree; a clinicopathological and immunohistochemical study. Histopathology 1988; 12:623–31.

42. Hayashi S, Miyazaki M, Kondo Y et al. Invasive growth patterns of hepatic hilar ductal cancer. Cancer 1994; 73:2922–9.

43. Kitagawa Y, Nagino M, Kamiya J et al. Lymph node metastasis from hilar cholangiocarcinoma: audit of 110 patients who underwent regional and paraaortic node dissection. Ann Surg 2001; 233:385–92.

44. Bhuiya MR, Nimura Y, Kamiya J et al. Clinico-pathologic studies on perineural invasion of bile duct carcinoma. Ann Surg 1992; 215:344–9.

45. Bismuth H, Castaing D, Traynor O. Resection or palliation: priority of surgery in the treatment of hilar cancer. World J Surg 1988; 12:37–47.

46. Blumgart LH, Benjamin IS. Liver resection for bile duct cancer. Surg Clin North Am 1989; 69:323–37.

47. Hadjis NS, Adam A, Gibson R et al. Non-operative approach to hilar cancer determined by the atrophy-hypertrophy complex. Am J Surg 1989; 157:395–9.

48. Jarnagin WR, Fong Y, DeMatteo RP et al. Staging, resectability, and outcome in 225 patients with hilar cholangiocarcinoma. Ann Surg 2001; 234:507–19.

   Prospective analysis of demographics, imaging, surgical findings and survival in 225 patients with hilar cholangiocarcinoma. A modified preoperative T-staging system is proposed.

49. Blumgart LH, Hadjis NS, Benjamin IS et al. Surgical approaches to cholangiocarcinoma at confluence of hepatic ducts. Lancet 1984; 1:66–70.

50. Altemeier WA, Gall EA, Zinninger MM et al. Sclerosing carcinoma of the major intrahepatic bile ducts. Arch Surg 1957; 75:450.

51. Davis RI, Sloan MJH, Hood JM et al. Carcinoma of the extrahepatic biliary tract: a clinicopathological and immunohistochemical study. Histopathology 1988; 12:623–31.

52. Paganuzzi M, Onetto M, Marroni P et al. CA19-9 and CA50 in benign and malignant pancreatic and biliary disease. Cancer 1988; 61:2100–8.

53. Wongkham S, Sheehan JK, Boonla C et al. Serum MUC5AC mucin as a potential marker for cholangiocarcinoma. Cancer Lett 2003; 195:93–9.

54. Boonla C, Wongkham S, Sheenhan JK et al. Prognostic value of serum MUC5AC mucin in patients with cholangiocarcinoma. Cancer 2003; 98:1438–43.

55. Chen CY, Lin XZ, Tsao HC et al. The value of biliary fibronectin for diagnosis of cholangiocarcinoma. Hepatogastroenterology 2003; 50:924–7.

56. Goydos JS, Brumfield AM, Frezza E et al. Marked elevation of serum interleukin-6 in patients with cholangiocarcinoma: validation of utility as a clinical marker. Ann Surg 1998; 227:398–404.

57. Halliday AW, Benjamin IS, Blumgart LH. Nutritional risk factors in major hepatobiliary surgery. J Parent Ent Nutr 1988; 12:43–8.

58. Yeung EC, McCarthy P, Gompertz RH et al. The ultrasonographic appearances of hilar cholangiocarcinoma (Klatskin tumour). Br J Radiol 1988; 61:991–5.

59. Tio TL, Reeders JW, Sie LH et al. Endosonography in the clinical staging of Klatskin tumour. Endoscopy 1993; 25:81–5.

60. Wiersma MJ, Vilmann P, Giovannini M et al. Endosonography-guided fine-needle aspiration biopsy: diagnostic accuracy and complication assessment. Gastroenterology 1997; 112(4):1087–95.

61. Engels JT, Balfe DM, Lee JKT. Biliary carcinoma: CT evaluation of extrahepatic spread. Radiology 1989; 172:35–40.

62. Schwartz LH, Coakley FV, Sun Y et al. Neoplastic pancreaticobiliary duct obstruction: evaluation with breath-hold MR cholangiopancreaticography. Am J Roentgenol 1998; 170:1491–5.

63. Lee MG, Lee HJ, Kim MH et al. Extrahepatic biliary disease: 3D MR cholangiopancreatography compared with endoscopic retrograde cholangiopancreatography. Radiology 1997; 202:663–9.

64. Benjamin IS. Biliary tract obstruction. Surg Gastroenterol 1983; 2:105–20.

65. Yeh T, Jan Y, Tseng J et al. Malignant perihilar biliary obstruction: magnetic resonance cholangiopancreatography findings. Am J Gastroenterol 2000; 95:432–40.

66. de Groen PC, Gores GJ, LaRusso NF et al. Biliary tract cancers. N Engl J Med 1999; 341:1368–78.

67. Nimura Y, Shionoya S, Hayakawa N et al. Value of percutaneous transhepatic cholangioscopy (PTCS). Surg Endosc 1988; 2:213–19.

68. Wallner BK, Schumacher KA, Weidenmaler W et al. Dilated biliary tract: evaluation with MR cholangiography with a T2-weighted contrast-enhanced fast sequence. Radiology 1991; 181:805–8.

69. Desa LA, Akosa AB, Lazzara S et al. Cytodiagnosis in the management of extrahepatic biliary stricture. Gut 1991; 32:1188–91.

70. D'Angelica M, Fong Y, Weber S et al. The role of staging laparoscopy in hepatobiliary malignancy: prospective analysis of 401 cases. Ann Surg Oncol 2003; 10:183–9.

71. Weber SM, DeMatteo RP, Fong Y et al. Staging laparoscopy in patients with extrahepatic biliary carcinoma. Analysis of 100 patients. Ann Surg 2000; 235:392–9.

72. Keiding S, Hansen SB, Rasmussen HH et al. Detection of cholangiocarcinoma in primary sclerosing cholangitis by positron emission tomography. Hepatology 1998; 28:700–6.

73. Delbeke D, Martin WH, Sandler MP et al. Evaluation of benign vs malignant hepatic lesions with positron emission tomography. Arch Surg 1998; 133:510–16.

74. Kluge R, Schmidt F, Caca K et al. Positron emission tomography with [^{18}F]fluoro-2-deoxy-D-glucose for diagnosis and staging of bile duct cancer. Hepatology 2001; 33:1029–35.

75. Tamada K, Kanai N, Wada S et al. Utility and limitations of intraductal ultrasonography in distinguishing longitudinal cancer extension along the bile duct from inflammatory wall thickening. Abdom Imaging 2001; 26:623–31.

76. Itoh A, Goto H, Naitoh Y et al. Intraductal ultra-sonography in diagnosing tumor extension of cancer of the papilla of Vater. Gastointest Endosc 1997; 45:251–60.

77. Jewkes AJ, Macdonald F, Downing R et al. Labelled antibody imaging in pancreatic cancer, cholangiocarcinoma, chronic pancreatitis and sclerosing cholangitis. Eur J Surg Oncol 1991; 17:354–7.

78. Tan CK, Podila PV, Taylor JE et al. Human chol-angiocarcinomas express somatostatin receptors and respond to somatostatin with growth inhibition. Gastroenterology 1995; 108:1908–16.

79. Murata T, Nagasaka T, Kamiya J et al. P53 labeling index in cholangioscopic biopsies is useful for determining spread of bile duct carcinomas. Gastrointestinal Endosc 2002; 56:688–95.

80. Voyles CR, Bowley NJ, Allison DJ et al. Carcinoma of the proximal extrahepatic biliary tree. Radiological assessment and therapeutic alternatives. Ann Surg 1983; 197:188–93.

81. Pinson CW, Rossi RL. Extended right hepatic lobectomy, left hepatic lobectomy and skeletonisation resection for proximal bile duct cancer. World J Surg 1988; 12:52–9.

82. Longmire WP Jr, McArthur MS, Bastounis EA et al. Carcinoma of the extrahepatic biliary tract. Ann Surg 1973; 178:333–45.

83. Guthrie CM, Haddock G, de Beaux AC et al. Changing trends in the management of extrahepatic cholangiocarcinoma. Br J Surg 1993; 80:1434–9.

84. Baer HU, Stain SC, Dennison AR et al. Improvements in survival by aggressive resections of hilar cholangiocarcinoma. Ann Surg 1993; 27:20–7.

85. Pichlmayr R, Burckhardt R, Lauchert W et al. Radical resection and liver grafting as the two main components of surgical strategy in the treatment of proximal bile duct cancer. World J Surg 1988; 12:68–77.

86. Launois B, Lebeau G, Kiroff G et al. Survival after surgical resection of carcinoma in the upper third of the biliary tract. Dig Surg 1979; 7:106–10.

87. Tsuzuki Y, Ogata Y, Iida S et al. Carcinoma of the bifurcation of the hepatic ducts. Arch Surg 1983; 118:1147–51.

88. Nimura Y, Hayakawa N, Kamiya J et al. Hepatic segmentectomy with caudate lobe resection for bile duct carcinoma of the hepatic hilus. World J Surg 1990; 14:535–44.

89. Mizumoto R, Kawarada Y, Suzuki H. Surgical treatment of hilar carcinoma of the bile duct. Surg Gynecol Obstet 1986; 162:153–8.

90. Nimura Y, Kamiya J, Kondo S et al. Aggressive preoperative management and extended surgery for hilar cholangiocarcinoma: Nagoya experience. J Hepatobiliary Pancreat Surg 2000; 7:155–62.

Review of 177 patients with hilar cholangiocarcinoma. Curative resection was possible in 108 patients with most of these (100 patients) requiring liver resection with caudate lobectomy. The recurrence rates and survival rates are analysed.

91. Nagino M, Nimura Y, Hayakawa N et al. Diagnostic value of computed tomography for the detection of invasion of the caudate bile duct branch in carcinoma of the hepatic hilum. Nippon Geka Gakkai Zasshi 1988; 89:889–97.

92. Nimura Y, Hayakawa N, Kamiya J. Hilar cholangiocarcinoma: the surgical therapy. In: Serio G, Huguet C, Williamson RCN (eds) Hepatobiliary and pancreatic tumours. Edinburgh: Graffham Press, 1994; pp. 116–22.

93. Blumgart LH, Benjamin IS. Liver resection for bile duct cancer. Surg Clin North Am 1989; 69:323–37.

94. Fletcher MS, Dawson JL, Wheeler PG et al. Treatment of high bile duct carcinoma by internal radiotherapy with iridium-192 wire. Lancet 1981; 2:172–4.

95. Busse PM, Stone MD, Sheldon TA et al. Intraoperative radiation therapy for biliary tract carcinoma: results of a 5-year experience. Surgery 1989; 105:724–33.

96. Deziel DJ, Kiel KD, Kramer TS et al. Intraoperative radiation therapy in biliary tract cancer. Am J Surg 1988; 54:402–7.

97. McMasters KM, Tuttle TM, Leach SD et al. Neoadjuvant chemoradiation for extrahepatic cholangiocarcinoma. Am J Surg 1997; 174:605–9.

98. Pitt HA, Nakeeb A, Abrams RA et al. Perihilar cholangiocarcinoma. Postoperative radiotherapy does not improve survival. Ann Surg 1995 221:788–97; discussion 797–8.

99. Kamada T, Saitou H, Takamura A et al. The role of radiotherapy in the management of extrahepatic bile duct cancer: an analysis of 145 consecutive patients treated with intraluminal and/or external beam radiotherapy. Int J Radiat Oncol Biol Phys 1996; 34:767–74.

100. Longmire WP, Sanford MC. Intrahepatic cholangiojejunostomy with partial hepatectomy for biliary obstruction. Surgery 1948; 128:330–47.

101. Bismuth H, Castaing D, Traynor O. Resection or palliation: priority of surgery in the treatment of hilar cancer. World J Surg 1988; 12:37–47.

102. Guthrie CM, Banting SW, Garden OJ et al. Segment III cholangiojejunostomy for palliation of malignant hilar obstruction. Br J Surg 1994; 81:1639–41.

103. Jarnagin WR, Burke E, Powers C et al. Intrahepatic biliary enteric bypass provides effective palliation in selected patients with malignant obstruction at the hepatic duct confluence. Am J Surg 1998; 175:453–60.

The results obtained in 55 patients who underwent biliary enteric bypass for irresectable hilar cholangiocarcinoma/gallbladder cancer are analysed in this paper. The patients are divided into three groups depending on the site of the primary tumour and the type of bypass performed.

104. Terblanche J, Saunders SJ, Louw JH. Prolonged palliation in carcinoma of the main hepatic duct junction. Surgery 1972; 71:720–31.

105. Hatfield ARW. Palliation of malignant obstructive jaundice – surgery or stent? Gut 1990; 31:1339–40.

106. Prat F, Chapat O, Ducot B et al. A randomised trial of endoscopic drainage methods for inoperable malignant strictures of the common bile duct. Gastrointest Endosc 1998; 47:1–7.

107. Lammer J, Hausegger KA, Fluckiger F et al. Common bile duct obstruction due to malignancy: treatment with plastic versus metal stent. Radiology 1996; 201:167–72.

Randomised trials demonstrating improved long-term patency with metallic stents in all forms of malignant biliary obstruction.

108. Kaassis M, Boyer J, Dumas R et al. Plastic or metal stents for malignant stricture of the common bile duct? Results of a randomized prospective study. Gastrointest Endosc 2003; 57:178–82.

109. Adam A, Chetty N, Roddie N et al. Self-expanding stainless steel endoprosthesis for treatment of malignant bile duct obstruction. Am J Roentgenol 1991; 156:321–5.

110. Dooley JS. External bile drainage – the state of the art. J Hepatol 1985; 1:681–6.

111. Casola G, O'Laoide R. Hilar cholangiocarcinoma: percutaneous approach. In: Serio G, Huguet C, Williamson RCN (eds) Hepatobiliary and pancreatic tumours. Edinburgh: Graffham Press, 1994; pp. 123–66.

112. Becker CD, Glattli A, Mailbach R et al. Percutaneous palliation of malignant obstructive jaundice with Wallstent endoprosthesis: follow-up and reintervention in patients with hilar and non-hilar obstruction. J Vasc Interv Radiol 1993; 4:597–604.

113. Cremer M, Deviere J, Sugai B et al. Expandable biliary metal stents for malignancies: endoscopic insertion and diathermic cleaning for tumor ingrowth. Gastrointest Endosc 1990; 36:451–7.

114. Bueno JT, Gerdes H, Kurtz RC. Endoscopic management of occluded biliary Wallstents: A cancer centre experience. Gastrointest Endosc 2003; 58:879–84.

115. Ghosh S, Palmer KR. Prevention of biliary stent occlusion using cyclical antibiotics and ursodeoxycholic acid. Gut 1994; 35:1757–9.

116. Huibregtse K, Carr-Locke DL, Cremer M and the European Wallstent Study Group. Biliary stent

occlusion – a problem solved with self-expanding metal stents? Endoscopy 1992; 24:391–4.

117. Cheng JL, Bruno MJ, Bergman JJ et al. Endoscopic palliation of patients with biliary obstruction caused by nonresectable hilar cholangiocarcinoma: efficacy of self-expandable metallic Wallstents. Gastrointest Endosc 2002; 56:33–9.

118. Rerknimitr R, Fogel EL, Kalayci C et al. Microbiology of bile in patients with cholangitis or cholestasis with or without plastic biliary endoprosthesis. Gastrointest Endosc 2002; 56:885–9.

119. Hochwald SN, Burke EC, Jarnagin WR et al. Association of preoperative biliary stenting with increased postoperative infectious complications in proximal cholangiocarcinoma. Arch Surg 1999; 134:261–6.

120. Hodul P, Creech S, Pickelman J et al. The effect of preoperative biliary stenting on postoperative complications after pancreatico-duodenectomy. Am J Surg 2003; 186:420–5.

121. Fletcher MS, Brinkley D, Dawson JL et al. Treatment of hilar carcinoma by bile drainage combined with internal radiotherapy using ^{192}iridium wire. Br J Surg 1983; 70:733–65.

122. Meyers WC, Scott Jones R. Internal radiation for bile duct cancer. World J Surg 1988; 12:99–104.

123. Urban MS, Siegel JH, Pavlou W et al. Treatment of malignant biliary obstruction with a high-dose rate remote afterloading device using a 10F nasobiliary tube. Gastrointest Endosc 1990; 36:292–6.

124. Levitt MD, Laurence BH, Cameron F et al. Transpapillary iridium-192 wire in the treatment of malignant bile duct obstruction. Gut 1988; 29:149–52.

125. Vallis KA, Benjamin IS, Munro AJ et al. External beam and intraluminal radiotherapy for locally advanced bile duct cancer: role and tolerability. Radiother Oncol 1996; 41:61–6.

126. Gonzalez Gonzalez D, Gouma DJ, Rauws EA et al. Role of radiotherapy, in particular intraluminal brachytherapy, in the treatment of proximal bile duct carcinoma. Ann Oncol 1999; 10(Suppl. 4): 215–20.

127. Bowling TE, Galbraith SM, Hatfield ARW et al. A retrospective comparison of endoscopic stenting and radiotherapy in non-resectable cholangio-carcinoma. Gut 1996; 39:852–5.

128. Oberfield RA, Rossi RL. The role of chemotherapy in the treatment of bile duct cancer. World J Surg 1988; 12:105–8.

129. Isacoff WH, Botnick L, Tompkins R. Treatment of patients with advanced tumours of the bile ducts with continuous infusion of 5-FU in conjunction with calcium leucovorin, mitomycin-C and dipyridamole. ASCO Proceedings March 1993; 12:225.

130. Ellis PA, Norman A, Hill A et al. Epirubicin, cisplatin and infusional 5-fluorouracil (5-FU) (ECF) in hepatobiliary tumours. Eur J Cancer 1995; 31A(10):1594–8.

131. Sanz-Altamira PM, Ferrante K, Jenkins RL et al. A phase II trial of 5-fluorouracil, leucovorin, and carboplatin in patients with unresectable biliary tree carcinoma. Cancer 1998; 82:2321–5.

132. Smith GW, Bukowski RM, Hewlett JS et al. Hepatic artery infusion of 5-fluorouracil and mitomycin C in cholangiocarcinoma and gallbladder carcinoma. Cancer 1984; 54:1513–16.

133. Pass HI. Photodynamic therapy in oncology: mechanisms and clinical use. J Natl Cancer Inst 1993; 85:443–56.

134. Berr F, Wiedmann M, Tannapfel A et al. Photodynamic therapy for advanced bile duct cancer: Evidence for improved palliation and extended survival. Hepatology 2000; 31:291–8.

135. Pichlmayr P, Weimann A, Klempnauer J et al. Surgical treatment in proximal bile duct cancer: A single-centre experience. Ann Surg 1996; 224:628–38.

136. Meyer CG, Penn I, James L. Liver transplantation for cholangiocarcinoma: results in 207 patients. Transplantation 2000; 69:1633–7.

137. De Vreede I, Steers JL, Burch PA et al. Prolonged disease-free survival after orthotopic liver transplantation plus adjuvant chemoirradiation for cholangiocarcinoma. Liver Transplantation 2000; 6:309–16.

138. Jeyarajah DR, Klintmalm GB. Is liver transplantation indicated for cholangiocarcinoma? J Hepatobiliary Pancreat Surg 1998; 5:48–51.

139. Gompertz RH, Benjamin IS, Blumgart LH. Resection for hilar cholangiocarcinoma: does clearance matter? Gut 1988; 29:A736–7.

140. Little JM. Editorial comment: Hilar biliary cancer – are we getting it right? Hepatobiliary Surg 1989; 1:93–6.

141. Benjamin IS. Surgical possibilities for bile duct cancer: standard surgical treatment. Ann Oncol 1999; 10(Suppl. 4):239–42.

142. Misra S, Chaturvedi A, Misra NC et al. Carcinoma of the gallbladder. Lancet Oncol 2003; 4:167–76.

> Excellent review article on gallbladder cancer: epidemiology, aetiology, pathology, modes of presentation, investigations and treatment options are discussed.

143. Antonakis P, Alexakis N, Mylonaki D et al. Incidental finding of gallbladder carcinoma detected during or after laparoscopic cholecystectomy. Eur J Surg Oncol 2003; 29:358–60.

144. Lazcano-Ponce EC, Miquel JF, Munoz N et al. Epidemiology and molecular pathology of gallbladder cancer. CA Cancer J Clin 2001; 51:349–64.

145. Lowenfels AB, Walker AM, Althaus DP et al. Gallstone growth, size and risk of gallbladder cancer: an interracial study. Int J Epidemiol 1989; 18:50–4.

146. Caygill CP, Hill MJ, Braddick M et al. Cancer mortality in chronic typhoid and paratyphoid carriers. Lancet 1994; 343:83–4.

147. Nath G, Singh H, Shukla VK. Chronic typhoid carriage and carcinoma of the gallbladder. Eur J Cancer Prev 1997; 6:557–9.

148. Strom BL, Soloway RD, Rios-Dalenz JL et al. Risk factors for gallbladder cancer. An international collaborative case-control study. Cancer 1995; 76:1747–56.

149. Kubota K, Bandai Y, Noie T et al. How should polypoid lesions of the gallbladder be treated in the era of laparoscopic cholecystectomy? Surgery 1995; 117:481–7.

150. Chijiiwa K, Tanaka M. Polypoid lesions of the gallbladder: indications of carcinoma and outcome after surgery for malignant polypoid lesion. Int Surg 1994; 79:106–9.

151. Shinkai H, Kimura W, Muto T. Surgical indications for small polypoid lesions of the gallbladder. Am J Surg 1998; 175:114–17.

152. Caygill C, Hill M, Kirkham J et al. Increased risk of biliary tract cancer following gastric surgery. Br J Cancer 1988; 57:434–6.

153. Kapoor VK, Benjamin IS. Gallbladder and biliary-tract cancer. In: Badellino F, Gipponi M (eds) UICC flow charts for diagnosis and staging of cancer in developed and developing countries. Geneva: UICC, 1998; pp. 90–103.

154. Hemminiki K, Li X. Familial liver and gallbladder cancer: a nationwide epidemiological study from Sweden. Gut 2003; 52:592–6.

155. Zatonski WA, Lowenfels AB, Boyle P et al. Epidemiologic aspects of gallbladder cancer: a case-control study of the SEARCH Program of the International Agency for Research on Cancer. J Natl Cancer Inst 1997; 89:1132–8.

156. Kimura K, Ohto M, Saisho H et al. Association of gallbladder carcinoma and anomalous pancreaticobiliary ductal union. Gastroenterology 1985; 89:1258–65.

157. Chijiiwa K, Kimura H, Tanaka M. Malignant potential of the gallbladder in patients with anomalous pancreaticobiliary ductal junction. The difference in risk between patients with and without choledochal cyst. Int Surg 1995; 80: 61–4.

158. Hu B, Gong B, Zhou DY. Association of anomalous pancreaticobiliary ductal junction with gallbladder carcinoma in Chinese patients: an ERCP study. Gastrointest Endosc 2003; 57:541–5.

159. Joffe N, Antonioli DA. Primary carcinoma of the gallbladder associated with chronic inflammatory bowel disease. Clin Radiol 1981; 32:319–24.

160. Nevin JE, Moran TJ, Kay S et al. Carcinoma of the gallbladder. Cancer 1976; 37:141–8.

161. Fong Y, Heffernan N, Blumgart LH. Gallbladder carcinoma discovered during laparoscopic cholecystectomy – aggressive resection is beneficial. Cancer 1998; 83:423–7.

Report in 42 consecutive patients managed at a tertiary referral centre for gallbladder carcinoma discovered during or after laparoscopic cholecystectomy. An aggressive resectional approach in 20 patients appeared to be associated with a more favourable outcome.

162. Bach AM, Loring LA, Hann LE et al. Gallbladder cancer: can ultrasonography evaluate extent of disease? J Ultrasound Med 1998; 17:303–9.

163. Zissin R, Osadchy A, Shapiro-Feinberg M et al. CT of a thickened-wall gall bladder. Br J Radiol 2003; 76:137–43.

164. Koh T, Taniguchi H, Yamaguchi A et al. Differential diagnosis of gallbladder cancer using positron emission tomography with fluorine-18-labeled fluoro-deoxyglucose (FDG-PET). J Surg Oncol 2003; 84:74–81.

165. Nimura Y, Kamiya J. Cholangioscopy. Endoscopy 1998; 30:1282–8.

166. Kapoor VK, Benjamin IS. Resectional surgery for gallbladder cancer. Br J Surg 1998; 85:145–6.

Leading article about resection and outcome for gallbladder cancer.

167. Tsukada K, Kurosaki I, Uchida K et al. Lymph node spread from carcinoma of the gallbladder. Cancer 1997 ; 80:661–7.

168. Houry S, Haccart V, Huguier M et al. Gallbladder cancer: role of radiation therapy. Hepatogastroenterology 1999; 46:1578–84.

169. Takada T, Amano H, Yasuda H et al. Is postoperative adjuvant chemotherapy useful for gallbladder carcinoma? A phase III multicenter prospective randomized controlled trial in patients with resected pancreaticobiliary carcinoma. Cancer 2002; 95:1685–95.

170. Kondo S, Nimura Y, Kamiya J et al. Factors influencing postoperative hospital mortality and long-term survival after radical resection for stage IV gallbladder carcinoma. World J Surg 2003: 27:272–7.

171. Duffy JP, Hines OJ, Liu JH et al. Improved survival for adenocarcinoma of the ampulla of Vater. Arch Surg 2003; 138:941–50.

172. Halstead WS. Contributions to the surgery of the bile duct passages, especially of the common bile duct. Boston Med Surg J 1899; 141:645–54.

173. Offerhaus GJ, Giardiello FM, Krush AJ et al. The risk of upper gastrointestinal cancer in familial adenomatous polyposis. Gastroenterology 1992; 102:1980–2.

174. Crile G Jr. The advantages of bypass operation over radical pancreatoduodenectomy in the treatment of pancreatic carcinoma. Surg Gynecol Obstet 1970; 130:1049–53.

175. Kayahara M, Nagakawa T, Ohta T et al. Surgical strategy for carcinoma of the papilla of Vater on the basis of lymphatic spread and mode of recurrence. Surgery 1997; 121:611–17.

176. Klempnauer J, Ridder GJ, Maschek H et al. Carcinoma of the ampulla of Vater: determinants of long-term survival in 94 resected patients. HPB Surg 1998; 11:1–11.

177. Rattner DW, Fernandez-del Castilo C, Brugge WR et al. Defining criteria for local resection of ampullary cancer. Arch Surg 1996; 131:366–71.

178. Midwinter MJ, Beveridge CJ, Wilsdon JB et al. Correlation between spiral computed tomography, endoscopic ultrasonography and findings at operation in pancreatic and ampullary tumours. Br J Surg 1999; 86:189–93.

179. Traverso LW, Longmire WP. Preservation of the pylorus in pancreaticoduodenectomy. Ann Surg 1994; 192:306–10.

180. Grace PA, Pitt HA, Tompkins RK et al. Decreased morbidity and mortality after pancreatoduodenectomy. Am J Surg 1986; 151:141–9.

181. Braasch JW, Rossi RC, Wakins E Jr et al. Pyloric and gastric preserving pancreatic resection. Experience with 87 patients. Ann Surg 1986; 204:411–18.

182. Lillemoe KD, Cameron JL, Hardacre JM et al. Is prophylactic gastrojejunostomy indicated for unresectable periampullary cancer? A prospective randomised trial. Ann Surg 1999; 230:322–8.

183. Mehta VK, Fisher GA, Ford JM et al. Adjuvant chemoradiotherapy for 'unfavourable' carcinoma of the ampulla of Vater. Arch Surg 2001; 136:65–9.

184. Howe JR, Klimstra DS, Moccia RD et al. Factors predictive of survival in ampullary carcinoma. Ann Surg 1998; 228:87–94.

185. McPherson GAD, Benjamin IS, Blumgart LH. Improving renal function in obstructive jaundice without preoperative drainage. Lancet 1984; 1:511.

186. Nakayama T, Ikeda A, Okuda K. Percutaneous transhepatic drainage of the biliary tract. Gastroenterology 1978; 74:554–9.

187. Hatfield ARW, Tobias R, Terblanche J et al. Preoperative external biliary drainage in obstructive jaundice. Lancet 1982; 2:896–9.

188. McPherson GAD, Benjamin IS, Hodgson HIF et al. Preoperative percutaneous transhepatic biliary drainage: the results of a controlled trial. Br J Surg 1984; 71:371–5.

189. Pitt HA, Gomes AS, Lois JF et al. Does preoperative percutaneous biliary drainage reduce operative risk or increase hospital cost? Ann Surg 1985; 201:9–16.

190. Diamond T, Dolan S, Thompson RLE et al. Development and reversal of endotoxemia and endotoxin-related death in obstructive jaundice. Surgery 1990; 108:370–5.

191. Blumgart LH, Benjamin IS. Liver resection for bile duct cancer. Surg Clin North Am 1989; 69:323–37.

192. Voyles CR, Blumgart LH. A technique for construction of high biliary enteric anastomosis. Surg Gynecol Obstet 1982; 154:885–7.

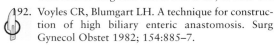

Technical paper describing the technique for hepatico-jejunostomy.

193. Krige JE, Bornman PC, Harris-Jones EP et al. Modified hepaticojejunostomy for permanent biliary access. Br J Surg 1987; 74:612–13.

194. Roddie ME, Benjamin IS. Transjejunal radiological intervention in hepatobiliary disease. Semin Intervent Radiol 1995; 12:55–62.

195. Al-Ghnaniem R, Benjamin IS. Long-term outcome of hepaticojejunostomy with routine access loop formation following iatrogenic bile duct injury. Br J Surg 2002; 89:1118–24.

This paper examines the long-term outcome in 48 patients following hepatico-jejunostomy and construction of an access loop for iatrogenic bile duct injury. The likelihood of needing the access loop for radiological intervention was found to be dependent on the Bismuth level.

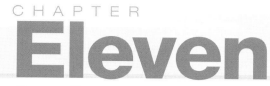

CHAPTER Eleven

Acute pancreatitis

Clement W. Imrie, C. Ross Carter and
Colin J. McKay

GENERAL DESCRIPTION

Acute pancreatitis is a common cause for emergency hospital admission, with approximately 40 cases per year for each 100 000 population in Scotland.[1] This figure is very similar to that reported from separate studies in Norway and Sweden.[2,3] For reasons that remain unexplained, the incidence continues to rise steadily, and there has been a slight but significant reduction in case mortality over the period 1985–94.[1] The two main causes of acute pancreatitis are gallstones and alcohol abuse, with gallstones being responsible for the majority of first attacks in the UK, Europe, Asia and USA. The relative proportion of cases due to gallstones varies between populations and depends on the intensity of investigation in addition to the prevalence of gallstone disease and alcohol abuse in the population under study. Many patients with suspected alcohol associated pancreatitis have coexistent cholelithiasis. Studies from Finland demonstrated an increasing proportion of alcohol-related acute pancreatitis corresponding to increasing alcohol consumption within that population,[4,5] whereas in Asia most cases are biliary in origin.[6] Less commonly, viral infection (particularly mumps and coxsackievirus B), trauma (including iatrogenic trauma), ampullary adenoma/carcinoma and primary hyperparathyroidism may be responsible. Many

drugs have been linked with acute pancreatitis especially azathioprine, asparaginase and steroids, but drug-induced acute pancreatitis appears to be relatively rare and usually runs a benign course.[7] In approximately 80% of patients, acute pancreatitis is a rapidly resolving condition requiring little more than analgesia and a short period of intravenous fluid resuscitation.

PATHOPHYSIOLOGY

The mechanism by which gallstones trigger an attack of acute pancreatitis has not been defined clearly. The bile reflux theory, proposed by Opie[8] in 1901, suggested that obstruction of the common bile duct/pancreatic duct common channel by a gallstone induced reflux of bile into the pancreatic duct causing acute pancreatitis. While there is no doubt that passage of and at least transient obstruction by a gallstone is the initial step in biliary acute pancreatitis, there is little evidence that bile reflux is involved. Studies in the opossum,[9] which has a long common channel between common bile duct and pancreatic duct, have demonstrated that obstruction of the pancreatic duct alone, obstruction of the pancreatic duct and common bile duct separately, and obstruction of the common channel all induce acute pancreatitis of similar severity.

Experimental models have shed some light on the mechanism by which pancreatic duct obstruction induces acute pancreatitis. Pancreatic duct obstruction has been shown to induce activation of pro-enzymes within the acinar cell by intracellular lysosomal enzymes.[10,11] These enzymes are normally segregated within the acinar cell but in the presence of duct obstruction, mixing of these enzymes occurs by a process termed colocalisation.[12] Hyperstimulation of pancreatic acinar cells with a cholecystokinin (CCK) analogue in vitro induces intracellular activation of trypsinogen by lysosomal enzymes, following which activated trypsin is released into the cytosolic compartment.[10] Recent evidence has demonstrated that these intracellular events are triggered by a rise in intracellular calcium.[13,14]

The mechanism of alcohol-induced acute pancreatitis is less clear, but alcohol has been shown to increase the sensitivity of acinar cells to CCK hyperstimulation, resulting in enhanced intracellular protease activation.[15] Alcohol also influences acinar cell calcium homeostasis, but several alternative theories have been proposed.

NATURAL HISTORY

Acute pancreatitis varies from a mild, self-limiting attack to a severe, life-threatening illness, and for this reason patients are often classified as having either mild or severe acute pancreatitis. This rather simplistic categorisation ignores the wide variety of clinical behaviour that can be observed in these patients but helps to focus attention on the subgroup of patients who develop complications. Several international consensus meetings have examined nomenclature of pancreatitis,[16–19] the Atlanta meeting clarifying the terminology used in acute pancreatic inflammation with the rejection of terms such as 'phlegmon' and 'infected pseudocyst' in favour of inflammatory mass and abscess.

Within this framework, different patterns of disease have emerged. Recent multicentre trials in acute pancreatitis have enabled the prospective study of severe acute pancreatitis, and several important points have emerged.

1. The majority of patients who develop severe acute pancreatitis have evidence of early

systemic organ dysfunction. It is exceptional for a patient to have no evidence of organ failure in the first week of illness and to subsequently develop a significant later local complication.

2. Most patients who develop organ failure have evidence of this at the time of admission or very shortly thereafter.[20,21]

3. While the tendency is for early organ dysfunction to recover without further problems, worsening organ failure is associated with a high mortality.[22,23]

These observations have important implications for patient management. The presence of early organ dysfunction identifies a high-risk group of patients who merit close observation for both early and late clinical complications. In particular, deteriorating organ failure carries a mortality of around 50% and should prompt early involvement of intensive care and consideration of transfer to a specialist unit if possible. The fact that organ dysfunction is present at or shortly after admission in the majority of patients in whom it develops means that efforts should be directed at early recognition of this rather than employing prediction systems of disease severity.

The majority of patients with severe early organ dysfunction will have pancreatic necrosis on computed tomography (CT) scan. A significant proportion (30–40%)[24] of patients with pancreatic necrosis will develop secondary pancreatic infection, usually in the 2nd to 3rd week after admission,[25] which may be associated with a deterioration in organ failure. Patients who have infected pancreatic necrosis complicated by multiple organ failure have a particularly poor prognosis, even with surgical intervention.

DIAGNOSIS

In the majority of patients the diagnosis of acute pancreatitis (AP) is relatively easy, characterised by a clinical presentation of sudden severe epigastric pain radiating through to the back, and usually associated with vomiting. The presence of other signs and symptoms, such as jaundice, tachycardia, tachypnoea, circulatory collapse and renal failure, are dependent partly on the underlying aetiology and mostly on the severity of the attack.

Most patients with AP present with sudden-onset severe upper abdominal pain, which can have a focus in the epigastrium, either right or left upper quadrant, or cover the upper abdomen. Vomiting is very frequently severe and contributes to dehydration and a tendency to renal failure. Tachypnoea is typical of the condition and is due to hypoxia, the early marker of respiratory compromise/failure. The diagnosis is usually supported by a raised total serum amylase (at least three times the upper limit normal). Serum amylase estimation may be inaccurate in association with hyperlipidaemia, where a raised urinary amylase can be diagnostic. Serum lipase may be marginally more accurate but is not frequently used in clinical practice.

Despite the apparent ease of diagnosis, about 30% of fatal attacks of acute pancreatitis are diagnosed at post-mortem, often in patients admitted initially to the medical wards with non-specific chest pain, in whom the diagnosis was not considered. For this reason a high index of suspicion is required, and a serum amylase should be a routine investigation in all patients admitted with lower left-sided chest pain as well as the more usual locations described. Plain abdominal radiographs are of little value, but CT can confirm the diagnosis where doubt exists, or in patients with delayed presentation.

AETIOLOGY

Gallstones are the most common aetiological factor and can be responsible for an attack even in those with a strong alcohol history. Stones are usually small, and therefore pass more easily from the gallbladder, where they are formed, into the common duct, where they are very likely to be held up at the lower end because of its tapering shape. The average diameter of the central portion of the common bile duct (CBD) is 6–7 mm, while the normal diameter at the ampullary area is 2–3 mm. Transient hold-up or impaction in the ampullary area is associated with 35–65% of episodes of acute pancreatitis in most prospective studies.[26] It is important to be aware that biliary sand or sludge may be sufficient to trigger an episode of acute pancreatitis, and that in a proportion of patients the stone material is too small to be detected by standard ultrasonic scanning. Indeed, most patients initially labelled

as suffering idiopathic acute pancreatitis prove ultimately to have this aetiology.

The next most common aetiology is alcohol abuse. Genetic vulnerability has been proposed as a contributory factor in view of the large numbers who abuse alcohol and do not suffer pancreatitis. As yet, however, no firm evidence has emerged to support this theory. Alcohol is the most common aetiology in prospective studies from Helsinki in Finland[5] and from the famous pioneer studies of Ranson[27] in New York City. In each of these groups approximately 75–80% of patients had alcohol abuse as the aetiology, and the median age of patients tended to be around 40 years compared with studies of a predominantly biliary aetiology, in which the median age is usually around 53 years.

In most prospective studies the combination of biliary and alcohol aetiologies accounts for 75–90% of patients, with less common aetiologies, such as viral infection (predominantly coxsackie B and mumps), ampullary pathology in the form of adenoma or carcinoma, hyperlipaemia, hyperparathyroidism and drug-related causes,[28] accounting for 5–10% of patients. In children, viral causes and blunt abdominal trauma account for the majority of cases of acute pancreatitis. Prodromal diarrhoea is often a feature of viral pancreatitis and is unusual in other aetiologies.

Prospective studies indicate that 1–3% of patients having diagnostic endoscopic retrograde cholangio-pancreatography (ERCP) may develop clinical and biochemical signs of acute pancreatitis, while the incidence associated with therapeutic ERCP rises to 4–5%.[29] Risk factors for ERCP-induced acute pancreatitis are female sex, sphincter of Oddi dysfunction (SOD), normal serum bilirubin levels and a history of recurrent pancreatitis. Procedure-related factors include pancreatic duct contrast injection, balloon dilatation of the sphincter, operator inexperience and the use of needle-knife sphincterotomy.[30] A recent randomised trial from our unit, of postprocedural diclofenac, has suggested that this may be may be helpful in preventing pancreatitis in high-risk patients.[31]

Pancreas divisum is a condition in which malunion of the pancreatic ducts from the ventral and dorsal buds of the pancreas results in complete or partial separation of the duct systems of Wirsung (main) and Santorini (accessory). This has variously been reported to occur in 0.3–5.8% of patients in endoscopy series and 5–14% in autopsy studies.[32] A small group of patients with pancreas divisum may be prone to attacks of acute pancreatitis due to poor outflow of the accessory duct system, but this remains controversial and in the majority of patients there is no association with acute pancreatitis.

A wide range of genetic mutations has been identified in patients with recurrent or chronic pancreatitis. The most common of these are the R122H, N29I, and A16V mutations of the cationic trypsinogen gene. Other mutations of this gene and mutations of other genes, in particular of the cystic fibrosis gene (CFTR) and intracellular trypsin inhibitor (SPINK1) have been described. Genetic testing is available for the three most common trypsinogen gene mutations but no specific treatment is available. The clinical course of this type of hereditary pancreatitis progresses to chronic pancreatitis, and there is a documented increase in the risk of pancreatic cancer, which may be as high as 40%.[33]

ASSESSMENT OF SEVERITY

Acute pancreatitis varies in severity, and can be described as either mild or severe. The Atlanta definitions of these are given in **Box 11.1**.

Multifactorial scoring systems

The variability of clinical behaviour seen in acute pancreatitis has stimulated numerous attempts to predict the severity of disease. Unfortunately, the accuracy of predictive systems has often been overstated. Most patients with severe attacks of acute pancreatitis have some evidence of systemic organ dysfunction at the time of presentation. It is recognition of this rather than the use of prediction systems that is important. Perhaps the best example of this shift in emphasis is to look at the commonly used multiple factor scoring systems (**Box 11.2**).[27,34] In both, hypoxia is simply one factor of prognostic significance but, by currently accepted criteria, is already indicative of severe acute pancreatitis.[19] It is also important to recognise that predicted severe acute pancreatitis, defined as three or more positive

Box 11.1 • 1992 Atlanta Conference – Classification of Pancreatitis meeting

Acute pancreatitis

An acute inflammatory process of the pancreas, with variable involvement of other regional tissues or remote organ systems.

Mild acute pancreatitis

Mild acute pancreatitis is associated with minimal organ dysfunction and an uneventful recovery. The predominant feature is interstitial oedema of the gland.

Severe acute pancreatitis

Severe acute pancreatitis is associated with organ failure and/or local complication such as necrosis (with infection), pseudocyst or abscess. Most often this is an expression of the development of pancreatic necrosis although patients with oedematous pancreatitis may manifest clinical features of a severe attack.

Box 11.2 • Modified Glasgow criteria. The presence of three or more criteria-severe disease.[34]

Within 48 h of admission:

- P_aO_2 <60 mmHg
- Albumin <32 g/L
- Calcium <2.00 mmol/L (unadjusted)
- WBC >15 × 10^9/L
- AST/ALT >200 U/L
- LDH >600 U/L
- Glucose >10 mmol/L (in the absence of diabetes)
- Urea >16 mmol/L (not responding to therapy)

criteria, is not synonymous with severe pancreatitis. In three prospective studies, the Glasgow predictive system had a positive predictive value of only 46–60%, with a sensitivity of 50–70%.[35] Therefore using this system, between half and a third of severe attacks will be missed and approximately half of those predicted to have severe pancreatitis would have an uncomplicated attack. It is also important to appreciate that such systems require 48 hours for full evaluation, by which time clinical assessment is almost as accurate. Nonetheless, predictive systems remain useful for comparison of results between centres and for selection of patients for clinical trials. Most widely used for these purposes in recent years has been the APACHE II score, which has been compared with the older pancreatic multiple factor scoring systems and clinical assessment in two prospective studies.[35,36] The APACHE II system uses 12 routinely available physiological and biochemical measurements, coupled with a score for age and pre-existing health, and has the advantage over the Glasgow and Ranson systems that it can be used within 24 h of admission. However, the low positive predictive value of the admission APACHE II score[37] means that the main use of the APACHE II score in acute pancreatitis is for stratification of patients for clinical trials. It is also useful for comparison of results between centres and can be used to monitor the course of an individual illness.

C-reactive protein (CRP)

This acute-phase reactant is easily and cheaply measured in most hospitals. It is a reliable and simple test, which has the disadvantage that it takes around 36 hours after onset of acute pancreatitis for peak serum levels to occur.[38,39] Normal levels of CRP in the peripheral blood are <6 mg/L. Patients with mild acute pancreatitis rarely have levels above 100 mg/L. In contrast patients who have clinically severe acute pancreatitis usually demonstrate levels over 200 mg/L, with a practical cut-off being 150 mg/L. The inherent delay in the CRP response makes it impractical for use as an early predictor of outcome but it is useful for monitoring the clinical course and, like APACHE II, may be used to help stratify disease severity.

Interleukin 6

Interleukin 6 (IL-6) is a proinflammatory cytokine induced by stimuli such as tumour necrosis factor (TNF) and interleukin 1 (IL-1). Whereas TNF and IL-1 are rarely found in appreciable quantities in the systemic circulation, the great majority of patients with severe acute pancreatitis have raised levels of IL-6 within 24 h of admission. Interleukin 6 is largely responsible for the induction of hepatic acute-phase protein production and is detectable 12–24 h before the rise in serum CRP. IL-6 shows

promise as a predictor of disease severity, and two studies have indicated the likely benefit of interleukin 6 when compared with CRP or phospholipase A.[40] At present, however, it is only measured in the research setting.

Trypsinogen activation peptide (TAP)

When trypsinogen is activated to form trypsin a small peptide molecule is split off (trypsinogen activation peptide, TAP). A pilot study in 1990 indicated the potential for the measurement of urinary TAP levels as an early predictor of severe acute pancreatitis.[41] More recently a commercially developed enzyme assay has been produced, and the initial clinical study of this was encouraging.[42] A follow-up study showed that admission levels of urinary TAP did not aid clinical management.[43]

Leucocyte (PMN) elastase

Polymorph neutrophil elastase is chemically different from pancreatic elastase, and high levels occur in acute pancreatitis as a manifestation of leucocyte activation. Once again pilot studies in both Spain and Germany have suggested the potential benefit of a fast commercial assay for this enzyme,[44,45] but this is not yet a practical approach.

Repeated clinical assessment

In the absence of clinically useful predictive systems, our own practice is to monitor patients for the development of systemic organ dysfunction by repeated clinical and biochemical assessment. The presence of a systemic inflammatory response syndrome (SIRS) (defined as two or more of the following: fever, tachycardia, tachypnoea, or leucocytosis; **Box 11.3**) identifies patients at risk of multiple organ dysfunction syndrome (MODS), particularly when three or four SIRS criteria are present or when SIRS persists for 48 h or more after admission. Patients without SIRS at admission are at very low risk. The development of systemic organ dysfunction (usually clinically manifest as hypoxaemia) mandates careful monitoring in a high-dependency or intensive care unit (ICU)

Box 11.3 • Definitions of SIRS and MODS

Systemic inflammatory response syndrome (SIRS)[46]

A response to a variety of severe clinical insults, manifested by two or more of the following conditions:

- Temperature >38 or <36°C
- Heart rate >90 beats/min
- Respiratory rate >20/min or P_aCO_2 <32 mmHg (<4.3 kPa)
- WBC >12 000 cells/mm^3, <4000 cells/mm^3, or >10% immature (band) forms

Multiple organ dysfunction syndrome (MODS)[46]

The presence of altered organ function in an acutely ill patient such that homeostasis cannot be maintained without intervention.

---

environment, and worsening respiratory dysfunction or involvement of other systems is associated with a poor prognosis.

IMAGING

Ultrasound (US)

All patients with acute pancreatitis should have an ultrasonic assessment of the biliary tree within 24 h of admission.[47] In those with gallstones, the majority will have mild disease, and this will facilitate definitive treatment of cholelithiasis prior to discharge. In patients with severe acute pancreatitis the presence of gallstones may be an indication for early ERCP.

In the emergency situation, ultrasonography can be difficult due to a number of factors, including the presence of intraluminal bowel gas, or lack of patient cooperation. Therefore, in patients with a negative initial ultrasound, and no other obvious aetiological factor, the ultrasound should be repeated, prior to discharge, by an experienced radiologist using optimum equipment before a diagnosis of idiopathic acute pancreatitis is made. It must be remembered that the limit of resolution of normal ultrasound is a 4 mm stone. Stones of this size and smaller can cause acute pancreatitis.

Owing to simplicity and the lack of radiation, ultrasound-guided rather than CT-guided fine-

needle aspiration of pancreatic and peripancreatic collections has been advocated,[48] particularly in Europe. Our own preference is to use a CT-guided technique as this allows accurate route selection to avoid inadvertent puncture of the bowel and the increased likelihood of iatrogenic introduction of infection.

All patients should have an ultrasound of their biliary tree within 24 h of admission, regardless of the suspected aetiology. The diagnosis of idiopathic acute pancreatitis requires, at least, a second negative ultrasound performed under optimal conditions.

CT scanning

CT scanning is a useful adjunct to clarify the diagnosis from intestinal perforation, gut ischaemia, or dissecting aortic aneurysm. In patients with severe acute pancreatitis, particularly when complicated by MODS, early CT not only helps to exclude other pathology but if carried out with intravenous contrast will detect evidence of pancreatic necrosis. Such patients may benefit from prophylactic antibiotics. The use of high-dose iodinated contrast raises a theoretical potential for exacerbating renal compromise, found in experimental studies,[49] but this is as yet unproven in the clinical context.

Dynamic contrast-enhanced CT can be used to assess disease severity[50] and predict the potential for complications.[51] Although not widely used for this purpose clinically in Britain, it is more popular in the USA, Germany and Finland, and can be useful in comparing patient groups in studies. The CT Severity Index (CTSI)[51] evolved from the earlier CT grade, and combines a score for the radiological pancreatic and peripancreatic abnormalities with a weighting for the extent of necrosis (**Table 11.1**).

Magnetic resonance/MRCP

Magnetic resonance imaging (MRI) offers a realistic alternative to contrast-enhanced CT in the assessment of patients with acute pancreatitis. The avoidance of cumulative radiation exposure and potentially nephrotoxic iodinated contrast media, combined with the excellent contrast sensitivity and spatial resolution would make it an attractive alternative. Axial T1- and T2-weighted scans produce

Table 11.1 • CT Severity Index of Balthazar[51]

Score	CT grade score
0	A = Normal pancreas
1	B = Pancreatic enlargement +/− small (<3 cm) intrapancreatic fluid collection/necrosis
2	C = Inflammation extending into the peripancreatic tissues
3	D = More extensive peripancreatic inflammation but not more than one fluid collection
4	E = Marked pancreatic/peripancreatic inflammation with multiple/extensive fluid collections or abscess

Score	Necrosis score
0	None
2	30%
4	50%
6	>50%

CTSI score (0–10) = CT score (0–4) + Necrosis score (0–6).

images analogous to those of CT. Gadolinium contrast enhancement can infer viability and improve anatomical definition. Heavily T2-weighted image acquisition, using a single breath hold and a long repetition (TR) and echo (TE) time, results in little signal being produced by solid tissue, and a high signal from static fluid in the biliary and pancreatic ducts, enabling images anatomically comparable to those of ERCP to be produced.

Whilst technically feasible in most centres, the magnetic resonance environment is unsuitable for patients requiring significant circulatory or respiratory support, and at present, few centres have the capability to perform MR-guided intervention. Contrast-enhanced CT therefore remains the imaging modality of choice for assessment and intervention in severe acute pancreatitis. However, MR has a role in the follow-up of acute inflammatory collections, and the exclusion of choledocholithiasis in suitable patients (**Fig. 11.1**).

Endoscopic ultrasound

Endoscopic ultrasound (EUS) has rapidly emerged as an important tool in diagnostic and therapeutic

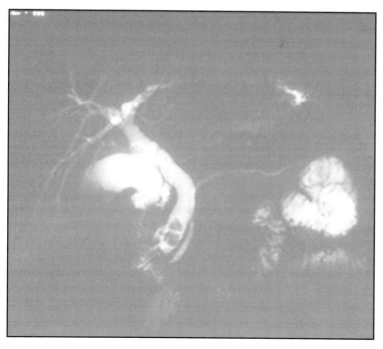

Figure 11.1 • MRCP confirming choledocholithiasis.

algorithms in patients with acute pancreatitis. Its main areas of use – diagnosis of microlithiasis in idiopathic pancreatitis and linear EUS-guided drainage of peripancreatic collections – are discussed in the relevant sections below.

MANAGEMENT

Initial management

Several guideline documents outlining the management of acute pancreatitis have been published in the last five years.[47,52,53] Initial management of patients presenting with acute pancreatitis should be directed at fluid resuscitation and pain relief, plus careful assessment for incipient or established respiratory or renal insufficiency and provision of adequate facilities for monitoring of the patient. The intravenous fluid requirements may be in excess of 6 L in the first 24 h, and careful monitoring of the urine output is mandatory. If there is a poor response to initial fluid resuscitation, or if renal impairment is present, further fluid administration should be guided by monitoring of central venous pressure. Respiratory dysfunction is a hallmark of the disease and should be treated with humidified oxygen. Continuous monitoring of oxygen saturation is required in these patients in order to detect evidence of worsening respiratory insufficiency. It should be appreciated that any deterioration in a patient's clinical condition is an ominous sign and necessitates the involvement of the intensive care team at an early stage. As many as half of all deaths from acute pancreatitis occur in less than 7 days from disease onset, and the majority of these occur within 72 h of admission.[1] There is evidence that patients managed in specialist institutions have a reduced risk of early death, and this may be an indication that management of early MODS could be improved.

Supportive management

All patients with severe pancreatitis should be managed within a high-dependency/ICU environment with the potential for inotropic, ventilatory or renal dialysis support. Where possible, these patients should be managed by a designated multidisciplinary team who have an interest in pancreatico-biliary pathology. Facilities should be available for patients to undergo ERCP/sphincterotomy when indicated (see below). Management of these patients is complex and should be discussed with a specialist unit at an early stage.

Specific measures will be determined by the clinical situation. However, our therapeutic aims are guided to the correction of intravascular hypovolaemia rather than early aggressive inotropic support, often ignoring significant interstitial fluid overload. Acute dialysis for acidosis has not been shown to improve outcome but is required for established renal failure. Currently no specific therapy to reverse respiratory compromise exists other than ventilatory support.

Specific medical management

There have been many attempts to introduce specific medical treatments for acute pancreatitis and these broadly fall into the following categories.

PREVENTION OF INFECTION

In patients who survive the early, systemic complications of acute pancreatitis, secondary infection of pancreatic necrosis is the most important late complication. Infection occurs in 30–40% of patients, with a minimum 30% pancreatic necrosis,[24] and is responsible for the majority of late deaths from acute pancreatitis. Secondary infection manifests as escalating sepsis or a deterioration in organ failure scores, usually in the second (36%) and third (71%) weeks of the illness.[25] Sterile necrosis should, in general, be treated without surgery.[54–56]

Advocates of antibiotic prophylaxis cite experimental evidence using in vivo models of acute pancreatitis, confirming reduced bacterial counts in pancreatic and peripancreatic tissues.[57–59] However, these studies assessed short-term colonisation of non-necrotic material, which is not analogous to the human situation. Potentially stronger evidence comes from the Mithofer study,[60] which followed an acute pancreatitic model for 3 weeks, and showed a reduction in both late complications and mortality rates in antibiotic-treated animals.

In the 1970s three studies assessed the role of antibiotics in acute pancreatitis using ampicillin and none showed any benefit.[61–63] The inclusion of all grades of severity of acute pancreatitis reduced the power of these studies, and ampicillin has since been shown to penetrate poorly into pancreatic tissue. In the last decade there has been considerable interest in the potential role of antibiotic prophylaxis in patients with pancreatic necrosis and five recent randomised trials have addressed this issue.

In 1993 Pederzoli and colleagues[64] reported the results of a multicentre Italian study, which recruited 74 patients with necrotising pancreatitis. Patients were randomised to receive imipenem, 0.5 g 8-hourly for 14 days, or standard treatment (some of the control group also received either ampicillin or an aminoglycoside for 'non-pancreatic' infective complications). The use of imipenem was associated with a reduction in secondary pancreatic infection from 30% to 12% and a reduction in extrapancreatic sepsis from 49% to 15%. Three deaths occurred in each group. Despite negative fine needle aspirate (FNA) cultures, pancreatic sepsis was, however, clinically suspected in nearly 60% of the treated group, and there was no beneficial effect on organ dysfunction, operation rate or mortality.

In a single-centre study of similar design, Sainio and colleagues[5] randomised 60 young patients (median age 40 years) with mainly alcohol-induced pancreatic necrosis to receive cefuroxime, 1.5 g three times daily until full clinical recovery, or standard treatment. This study, commonly interpreted as further evidence in support of antibiotic therapy, had findings that contrasted sharply with those of the Italian trial.[64] No difference was observed in the incidence of secondary pancreatic infection but there was a significant reduction in mortality associated with cefuroxime prophylaxis. Two of the deaths in the control group were due to an early fulminant course, and therefore unlikely to be related to infection. No patient in the control group had a positive FNA prior to starting antibiotics, which occurred in 70% at a median of 6.1 days post admission. Finally, the majority of those in the cefuroxime arm required a change in antibiotics to imipenem, vancomycin and fluconazole.

Two other smaller randomised studies have compared intravenous antibiotics to a control arm. In a study from France,[65] patients with alcohol-induced acute pancreatitis associated with peripancreatic fluid collections were randomised to no antibiotics or ceftazidime 2 g 8-hourly, amikacin 7.5 mg/kg/12 h, and metronidazole 500 mg 8-hourly for 10 days. Seven infections occurred in the control group and none in the treatment arm. Sepsis-associated organ dysfunction was only found in three patients in the control group. Schwarz and colleagues from Ulm[66] reported a study of 26 patients with CT-proven necrotising pancreatitis. Thirteen received ofloxacin 200 mg 12-hourly and metronidazole 500 mg 12-hourly, while the control group had antibiotics initially withheld. Fine needle aspiration cytology (FNAC) was performed on patients on days one, three, five, seven and ten. The mortality of treated patients was zero and two died in the control group (mortality 15%).

A fifth randomised, 6-year, multicentre study, reported by Bassi and colleagues,[67] compared imipenem and pefloxacin, in patients with acute necrotising pancreatitis. Pefloxacin, which has limited activity against the range of organisms commonly associated with infected pancreatic necrosis, was associated with more secondary pancreatic infection than imipenem. The imipenem group had a 10% infection rate, which is similar to the 12% found in the earlier 1993 study by the same group from Verona[64] using the same antibiotic prophylaxis.

As the majority of secondary pancreatic infections are Gram-negative in origin, it is widely believed that the source of these organisms is translocation from the intestinal tract. Luiten and colleagues[68] assessed the effect of selective gut decontamination (SD) using oral and rectal colistin, amphotericin and norfloxacin, and in addition those in the SD group received intravenous (i.v.) cefotaxime. Although this i.v. cephalosporin was only given for a few days to cover the period until the orally administered drugs had reduced the endogenous flora, this does blur the scientific credibility of suggesting selective decontamination alone to be an effective treatment. Treatment was continued until full resolution of organ dysfunction was achieved.

In this study there were 102 patients treated in 16 hospitals over a 3-year period, and there was an almost total elimination of Gram-negative sepsis. A high mortality rate was found in the treatment group (22%) and the control group (35%), with no difference in early mortality (six patients in each group died due to multiorgan failure). There were three deaths due to Gram-negative sepsis in the treatment group compared to ten in the control group ($P = 0.07$). The main finding of the study was therefore a reduction in the need for surgical intervention, and there was also a trend towards reduced mortality in the SD group. An incidental finding was the lowering of fungal infection in the treatment group, with only two patients having this problem compared to ten in the control group. Unfortunately, little information is given regarding the time and clinical course from symptom onset to randomisation, and at least 10% of patients were randomised at or following a laparotomy.

Since then, two further studies[69,70] have been presented in patients with objectively graded severe acute pancreatitis, but as yet these have only been published in abstract form. The Ulm group[69] coordinated a study and reported their results from a randomised trial of ciprofloxacin and metronidazole versus placebo in 105 patients with severe acute pancreatitis. Antibiotic prophylaxis was not associated with a reduction in infected pancreatic necrosis or in the incidence of systemic complications. In contrast, Delcenserie and colleagues[70] reported a randomised trial of prophylactic ciprofloxacin in 81 patients with either peripancreatic fluid collections or necrosis. Patients were randomised to one of three groups: placebo, ciprofloxacin (7 days) or ciprofloxacin (21 days). Antibiotics were associated with a significant reduction in pancreatic and non-pancreatic septic complications, but mortality was highest in the patients receiving prolonged prophylaxis (21 days).

In 1999 we reported concern at the widespread adoption of a broad-spectrum prophylactic antibiotic policy. Our study of 60 patients with infected necrosis found the incidence of fungal infection had increased following the introduction of prophylactic antibiotics in 1993–94.[71] Furthermore, fungal infection at the initial surgical procedure for infected pancreatic necrosis was also associated with a 57% mortality. Sarr's group[72] at the Mayo Clinic described similar findings in 57 patients collected in a 12-year period (1983–95). Fungal infection was present in 7 and bacteria in 50 patients. They also reported higher mortality in patients with fungal infection (43% vs. 20%) and found that an average of four antibiotics were given to patients with fungal infection. Both the total hospital stay and

days in intensive care were extended for those with fungal infection. A recent study from Belgium also reported a 37% incidence of fungal infection in 46 patients with infected pancreatic necrosis.[73]

Until recently there was a general acceptance of a role for prophylactic antibiotics in patients with prognostically severe acute pancreatitis, and a UK survey confirmed that nearly 90% of surgeons treating patients with acute pancreatitis regularly used prophylactic antibiotics.[74] At present there are no data to guide decisions on the optimal timing and duration of antibiotic treatment. The selection of patients for antibiotic prophylaxis is also difficult, as CT scans to detect the presence of pancreatic necrosis are not performed routinely early in acute pancreatitis. From published data it appears that systemic antibiotics are as effective as selective gut decontamination in prophylaxis of secondary pancreatic infection and have the benefit of ease of administration. However, questions remain as to whether this will translate into a reduction in overall mortality or if a reduction in mortality from Gram-negative sepsis will be matched by an increase in mortality from fungal infection and resistant bacterial strains. A summary of the main publications concerning infection in severe acute pancreatitis is shown in **Table 11.2**, which illustrates the rising incidence of fungal infection since 1993.

Prophylactic antibiotics can reduce the risk of infected pancreatic necrosis but may not influence mortality. If used they should be restricted to patients with proven pancreatic necrosis. Appropriate intravenous antibiotics appear to be as effective as selective gut decontamination.

NUTRITIONAL SUPPORT

Although Navarro and colleagues[77] have shown in a randomised controlled study that nasogastric suction alone is of no benefit in mild or moderate disease, until recently the usual management of patients with acute pancreatitis involved a period of gut rest until symptoms begin to resolve. The potential for a long period of starvation led to the use of total parenteral nutrition (TPN) in those with severe disease. Clinical trials in other conditions such as trauma and sepsis, however, have shown a reduction in septic complications associated with

Table 11.2 • Pancreatic necrosis, fungal infection and benefit of antibiotics

Authors (year of publication)	Patients with infected necrosis	Patients with fungal infection	Percent fungal infection	Antibiotic advantage Infection	Mortality
Warshaw et al. (1985)[75]	45	3	6.7	–	–
Beger et al. (1986)[25]	45	3	6.7	–	–
Bradley (1993)[76]	71	4	5.6	–	–
Pederzoli et al. (1993)[64]	15	4	27	+ve	–
Sainio et al. (1995)[5]	10	1	10	–	+ve
Luiten et al. (1995)[68]*	29	12	41	+ve	–
Farkas et al. (1996)[77]	123	21	17	–	–
Delcenserie et al. (1996)[65]	7	?	?	+ve	–
Schwarz et al. (1997)[66]	15	?	33	–	–
Bassi et al. (1998)[67]	13	4	31	?	?
Rau et al. (1998)[48]	29	3	10	–	–
Eatock et al. (1999)[71]	60	25	42	?	–ve
Grewe et al. (1999)[72]	57	7	12	?	–ve

*Selective decontamination of the GI tract.

nasojejunal feeding compared with TPN,[79] and there have now been several studies of this approach in acute pancreatitis.

In an uncontrolled pilot study of 21 patients with severe acute pancreatitis, Nakad and his colleagues[80] from Brussels demonstrated the feasibility of utilisation of a double-lumen nasogastrojejunal tube in all but one of the 21 patients studied. McClave and his colleagues[81] randomised 32 patients with mild or moderate acute pancreatitis to either TPN or nasojejunal feeding and showed no difference between the groups. However, enteral feeding was associated with signifiantly lower costs and lower morbidity.

The largest clinical study, from the city of Patras in Greece,[82] involved 38 patients with severe acute pancreatitis. Eighteen were randomised to nasojejunal feeding and 20 patients to intravenous feeding. Gallstones were the predominant aetiology occurring in 30 patients while 5 suffered from alcohol abuse. Objective evidence of severity of acute pancreatitis was present with the mean Glasgow score being over 4 and the mean APACHE II score being over 11.5 while CRP mean values were over 280 mg/L. As expected there was a greater incidence of hyperglycaemia in the intravenous feeding group, and infective complications occurred in twice as many patients. In each group the average stay in intensive care was 12 days and the total in-hospital stay was 40 days. There was no difference in these aspects and mortality was also unaffected. The cost of nutritional therapy was £30 UK per day in the enterally fed group and £100 per day in those fed parenterally. Similarly, a study from Virginia found early enteral nutrition to be associated with less septic complications than TPN, with an estimated $2300 saving per patient fed.[83]

Another study, from Leeds,[84] investigated the place of early enteral feeding in a group of 34 patients, of whom 13 had objective evidence of severe acute pancreatitis. Sixteen patients were randomised to enteral feeding and 18 to intravenous feeding: no deaths occurred in the enterally fed group, but two occurred in the parenterally fed patients. Although this was a small study, examination of the markers of systemic inflammatory response at the onset of hospitalisation compared to 1 week after admission showed that the inflammatory response was less in the enterally fed group and fewer developed multiorgan failure. In addition, IgM anticore endotoxin antibodies rose in the intravenously fed patients but not in those fed enterally. The anti-oxidant capacity was also enhanced in the group fed enterally but decreased in the intravenously fed patients.

All of these studies utilised enteral feeding distal to the duodeno-jejunal flexure. This was due to the belief that the delivery of nutrients proximal to the this flexure will cause release of CCK and exacerbate the inflammatory process within the pancreas as a result of stimulation of exocrine pancreatic secretion.[85] However, our own group investigated the possibility of proximal (nasogastric) feeding in patients with acute pancreatitis. In 1998 we reported the results of a pilot study[86] involving 26 patients with predicted severe acute pancreatitis, in whom enteral feeding was commenced by fine-bore nasogastric tube as soon after presentation as possible. The method proved successful in 22 of the 26 patients, and we could find no evidence of either exacerbation of pain or an increase in markers of disease severity associated with the introduction of enteral feeding. We have also reported a randomised comparison of nasogastric versus nasojejunal feeding and found no evidence that the nasogastric route was associated with increased morbidity.[87]

A further consideration in the decision to implement enteral feeding is the potential for improving gut permeability. There has been interest in the role of the intestine in the pathophysiology of multiple organ failure in critical illness, with loss of gut barrier function potentially leading to endotoxaemia and SIRS. Enteral nutrition is associated with improved gut barrier function, and there is evidence that supplementing the enteral formula with key nutrients may have additional effects on the immune system. There have been several trials comparing so called 'immunonutrition' with standard enteral feed in critically ill patients, with promising results.[88,89]

This approach has not yet been assessed in acute pancreatitis. However, one study has compared early enteral nutrition to a 'nil by mouth' regime and found no evidence of a reduction in markers of the inflammatory response; neither was there any evidence of improved gut permeability in the enterally fed group.[90]

In summary, current evidence would suggest that nutritional support where required in acute

pancreatitis should be given enterally. It is not yet established that early enteral feeding in itself influences the outcome from an attack of acute pancreatitis.

There is no evidence that the early introduction of enteral nutritional support is detrimental in acute pancreatitis. Enteral feeding is therefore the preferred method of nutritional support in patients with severe acute pancreatitis, TPN being reserved for those in whom the enteral route is not tolerated.

INHIBITION OF PANCREATIC SECRETION

It was formerly considered important in the treatment of acute pancreatitis to 'rest the pancreas', and the standard approach of withholding diet until clinical resolution was based on this philosophy. Pharmacological attempts to suppress pancreatic function have included intravenous glucagon, somatostatin and, more recently, the somatostatin analogue octreotide. There have now been five randomised trials of octreotide in the management of acute pancreatitis reported in the literature.[91–95]

Two of these were appropriately designed placebo-controlled trials. The West of Scotland study,[94] in contrast to the previous optimistic reports, showed no evidence of a beneficial effect of continuous i.v. octreotide (50 μg/h) on outcome. A multicentre trial from Germany[95] recruited 302 patients from 32 hospitals but failed to demonstrate any effect of subcutaneous 8-hourly octreotide (max. 600 μg/24 h) on a number of clinical endpoints. Following this report, there can be no justification for the use of octreotide in the treatment of acute pancreatitis.

Octreotide is of no benefit in the treatment of patients with acute pancreatitis.

INHIBITION OF PANCREATIC ENZYMES

Several studies evaluated the concept of supporting the endogenous antiprotease defence mechanisms. Double-blind randomised trials of i.v. aprotinin (Trasylol) and gabexate mesilate[96,97] and a meta-analysis[98] showed no advantage over placebo. Intraperitoneal aprotinin also failed to show any benefit.[99] The use of both low- and high-dose fresh frozen plasma (FFP) proved unhelpful.[100,101]

The antiproteases aprotinin and gabexate mesilate, or FFP are of no benefit in the treatment of acute pancreatitis.

INHIBITION OF THE INFLAMMATORY RESPONSE

Anticytokine therapy: lexipafant

In recent years there has been much interest in the potential use of the platelet-activating factor (PAF) antagonist, lexipafant, in the treatment of patients with acute pancreatitis. PAF is an inflammatory mediator released from many inflammatory cells and is considered to play an important role in the priming and amplification of the inflammatory response. Lexipafant is a PAF receptor antagonist that had shown promise in studies in experimental pancreatitis. Two phase II clinical trials reported a reduction in organ failure scores following lexipafant treatment.[20,102] A common finding in both studies was that no patients in the treatment groups developed significant organ failure following admission to hospital.

These encouraging results led to a multicentre UK study,[103] which recruited 290 patients with predicted severe attacks from 78 hospitals. There was a significant reduction in organ failure scores at day 3 in the treatment group but by day 7, at completion of the trial infusion, there was no difference between the groups. Of further concern was the fact that there was no difference in the incidence of newly developed organ failure. There was also no difference in mortality overall, but a subgroup analysis, comparing mortality in the 70% of patients entering the study within 48 h of symptom onset, found a significant reduction in mortality with lexipafant treatment.

There followed an international multicentre study that recruited 1518 patients randomised to receive lexipafant 100 mg daily, lexipafant 10 mg daily, or placebo. This study recruited only those patients with symptoms of less than 48 h duration, and again was restricted to those with predicted severe attacks. The mortality rate in the placebo, lexipafant 10 mg and lexipafant 100 mg groups was 8.1%, 8.3% and 7.7%, respectively. Not only was there no difference in mortality between groups, the incidence of local complications, length of ICU stay, hospital stay and change in organ failure scores were all similar in the three study groups.

The potential for other agents that modify the inflammatory response or influence outcome in acute pancreatitis has only been assessed in experimental models and evidence from large studies in patients with sepsis is not encouraging.

 There is currently no evidence to support the use of agents designed to inhibit the inflammatory response.

ROLE OF ERCP

In the absence of an effective medical therapy, the main therapeutic question in the early phase of acute pancreatitis relates to the necessity for ERCP and sphincterotomy. As many as 10% of all patients with gallstone-associated acute pancreatitis will develop ascending cholangitis, and this group stand to benefit from ERCP, sphincterotomy and duct drainage.[104] Experimental studies indicate that the duration of biliary and pancreatic obstruction also relates to the severity of acute pancreatitis, and that early decompression can lessen the degree of pancreatic injury.[9]

There have now been four randomised trials reported that have addressed this issue. In the first study, from the UK, 121 patients with gallstone pancreatitis were randomised to receive conservative treatment or ERCP with endoscopic sphincterotomy within 72 h of admission.[105] In this study, there was no procedure-related morbidity, confirming the safety of this procedure in expert hands. When the subgroup with predicted severe pancreatitis was examined, there was a reduction in morbidity and a trend towards a reduction in mortality in the ERCP group. A subsequent study from Hong Kong[106] found a marked reduction in the incidence of biliary sepsis in the patients randomised to ERCP, and once again the effect was most obvious in the predicted severe group. These studies have been criticised for including patients with possible cholangitis, and the Hong Kong study in particular, where bile duct stones and cholangitis are common, may reflect the effect of early endoscopic sphincterotomy on patients with coexisting cholangitis and acute pancreatitis.

A multicentre German study randomised 238 patients to early ERCP or no treatment.[107] In this study, patients with jaundice were excluded (bilirubin >90 μmol/L) and no benefit from ERCP was seen, lending weight to the suggestion that

ERCP and endoscopic sphincterotomy is of little value in the absence of jaundice or cholangitis. Conversely, an unexplained increase in respiratory complications was observed in the ERCP group. This study has come in for much criticism, mainly because 19 of the 22 centres recruited fewer than two patients per year to the study, suggesting either significant selection bias or limited experience with ERCP in acute pancreatitis in the majority of centres. The mortality of the predicted severe ERCP group was also much higher than in the Leicester and Hong Kong studies.

In another study from Poland,[108] 280 patients with acute pancreatitis underwent early ERCP. Patients with bile duct calculi underwent endoscopic sphincterotomy while the remainder were randomised to sphincterotomy or no treatment. Significant reductions in morbidity and mortality were seen in the group randomised to endoscopic sphincterotomy, suggesting that this is beneficial even in the absence of bile duct stones. Unfortunately this study, which was presented 10 years ago, has never been published in a peer-reviewed journal and it is therefore impossible to make recommendations based on its findings.

At the present time, the evidence (Table 11.3) strongly supports early ERCP for all patients with gallstone pancreatitis who are jaundiced or in whom there is a suspicion of cholangitis. Some argue that urgent ERCP and sphincterotomy may be valuable in **all** predicted severe patients with gallstone-associated acute pancreatitis within 48 h

of admission, but a further large randomised study of the role of early ERCP and sphincterotomy in severe gallstone acute pancreatitis would be needed, before firm recommendations can be given.

DEFINITIVE MANAGEMENT ISSUES

The last decade has witnessed radical changes in the understanding and management principles of patients with acute pancreatitis. Traditional management involved a dogmatic surgical approach driven by biochemical, radiological and bacteriological factors rather than an individual patient's presentation and clinical features. A more flexible approach is emerging based on the observed dynamic pattern of organ dysfunction with time, the involvement of a multidisciplinary team, and modification of the traditional indications for surgical intervention. The definitive management issues may be considered as being (i) those designed to prevent further attacks once a mild attack has subsided, and (ii) those specifically related to the management of early and late complications.

Prevention of recurrent acute pancreatitis

MANAGEMENT OF GALLSTONES

The timing of cholecystectomy will obviously depend on the clinical situation. In patients

Table 11.3 • Randomised controlled trials (RCTs) of early endoscopic retrograde cholangiopancreatography (ERCP)/endoscopic sphincterotomy (ES) in patients with severe acute pancreatitis (AP)

RCT	Leicester[105]*		Hong Kong[106]		Germany[107]	
	ES	**Controls**	**ES**	**Controls**	**ES**	**Controls**
Predicted severe	22*	24	30*	28	26	20
Attempted early ERCP	22	–	30	–	26	–
Successful ERCP	19	–		–	?	–
Number undergoing ES	12		19		?	
No. deaths from AP (%)	0 (0)	5 (21)	5 (17)	9 (32)	10[‡] (38)	4 (20)
Deaths (all causes)	1[†]	5	5	9	14	7

*Confirmed gallstones.
[†]Death in a patient who did not have ES (no stone in main bile duct).
[‡]It is unclear from the text whether the deaths were all within the severe group.

recovering from mild acute biliary pancreatitis, definitive management of the gallstones to prevent a further attack should be achieved during the same admission, and **no later than 4 weeks** following discharge from hospital.[47] This will normally involve a cholecystectomy (laparoscopic or open) with intraoperative cholangiography, or alternatively duct imaging followed by cholecystectomy. Elderly or unfit patients considered inappropriate for elective surgery may be managed by an ERCP with sphincterotomy as definitive treatment although this may not be as effective as definitive surgery.

In the open surgical era, operative cholangiography was considered a routine skill, and cholecystectomy is still considered a general surgical procedure. A laparoscopic approach to cholecystectomy, coupled with subspecialisation, has resulted in many surgeons caring for patients with acute pancreatitis being unable to image adequately the bile duct intraoperatively. Preoperative bile duct imaging consequently became commonplace, most often by ERCP. However, the role of diagnostic preoperative ERCP in the absence of common bile duct dilatation or stones, and with normal liver function tests, must be questioned due to the inherent risks of the procedure and the more general availability of non-invasive methods of bile duct stone detection (MR/MRCP or EUS). Debate continues regarding what to do with stones identified at operative cholangiography (OC). At open surgery duct exploration should be performed. Laparoscopic common bile duct exploration, either transcystic or transmural, is appropriate where local expertise exists, particularly with significant duct dilatation. Postoperative ERCP and stone extraction during the same admission is a further option, and may be preferred where the bile duct is of normal calibre.

In severe acute pancreatitis, interval cholecystectomy should be performed when the inflammatory process has subsided, and the procedure made potentially easier. Occasionally the urgency may be lessened if the patient undergoes an ERCP with sphincterotomy early in the course of the disease. The decision on timing can be difficult, particularly in the presence of postinflammatory fluid collections, which may in themselves require intervention. The need for cholecystectomy and intraoperative cholangiography should be considered during any open surgical procedure performed for a complication

of acute pancreatitis, as a significant proportion of patients diagnosed as having alcohol-induced or idiopathic acute pancreatitis have undiagnosed cholelithiasis. However, the place of routine cholecystectomy in all patients undergoing an open procedure for pancreatitis remains controversial.

Mild gallstone pancreatitis without complications should have definitive management of lithiasis, ideally within the same admission. Cholecystectomy with biliary duct imaging, or ERCP with sphincterotomy are acceptable alternatives.

All patients require an adequate cholangiogram, usually by operative cholangiography or ERCP prior to discharge, but should this fail, provided there is no direct evidence of choledocholithiasis, non-invasive biliary imaging by MRCP/EUS would be acceptable prior to discharge back to the primary health care team.

INVESTIGATION OF NON-GALLSTONE-ASSOCIATED PANCREATITIS

Following resolution of an attack of acute pancreatitis, an assessment of potential aetiological factors is an important aspect of care, and a diagnosis of idiopathic pancreatitis should be made in less than 20% of patients.[47] Most cases are attributable to cholelithiasis, alcohol ingestion, mechanical ductal obstruction due to stricture or tumour, medications or metabolic derangements. Evaluation of the initial acute attack should include an adequate history (alcohol, drugs, family), biochemical tests (LFTs, lipids (hypertriglyceridaemia), hypercalcaemia), and biliary ultrasound (repeated before discharge if initially normal). If the patient presents with a second idiopathic attack, repeat transcutaneous ultrasound followed by EUS (microlithiasis) would be appropriate. If the ultrasound results appear normal, then axial imaging (CT or MR/MRCP) and possibly ERCP may be appropriate to exclude a mechanical cause. A cholecystectomy or biliary sphincterotomy is justified in patients with recurrent idiopathic pancreatitis in whom microlithiasis or biliary sludge is identified, non-pancreatic sources of hyperamylasaemia, or macroamylasaemia should be considered. Attacks that recur despite the above measures should be assessed in a unit with access to biliary manometry, genetic testing, and pancreatic functional assessment.

Peripancreatic fluid collections

MANAGEMENT OF AN EARLY FLUID COLLECTION

Up to 25% of patients with acute pancreatitis will develop a fluid collection in the peripancreatic area identifiable on CT scan. These collections may later develop into pseudocysts, pancreatic abscess, or abscess associated with necrosis. The management of these is discussed below. The majority of simple fluid collections within the first weeks will resolve spontaneously, and we would counsel against aspiration, and especially against external drainage as this commonly leads to the development of secondary infection.[109]

Acute fluid collections occur early in the course of acute pancreatitis, are located in or near the pancreas, and always lack a wall of granulation or fibrous tissue. Most resolve spontaneously.

MANAGEMENT OF PSEUDOCYST

The management approach to pseudocyst is often discussed as a single entity regardless of the aetiology and presentation. Pseudocysts consequent on chronic pancreatitis usually result from fibrosis/stricturing with secondary proximal ductal disruption, rarely settle spontaneously and contain clear fluid, whereas acute pseudocysts result from organisation of acute peripancreatic fluid collections or parenchymal necrosis that involves the ductal system and normally contain solid components. They may or may not communicate with the duct system. Management is determined by an understanding of the anatomy (CT), the ductal morphology (ERCP), the presence or absence of solid material (MR/EUS) and the clinical condition of the patient. As a general rule, definitive management should be delayed until all organ dysfunction has resolved and can often be performed simultaneously with management of cholelithiasis (see above).

Asymptomatic pseudocysts do not require treatment. Acute pseudocysts are most commonly retrogastric (**Fig. 11.2**), and may or may not link to a disrupted pancreatic duct. Three-quarters will be associated with a mild to moderate hyperamylasaemia.[110] In symptomatic cysts, a conservative policy may be warranted for up to 12 weeks from the onset of acute pancreatitis as up to 50% of these may resolve.[111] This policy is not, however, without risk as pseudocyst rupture or abscess formation[112] may occur. The likelihood of resolution is related at least in part to pseudocyst size, and if conservative treatment fails the options are percutaneous, endoscopic or surgical drainage. Where duct integrity is not compromised percutaneous or internal EUS-guided aspiration/drainage is appropriate. The technique of endoscopic cystgastrostomy was first described by Baron et al.,[113] initially by blind puncture of a cyst bulging into the stomach wall using side-viewing endoscopes. This has been subsequently refined using endoscopic ultrasound guidance. Where disruption of the pancreatic duct has occurred, transpapillary duct stenting can aid resolution. Strictures within the pancreatic duct system are less common than with chronic pseudocysts but when present should be managed by stricture dilatation prior to stenting. The presence of necrosis should be considered a relative contraindication to simple drainage techniques as drain blockage and secondary infection are common. Endoscopic techniques may, however, form part of an overall management strategy. Open or laparoscopic surgical drainage with a cystgastrostomy or cyst-jejunostomy is usually reliable in those cases inaccessible to the endoscope or where local expertise is unavailable, and has the advantage of simultaneous cholecystectomy and effective clearance of any associated necrotic material.

An acute pseudocyst is a collection of pancreatic juice enclosed in a wall of fibrous or granulation tissue that arises following an attack of acute pancreatitis. Formation of pseudocyst requires 4 or more weeks from the onset of acute pancreatitis.

PANCREATIC DUCT FISTULA

This complication most commonly follows prior intervention for pseudocyst or infected necrosis, and manifests as persistent drainage of amylase-rich opalescent fluid, in the absence of significant sepsis. Management is similar to that of a communicating pseudocyst, initially by transpapillary stenting where possible. Intraperitoneal rupture of a pseudocyst can result in pancreatic ascites or pleural effusion. More invasive management of a persistent fistula, either inaccessible or failing to respond to ductal stenting, should be delayed until the patients has

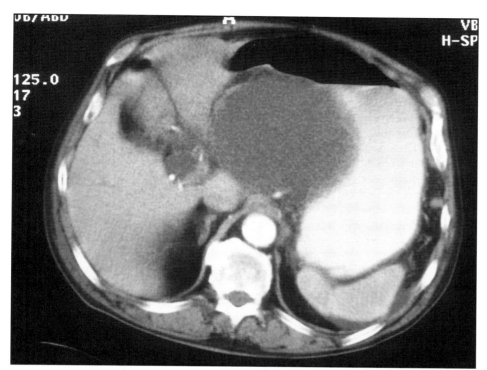

Figure 11.2 • Postinflammatory pancreatic pseudocyst.

made a full recovery, and often requires surgical resection (distal pancreatectomy) of an isolated functional tail following central glandular necrosis.

Management of necrosis

Management strategies for pancreatic necrosis are in the process of evolution and the indications for intervention blurred. Until the mid-1990s, treatment was initially supportive, but radical surgical intervention was recommended for all patients developing secondary infection, or those with extensive necrosis failing to respond to conservative measures. It has been recognised for some time that the outcome for patients undergoing major surgery whilst in established multiorgan failure is poor, and that heroic surgery often preceded a terminal decline. It is not the necrosis itself that drives the organ dysfunction, but rather uncontrolled sepsis. The traditional surgical approach of radical debridement evolved because the associated necrosis tended to lead to problems with inadequate drainage and recurrent or uncontrolled sepsis. Contemporary management aims to primarily control the sepsis to

allow recovery of organ function, the necrosis itself being a secondary issue. This may be achieved by a variety of percutaneous, endoscopic, laparoscopic or open procedures, several techniques often being employed in an individual patient's management. Consequently the universal application of a single technique to a consecutive series of patients is gradually changing to a more flexible approach, based on the individual needs of the patient at the time of intervention.

MANAGEMENT OF PANCREATIC OR PERIPANCREATIC NECROSIS

The necrotic process associated with pancreatitis tends to involve both the pancreatic parenchyma and surrounding adipose tissue. Indeed, significant quantities of necrotic peripancreatic tissue can be present with an essentially viable gland. Complications relate to the extent of the necrotic process, and in particular the extent of parenchymal necrosis. Early aggressive debridement in the absence of infection has been advocated.[114] However, mortality in this series was 25% overall, and the only randomised study of early versus late (>12 days) necrosectomy was discontinued as a result of the mortality rate in the early treatment group (56% vs. 27%).[115] The general principle is now to withhold surgery in the early phase of disease, operating for complications ideally once the acute inflammatory insult has subsided.

Most centres report the overall mortality in patients with necrosis associated with severe acute pancreatitis to be around 10% for those with sterile necrosis and 25–30% should secondary infection occur.[116-118] Some of these series only report the results from patients undergoing surgical intervention and not the outcome of the overall group. Many patients with proven necrosis, particularly those with severe MODS in the first week, may never undergo surgical intervention.

MANAGEMENT OF STERILE NECROSIS

The development of retroperitoneal necrosis secondary to acute pancreatitis is not in itself an indication for surgery. Both Bradley and Buchler and colleagues have shown that necrosis can be treated adequately.[54,56,119] There is undoubtedly a relationship between the extent of necrosis and the development of secondary infection necessitating surgery. There is also debate regarding the role of debridement in patients failing to respond to conservative treatment. Early debridement does not improve outcome; however, some specialists advocate debridement in patients with static organ dysfunction after several weeks. Uomo and colleagues have shown that surgical intervention may have a detrimental effect on outcome.[120] In addition, the majority of postinflammatory fluid

collections associated with a significant quantity of sterile necrosis will organise into a postinflammatory pseudocyst, which can be managed with relatively low morbidity and mortality as described above. Our own policy therefore is to avoid surgery where possible in these patients and to delay any intervention until the quiescent phase (>6 weeks) of the acute illness, to avoid undue exacerbation of the inflammatory response. The management of these patients is discussed in the section dealing with fluid collections associated with necrosis.

IDENTIFICATION OF INFECTION/ROLE OF FNAC

In the 1990s the identification of secondary infection within necrosis was considered the cornerstone of management. It was known that sterile necrosis could generally be managed by continued conservative management, whereas infected necrosis mandated surgical intervention. The mortality in patients with multiorgan failure undergoing radical debridement led to an approach whereby a conservative policy was followed unless infection was proven to be present. Patients with a significant quantity of retroperitoneal necrosis usually have evidence of SIRS, and therefore the clinical discrimination between infected and non-infected necrosis can be difficult. In patients with a secondary deterioration in organ failure scores or systemic signs of infection, a CT- or US-guided FNAC[121,122] of the pancreatic or peripancreatic area was performed (**Fig. 11.3a,b**), the confirmation of infection changing the management approach. Occasionally, despite negative culture, the clinical picture is

(a)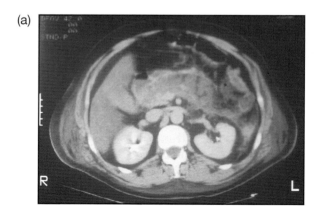

(b)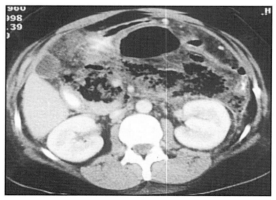

Figure 11.3 • **(a)** Acute pancreatitis with necrosis. **(b)** Retroperitoneal gas.

sufficiently convincing to warrant surgery, and in these infection of the necrotic tissue was often confirmed postoperatively. This remains the policy in many centres.

Our own approach has progressed from one based on the presence/absence of infection to one based on organ dysfunction. Infected collections, even those containing gas, may be observed provided the patient is clinically well and recovering with conservative treatment. Patients with profound organ dysfunction in whom we suspect secondary infection will undergo percutaneous drainage of peripancreatic collections, with later staged percutaneous or open management of the necrosis as clinically appropriate.

We no longer perform routine diagnostic FNAC but this is occasionally performed in order to exclude infection in patients with sepsis syndrome, in order to justify continued conservative management. CT-guided percutaneous drainage and staged intervention has therefore superseded our previous algorithm of diagnostic FNAC followed by surgery if positive. Decision-making in these patients is extremely difficult and is best carried out within an experienced multidisciplinary team.

Management of pancreatic sepsis

Secondary pancreatic or peripancreatic infection is a frequent complication of severe acute pancreatitis. The clinical consequences and management strategy vary according to the duration between the initial presentation and the onset of infection, the clinical condition of the patient, and the amount of solid necrotic material present. The morbidity and mortality associated with intervention for true infected necrosis (up to 6 weeks following presentation) is very different to that associated with drainage of a well-demarcated infected pseudocyst (abscess) presenting at a later stage. These require different approaches and should be considered as separate entities on a spectrum of pancreatic sepsis. Many series, however, report results on all-comers and are inevitably heavily biased by patient selection.

MANAGEMENT OF INFECTED NECROSIS

Infected pancreatic necrosis has been described as the most feared surgical complication of acute pancreatitis. It occurs in 8–12% of patients with acute pancreatitis, and up to 70% with necrotising pancreatitis,[123] and in these patients mortality without intervention approaches 100%.[123] The management of infected necrosis requiring intervention within 4 or 5 weeks of presentation should be considered a separate entity from a pancreatic abscess containing some necrotic material, which presents later (6–12 weeks) and from which recovery is the norm.

Fifty years ago, surgical exploration in severe acute pancreatitis was almost universally fatal.[124] In 1963 Watts[125] described the survival of one patient following a total pancreatectomy. Further experience of resective procedures for necrosis, however, confirmed the morbidity and mortality to be prohibitive.[126]

Surgical teaching was that without adequate clearance of all necrotic material, death was inevitable, and any delay in surgical intervention resulted in higher mortality once infection had occurred.[127] Until the 1970s, standard management of this condition involved partial or total resective procedures but the mortality was often >50%.[128] Open surgical debridement of devitalised tissue and simple postoperative drainage was associated with a more favourable outcome,[75] but the requirement for repeated surgical intervention remained, mainly due to recurrent sepsis. This has led to the development of a variety of techniques,[117,129] described below, aimed at preventing recurrent sepsis in the pancreatic bed. This aggressive surgical policy, coupled with optimum intensive care management, has resulted in an improvement in survival, although even in specialist units, the mortality for true infected necrosis remains between 20 and 25%.

Methods of necrosectomy

Laparotomy/debridement By the 1970s the technique of pancreatic debridement had grown in popularity, and involved a wide exposure of the abdomen, usually through a bilateral subcostal/rooftop incision. Both colonic flexures are mobilised to expose the retroperitoneum and the lesser sac entered via the gastrocolic omentum, or occasionally the transverse mesocolon. The retroperitoneum is opened, and pus is aspirated widely, opening the anterior aspect of the abscess cavity and allowing necrotic material to be removed by a blunt 'finger' dissection technique, leaving all viable tissue. Tissue

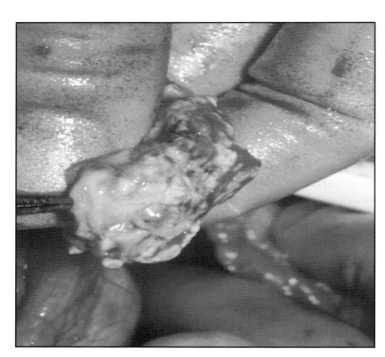

Figure 11.4 • Solid necrotic material removed at necrosectomy by blunt finger dissection.

that will not come away by finger teasing should be left in situ to demarcate. Blind resection of a dusky pancreatic tail should be avoided as much of the central gland may be viable. The procedure may also include a cholecystectomy, operative cholangiogram and a feeding jejunostomy. Whilst there has been debate regarding the optimal postoperative management of the necrotic cavity, blunt finger debridement (**Fig. 11.4**) remains the most widely adopted technique for removal of the necrotic tissue.

Several methods can be used in **postoperative management of the debridement cavity** after laparotomy.

1. **Drainage/'closed packing'.** Simple drainage, often with multiple retroperitoneal tube drains, has been the conventional approach to the postoperative management of the debrided pancreatic and peripancreatic bed. Whilst mortality was less than with resective procedures, multiple second-look laparotomies were often required for residual sepsis. The initial results reported by Warshaw and colleagues[75] showed respectable mortality figures of 24% using this technique. However,

over 40% of the patients treated had pancreatic abscess rather than true infected necrosis. Their technique has been modified[130] using multiple soft Penrose drains containing cotton gauze to pack the cavity following completion of the necrosectomy. These are subsequently removed at intervals allowing the cavity to collapse around the drains. Warshaw's reported mortality rate using this technique is the lowest in the literature (6.2%), although the series included patients with sterile necrosis (11%) and pancreatic abscess (39%), and only 14% had both sepsis syndrome and a positive culture requiring early intervention, which is indicative of the difficulties in interpreting the available literature.[75]

2. **Open packing.** Bradley and his colleagues from Atlanta have been the principal proponents of the open laparostomy technique.[129] In this, at the conclusion of the debridement, the lesser sac is packed with lubricated cotton gauze, and the abdomen left open, allowing planned re-explorations every few days until granulation tissue forms. Enteric fistula and secondary haemorrhage are not uncommon, and the technique is rarely performed as a first option.

Surgical packing and planned re-operation is, however, sometimes required to control blood loss from the retroperitoneum following the development of an intraoperative coagulopathy, a lavage system being created, following correction of the coagulopathy, at the time of subsequent pack removal.

3. **Limited lateral (retroperitoneal) approach/open laparostomy.** Fagniez and colleagues[131] described a similar technique utilising a limited loin/subcostal retrocolic approach for debridement of pancreatic and peripancreatic necrosis. However, the technique was associated with major morbidity (enteric fistula 45%, haemorrhage 40%, and colonic necrosis 15%), and has not gained popularity.

4. **Closed lavage.** Radical debridement combined with postoperative closed lavage, as described by Beger et al.,[117] is considered the current gold standard for the management of infected pancreatic necrosis, the aim of the lavage being the continuous removal of devitalised necrotic material and bacteria. Several (4–6) large-diameter tube drains are inserted in the lesser sac and throughout the abdomen, and the abdomen is closed. Continuous lavage is then commenced, our own preference being for continuous amulatory peritoneal dialysis (CAPD) dialysis fluid (Dianil 7, Baxter Healthcare, potassium free, iso-osmolar) warmed through a blood warmer and delivered at 500 mL/h. The lavage is continued, for around 3–4 weeks on average, until the return fluid is clear, and the patient has no residual signs of systemic sepsis. This technique has been adopted with minor variations by centres on both sides of the Atlantic.[118,132–134]

Minimally invasive approaches to infected necrosis Minimally invasive surgery has been consistently shown to be associated with a lesser activation of the inflammatory response than equivalent open surgery, and there is experimental evidence suggesting that local sepsis and the inflammatory response may be lessened by a minimally invasive rather than an open technique. It has been suggested that by minimising the massive inflammatory 'hit' of open pancreatic necrosectomy, a minimally invasive approach to the management of infected pancreatic necrosis may lessen the risk of multiple organ failure, and reduce respiratory and wound morbidity in these patients.

1. **Percutaneous drainage.** Freeny and his colleagues,[135] combining aggressive CT-guided percutaneous drainage with continuous post-drainage lavage, showed that nearly half the pancreatic abscesses may resolve. However, he required a median of four drains per patient and postoperative lavage lasting a mean of 87 days. More than half of these patients required subsequent surgical intervention for residual sepsis. Drain occlusion is common due to necrotic debris and small diameter drains.

2. **Endoscopic drainage.** In 1996, Baron et al.[113] described a variation on this approach, combining endoscopic cyst-gastrostomy with naso-cyst lavage, and reported good results in an initial series of 11 patients. Three-quarters of his patients had pseudocysts rather than abscesses (only 28% were infected at the time of drainage), at a median of 7 weeks following the onset of their illness. Postprocedure infection of the necrotic tissue occurred in 38% of their patients, requiring further intervention and highlighting the need for removal of necrotic tissue from the abscess cavity.[136] Solid debris preventing drainage was again a problem, and 60% of those patients successfully drained developed further collections in the subsequent 2 years.[137]

Minimally invasive approaches to the management of necrosis Simple percutaneous or endoscopic drainage alone rarely result in complete resolution; however, they may have a useful role as a temporising measure in the hope of finding a 'window of opportunity' in which to perform more definitive intervention. Careful drain management is required to recognise drain blockage early and prevent recurrent sepsis. As a result of the difficulties in maintaining drain patency, we in Glasgow have developed a technique[138] to allow minimally invasive drainage, and in addition removal of the necrotic component. This involves the intraoperative dilatation of a previously placed CT-guided percutaneous drain tract, and subsequent necrosectomy using a urological rigid rod lens system. Complete resolution of sepsis and necrosis can occur without recourse to further surgery, and the need for postoperative organ support is lessened compared to the open procedures.[139] However, whether this technique can reduce overall mortality remains open to question. The principle of tract dilatation and minimally invasive necrosectomy has also been used with the endoscopic approach. Seifert et al.[140] have reported the dilatation of the endo-cyst-gastrotomy tract, allowing insertion of the endoscope into the retro-peritoneum, and subsequent piecemeal debridement.

Summary

In the last 20 years the technique of open surgical debridement has included necrosectomy with simple drainage, second-look procedures, open laparostomies, necrosectomy with packing, or with postoperative lavage. Minimally invasive approaches, either endoscopic or percutaneous, have been associated with low rates of resolution due to the inability to remove the necrotic debris, and should be discouraged except as a temporising procedure in the occasional patient with severe organ dysfunction in whom a delayed necrosectomy is planned. Our own percutaneous necrosectomy technique is in its early stages, as is the endoscopic approach.

The management of infected necrosis has changed radically in the last few years. A flexible approach has emerged, often combining several techniques in a single patient, weighing up the risks of intervention against the need for adequate control of sepsis.

Our own preference is to reserve open exploration for patients with secondary complications or extensive necrosis once organ failure has resolved. In these we perform a radical retroperitoneal debridement, with vigorous postoperative lavage. Packing of the abdomen is normally reserved for patients with significant intraoperative bleeding, in whom a lavage system is created at the time of pack removal.

Patients with significant organ failure undergo initial percutaneous drainage, with tract dilatation and cavity lavage, if appropriate, until the organ failure has resolved.

MANAGEMENT OF PANCREATIC ABSCESS

A pancreatic abscess is a circumscribed intra-abdominal collection of pus, usually in proximity to the pancreas, that contains little or no pancreatic necrosis and arises as a consequence of acute pancreatitis.

Pancreatic abscess usually results from secondary infection of a postinflammatory pseudocyst. The endoscopic technique of Baron described above has been used in this situation with reasonably good effect, but there is a significant risk of haemorrhage from blind puncture of the abscess wall. As a result, Giovannini modified the technique to an EUS-guided puncture, and reported resolution of sepsis in nearly 90% of cases.[141] Problems with ultimate resolution due to residual necrosis have led to some specialists favouring a more formal approach to drainage of the cavity. Most prefer internal drainage through the back wall of the stomach, rather than by the open necrosectomy, which may be associated with a prolonged recovery. Therefore, in patients thought unlikely to resolve through percutaneous or endoscopic drainage, a cyst-gastrostomy may be performed, which involves creating a formal 5–10-cm surgical fistula between the abscess cavity and the back wall of the stomach, draining the cyst into the back wall of the stomach, with formal clearance of any associated necrotic tissue. This transgastric procedure may be performed either through a laparotomy incision or laparoscopically. Cholecystectomy, if required for definitive gallstone control, should be performed simultaneously. This mode of management is only appropriate once the cyst/abscess wall has matured for a minimum of 6–8 weeks following the acute attack and where the cyst/abscess is located in the retrogastric area.

Open or laparoscopic surgical exploration of the abscess is the treatment of choice, allowing adequate drainage and debridement of any associated necrosis. In the absence of necrosis, or when the patient is deemed unfit for exploration, percutaneous or endoscopic drainage, combined with lavage, may be successful.

Specific late complications

HAEMORRHAGE

Rarely, life-threatening haemorrhage may occur acutely into pancreatic necrosis within the first week following presentation, and requires mesenteric embolisation or surgical exploration. However, a relatively common problem following prior necrosectomy is postoperative reactionary haemorrhage, due to a combination of a large raw surface, partly controlled sepsis and exposed major vessels. Urgent operative intervention and surgical control may be required, sometimes necessitating ligation of proximal visceral vessels. However, the combination of haemorrhage and subsequent laparotomy frequently precipitate escalating organ failure and death. Angiography and embolisation, with endovascular metal coils, is therefore the treatment of choice.

SEGMENTAL PORTAL HYPERTENSION AND GASTROINTESTINAL HAEMORRHAGE

Splenic vein thrombosis is associated with up to 15% of patients dying with acute pancreatitis.[142] In those patients with thrombosis that survive the acute attack, the splenic venous drainage diverted through the short gastric vessels may result in patients developing large venous collaterals. Short gastric and lienocolic varices may make surgery on late complications of an acute pancreatitic episode hazardous. When necessary, splenectomy is curative. Despite the frequency of venous collaterals on

follow-up CT, late gastrointestinal haemorrhage through gastric varices is in practice rare. Ulcer-associated gastrointestinal haemorrhage is no more common than with other acute illnesses, and prophylactic use of proton pump inhibitors has probably reduced the incidence of bleeding from oesophageal or gastric erosions or peptic ulceration. The majority of patients can be controlled using endoscopic methods with adrenaline (epinephrine) injection combined with heater probe coagulation or sclerosants. Any bleeding, either enteric or through drains, should raise suspicion of a pseudoaneurysm of a major vessel.

PANCREATIC DUCT STRICTURE

Pancreatic duct stricture (**Fig. 11.5**) can occur following resolution of an attack of acute pancreatitis as a result of local tissue damage and fibrotic repair. It may be present on its own, or in association with a duct disruption causing a pseudocyst or pancreatic fistula. Isolated pancreatic duct stricture can result in recurrent attacks of abdominal pain, sometimes with hyperamylasaemia and with dilatation of the distal duct system. Management of the stricture may be by simple dilatation and temporary stenting, by surgical resection of the stricture along with the pancreatic

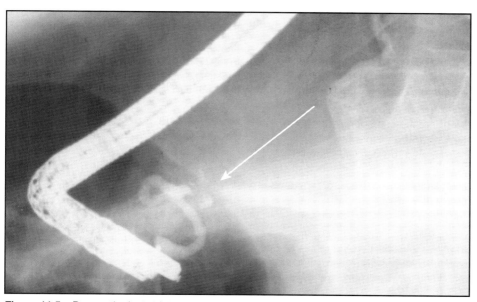

Figure 11.5 • Pancreatic duct stricture.

tail, or by surgical drainage of the pancreatic duct system into a Roux loop.

GASTRIC OUTLET OBSTRUCTION

Gastric outlet obstruction resulting in persistent vomiting or high-volume gastric aspirates from nasogastric suction may complicate up to 10% of patients with severe acute pancreatitis. The recent trend towards nasojejunal intubation has rendered this complication less troublesome, and the majority of patients can be treated by nasoenteric feeding until the local oedema/ileus settles. Occasionally a gastroenterostomy is required for longstanding gastric stasis.

• Key points

Eight-five percent of episodes of acute pancreatitis are mild and settle spontaneously on conservative management.

Patients with any evidence of organ dysfunction after initial resuscitation should be managed within an HDU/ITU environment.

Discussion with, but not necessarily transfer to, a Regional Centre is appropriate for patients with severe disease. The mainstay of early management is aggressive resuscitation and organ support where necessary and can often be carried out locally. Transfer may be required for the small percentage requiring subsequent intervention.

There is no evidence that outcome is improved by any pharmacological intervention.

ERCP and sphincterotomy is indicated only in patients with coexistent cholangitis.

The evidence for/against the use of prophylactic antibiotics is equivocal, and antibiotics, if given, should probably be restricted to those with proven necrosis on CT and for a time-limited course.

Nutritional support should be by the enteral route where tolerated.

Intervention is indicated for infected necrosis, the aim being sepsis control. Drainage may be achieved through a variety of percutaneous, endoscopic or surgical methods as determined by the individual clinical presentation and comorbidity.

REFERENCES

1. McKay CJ, Evans S, Sinclair M et al. High early mortality rate from acute pancreatitis in Scotland, 1984–1995. Br J Surg 1999; 86:1302–5.

   Authors' own review providing clear information on demographic presentation and outcome.

2. Appelros S, Borgstrom A. Incidence, aetiology and mortality rate of acute pancreatitis over 10 years in a defined urban population in Sweden. Br J Surg 1999; 86:465–70.

3. Halvorsen F-A, Ritland S. Acute pancreatitis in Buskerud County, Norway: Incidence and etiology. Scand J Gastroenterol 1996; 31:411–14.

4. Mero M. Changing aetiology of acute pancreatitis. Annales Chir Gynaecol 1982; 71:126–9.

5. Sainio V, Kemppainen E, Puolakkainen P et al. Early antibiotic treatment in acute necrotising pancreatitis. Lancet 1995; 346:663–7.

6. Fan ST, Choi TK, Lai ECS et al. Prediction of severity of acute pancreatitis: an alternative approach. Gut 1989; 30:1591–5.

7. Lankisch, PG. Epidemiology of acute pancreatitis. In: Buchler MW, Uhl W, Friess H et al. (eds) Acute pancreatitis: novel concepts in biology and therapy. Oxford: Blackwell Science, 1999; pp. 145–54.

8. Opie EL. The etiology of acute hemorrhagic pancreatitis. Bull Johns Hopkins Hosp 1901; 12:182–8.

9. Runzi M, Saluja A, Lerch MM et al. Early ductal decompression prevents the progression of biliary pancreatitis: An experimental study in the opossum. Gastroenterology 1993; 105:157–64.

10. Hofbauer B, Saluja AK, Lerch MM et al. Intra-acinar cell activation of trypsinogen during caerulein-induced pancreatitis in rats. Am J Physiol 1998; 275:G352–G362.

11. Ohshio G, Saluja A, Steer ML. Effects of short-term pancreatic duct obstruction in rats. Gastroenterology 1991; 100:196–202.

12. Steer ML. Early events in acute pancreatitis. Baillière's Best Pract Clin Gastroenterol 1999; 13(2):213–25.

13. Saluja AK, Bhagat L, Lee HS et al. Secretagogue-induced digestive enzyme activation and cell injury in rat pancreatic acini. Am J Physiol 1999; 276:G835–G842.

14. Raraty MGT, Petersen OH, Sutton R et al. Intracellular free ionized calcium in the pathogenesis of acute pancreatitis. Baillière's Best Pract Clin Gastroenterol 1999; 13(2):241–51.

15. Katz M, Carangelo R, Miller LJ et al. Effect of ethanol on cholecystokinin-stimulated zymogen conversion in pancreatic acinar cells. Am J Physiol 1996; 270:G171–G175.

16. Sarles H. Proposal adopted unanimously by the participants of the symposium on pancreatitis at Marseilles, 1963. Bibl Gastroenterol 1965; 7:VII–VIII.

17. Sarner M, Cotton P. Classification of pancreatitis. Gut 1984; 25:756–9.

18. Singer P, Gyr K, Sarles H. Revised classification of pancreatitis. Gastroenterology 1985; 89:683–5.

19. Bradley EL, International Symposium on Acute Pancreatitis AAS1. A Clinically Based Classification System for Acute Pancreatitis. Arch Surg 1993; 128:586–90.

20. McKay CJ, Curran F, Sharples C et al. Prospective placebo-controlled randomized trial of lexipafant in predicted severe acute pancreatitis. Br J Surg 1997; 84:1239–43.

21. Johnson CD, Kingsnorth AN, Imrie CW et al. Double blind, randomised, placebo controlled study of a platelet activating factor antagonist, lexipafant, in the treatment and prevention of organ failure in predicted severe acute pancreatitis. Gut 2002; 48:62–9.

22. Buter A, Imrie CW, Carter CR et al. Dynamic nature of early organ dysfunction determines outcome in acute pancreatitis. Br J Surg 2002; 89:298–302.

23. Isenmann R, Rau B, Beger HG. Early severe acute pancreatitis: characteristics of a new subgroup. Pancreas 2001; 22:274–8.

24. Beger HG, Rau B, Mayer J et al. Natural course of acute pancreatitis. World J Surg 1997; 21:130–5.

25. Beger HG, Bittner R, Block S et al. Bacterial contamination of pancreatic necrosis. A prospective clinical study. Gastroenterology 1986; 91:433–8.

26. Banerjee AK, Kaul A, Bache E et al. An audit of fatal acute pancreatitis. Postgrad Med J 1995; 71:472–5.

27. Ranson HJC, Rifkind KM, Roses DF et al. Prognostic signs and the role of operative management in acute pancreatitis. Surg Gynaecol Obstet 1974; 139:69–81.

28. Underwood TW, Frye CB. Drug induced pancreatitis. Clin Pharm 1993; 12:440–8.

29. Parsons WG, Carr-Locke DL. Endoscopic retrograde cholangiopancreatography. In: Beger HG, Warshaw AL, Buchler MW et al. (eds) Pancreas. Oxford: Blackwell Science, 1998; pp. 231–46.

30. Freeman ML, DiSario JA, Nelson DB et al. Risk factors for post-ERCP pancreatitis: a prospective, multicenter study. Gastrointest Endosc 2001; 54:425–34.

31. Murray B, Carter R, Imrie C et al. Diclofenac reduces the incidence of acute pancreatitis after endoscopic retrograde cholangiopancreatography. Gastroenterology 2003; 124:1786–91.

32. Davenport M, Howard ER. Acute pancreatitis associated with congenital abnormalities. In: Beger HG, Warshaw AL, Buchler MW et al. (eds) Pancreas. Oxford: Blackwell Science, 1998; pp. 343–54.

33. O'Reilly DA, Kingsnorth AN. Hereditary pancreatitis and mutations of the cationic trypsinogen gene. Br J Surg. 2000; 87:708–17.

34. Blamey SL, Imrie CW, O'Neill J et al. Prognostic factors in acute pancreatitis. Gut 1984; 25:1340–6.
Author's own early work on prognostic scoring system.

35. Corfield AP, Cooper MJ, Williamson RCN. Prediction of severity in acute pancreatitis: Prospective comparison of three prognostic indices. Lancet 1985; 2:403–7.

36. Wilson C, Heath DI, Imrie CW. Prediction of outcome in acute pancreatitis: A comparative study of APACHE II, clinical assessment and multiple factor scoring systems. Br J Surg 1990; 77:1260–4.
Author's own early work on prognostic scoring system.

37. Dominguez-Munoz JE, Carballo F, Garcia MJ et al. Evaluation of the clinical usefulness of APACHE II and SAPS systems in the initial prognostic classification of acute pancreatitis: A multicenter study. Pancreas 1993; 8:682–6.

38. Puolakkainen P, Valtonen V, Paananen A et al. C-reactive protein (CRP) and serum phospholipase A2 in the assessment of the severity of acute pancreatitis. Gut 1987; 28:764–71.

39. Wilson C, Heads A, Shenkin A et al. C-reactive protein, antiproteases and complement factors as objective markers of severity in acute pancreatitis. Br J Surg 1989; 76:177–81.

40. Viedma JA, Perez-Mateo M, Dominguez-Munoz JE et al. Role of interleukin-6 in acute pancreatitis. Comparison with C-reactive protein and phospholipase A2. Gut 1992; 33:1264–7.

41. Gudgeon AM, Heath DI, Hurley P et al. Trypsinogen activation peptides assay in the early prediction of severity of acute pancreatitis. Lancet 1990; 335:4–8.

42. Kemppainen E, Mayer J, Puolakkainen P et al. Plasma trypsinogen activation peptide in patients with acute pancreatitis. Br J Surg 2001; 88:679–80.

43. Johnson CD, Lempinen M, Imrie CW et al. Urinary trypsinogen activation peptide as a marker of severe acute pancreatitis. Br J Surg 2004; 91:1027–33.

44. Dominguez-Munoz JE, Carballo F, Garcia MJ et al. Clinical usefulness of polymorphonuclear elastase in predicting the severity of acute pancreatitis: results of a multicentre study. Br J Surg 1991; 78:1230–4.

45. Uhl W, Beger HG. Prediction of severity in acute pancreatitis. HPB Surg 1991; 5(1):61–4.

46. Bone RC, Balk RA, Cerra FB et al. Definitions for sepsis and organ failure and guidelines for the use of innovative therapies in sepsis. The ACCP/SCCM Consensus Conference Committee. American College of Chest Physicians/Society of Critical Care Medicine. Chest 1992; 101:1644–55.

47. Glazer G, Mann DV. United Kingdom Guidelines in the management of acute pancreatitis. Gut 1998; 42:S1–S13.

    Current UK guideline document on management of acute pancreatitis.

48. Rau B, Pralle U, Mayer JM et al. Role of ultra-sonographically guided fine-needle aspiration cytology in the diagnosis of infected pancreatic necrosis. Br J Surg 1998; 85:179–84.

49. Foitzik T, Bassi DG, Schmidt J et al. Intravenous contrast medium accentuates the severity of acute necrotizing pancreatitis in the rat. Gastroenterology 1994; 106:207–14.

50. Balthazar EJ, Ranson JHC, Naidich DP et al. Acute pancreatitis: prognostic value of CT. Radiology 1985; 156:767–72.

51. Balthazar EJ, Robinson DL, Megibow AJ et al. Acute pancreatitis: Value of CT in establishing prognosis. Radiology 1990; 174:331–6.

52. Dervenis C, Johnson CD, Bassi C et al. Diagnosis, objective assessment of severity, and management of acute pancreatitis. Santorini consensus conference. Int J Pancreatol 1999; 25:195–210.

53. Uhl W, Warshaw A, Imrie C et al. IAP Guidelines for the Surgical Management of Acute Pancreatitis. Pancreatology 2003; 2:565–73.

    International guidelines on the management of acute pancreatitis.

54. Bradley EL III, Allen K. A prospective longitudinal study of observation versus surgical intervention in the management of necrotizing pancreatitis. Am J Surg 1991; 161:19–25.

55. Rau B, Pralle U, Uhl W et al. Operative vs non-operative management in sterile necrotizing pancreatitis. HPB Surg 1997; 10:188–91.

56. Buchler MW, Gloor B, Muller CA et al. Acute necrotizing pancreatitis: treatment strategy according to the status of infection. Ann Surg 2000; 232:619–26.

57. Foitzik T, Hotz HG, Kinzig M et al. Improvement of pancreatic capillary blood flow does not augment the pancreatic tissue concentration of imipenem in acute experimental pancreatitis. Eur Surg Res 1996; 28:395–401.

58. Araida T, Frey CF, Ruebner B et al. Therapeutic regimens in acute experimental pancreatitis in rats: Effects of a protease inhibitor, a beta-agonist, and antibiotic. Pancreas 1995; 11:132–40.

59. Widdison AL, Karanjia ND, Reber HA. Anti-microbial treatment of pancreatic infection in cats. Br J Surg 1994; 81:886–9.

60. Mithofer K, Fernandez-Del Castillo C, Ferraro MJ et al. Antibiotic treatment improves survival in experimental acute necrotizing pancreatitis. Gastroenterology 1996; 110:232–40.

61. Howes R, Zuidema GD, Cameron JL. Evaluation of prophylactic antibiotics in acute pancreatitis. J Surg Res 1975; 18:197–200.

62. Craig RM, Dordal E, Myles L. The use of ampicillin and acute pancreatitis. Ann Intern Med 1975; 83:831–2.

63. Finch WT, Sawyers JL, Schencker S. A prospective study to determine the efficacy of antibiotics in acute pancreatitis. Ann Surg 1976; 183:667–71.

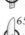

64. Pederzoli P, Bassi C, Vesentini S et al. A randomized multicenter clinical trial of antibiotic prophylaxis of septic complications in acute necrotizing pancreatitis with imipenem. Surg Gynecol Obstet 1993; 176:480–3.

65. Delcenserie R, Yzet T, Ducroix JP. Prophylactic antibiotics in treatment of severe acute alcoholic pancreatitis. Pancreas 1996; 13:198–201.

66. Schwarz M, Meyer H, Isenmann R et al. Antibiotic prophylaxis for reduction of complications in acute necrotizing pancreatitis. Zentralblatt Chir 1997; 123:28–31.

67. Bassi C, Falconi M, Talamini G et al. Controlled clinical trial of pefloxacin versus imipenem in severe acute pancreatitis. Gastroenterology 1998; 115:1513–7.

    Key studies that have failed to demonstrate convincing evidence for routine use of prophylactic antibiotics in acute pancreatitis.

68. Luiten EJT, Hop WCJ, Lange JF et al. Controlled clinical trial of selective decontamination for the treatment of severe acute pancreatitis. Ann Surg 1995; 222:57–65.

69. Isenman R, Kron M, Sander S et al. Ciprofloxacin/ Metronidazole in patients with severe acute pancreatitis – results of a double blind placebo controlled multicentre trial. Pancreas 2002; 25:433 (abstr.).

70. Delcenserie R, Delion-Lozinguez MP, Nord CHU et al. Prophylactic ciprofloxacin treatment in acute necrotising pancreatitis: a prospective randomised multicentre clinical trial. Gastroenterology 2003; 120:A-25–119.

71. Eatock FC, Brombacher GD, Hood J et al. Fungal infection of pancreatic necrosis is associated with increased mortality. Br J Surg 1999; 86:78 (abstr.).

72. Grew, M., Tsiotos GG, Luque-de Leon E et al. Fungal infection in acute necrotising pancreatitis. J Am Coll Surg 1999; 188:408–13.

275

73. De Waele JJ, Vogelaers D, Blot S et al. Fungal infections in patients with severe acute pancreatitis and the use of prophylactic therapy. Clin Infect Dis 2003; 37:208–13.

Three studies highlighting the risk of fungal infection in acute necrotising pancreatitis.

74. Powell JJ, Campbell E, Johnson CD et al. Survey of antibiotic prophylaxis in acute pancreatitis in the UK and Ireland. Br J Surg 1999; 86:320–2.

75. Warshaw AL, Jin G. Improved survival in 45 patients with pancreatic abscess. Ann Surg 1985; 202:408–15.

76. Bradley EL III. A fifteen year experience with open drainage for infected pancreatic necrosis. Surg Gynaecol Obstet 1993; 177:215–22.

77. Farkas G, Marton J, Mandi Y et al. Surgical strategy and management of infected pancreatic necrosis. Br J Surg 1996; 83:930–3.

78. Navarro S, Ros E, Aused R et al. Comparison of fasting, nasogastric suction and cimetidine in the treatment of acute pancreatitis. Digestion 1984; 30:224–30.

79. Moore EE, Moore FA. Immediate enteral nutrition following multisystem trauma: a decade perspective. J Am Coll Nutr 1991; 10:633–48.

80. Nakad A, Piessevaux H, Marot J-C et al. Is early enteral nutrition in acute pancreatitis dangerous? About 20 patients fed by an endoscopically placed nasogastrojejunal tube. Pancreas 1998; 17:187–93.

81. McClave SA, Greene LM, Snider HL et al. Comparison of the safety of early enteral vs parenteral nutrition in mild acute pancreatitis. J Parenteral Enteral Nutr 1997; 21:14–20.

82. Kalfarentzos F, Kehagias J, Mead N et al. Enteral nutrition is superior to parenteral nutrition in severe acute pancreatitis: Results of a randomized prospective trial. Br J Surg 1997; 84:1665–9.

83. Abou-Assi S, Craig K, O'Keefe SJ. Hypocaloric jejunal feeding is better than total parenteral nutrition in acute pancreatitis: results of a randomized comparative study. Am J Gastroenterol 2002; 97:2255–62.

84. Windsor ACJ, Kanwar S, Li AGK et al. Compared with parenteral nutrition, enteral feeding attenuates the acute phase response and improves disease severity in acute pancreatitis. Gut 1998; 42:431–5.

85. Cassim MM, Allardyce DB. Pancreatic secretion in response to jejunal feeding of elemental diet. Ann Surg 1974; 180:228–31.

86. Eatock FC, Brombacher GD, Steven A et al. Challenging surgical dogma: Nasogastric feeding in severe acute pancreatitis may be practical and safe. Int J Pancreatol 2000; 28:25–31.

87. Eatock FC, Chang P, Menezes N et al. A randomized study of early nasogastric versus nasojejunal feeding in severe acute pancreatitis. Am J Gastroenterol 2005; 100:432–9.

Six studies providing evidence for use of enteral rather than intravenous nutrition in patients requiring nutritional support with acute pancreatitis.

88. Bower RH, Cerra FB, Bershadsky B et al. Early enteral administration of a formula (Impact) supplemented with arginine, nucleotides, and fish oil in intensive care unit patients: results of a multicenter, prospective, randomized, clinical trial. Crit Care Med 1995; 23:436–49.

89. Galban C, Montejo JC, Mesejo A et al. An immune-enhancing enteral diet reduces mortality rate and episodes of bacteremia in septic intensive care unit patients. Crit Care Med 2000; 28:643–8.

90. Powell JJ, Murchison JT, Fearon KC et al. Randomized controlled trial of the effect of early enteral nutrition on markers of the inflammatory response in predicted severe acute pancreatitis. Br J Surg 2000; 87:1375–81.

91. Paran H, Neufeld D, Mayo A et al. Preliminary report of a prospective randomized study of octreotide in the treatment of severe acute pancreatitis. J Am Coll Surg 1995; 181:121–4.

92. Beechey-Newman N. Controlled trial of high-dose octreotide in treatment of acute pancreatitis. Evidence of improvement in disease severity. Dig Dis Sci 1993; 38:644–7.

93. Karakoyunlar O, Sivrel E, Tanir N et al. High dose octreotide in the management of acute pancreatitis. Hepatogastroenterology 1999; 46:1968–72.

94. McKay C, Baxter J, Imrie C. A randomized, controlled trial of octreotide in the management of patients with acute pancreatitis. Int J Pancreatol 1997; 21:13–19.

95. Uhl W, Buchler MW, Malfertheiner P et al. and German Pancreatitis Study group. A randomised double blind multicentre trial of octreotide in moderate to severe acute pancreatitis. Gut 1999; 45:97–104.

Five studies showing no evidence for use of inhibition of secretion in acute pancreatitis.

96. Pederzoli P, Cavallini G, Falconi M et al. Gabexate mesilate vs aprotinin in human acute pancreatitis (GA.ME.P.A.): A prospective, randomized, double-blind multicenter study. Int J Pancreatol 1993; 14:117–24.

97. Trapnell JE, Rigby CC, Talbot CH. Controlled trial of Trasylol in the treatment of acute pancreatitis. Br J Surg 1974; 61:177–180.

98. Messori A, Rampazzo R, Scroccaro G et al. Effectiveness of Gabexate Mesilate in acute pancreatitis. A meta-analysis. Dig Dis Sci 1995; 40:734.

99. Larvin M, Wilson C, Heath D et al. A prospective multcenter randomised trial of intraperitoneal anti-protease therapy for acute pancreatitis. Gastroenterology 1992; 102:274 (abstr.).

100. Leese T, Holliday M, Heath D et al. Multicentre clinical trial of low volume fresh frozen plasma therapy in acute pancreatitis. Br J Surg 1987; 74:907–11.

101. Leese T, Holliday M, Watkins M et al. A multicentre controlled clinical trial of high-volume fresh frozen plasma therapy in prognostically severe acute pancreatitis. Ann R Coll Surg Engl 1991; 73:207–14.

102. Kingsnorth AN, Galloway SW, Formela LJ. Randomised, double blind, phase II trial of Lexipafant, a platelet activating factor antagonist, in human acute pancreatitis. Br J Surg 1995; 82:1414–20.

103. Imrie CW, McKay CJ. The possible role of platelet activating factor antagonist therapy in the management of severe acute pancreatitis. In: Neoptolemos JP, Tytgat GNJ (eds) Clinical gastroenterology, vol. 11. Best Practice and Research in Clinical Gastroenterology. Baillière Tindall, 1999; pp. 357–64.

104. Neoptolemos JP, Carr-Locke DL, Leese T et al. Acute cholangitis in association with acute pancreatitis: Incidence, clinical features and outcome in relation to ERCP and endoscopic sphincterotomy. Br J Surg 1987; 74:1103–6.

105. Neoptolemos JP, London NJ, James D et al. Controlled trial of urgent endoscopic retrograde cholangiopancreatography and endoscopic sphincterotomy versus conservative treatment for acute pancreatitis due to gallstones. Lancet 1988; 2:979–83.

106. Fan S-T, Lai ECS, Mok FPT et al. Early treatment of acute biliary pancreatitis by endoscopic papillotomy. New Engl J Med 1993; 328:228–32.

107. Folsch UR, Nitsche R, Ludtke R et al. Early ERCP and papillotomy compared with conservative treatment for acute biliary pancreatitis. New Engl J Med 1997; 336:237–42.

Three trials supporting the use of ERCP and sphincterotomy/duct drainage in patients suspected of having cholangitis and acute pancreatitis.

108. Nowak A, Nowakaowska-Dulawa E, Marek T et al. Final results of the prospective randomised controlled study on endoscopic sphincterotomy versus conventional management in acute biliary pancreatitis. Gastroenterology 1995; 108:A380.

109. Imrie CW, Shearer MG. The diagnosis and management of pancreatic pseudocyst. In: Johnson CD, Imrie CW (eds) Pancreatic disease. London: Springer-Verlag, 1991; pp. 299–309.

110. Imrie CW, Buist LJ, Shearer MG. Importance of cause in the outcome of pancreatic pseudocysts. Am J Surg 1988; 156:159–62.

111. Shearer MG, Imrie CW. Spontaneous resolution of pancreatic pseudocysts. Digestion 1990; 46:177–8 (abstr.).

112. Bradley EL III, Clements JL, Gonzales AC. Natural history of pancreatic pseudocysts: a unified concept of management. Am J Surg 1979; 137:135–41.

113. Baron TH, Thaggard WG III, Morgan DE et al. Endoscopic therapy for organised pancreatic necrosis. Gastroenterology 1996; III:755–64.

Original report describing the use of endoscopic cyst-gastroscopy.

114. Rattner DW, Legermate DA, Lee MJ et al. Early surgical debridement of symptomatic pancreatic necrosis is beneficial irrespective of infection. Am J Surg 1992; 163:105–9.

115. Meir J, Luque-de Leon E, Castillo A et al. Early versus late necrosectomy in severe necrotising pancreatitis. Am J Surg 1997; 173:71–5.

116. Karimgani I, Porter KA, Langevin RE et al. Prognostic factors in sterile pancreatic necrosis. Gastroenterology 1992; 103:1636–40.

117. Beger HG, Buchler M, Bittner R et al. Necrosectomy and postoperative local lavage in necrotizing pancreatitis. Br J Surg 1988; 75:207–12.

118. Buchler MW, Gloor B, Muller CA et al. Acute necrotizing pancreatitis: treatment strategy according to the status of infection. Ann Surg 2000; 232:619–26.

119. Buchler P, Reber HA. Surgical approach in patients with acute pancreatitis. Is infected or sterile necrosis an indication – in whom should this be done, when, and why? Gastroenterol Clin North Am 1999; 28:661–71.

120. Uomo G, Visconti M, Manes G et al. Nonsurgical treatment of acute necrotizing pancreatitis. Pancreas 1996; 12:142–8.

121. Banks PA, Gerzof SG, Chong FK et al. Bacteriologic status of necrotic tissue in necrotizing pancreatitis. Pancreas 1990; 5:330–3.

122. Rau B, Pralle U, Mayer JM et al. Role of ultrasonographically guided fine-needle aspiration cytology in the diagnosis of infected pancreatic necrosis. Br J Surg 1998; 85:179–84.

123. Rau B, Uhl W, Buchler MW et al. Surgical treatment of infected necrosis. World J Surg 1997; 21:155–61.

124. Moynihan B. Acute pancreatitis. Ann Surg 1925; 81:132–42.

125. Watts CT. Total pancreatectomy for fulminant pancreatitis. Lancet 1963: 2:384–9.

126. Alexander JH, Guerreri MT. Role of total pancreatectomy in the treatment of necrotising pancreatitis. World J Surg 1981; 5:369–77.

127. De Beaux AC, Palmer KR, Carter DC. Factors influencing morbidity and mortality in acute

pancreatitis; an analysis of 279 cases. Gut 1995; 37:121–6.

128. Hollender LF, Meyer C, Keller D. Planned operations for necrotising pancreatitis: the continental experience. In: Howard JM, Jordan GL, Reber HA (eds) Surgical diseases of the pancreas. Philadelphia: Lea & Febiger, 1986; pp. 450–60.

129. Bradley EL III. Management of infected pancreatitis necrosis by open drainage. Ann Surg 1987; 206:542–50.

130. Fernandez-Del CC, Rattner DW, Makary MA et al. Debridement and closed packing for the treatment of necrotizing pancreatitis. Ann Surg 1998; 228:676–84.

131. Fagniez PL, Rotman N, Kracht M. Direct retroperitoneal approach to necrosis in severe acute pancreatitis. Br J Surg 1989; 76:264–7.

132. Branum G, Galloway J, Hirchowitz W et al. Pancreatic necrosis: results of necrosectomy, packing, and ultimate closure over drains. Ann Surg 1998; 227:870–7.

133. Isenmann R; Rau B; Zoellner U et al. Management of patients with extended pancreatic necrosis. Pancreatology 2001; 1:63–8.

134. Larvin M, Chalmers AG, Robinson PJ et al. Debridement and closed cavity irrigation for the treatment of pancreatic necrosis. Br J Surg 1989; 76:465–71.

135. Freeny PC, Hauptmann E, Althaus SJ et al. Percutaneous CT-guided catheter drainage of infected acute necrotizing pancreatitis: Techniques and results. Am J Roentgenol 1998; 170:969–75.

136. Morgan DE, Smith JK, Baron TH et al. Pancreatic fluid collections prior to drainage: evaluation of MR imaging compared with CT and US. Radiology 1997; 203:773–8.

137. Adkisson KW, Morgan DE, Baron TH. Long term outcome following successful endoscopic drainage of organised pancreatic necrosis (OPN): Skunkpoking revisited. Gastrointest Endosc 1997; 45:514 (abstr.).

138. Carter CR, McKay CJ, Imrie CW. Percutaneous necrosectomy and sinus tract endoscopy in the management of infected pancreatic necrosis: An initial experience. Ann Surg 2000; 232:175–80.

Authors' original description of percutaneous necrosectomy in the management of infected pancreatic necrosis.

139. Connor S, Ghaneh P, Raraty M et al. Minimally invasive retroperitoneal pancreatic necrosectomy. Dig Surg 2003; 20:270–7.

140. Seifert H, Faust D, Schmitt T et al. Transmural drainage of cystic peripancreatic lesions with a new large-channel echo endoscope. Endoscopy 2001; 33:1022–6.

141. Giovannini M, Moutardier V, Pesenti C et al. Endoscopic ultrasound-guided bilioduodenal anastomosis: a new technique for biliary drainage. Endoscopy 2001; 33:898–900.

142. Renner IG, Savage WT, Pantoja JL et al. Death due to acute pancreatitis – a retrospective analysis of 405 cases. Dig Dis Sci 1985; 30:1005–18.

C H A P T E R

Twelve
Chronic pancreatitis

Philippus C. Bornman

INCIDENCE

The incidence of chronic pancreatitis is on the rise in industrialised countries, where alcohol is the predominant aetiological factor. However, accurate epidemiological studies on the frequency of the disease are sparse[1] due to the difficulties in confirming the diagnosis during the early stages of the disease, differences in classification (e.g. acute flare-ups in chronic pancreatitis may be recorded as acute pancreatitis), and lack of systematic post-mortem data. The only prospective study, performed in the city of Copenhagen,[2] noted an incidence of 13 per 100 000 inhabitants, which is in keeping with retrospective studies in Europe and North America. In England and Wales, the number of patients discharged from hospital with a diagnosis of chronic pancreatitis increased four-fold in men and two-fold in women between two comparable 5-year periods in the 1960s and 1980s.[3] However, in a more recent study amongst the population of Rochester, Minnesota, there was a disproportionate increase amongst women.[4]

There has been a close correlation between alcohol consumption per head of the population and the number of patients discharged from hospital with a diagnosis of chronic pancreatitis 6 years later[3] (**Fig. 12.1**). A linear correlation between alcohol consumption and the logarithmic risk of chronic pancreatitis has also been demonstrated.[5]

AETIOLOGY

Alcohol is recognised as the prime aetiological factor in chronic pancreatitis, accounting for 60–70% of cases of chronic pancreatitis in the Western world. Owing to their larger consumption of alcohol, men are more commonly affected than women. In terms of risk there also appears to be a racial difference. Compared with white patients, black patients are two to three times more likely to be hospitalised for chronic pancreatitis than for alcoholic cirrhosis.[6] In contrast to research in patients with liver disease, no precise level of daily alcohol consumption has been demonstrated above which chronic pancreatitis is more likely to develop. Individual sensitivity to the toxic effects of alcohol must vary greatly since not all alcoholics develop clinical pancreatitis, although distinct morphological changes in the pancreas have been recorded at autopsy in 19–58% of cases.[7,8] In patients with alcohol-associated chronic pancreatitis, the average daily intake of pure alcohol generally exceeds 60–80 g, although, as in liver disease, women may have a lower threshold, with no clear correlation to the amount of alcohol consumption.[9] The interval between the commencement of regular alcohol consumption and the clinical manifestations of chronic pancreatitis averages only 12 years in women and 18 years in men.[5] Tobacco has been identified as an additional risk factor[10] but it is difficult to separate its role

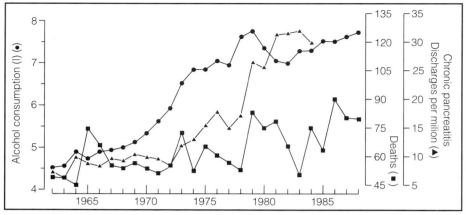

Figure 12.1 • Changes in annual alcohol consumption (litres per head of population), hospital discharges for chronic pancreatitis per million of population, and total number of deaths from chronic pancreatitis in England and Wales, 1960–88. Reproduced from Johnson CD, Hosking S. Gut 1991; 32:1401–5, with permission of the publishers.

from that of alcohol. The frequency of consumption and type of alcoholic beverage has no bearing on the risk of developing chronic pancreatitis.[11]

Alcohol has been identified as the most common cause of chronic pancreatitis, and patients in whom alcohol has been identified as a causative agent should be advised to abstain from its use.

Nutritional factors

It has been suggested that the development of alcoholic pancreatitis may be associated with an increased dietary intake of protein and fat. However, various studies have implicated a higher than normal, normal or lower than normal intake of calories, fat and protein, and an insufficient intake of the trace elements zinc and selenium.[12] There is a substantial body of evidence that in patients with chronic pancreatitis, advanced levels of free radical production, cytochrome P450 induction and antioxidant deficiencies, in particular selenium, exist.[13] It remains uncertain, however, whether selenium deficiency per se is an aetiological factor or the result of poor nutritional status associated with chronic pancreatitis and alcoholism. In one study,[14] the antioxidant profiles of patients with recurrent acute pancreatitis did not differ from those of controls, suggesting that these attacks are not an intermediate state between normality and chronic pancreatitis.

Tropical pancreatitis

There seems to be a link between nutrition and the development of tropical pancreatitis, a disease in which alcohol has no role. This particular form of pancreatitis is noted for the calcific changes in the pancreas and is reported in a number of countries situated within 15° of the Equator.[15] The first report on this distinct entity came from Indonesia in 1955 and described 18 cases of chronic pancreatitis with extensive calcification in young, non-alcoholic patients.[16] Similar reports came from Asia, Africa, South America and in particular the south-western state of Kerala in India.[17] Tropical pancreatitis is a disease of the young, with a male to female ratio ranging from 1.6 to as high as 5:1 in some studies. Its main clinical features include abdominal pain with distension, pancreatic calcification, diabetes mellitus, steatorrhoea related to exocrine insufficiency, and early death.[18,19] The main pancreatic duct is usually grossly dilated and contains large stones (**Fig. 12.2**). There is a higher incidence of pancreatic cancer amongst these patients, with an average age of onset of 45 years.[20] Protein-calorie malnutrition or childhood kwashiorkor was thought to be the main aetiological factor, but malnutrition is more likely to be the result of the disease. The disease is not seen in all areas where protein-energy malnutrition is prevalent, and this has further raised doubts as to whether malnutrition is truly an

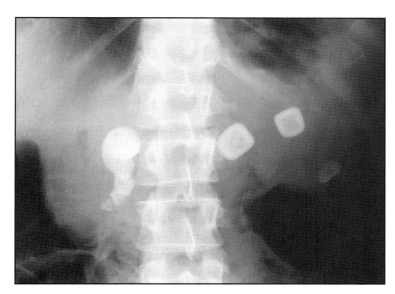

Figure 12.2 • Plain abdominal radiograph showing large pancreatic duct calculi in a patient with tropical pancreatitis.

initiating factor in the pathogenesis of tropical pancreatitis. However, reduced protein intake (less than 40 g/d) and a low-fat diet (less than 24 g/d) may be contributing factors.[21,22] Familial aggregation and vertical transmission have suggested a genetic element for the disease. Although no specific genetic marker has been identified thus far,[23] a genetic predisposition linked to the cystic fibrosis transmembrane conductance regulator (CFTR) has been implicated.[24]

Epidemiological studies have also implicated toxic cyanogenetic glycosides in cassava agents (*Manihot esculenta*),[24] which could theoretically cause pancreatic injury by interfering with the action of free radical scavengers such as superoxide dismutase. A cassava-rich diet may also be deficient in methionine and trace elements such as zinc and selenium, leading to impaired detoxification of cyanogens and increased production of free radicals. A recent study, however, could not show a clear association between cassava consumption and tropical pancreatitis syndrome.[25]

The management of tropical pancreatitis is similar to other forms of chronic pancreatitis, namely controlling brittle diabetes mellitus, nutritional support and pancreatic replacement, and endoscopic or surgical pancreatic duct drainage procedures for intractable pain. The higher risk for developing pancreatic cancer also demands close surveillance.

Obstructive pancreatitis

A form of chronic pancreatitis has been described where ductal obstruction has been implicated as the major predisposing factor. Common causes include congenital abnormalities such as pancreas divisum or acquired strictures as a consequence of complicated acute pancreatitis, neoplasia or trauma. Obstructive pancreatitis differs from alcoholic pancreatitis in that the epithelium of the obstructed ducts is usually preserved and the obstructive pancreas shows uniform chronic inflammatory changes rather than the patchy involvement that characterises alcoholic chronic pancreatitis. Intraductal protein plugs are not commonly found and progression to calcification and stone formation is an unusual finding.

Pancreas divisum, in which the dorsal and ventral pancreatic ducts fail to fuse, is the commonest congenital abnormality of the pancreas. It is thought that pancreatitis may develop due to the impaired passage of juice through the small minor papillae from the larger dorsal pancreas. Autopsy and endoscopic retrograde cholangiopancreatography (ERCP) studies have shown a prevalence rate of up to 7% of the population.[12] In some studies[26,27] a very high incidence (26–50%) of this anomaly was demonstrated in patients with acute idiopathic pancreatitis. However, the association between pancreatitis, in particular chronic pancreatitis, and pancreas divisum remains at best tenuous.[28]

A recently described condition, mucinous ductal ectasia, is associated with secretion of copious amounts of mucus, and this pathology has been incorporated amongst the group of causes for obstructive pancreatitis. This condition has a malignant potential of 20–30%.[29]

Hypercalcaemia

Hypercalcaemia associated with hyperparathyroidism and chronic renal failure can give rise to both acute and chronic pancreatitis. Since the early detection of hypercalcaemia on routine blood testing, chronic pancreatitis is nowadays an infrequent complication of hyperparathyroidism.[30]

Hereditary chronic pancreatitis

Hereditary diseases of the pancreas are divided into those presenting with mainly exocrine pancreatic insufficiency and those with acute or chronic pancreatitis as the first manifestation. Those diseases associated with pancreatitis include cystic fibrosis, alpha-antitrypsin deficiency, inborn errors of metabolism and hereditary pancreatitis.

Hereditary pancreatitis is inherited as an autosomal dominant trait with apparently complete penetrance but variable expression,[31] and it does not normally become manifest until the age of 5 to 15 years. The onset of the disease may be delayed to the third and fourth decades of life in some patients. Genetic studies have shown a linkage between hereditary pancreatitis phenotype and chromosome 7q.[32,33] It is now also established that cationic trypsinogen mutations seem to play a central role in the common autosomal dominant form of the disease, and that the key molecule in human pancreatitis seems to be cationic trypsin with unique properties promoting autoactivation and stabilisation.[34]

Thus, prematurely activated trypsinogen can lead to activation of the pancreatic enzyme cascade and result in autodigestion. The diagnosis should be suspected if several members of a family develop chronic pancreatitis without obvious reason. Patients with hereditary chronic pancreatitis have a 53-fold

increased risk of developing pancreatic cancer[35] and should enter a closer surveillance programme.[36]

Patients with unexplained pancreatitis or chronic pancreatitis for which no causative factor has been identified or with a history in a first- or second-degree relative should be suspected of having hereditary pancreatitis and should undergo genetic study.

Patients with hereditary pancreatitis are at a substantially increased risk of developing pancreatic ductal adenocarcinoma, and this risk is greatest after 40 years of age.

Patients at increased risk should be advised regarding the need to eliminate concomitant risk factors such as smoking and alcohol ingestion.

Patients should be offered pancreatic cancer surveillance and the imaging modality should be dictated by local practice and expertise.

Biliary tract disease

Although gallstone disease is the most frequent cause of acute pancreatitis in many industrialised countries, it is not clear whether patients experiencing recurrent episodes of acute gallstone pancreatitis proceed to the development of chronic pancreatitis. As many as half of patients with gallstones have an abnormal pancreatogram, and 1 in 6 have changes resembling those of chronic pancreatitis.[37] However, the significance of these abnormal findings is uncertain and it is felt that except in the context of obstructive pancreatitis as a sequela of severe pancreatitis, choledocholithiasis is not a cause of chronic pancreatitis. It should be noted, however, that chronic pancreatitis not infrequently causes biliary stasis leading to the formation of stones in the common bile duct.

Idiopathic chronic pancreatitis

In 10–30% of patients, no obvious aetiological factor is identified. Idiopathic chronic pancreatitis has an equal sex distribution, and in the absence of a defined aetiology, many of these patients are often wrongly labelled as having alcohol-associated disease. Recent evidence suggests that cystic fibrosis transmembrane conductance regulator (CFTR) gene mutations occur in 20–33% of patients with idiopathic chronic and acute recurrent pancreatitis.[38,39]

This would support the hypothesis that recurrent attacks of pain are due to recurrent episodes of inflammation and necrosis caused by intra-pancreatic activation of trypsin.[40]

There are two distinct forms of idiopathic chronic pancreatitis, namely early-onset (<35 years), which pursues a long and often severe, painful clinical course with slow development of morphological and functional pancreatic damage, and a late-onset type with a mild and often painless clinical course with associated weight loss, exocrine and endocrine insufficiency, and pancreatic calcification.[41] Pancreatic atrophy, functional impairment and morphological change (including calcification) is an accepted feature of ageing, but it remains unclear whether some patients with late-onset chronic pancreatitis represent an exaggeration of this process.

Other factors

Rare causes of chronic pancreatitis include previous abdominal radiotherapy,[42] drug-induced (phenacetin, antihypertensive and anticonvulsant drugs) and possibly stress-induced related to increased energy expenditure during work amongst low social classes.[43]

PATHOGENESIS

The precise mechanism by which alcohol induces chronic pancreatitis remains uncertain. One theory suggests that the initial step is a primary effect of alcohol on pancreatic exocrine secretion. Chronic alcohol intake decreases pancreatic bicarbonate and water secretion, which results in an increase in protein secretion. There is a disturbed diffusion barrier with increased permeability between interstitial spaces[44] with enhanced diffusion of calcium and proteins into the ducts,[45] where calcium precipitates in the alkaline juice. The increased viscosity of the pancreatic juice, activation of enzyme and a reduction in the amount of substances (lithostathines and citrate) that keep protein soluble may contribute to the formation of protein plugs and their calcification (**Fig. 12.3**). It is thought that a non-inherited or acquired defect of the biosynthesis of lithostathine leads to an increase secretion of the abnormal form of this protein (H$_2$ lithostathine), previously called pancreatic stone protein (PSP). This protein forms an organic matrix at the neutral pH of pancreatic juice, and with another pancreatic protein, GP2, and calcium carbonate, precipitates with resulting stone formation.[46,47] There is evidence that eosinophilic protein precipitates have been found in the pancreatic secretions before histological damage to acinar and ductal cells is evident. Levels of messenger RNA encoding for lithostathine are lower in the juice of patients with chronic calcific pancreatitis than in controls, regardless of the aetiology of the disease.[48,49] There is not universal support for this particular theory and some investigators have been able to identify differences in lithostathine concentrations in groups of patients with chronic pancreatitis, pancreatic neoplasia and non-pancreatic disease.[50] Other factors may favour calcification of protein in the pancreatic ductules. In alcohol-induced chronic pancreatitis, the pancreatic juice may be more viscous due to increased protein secretion, increased secretion of calcium by acinar cells, and a decreased concentration of citrate in pancreatic juice.[51,52]

A second theory has been proposed that suggests that acinar cell damage may be due primarily to ductular obstruction by protein precipitates secondary to fatty degeneration of pancreatic cells. There may be associated loss of zymogen content and periacinar fibrosis.[53–55] It has also been suggested that alcohol may lead to the production of toxic metabolites of lipid metabolism within pancreatic cells, thereby precipitating the development of chronic pancreatitis.[56]

A third hypothesis, from Klöppel and Maillet,[57,58] postulates a sequence of interstitial fat necrosis during acute attacks leading to perilobular fibrosis and distortion of interlobular ducts. This results in impairment of normal flow of pancreatic secretions, which then predisposes to precipitation of protein plugs and their calcification.

Finally, impaired hepatic detoxification has been implicated; this may generate toxic free radicals and reactive intermediates, which are excreted in bile and reflux into the pancreatic duct system.[59] The process may be initiated by the induction of hepatic mixed function oxidases by alcohol. This theory offers an explanation for the varied genetic susceptibility to alcohol while stressing the potential

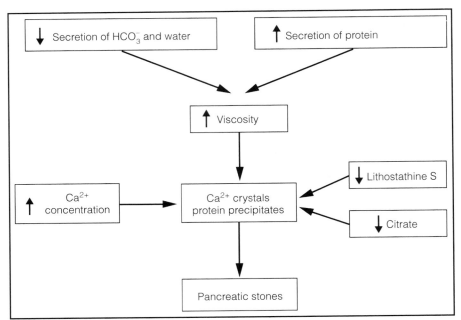

Figure 12.3 • Factors implicated in the calcification of chronic pancreatits.

importance of toxic factors in the pathogenesis of chronic pancreatitis.

PATHOLOGY

According to the Marseille classification[60] chronic pancreatitis is morphologically characterised by an irregular sclerosis with destruction and permanent loss of exocrine parenchyma, which may be focal, segmental or diffuse. Oedema and acute inflammation often coexist during acute flare-ups with or without associated necrosis. These changes may be associated with varying degrees of dilatation of the main and side ducts associated with protein plugs and calcification. Intrapancreatic and peripancreatic cysts are common and frequently communicate with the ductal system. There is a general belief that duct dilatation is the result of obstruction by fibrotic strictures and intraductal stones, but the causal relationship remains difficult to prove. It is possible that duct ectasia may develop simultaneously with progressive parenchymal destruction.

However, there is a subgroup of patients in whom the pancreas is densely sclerosed without duct dilatation.[61] Focal (segmental) pancreatitis is also a recognised entity, sometimes associated with

pancreas divisum or groove pancreatitis,[62] where the inflammatory process is confined to the groove between the duodenum, common bile duct and head of the pancreas. These may mimic carcinoma of the pancreas.

Calcification usually indicates advanced disease, and in an appreciable proportion of cases (20–30%) there is an inflammatory mass of the head complicated by bile duct and duodenal obstruction (**Fig. 12.4**). Splenic vein thrombosis with segmental portal hypertension is also a recognised complication.

Perineural disintegration and eosinophilic infiltration are typical features and are associated with an increase in mean nerve diameter.[63] These changes may account for pain being the predominant feature of chronic pancreatitis, possibly caused by abnormally large amounts of serotonin and calcitonin gene-related peptide.[64,65]

It may be difficult to exclude the presence of carcinoma, and the two conditions may coexist. There is some conflicting evidence whether patients with non-hereditary chronic pancreatitis are at increased risk of developing pancreatic cancer. Lowenfels et al.[66] showed a 16-fold increased risk, while a more recent Swedish cohort study[67] could

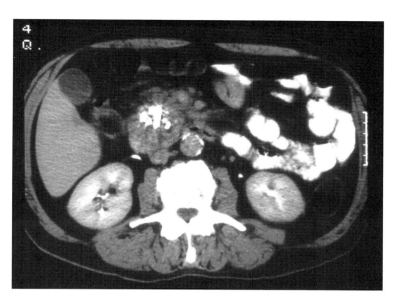

Figure 12.4 • CT scan showing a grossly enlarged and calcified head of pancreas.

not provide strong support for a causal association between pancreatitis and pancreatic cancer.

CLINICAL FEATURES

Pain is the most important cause of disability in chronic pancreatitis and is responsible for most of the poor quality of life in these patients. The pain presents a heterogeneous pattern ranging from relapsing episodes to persistent pain of varying intensity. There is also a small subgroup of patients in which the disease is painless throughout its course, and in these the clinical emphasis is on pancreatic insufficiency. Initially the pain is episodic in nature with pain-free intervals of varying periods. In alcohol-induced pancreatitis the recurrent attacks are closely linked to alcohol binges, but with time the pain becomes more persistent and the beneficial effect of alcohol withdrawal becomes less evident.[68]

The pathogenesis of pain in chronic pancreatitis remains an enigma. The cause of pain is almost certainly multifactorial and may vary at different stages of the disease process. Causal factors may include:

- the release of excessive oxygen-derived free radicals[69]
- tissue hypoxia and acidosis[70]

- inflammatory infiltration with influx of pain transmitter substances (calcitonin gene-related peptide, substance P and growth-associated protein-43) into damaged nerve ends[71]
- development of pancreatic ductal and tissue fluid hypertension due to morphological changes of the pancreas – the so-called 'compartmental syndrome'.[72]

There appear to be three pain patterns: early onset idiopathic, late-onset idiopathic and alcoholic. The mean age of onset in these three groups of patients is 21, 45 and 55 years, and the incidence of pain is 100%, 50% and 75%, respectively.[41] While there is a tendency for pain to decrease with time this is by no means predictable nor does this necessarily correspond to the development of endocrine and exocrine insufficiency (burnout syndrome). As for the non-alcoholic group, alcohol-induced pancreatitis also appears to comprise mild and severe types.[73] Those with mild pain experience intermittent attacks with pain-free intervals responding to conservative treatment and tend to improve with time, whereas those with severe and persistent pain do not burn out and often require surgery for pain relief and complications.

Pain is generally felt centrally in the epigastric region or subcostally with radiation to the back or shoulder tip, and is often eased by leaning forward or lying down to one side with knees pulled up, the so-called 'jack-knife' position. Some patients note that the pain is exacerbated by meals or the ingestion of certain foods such as those high in fat. Application of a hotwater bottle or a hot bath may ease the pain. Most patients with the severe form of the disease will eventually require high doses of opiates, and fear of addiction is a recurring anxiety in management. Loss of sleep, time off work and the need for admission to hospital are useful pointers to severity, and it is important to establish whether the pain does significantly impair the patient's quality of life. Assessment of pain can be difficult in these patients, some of whom remain addicted to alcohol and have manipulative personalities.

Progressive pancreatic insufficiency (dysfunction) is a frequent late manifestation of the disease, presenting usually 10–15 years after the clinical onset of the disease. Reports differ on which of diabetes and steatorrhoea presents first. Endocrine and exocrine insufficiency may contribute to the weight loss often observed in these patients, although anorexia, nausea and vomiting may be implicated.

Patients should be questioned carefully regarding the passage of pale bulky or oily stools, which may be offensive in smell and difficult to flush away. Some patients are incapacitated socially because of this symptom. There is some evidence that functional impairment and calcification is associated with relief from pain,[74] but this is not generally accepted.[41,68] In patients who develop diabetes there may be a transition from diet control to the use of oral hypoglycaemic agents and ultimately to the use of insulin. Patients with diabetes mellitus and chronic pancreatitis are less inclined to the development of retinopathy and diabetic neuropathy, probably due to their shorter life expectancy. Vascular diseases, however, are common with heavy smoking as a major contributing factor.

While duodenal obstruction due to inflammation in the head of the pancreas is uncommon, jaundice is encountered frequently in advanced cases as a complication of an inflammatory mass or cyst formation in the head. Rarely, haemorrhage from gastro-oesophageal varices may arise as a consequence of splenic vein thrombosis, or major bleeding may occur from a false aneurysm due to erosion of a pancreatic vessel by adjacent pancreatic

enzyme-rich fluid collections. When these collections communicate with the pancreatic duct, haemorrhage will occur via the pancreatic duct and presents as an upper gastrointestinal haemorrhage, often referred to as haemosuccus pancreaticus. There is often a delay in diagnosis of this condition; many patients present with recurrent episodes of upper gastrointestinal bleeding with repeated negative forward-viewing upper gastrointestinal endoscopies. The diagnosis should be suspected when pain is associated with an upper gastrointestinal bleeding against a background of chronic pancreatitis. A side-viewing duodenoscope may detect blood coming from the ampulla but angiography is the most definitive investigation to confirm the diagnosis.[75]

Examination may be unrewarding and there are no specific features of chronic pancreatic disease. Evidence of weight loss and malnutrition may be present, and mottled burn marks, so-called erythema ab igne (**Fig. 12.5**), may be associated with the use of heat pads or hotwater bottles. The patient should be examined for evidence of jaundice, a palpable abdominal mass and splenomegaly, which may indicate splenic vein thrombosis. Stigmata of chronic liver disease are unusual in patients with known alcohol-associated pancreatitis. Ascites due to disruption of a pancreatic duct with or without a pseudocyst may have an insidious onset and is often attributed to liver decompensation or chronic lung disease when presenting with an isolated pleural effusion. The diagnosis is confirmed when the serum and, in particular, ascitic fluid/amylase levels are very high. Similarly, sampling of the pleural effusion will reveal fluid with an amylase-rich content.

INVESTIGATIONS

Biochemical and haematological investigation

In chronic pancreatitis, serum amylase levels are usually normal or may be only slightly raised. With biliary tract obstruction liver function tests may demonstrate an obstructive jaundice pattern or, not infrequently an isolated and disproportionate increase of serum alkaline phosphatase levels. The presence of leucopenia and thrombocytopenia suggests that splenic vein thrombosis may have

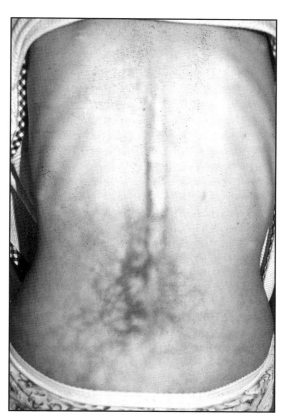

Figure 12.5 • Typical hotwater bottle marks (erythema ab igne) in the lower lumbar region.

resulted in hypersplenism, and the prothrombin time should be assessed in patients with cholestasis. A random blood glucose level should be measured to exclude diabetes mellitus.

Tests of pancreatic exocrine function

Few centres use pancreatic function tests routinely in diagnosis, which is generally based on the history and imaging of the pancreas. Function tests[76] (**Box 12.1**) may be helpful when chronic pancreatitis is suspected and the imaging studies are normal or show minimal change, but none of the available tests is sufficiently sensitive to exclude chronic pancreatitis when negative. The established direct tests involve measuring the concentrations of bicarbonate and enzymes in duodenal juice after stimulating the pancreas by a meal (Lundh test) or by exogenous secretin with or without cholecysto-

Box 12.1 • Pancreatic exocrine function tests.[76] From Lankisch PG. Int J Pancreatol 1993; 14:9–20, with permission.

Direct pancreatic function tests
Secretin-pancreozymin test
Lundh test
Indirect pancreatic function tests **Measurement of enzymes**
Serum pancreatic isoamylase
Serum immunoreactive trypsin
Faecal trypsin
Faecal chymotrypsin
Faecal elastase
Measurement of enzyme actions
NBT-PABA (bentiromide) test
Pancreolauryl test
Faecal fat analysis

kinin or caerulein (secretin-pancreozymin test). These tests are, however, time consuming, invasive and expensive. In addition, they are difficult to standardise and are therefore now used in very few centres. Indirect tests measure digestive capacity, since they are easier to standardise, non-invasive and more commonly undertaken. These include measurement of enzymes, including pancreatic isoamylase, immunoreactive trypsin and faecal levels of trypsin, chymotrypsin or elastase. Pancreatic function can also be assessed by measurement of enzyme actions and these include N-benzoyl-L-tyrosyl-para-aminobenzoic acid (NBT-PABA) (bentiromide) test, pancreolauryl test and faecal fat analysis. Function tests are a non-specific means of diagnosing exocrine insufficiency and cannot differentiate between chronic pancreatitis and pancreatic cancer.

Imaging studies

Plain abdominal radiography may demonstrate the presence of calcification within the pancreas. When diffuse the diagnosis is seldom in doubt but, when localised, other conditions such as pancreatic cancer should be considered. Ultrasound is employed normally to assess the presence of pancreatic enlargement, duct dilatation, cysts or pseudocysts. The demonstration of splenomegaly or biliary dilatation may indicate splenic vein thrombosis and/or biliary tract obstruction. Computed tomography (CT) provides better definition of morphological changes and extent of calcification, and gives a fair amount of information on main pancreatic duct changes (**Fig. 12.6**). CT also remains the best imaging modality to define the type and position of

cysts and their relationship to adjacent structures (**Fig. 12.7**). Endoscopic retrograde cholangio-pancreatography (ERCP) is the most effective method of detecting early chronic pancreatitis, and when combined with ultrasound and CT a sensitivity of 95–97% and specificity of 100% are obtained for the diagnosis of both chronic pancreatitis and pancreatic cancer.[77,78] However, in practice it may be difficult to confirm the diagnosis of cancer. Brush cytology at ERCP and fine-needle aspiration cytology have been disappointing and

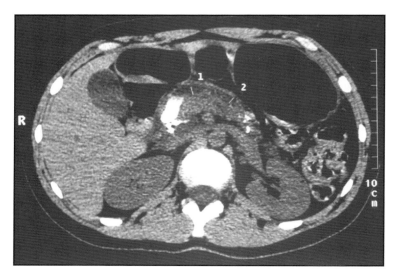

Figure 12.6 • CT scan showing a dilated main pancreatic duct with a large staghorn calculus in the pancreas head.

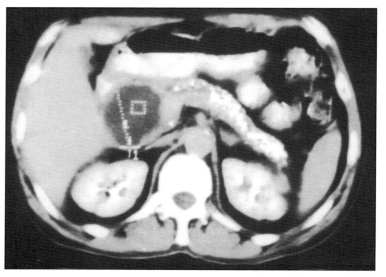

Figure 12.7 • CT scan showing an intrapancreatic cyst in the pancreas head with diffuse calcification in the body and tail.

there is an increasing tendency to resect in doubtful cases.[79]

Endoscopic ultrasound (EUS) with guided fine-needle aspiration (EUS-FNA) has been used increasingly in specialist centres in patients with suspicious pancreatic lesions. While this test has a high sensitivity in those patients with focal lesions with normal parenchyma (89–95%) the specificity in those with chronic pancreatitis is disappointingly low.[80,81]

According to the Cambridge classification,[82] severity related to ductal changes on ERCP is categorised as:

- mild (normal main duct and three or more abnormal side branches)
- moderate (abnormal main duct with more than three abnormal side branches)
- or severe (as in moderate disease but with additional features such as a large cavity, filling defect and severe duct dilatation or irregularity) (**Fig. 12.8**).

These morphological changes do not necessarily parallel the degree of functional impairment[83,84] nor the severity of symptoms.

Angiography is used only to locate a source of bleeding, particular when a false aneurysm is suspected, although dynamic CT and Doppler ultrasonography may similarly display vascular abnormalities. Barium studies are usually confined to patients with suspected duodenal stenosis or colonic obstruction. The new generation of magnetic resonance imaging (MRI) with magnetic resonance cholangiopancreatography (MRCP) images (**Fig. 12.9**) is about to replace ERCP as the investigation of choice for demonstrating pancreatic and biliary morphological changes, although detection of minimal ductal changes still eludes the current generation scans.

ERCP has been shown to be the most effective method of detecting early chronic pancreatitis and will differentiate between chronic pancreatitis and pancreatic cancer when combined with CT scan in most cases. CT scan and MRCP are the most appropriate means of demonstrating abnormalities associated with chronic pancreatitis.

MANAGEMENT

Pain control

The selected referral of severe cases to surgical practices may skew the perception that patients with chronic pancreatitis inevitably follow an

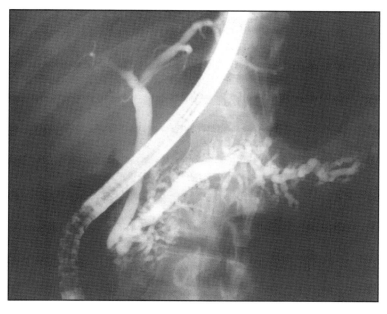

Figure 12.8 • Endoscopic retrograde pancreatogram in a patient with chronic pancreatitis showing irregular areas of narrowing and gross dilatation of the pancreatic duct system.

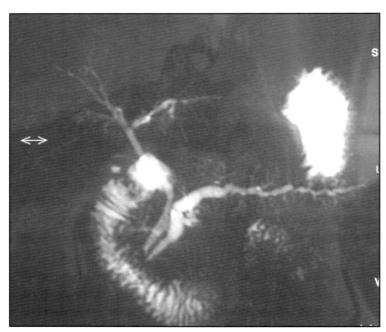

Figure 12.9 • MRCP showing clear delineation of both pancreatic and bile ducts.

intractable course with the emphasis on pain. On the contrary, in the majority of patients symptoms can be managed conservatively for long periods and in some cases indefinitely. Nonetheless, in about half of patients with established chronic pancreatitis medical treatment, including alcohol withdrawal, fails to control pain by non-narcotic analgesics or prevent the development of complications necessitating surgical intervention.

ALCOHOL WITHDRAWAL

Patients will require considerable support, which may include counselling, self-help groups and, where necessary, psychiatric treatment. The clinician will need to develop a strong rapport with the patient. Some patients will attempt to conceal continuing alcohol abuse, and others, in whom there may be doubt regarding the contribution of alcohol to their symptoms, may show considerable resentment over the stigma of an alcohol-related disease. Serum levels of carbohydrate-deficient transferrin may be useful to determine recent or continued alcohol abuse.[85]

The time-honoured view that continued alcoholism is largely responsible for pain and for failures after surgery has been questioned recently. While it would appear that alcohol plays an important role

in precipitating acute attacks during the early stages of the disease,[86–88] the association is less convincing amongst patients with advanced disease.[89–91] Explanations for these paradoxical findings may include an unreliable history of continued alcoholism, progressive functional impairment conferring immunity against pain, and the possibility that the higher mortality associated with continued alcoholism may obscure any significant correlation between abstinence and pain relief.[92]

Acute exacerbations of chronic inflammation may produce episodes of severe abdominal pain, often necessitating admission to hospital. The surgeon should resist the temptation to abandon conservative treatment in favour of operation in the face of such acute exacerbations. In the majority of cases, symptoms can be brought under control by hospitalisation and with adequate pain control and enteral or intravenous nutritional support.

MEDICATION

Non-opioid analgesics such as aspirin and paracetamol (acetaminophen) are more effective in the relief of muscular skeletal pain than in the treatment of visceral pain. Opioid drugs such as dihydrocodeine (DF118) and codeine (30 mg every 6 h) are suitable for patients with mild to moderate pain but often give rise to constipation, nausea and dizziness. Sublingual buprenorphine (200–400 µg every 6–8 h) can be used for more severe pain and has less risk of dependence than morphine. Due to the opioid agonist and antagonist properties of buprenorphine, withdrawal symptoms, including pain, may arise in patients dependent on other opioids. A slow-release morphine preparation (MST Continus: starting dose 10–20 mg twice daily) is often the best option for long-term relief. Tramadol, which has a mild opioid receptor affinity with less constipation effects, has recently been introduced for chronic pain states[93] but its role in chronic pancreatitis requires further evaluation. Non-steroidal analgesics may be of value in the short term, but these may increase the risk of gastrointestinal ulceration and bleeding complications. Antidepressants such as amitriptyline and selective serotonin reuptake inhibitors (SSRIs) may be effective adjuvants to non-opioid and opioid analgesic medications.

COELIAC PLEXUS BLOCK

Most series[94–96] on imaging-guided percutaneous coeliac plexus blockade, using a variety of neurolysis agents (e.g. ethanol or phenol), have reported disappointing results for pain control. The reason for the poor results may be due to late referral when most of these patients have been on long-term narcotic analgesics. Variations in the anatomy of the coeliac plexus may be another reason for failure even with CT-guided injections. EUS-guided coeliac plexus blockade via the posterior wall of the stomach is a recent addition to the list of image-guided techniques. It is purported to be safer than the posterior translumbar/retrocrural approaches particularly with respect to the risk of paraplegia.

In a larger prospective audit on EUS-guided coeliac plexus block,[97] significant improvement in overall pain scores was achieved in 50 (55%) of 90 patients. The follow-up, however, was less than a year, and patients younger than 45 years and those who had previously had pancreatic surgery did not benefit from this treatment.

VIDEO THORACOSCOPIC SPLANCHNICECTOMY

The emergence of minimal access surgery has rekindled interest in splanchnicectomy for pain control in chronic pancreatitis, particularly in patients with small-duct disease. It has been argued that, unlike coeliac ganglion blocks, splanchnicectomy provides a more complete interruption of the sympathetic nerves that constitute the main pathways for afferent transmission of pancreatic pain. Bilateral thoracoscopic splanchnicectomy is usually recommended, with division of the greater and lesser splanchnic nerves. The procedure is done under general anaesthesia using either a standard or double-lumen endotracheal tube. The patient is positioned in the prone position (Fig. 12.10). A pneumothorax is introduced with a Veress needle, keeping the pressure below 5 mmHg. This is usually sufficient to expose the operating field. Two ports are used, with the camera port placed in the seventh intercostal space in the posterior axillary line. The dissection port is placed in the fifth intercostal space in the posterior axillary line. The parietal pleura is dissected medial to the main sympathetic chain from the fifth intercostal space to the diaphragmatic recess. All branches along this course are isolated and divided with a hook-diathermy dissector (Fig. 12.11). The pneumothorax is evacuated with a combination of suction and positive end-expiratory pressure. The procedure is then repeated on the contralateral side. Postoperative chest radiograph is done when there is any doubt about a residual pneumothorax.

Morbidity and mortality for this procedure are low, and recent series with short- to medium-term follow-up have reported pain relief with variable and sometimes conflicting results[98–101] (Table 12.1). For example, some reports claim good results

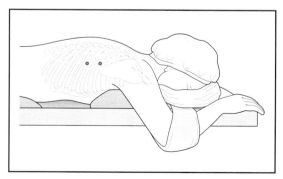

Figure 12.10 • Patient positioned in prone position with port placement in seventh and fifth intercostal spaces, posterior axillary line.

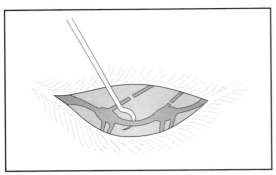

Figure 12.11 • Incision of parietal pleura and division of all sympathetic branches coming off medially from the sympathetic chain.

regardless of the presence of dilated pancreatic ducts or an inflammatory mass in the pancreatic head,[101] while others[98,102] have had disappointing results in these patients. Interpretation of the results is also difficult due to the heterogeneity of the patients (e.g. alcoholic and non-alcoholic), criteria used for successful outcome, and variations in technique. It should also be noted that while initial pain relief is encouraging, there is often a steady decline in the success rate with time,[101] and that a large percentage of patients remain dependent on opiates, albeit on smaller dosages.[103] Not many studies provide long-term results, which are the ultimate test for success in the treatment of chronic pancreatitis. Nonetheless, since thoracoscopic splanchnicectomy is a relatively minor operation it would seem reasonable to offer it to patients with small-duct disease before considering major pancreatic resection operations.

 Coeliac blockade and thoracoscopic splanchnicectomy have yet to be shown to be effective in the long-term control of pain in chronic pancreatitis.

Patients are often advised to avoid fat-rich diets and large meals, as these may give rise to pain. Avoidance of a high-fat, high-protein diet should restrict cholecystokinin release and physiological stimulation of the pancreas. Elemental diets, although theoretically beneficial, are no longer employed routinely. There has been considerable debate as to whether lumenal proteases reduce pancreatic exocrine secretion by a negative feedback mechanism and whether oral enzyme supplements reduce pancreatic pain in addition to combating steatorrhoea.

Unfortunately, the initial optimism regarding pancreatic replacement therapy[104–106] has not been substantiated by further studies published in full,[107–109] two of which were placebo-controlled.[108,109] Furthermore, similar disappointing results have been reported with the use of octreotide,[110,111] the most potent suppressing agent of pancreatic secretion.

Management of complications

BILIARY OBSTRUCTION

Obstruction of the biliary tree is common in cases with advanced disease with calcification and when an inflammatory mass is present in the head. The stenosis involves the retropancreatic portion of the common bile duct and is usually the tapering type rather than the abrupt cut-off seen in malignant obstruction (**Fig. 12.12**). Obstruction can be caused by oedema, an intrapancreatic pseudocyst or fibrosis, but is seldom complete. The natural history of the obstruction will vary according to the underlying pathology. Jaundice is usually transient when caused by oedema during acute flare-ups. About 20% of patients will present with asymptomatic

Table 12.1 • Reported series on thoracoscopic splanchnicectomy

Reference	Year	N	Opioid use	Success rate (%)	Median follow-up (months)
Maher et al.[98]	1996	15	11	79	18
Ihse et al.[99]	1999	21	14	50 reduction	42
Moodley et al.[100]	1999	17	4	94	12 (mean)
Buscher et al.[101]	2002	44	36	46	36

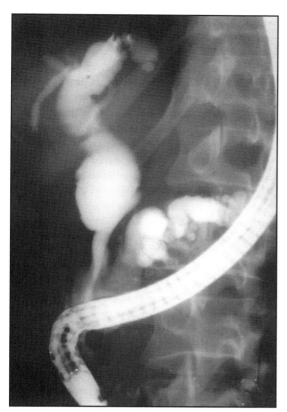

Figure 12.12 • ERCP showing tapering-type stricture of the distal bile duct and a grossly dilated main pancreatic duct.

common duct stenosis, detected only by an isolated raised alkaline phosphatase level or during ERCP when patients are investigated for pain. In such patients, deterioration of liver function and the development of secondary biliary cirrhosis is exceptional.[112–116] Nevertheless, if biliary obstruction persists for longer than 3 weeks, relief should be sought before hepatic sequelae result. Endoscopic insertion of a stent is indicated only as a temporary measure in high-risk patients when associated with cholangitis, since prolonged stenting leads to recurrent blockage,[117–120] sepsis and possible secondary sclerosing cholangitis. Metal stents in particular should be avoided unless surgery is contraindicated.[121]

If biliary obstruction is the only complication of chronic pancreatitis, some form of bilioenteric bypass is indicated. Cholecysto-jejunostomy is a poor option as a long-term drainage procedure.

Choledocho-duodenostomy or hepatico-jejunostomy utilising a long Roux-en-Y loop can be undertaken although most surgeons prefer the latter since this will avoid the possible risk of reflux of enteric contents into the biliary tree. It remains uncertain whether isolated biliary obstruction is an important cause of pain since most patients who require biliary drainage will also undergo a pancreatic drainage procedure for pain. Some surgeons, however, will argue in favour of some form of resection when severe pain is present or if there is an inflammatory mass of the pancreas head.

DUODENAL OBSTRUCTION

Some degree of duodenal obstruction is commonly found in chronic pancreatitis during endoscopy or in upper gastrointestinal radiology but this is seldom a cause of overt gastric outlet obstruction. If isolated duodenal obstruction occurs, this is best managed by mobilisation of the duodenum by Kocher's manoeuvre, which may suffice if there is a distinct fibrotic band across the duodenum. Failing this a duodeno-duodenostomy is preferred to a gastro-jejunostomy and vagotomy with its attendant sequelae. Many of these patients will also have severe pain with or without biliary obstruction, in which case it is probably better to perform some form of resection. A colonic stricture may mimic carcinoma but once this diagnosis has been excluded by colonoscopy, expectant conservative treatment should be pursued. Surgical intervention for this complication is exceptional.

PSEUDOCYST

Pancreatic and peripancreatic collections occur in some 25–30% of patients with chronic pancreatitis and are frequently associated with gross pancreatic duct abnormalities. Postnecrotic peripancreatic collection rarely occurs in patients with established chronic pancreatitis. These cysts are mostly intrapancreatic when present in the head due to obstruction of side ducts or necrosis, or are situated in the lesser sac region and are extrapancreatic as a complication of duct disruption. In both instances there is a high incidence of communication with the pancreatic duct system. Most of these cysts are mature by the time the diagnosis is made and spontaneous resolution is much less likely than in cases of acute postnecrotic collections.

Non-operative treatment options and in particular endoscopic drainages have enjoyed increasing support in the management of pseudocysts. In the context of chronic pancreatitis, simple aspiration or the placement of external drainage catheters is usually inappropriate due to a high failure rate or the development of an external fistula.[122]

Various techniques have been employed including transgastric or transduodenal drainage with a needle knife papillotomy with the placement of a stent, or transpapillary stent drainage. The overall success rates are encouraging (65–95%) with an associated complication rate of 10%.[123,124] However, long-term results are awaited in terms of recurrence and the need for more formal surgical drainage for pain from associated morphological abnormalities of the pancreas. Nonetheless, this relatively simple method is a worthwhile first option before surgery is contemplated.

It should be stressed that the indications for endoscopic drainage of pseudocysts should not differ from those for surgery, namely those of persistent pain and/or obstruction to the bile duct and duodenum. Unlike post-acute necrotic collections, size has little relevance to the need for intervention. Asymptomatic collections may be observed but there remains a concern that activated pancreatic enzymes may erode into an artery resulting in serious bleeding complications.

Selection for endoscopic drainage should adhere to the following strict guidelines. Only cysts which are clearly bulging into the bowel lumen and with a wall thickness of less than 10 mm are suitable for endoscopic drainage. Using these criteria, 30–40% of cysts in chronic pancreatitis are suitable for this treatment.[124] CT scanning is essential to determine cyst wall thickness, the relationship of the cyst to the bowel wall, and the presence of ascites, which may indicate communication with the peritoneal cavity. CT may also be helpful in excluding the possibility of a cystic tumour. Endoscopic ultrasonography may provide useful additional information in selecting the site of drainage when a bulge is less prominent.[125] ERCP during endoscopic drainage may be difficult due to distortion of the stomach and duodenum. While providing useful information regarding ductal morphology for future management, the demonstration of a leak or pancreatic duct obstruction has no relevance to the

immediate management of the cyst. A diathermy needle knife is used to create a fistula between the gut lumen and the cyst. Using an exchangeable system the needle knife is replaced by a guidewire while the sheath remains within the cyst cavity to avoid losing access. Some authors recommend dilating the tract before placing a pigtail stent. If the cyst cavity is large and contains necrotic material, it is advisable to place a nasocystic catheter for lavage, which reduces the risk of secondary infection. This can be removed once repeat imaging has confirmed collapse of the cyst cavity. It is usually recommended that the pigtail stent should remain in place for about 2–3 months to avoid early closure of the tract with recurrent pseudocyst formation.

The transpapillary route for pseudocyst drainage is usually reserved for pseudocysts in the region of the head but away from the bowel wall. The stent is placed either within the cavity or further up into the upstream duct. The risk of bleeding and perforation is less than for the transmural approach but secondary infection remains a potential problem.

Surgical drainage is achieved by anastomosing the stomach, duodenum or a Roux-en-Y limb of jejunum at the lowest point of the cyst wall. This latter method has been most popular in Europe. For cysts situated near the tail of the pancreas, resection is often considered. Resection should always be performed when there is a concern about the possibility of a cystic neoplasm.

Endoscopic pseudocyst drainage has been shown to be an effective option in patients with chronic pancreatitis before surgery is contemplated.

Surgery remains the definitive treatment for pseudocysts and allows additional drainage procedures or resection when there is pancreatic duct obstruction and dilatation.

PANCREATIC ASCITES

Pancreatic ascites and pleural effusion are rare but potentially serious complications of chronic pancreatitis and result from rupture of a pseudocyst or pancreatic duct. Such patients are generally malnourished and hypoalbuminaemia is invariably present, due in part to massive protein losses into the peritoneal cavity. Treatment consists of paracentesis, pleural aspiration and intravenous or enteral nutritional support. The success rate of conservative treatment is of the order of 50–60%. There is no convincing proof that the administration of a somatostatin analogue adds to the success of conservative treatment.[126] It is unwise to continue with conservative treatment beyond 2–3 weeks as it is unlikely that the ascites will resolve spontaneously. There is also the added risk of sepsis, often related to central line placement. When intervention is considered, ERCP should be undertaken to identify the site of the leak or an associated pancreatic duct obstruction. In more recent times, there have been reports of successful treatment by endoscopic stenting, which facilitates resolution of the ascites.[127] Pleural effusions will settle once the abdominal cause has been eradicated. Surgical treatment is now reserved for failures of conservative and or endoscopic treatment. Drainage at the site of the leak with a Roux-en-Y limb of jejunostomy with or without a pancreatic duct drainage procedure would usually suffice but occasionally a distal pancreatic resection may be appropriate.

GASTROINTESTINAL BLEEDING

Portal hypertension

Some involvement of the portal venous system is encountered in about 10% of patients presenting with chronic pancreatitis.[128] Involvement ranges from compression to frank occlusion with thrombosis. Splenic vein thrombosis causing segmental portal hypertension is the commonest manifestation and the resulting splenomegaly produces hypersplenism and the formation of gastric and oesophageal varices. Thrombosis confined to the splenic vein is best dealt with by distal pancreatectomy and splenectomy before bleeding occurs.[128] Portal or superior mesenteric venous thrombosis resulting in portal hypertension and cavernous transformation of the peripancreatic veins is considered to be a contraindication to any procedure on the pancreas itself.

Pseudoaneurysms

Erosion of peripancreatic arteries adjacent to pancreatic or peripancreatic enzyme-rich fluid collections may lead to false aneurysms, which may rupture directly into the pancreatic duct, peritoneum or retroperitoneum. When this is suspected contrast-enhanced CT scan will usually demonstrate the false aneurysm but angiography, with an attempt at embolisation, is recommended as the first step in the management. When the head of the pancreas is involved angiographic embolisation is the treatment of choice to avoid the hazards of major pancreatic resection. This is usually successful for smaller feeding vessels but collateral circulation or large vessel involvement may hamper successful embolisation,[75] in which case surgery in the form of a Frey-type procedure may be the safest option. For aneurysms in the body and tail region, distal pancreatectomy remains the treatment of choice.

SURGICAL OPTIONS FOR PAIN

Patient selection is as important as the choice of the operative procedure. The decision to undertake surgery should only be made when a full and thorough evaluation of the patient has been made, and the surgeon should not be pressurised into offering surgery until after all factors are considered. The patient must understand the risks of intervention and be aware that pain may not be relieved. It should also be emphasised that surgical intervention will not reverse the progressive loss of endocrine and exocrine pancreatic function. The timing of surgery is particularly problematic and it is often difficult to find the balance between avoiding resection operations, which may compromise pancreatic function, and the risk of opioid addiction when conservative treatment is prolonged.

Surgical treatment has to a large extent been tailored according to parenchymal and pancreatic ductal morphological changes of the pancreas, and can be divided into pancreatic drainage procedures and some form of resection. Modern imaging, in particular CT scan, ERCP and more recently MRCP, has facilitated the selection of the appropriate operations.

Since the 1950s numerous surgical approaches have been devised ranging from transduodenal sphincteroplasty to total pancreatectomy. Some have fallen into disrepute (e.g. transduodenal sphincteroplasty or caudal pancreatico-jejunostomy, the so-called Duval procedure),[129] while more recently pylorus- or duodenal-preserving resections of the head have been devised in an attempt to minimise malabsorption and glucose tolerance.

Pancreatic duct drainage procedures

Most surgeons will select some form of drainage procedure when the pancreatic duct is dilated. It is generally recommended that the operation should only be performed in patients with pancreatic ducts larger than 7–8 mm in diameter, although others have challenged this restriction.[130] More recently Izbicki et al.[131] have introduced a modified V-shaped excision of the ventral pancreas with a pancreatico-jejunostomy for ducts smaller than 3 mm in size. In a small series of 13 patients complete pain relief was achieved in 12 with a median follow-up of 30 months.

The most commonly performed drainage operation is a lateral pancreatico-jejunostomy, which is a modification of the Puestow procedure[132] as described by Partington and Rochelle.[133] Unlike the Duval[129] and Puestow[132] procedures this modified lateral pancreatico-jejunostomy preserves the spleen, and drainage is extended well towards the tail (**Fig. 12.13**). The duct should be opened to within 1–2 cm of the splenic hilus and extended to the head of the gland and, when necessary, into the uncinate process. Intraoperative ultrasonography may be used to locate the duct. Mucosa-to-mucosa apposition can be used as a one-layer continuous suture if the gland overlying the anterior aspect of the duct is thin. However, for most cases, anastomosis to the cut edge is performed when the duct is deeply embedded in an enlarged and inflamed pancreatic parenchyma. It is important to orientate the Roux limb so that its blind end is placed towards the tail of the pancreas, allowing the possibility of using the same limb for anastomosis to the biliary system. Pseudocysts can also be drained into the same Roux limb without any increase in morbidity or mortality.

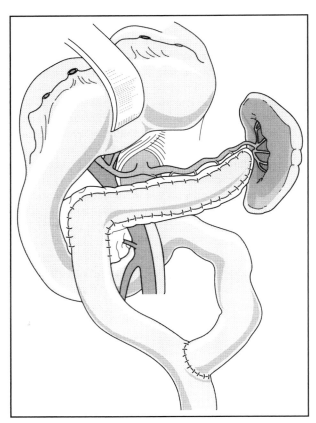

Figure 12.13 • Longitudinal pancreatico-jejunostomy. The pancreatic duct system is opened as widely as possible and anastomosed to a Roux limb of jejunum. Intestinal continuity is restored by an end-to-end jejuno-jejunal anastomosis. The same Roux limb can also be used to drain cystic collections or an obstructed bile duct, and to bypass an obstructed duodenum.

Although several series have shown encouraging results, with pain relief in up to 93%, there are other studies where the success rate is appreciably less (**Table 12.2**),[134–139] and these patients not infrequently require further surgery.[140] Drainage procedures in chronic pancreatitis are based on the concept that ductal obstruction leads to ductal hypertension due to fibrotic strictures and obstructions or stones. A number of studies, however, have shown poor correlation between pain, pancreatic duct obstruction and pressures.[68] The concept of a compartmental syndrome has recently been introduced, and some would argue that in addition to main pancreatic duct decompression, pain relief achieved with this operation is due, at least in part, to a fasciotomy effect relieving tissue pressure.[72]

It has been argued by some[141] that if the head of the pancreas is enlarged by more than 3 cm, it is unlikely that a standard longitudinal pancreatico-jejunostomy will be successful due to side duct obstruction leading to an inflammatory mass. Frey[142] has therefore modified the longitudinal pancreatico-jejunostomy to include partial excision of the head of the gland (**Fig. 12.14**), removing cysts and alleviating side duct obstruction or other areas of necrosis and scarring. A 25-mm rim of pancreatic tissue is left between the superior mesenteric vein and the core incision. A similar sliver of pancreatic tissue is preserved along the inner aspect of the duodenum and retroperitoneally. Once this core-out process is complete, the entire open pancreas is anastomosed to a Roux limb of jejunum.

There are no controlled data available to determine whether this more extensive drainage procedure is better than the standard lateral pancreatico-jejunostomy operation but when compared to the duodenal-preserving pancreatic head resection operation in a controlled study[143] the results were similar.

It is accepted that patients with chronic pancreatitis should be offered a surgical drainage procedure if pain is poorly controlled by medical therapy and endoscopic intervention has failed to confer long-term relief of symptoms.

There is no consensus on the optimal surgical drainage procedure but there is evidence to suggest that more extensive operations involving pancreatic head resection have a similar outcome to extended drainage procedures.

Pancreatic resection

Chronic pancreatitis generally affects the entire gland and the desire to remove the entire diseased pancreas has to be balanced against the problems posed by producing brittle insulin-dependent diabetes and total loss of exocrine function, which follow total pancreatectomy. When pancreatitis is confined to the body and tail of the gland a distal pancreatectomy would be appropriate. This procedure would be indicated for the presence of a pseudocyst behind ductal strictures in the body and tail region and when associated with a false aneurysm or segmental portal hypertension.[144] Distal pancreatectomy has not enjoyed a good reputation because of some series reporting poor pain relief, and the higher risk of developing diabetes mellitus postoperatively is a concern with more extensive resections. Less than 80% distal

Table 12.2 • Selected series of pancreatico-jejunostomy for chronic pancreatitis

Study (year)	No. of patients	Mean follow-up in years (range)	Pain relief (%)	Operative mortality (%)
Prinz and Greenlee (1981)[134]	100	7.9 (1–25)	82	4
Holmberg et al. (1985)[135]	51	8.2 (1–19)	85	0
Noguiera and Dani (1985)[136]	36	5.0	58	3
Bradley (1987)[137]	46	5.0	66	0
Adolff et al. (1991)[138]	105	6.5 (1–18)	93	2
Wilson et al. (1992)[139]	20	5.2	80	5

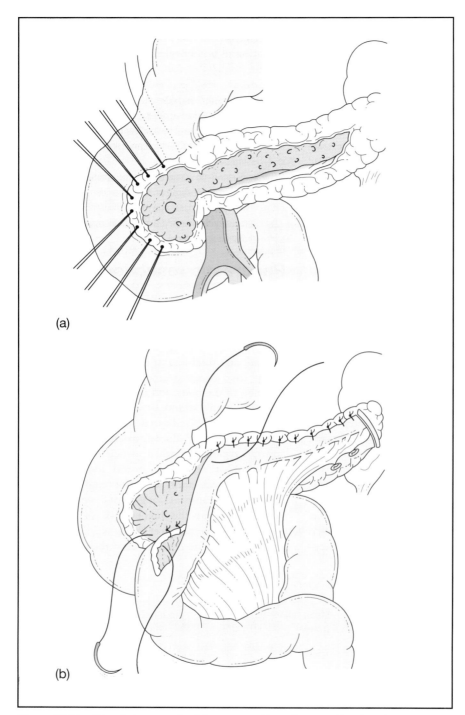

(a)

(b)

Figure 12.14 • Extended pancreatico-jejunostomy with coning out of head as described by Frey and Mikura.[142]

pancreatectomy is associated with a 19% incidence of new-onset diabetes mellitus, whereas this rises to 50–80% for an 80–95% distal pancreatectomy.[145] Up to 38% of patients will be troubled clinically by steatorrhoea on late follow-up. However, the results seem to be no different from other resections when patients are carefully selected based on ERCP and CT scanning.[146–148]

In up to 30% of patients with chronic pancreatitis, the head of the gland will be grossly enlarged by an inflammatory mass, often associated with bile duct stenosis and duodenal hold-up.[149] In these patients some form of pancreatic head resection is indicated even in the presence of gross pancreatic duct dilatation. The standard Whipple operation has now to a large extent been replaced by less radical resections, which include pylorus-preserving pancreatico-duodenectomy (**Fig. 12.15**) and duodenum-preserving pancreatic resection (**Fig. 12.16**) with the aim of reducing nutritional sequelae by preservation of the stomach, pylorus

and duodenum. These sequelae include rapid gastric emptying with poor mixing and digestion of fat and proteins, dumping, afferent loop syndrome and bile reflux. While concerns have been expressed of prolonged gastric outlet obstruction and increased risk of duodenal ulceration with the pylorus-preserving resection, recent reports[150,151] have allayed those fears to a large extent. Of interest, a recent study showed that pain relief after duodenal-preserving resections in patients with minimal or no enlargement of the pancreatic head was significantly less than in those with a distinct inflammatory mass.[152]

The duodenal-preserving pancreatic resection popularised by the Ulm group[149] was proposed to cause the least functional disturbances. However, one controlled study[153] and a recent review on the subject[154] were unable to give a clear verdict when the procedure was compared to the pylorus-preserving pancreatico-duodenectomy or the classic Whipple's resection.

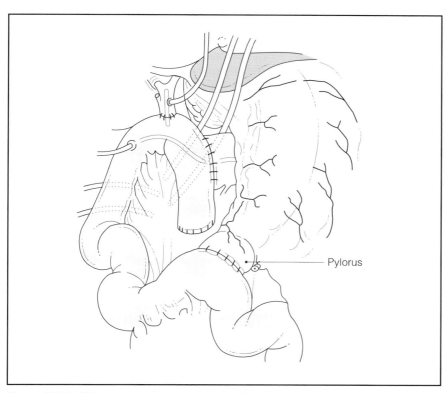

Pylorus

Figure 12.15 • Pylorus-preserving pancreato-duodenectomy.

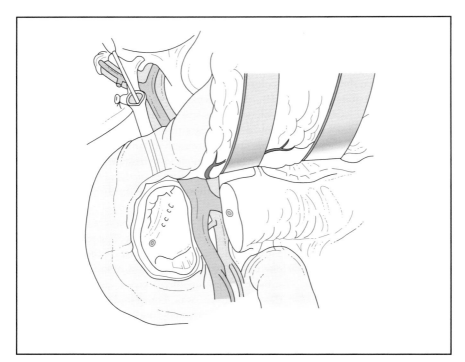

Figure 12.16 • Duodenal-preserving resection of pancreatic head as described by Beger and Imaizumi.[149]

These resection operations are technically demanding and should be preferably performed by specialist pancreatic surgeons. Operative mortality should be no more than 1–2%.[155] Good to excellent results are reported in up to 90% of patients although the postoperative incidence of diabetes in patients who underwent a standard Whipple resection is in excess of 50%, with late mortality rates of 20% reported by some.[155] Long-term results for the lesser resection operations are awaited to determine whether fewer of these complications occur. The results of the various resection operations are outlined in **Table 12.3**.

Generally, patients from lower socioeconomic backgrounds tolerate resections poorly, particularly when complicated by brittle diabetes and gross steatorrhoea with severe loss of weight, which may render them nutritional cripples. This is particularly true for total pancreatectomy, where rehabilitation of these patients may be made difficult if they come to the surgical procedure suffering from severe malnutrition from previous surgical intervention. In a review of 324 patients,[161] 31 patients (12.6%) died, and this was usually related to haemorrhage or sepsis. The morbidity of the operation is high, with as many as 40% of cases developing complications in the postoperative period.[162] Patients who develop septic complications tend also to develop multiple complications, and infection of the pancreatic bed is difficult to eradicate. Readmissions are also frequent for management of the metabolic effects of the operation. Some 15–30% of patients continue to experience significant discomfort or pain, and patients who continue to drink alcohol have worse results than those who abstain. Some workers have claimed better results with pancreatic segmental[163,164] or islet autotransplantation,[165] but more data are required to support these operations.

Pancreatic resection can be considered for localised disease but extensive resections are associated with considerable morbidity.

Endoscopic treatment

There have been conflicting reports on the efficacy of endoscopic treatment (sphincterotomy and stenting) with or without extracorporeal lithotripsy in relieving pain in patients with pancreatic duct obstruction due to fibrotic stenosis or stones.

Table 12.3 • Partial proximal pancreatic resection for pain in chronic pancreatitis

Study (year)	Type of resection	Number of patients	Mean follow-up (years) (%)	Pain relief (%)	Operative mortality (%)
Gall et al. (1989)[155]	Whipples	289	5.5	88	1
Rossi et al. (1987)[156]	Whipples	73 (20 PPW)	4.9	79	3
Moreaux (1984)[157]	Whipples	50	10.7	73	2
Traverso and Kozarek (1993)[158]	Whipples	28 (16 PPW)	2.6	88	0
Martin et al. (1996)[151]	PPW	78	5	92	2.2
Büchler et al. (1995)[153]	PPW	20	0.5	67	0
Beger and Büchler (1995)[159]	DPRPH	141	3.6	89	0.7
Bloechle et al. (1995)[160]	DPRPH	25	1.5	92	0
Büchler et al. (1995)[153]	DPRPH	20	0.5	94	0
Izibicki et al. (1995)[143]	DPRPH	20	1.5	95	0
Frey and Mikura (1994)[142]	Frey procedure	50	Not known	87	0

DPRPH = duodenal-preserving pancreatic resection pancreas head.
PPW = pylorus-preserving Whipple's.

Kozarek and Traverso[166] have recently analysed collected experiences of major publications from expert centres and indicated that symptomatic improvement varied greatly from 50 to 85% at 15–25 months.

A recent publication on a large multicentre study by specialised centres has reported encouraging results with a mean follow-up period of almost 5 years.[167] The study included 1018 patients treated with mainly strictures (47%), stones (18%) or a combination (32%). A long-term success rate of 86% was claimed although this figure was reduced to 65% in an intention-to-treat analysis. While there was no clear difference in the outcome in terms of morphological changes, those patients with intermittent pain fared better than those who had persistent pain. In contrast, another study of 80 patients with chronic pancreatitis found that only 43 (56%) could be treated successfully by extra-corporeal lithotripsy followed by endoscopic intervention.[168] Only patients with single stones had successful treatment but after a mean follow-up of 40 months (24–92) there was no discernible benefit in terms of either pain relief or prevention of progressive glandular insufficiency.

Endoscopic therapy is labour intensive, requires a high degree of expertise, and complications occur frequently. These include ERCP-induced acute pancreatitis, bleeding and perforation associated with endoscopic sphincterotomy, and stent-related complications such as occlusion, migration and sepsis.[169] There is also the concern that prolonged stenting may cause ductal and parenchymal injury.[170,171]

Interpreting the results of endoscopic treatment remains problematic. Most studies are retrospective, and assessments of pain severity are often poorly defined. Indeed, in several of the studies pain was intermittent and not severe, suggesting that the outcome may have been similar to conservative treatment.[73,172] Moreover, a poor correlation has been shown between the success of stone removal and pain relief.[173]

 The reported results of endoscopic therapy appear to be similar to surgical drainage procedures, and it would seem reasonable to offer this less invasive treatment in selected patients with dilated ducts with localised strictures and or stones.

Steatorrhoea

The place of pancreatic replacement therapy is more established for treating steatorrhoea. Fat malabsorption is the most important sequel of exocrine insufficiency in chronic pancreatitis, and as a general rule enzyme replacement is necessary when daily fat excretion exceeds 15 g and/or the patient is losing weight and/or has diarrhoea.[174] The treatment consists of a fat-reducing diet and pancreatic enzyme replacement therapy.

There are numerous pancreatic enzyme preparations available in the form of powder, tablets or capsules. All of the currently available pancreatic enzyme supplements consist of crude extracts of porcine pancreas, known in many countries as pancreatin. The enzymes are inactivated rapidly and irreversibly below pH 5 but more recently enteric-coated microspheres have been developed in which hundreds of individually coated microspheres are contained in a gelatine capsule. Capsules containing microspheres have the advantage of better mixing with the chyme. Under optimal conditions approximately 300 000 IU of lipase is required for each meal. Failure to respond may be due to poor compliance, incorrect diagnosis, incorrect prescription or choice of pancreatic enzyme preparations.

Gastric acid secretion may also influence absorption as lipase activity is inactivated in an acid milieu. This can be prevented by acid reduction with H_2 receptor antagonists, or proton pump inhibitors, or by the use of enteric-coated preparations.

As a general recommendation, pancreatic enzymes should be given in the form of multi-unit acid-protected dosages in patients with proven exocrine insufficiency and normal gastric acid secretion. In those patients who have had previous gastric resections, enzyme substitution should be with granules to ensure adequate mixing and simultaneous transport of enzymes with the chyme. A suggested treatment schema for exocrine pancreatic insufficiency is outlined in **Fig. 12.17**.[174]

Diabetic control may be difficult for patients on oral hypoglycaemic drugs or insulin, particularly if food intake is variable. Lack of endogenous glucagon contributes to a greater sensitivity to insulin and risk of hypoglycaemia, which is a major cause of death in the alcoholic group. Blood glucose control with insulin should therefore be monitored carefully and kept above normoglycaemic levels. However, diabetic ketoacidosis is uncommon in the patient with chronic pancreatitis, since there is usually sufficient insulin secretion to prevent the release of fatty acids from adipose tissue and their subsequent metabolism to ketone bodies in the liver.

CONCLUSION

Chronic pancreatitis has a mortality rate approaching 50% over 20–25 years.[175] Up to 20% of patients die of complications of the disease, whereas the remainder succumb to problems associated with alcohol abuse, tobacco smoking, malnutrition, infection, diabetes mellitus, insulin overdose and suicide. These patients are at greater risk of death from malignancy, many of which are related to smoking.

It is difficult to interpret the results of the various treatment options for chronic pancreatitis and in particular that of surgical and endoscopic interventions. Pancreatico-jejunostomy carries a lower operative mortality and morbidity than operations involving resection of the pancreas (**Table 12.4**).

Table 12.4 • Outcome following pancreatico-jejunostomy and resection for chronic pancreatitis[176]

	Pancreatico-jejunostomy	Distal pancreatectomy	Pancreatico-duodenectomy
No. of patients	228	102	278
Operative mortality (%)	4.3	8.2	5.3
Late mortality (%)	39	36	30
Insulin-dependent diabetes: preoperative (%) postoperative (%)	26 50	11 62	28 64

From Eckhauser FE et al. Surgery 1984; 96:599–607, with permission.

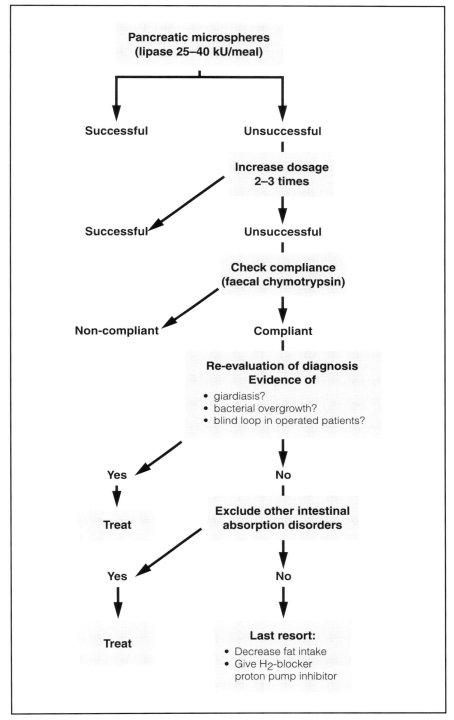

Figure 12.17 • Suggested treatment of exocrine pancreatic insufficiency. From Lankisch PG, Banks PA. Pancreatitis. Heidelberg: Springer-Verlag ©, 1998; 316–25, with permission of the publisher.

However, it should be recognised that the severity of the disease varies, and those patients who come to some form of resection usually have the more severe form of disease.[176] The generally quoted satisfactory control of pain in up to 75% of patients undergoing pancreatic surgery is similar to claims made in selected cases for endoscopic treatment. More recently medical treatment has focused on antioxidant therapy but the results of studies on this subject have yielded conflicting results.[177–180] The results of all forms of treatment should be interpreted with caution as most studies do not provide sufficient data on objective measurements of success,[181] with few addressing the important aspect of improving quality of life.

Considering the complexity of the disease process in chronic pancreatitis it is not surprising that lack of progress in the understanding of the pathogenesis of pain and the management thereof have frustrated the clinician in devising rational medical and surgical treatment strategies. There is a great need for standardising basic and clinical research methods to overcome the slow progress in the management of this debilitating disease.

• Key points

Alcohol is the most common causative agent in the development of pancreatitis and abstinence is associated with a more favourable prognosis.

Chronic pancreatitis is associated with a considerable mortality and patients succumb to the complications of the disease and associated socioeconomic factors.

Endoscopic intervention has gained an increasing role in the management of the complications of chronic pancreatitis.

Minimal access techniques for control of pain have yet to gain widespread acceptance.

Surgical options for the treatment of intractable pain now include extended drainage procedures, which have been shown to be as effective as more extensive resections.

There is a need to agree rational medical and surgical strategies for this debilitating disease.

REFERENCES

1. Worning H. Incidence and prevalence of chronic pancreatitis. In: Beger HG, Büchler M, Ditschuneit H et al. (eds) Chronic pancreatitis. Berlin/Heidelberg: Springer, 1990; pp. 8–14.

2. Copenhagen Pancreatitis Study. An interim report from a prospective epidemiological multicenter study. Scand J Gastroenterol 1981; 16:305–12.

3. Johnson CD, Hosking S. National statistics for diet, alcohol consumption and chronic pancreatitis in England and Wales 1960–1988. Gut 1991; 32:1401–5.

4. Riela A, Zinsmeister AR, Melton LJ et al. Trends in the incidence and clinical characteristics of chronic pancreatitis. Pancreas 1990; 5:727 (abstr.).

5. Durbec JP, Sarles H. Multicentre survey of the etiology of pancreatic diseases. Relationship between the relative risk of developing chronic pancreatitis and alcohol, protein, and lipid consumption. Digestion 1978; 18:337–50.

6. Lowenfels AB, Maisonneuve P, Grover H et al. Racial factors and the risk of chronic pancreatitis. Am J Gastroenterol 1999; 94:790–4.

7. Pitchumoni CS, Sonneshein M, Candido FM et al. Nutrition in the pathogenesis of alcoholic pancreatitis. Am J Clin Nutr 1980; 33:631–6.

8. Renner IG, Savage WT, Pantoja JL et al. Death due to acute pancreatitis: a retrospective analysis of 405 autopsy cases. Dig Dis Sci 1985; 30:1005–18.

9. Yen S, Hsieh CC, MacMahon B. Consumption of alcohol and tobacco and other risk factors for pancreatitis. Am J Epidemiol 1982; 116:407–14.

10. Bourliere M, Barhtet M, Berthezene P et al. Is tobacco a risk factor for chronic pancreatitis and alcoholic cirrhosis? Gut 1991; 32:1392–5.

11. Sarles H, Cros RC, Bidart JM. International Group for the Study of Pancreatic Diseases. A multicentre inquiry into the etiology of pancreatic diseases. Digestion 1979; 19:110–25.

12. Muller MK, Singer MV. Aetiology and pathogenesis of chronic pancreatitis. In: Trede M, Carter DC (eds) Surgery of the pancreas. Edinburgh: Churchill Livingstone, 1993.

13. Bowrey DJ, Morris-Stiff GJ, Puntis MCA. Selenium deficiency and chronic pancreatitis: Disease mechanism and potential for therapy. HPB Surg 1999; 11:207–16.

14. Morris Stiff GJ, Bowrey DJ, Oleesky D et al. The antioxidant profiles of patients with recurrent acute and chronic pancreatitis. Am J Gastroenterol 1999; 94:2135–40.

15. Pitchumoni CS. Special problems of tropic pancreatitis. Clin Gastroenterol 1984; 13:941–59.

16. Zuidema PJ. Calcification and cirrhosis of the pancreas in patients with deficient nutrition. Doc Med Geograph Trop Amsterdam 1955; 7:229–51.

17. Thomas PG, Augustine P, Ramesh H et al. Obervation and surgical management of tropical pancreatitis in Kerala and Southern India. World J Surg 1990; 14:32–42.

18. Nwokolo C, Oli J. Pathogenesis of juvenile tropical pancreatitis syndrome. Lancet 1980; i:456–9.

19. GeeVarghese PJ. Calcific pancreatitis. Causes and mechanisms in the tropics compared with those of the subtropics. Varghese, Bombay: St Joseph's Trivandrum, 1986.

20. Chari ST, Mohan V, Pitchumoni CS et al. Risk of pancreatic cancer in tropical calcifying pancreatitis: an epidemiologic study. Pancreas 1994; 9:62–6.

21. Ramesh H. Tropical pancreatitis. Ind J Gastroenterol 1997; 16:20–5.

22. Balakrishnan V, Sauniere JF, Haribaran M et al. Diet, pancreatic function and chronic pancreatitis in Southern India and France. Pancreas 1988; 3:30–5.

23. Mohan V, Chari ST, Hitman GE. Familial aggregation in tropical fibrocalculous pancreatic diabetes. Pancreas 1989; 4:690–3.

24. Pitchumoni CS. Chronic pancreatitis: A historical and clinical sketch of the pancreas and pancreatitis. Gastroenterologist 1998; 6:24–33.

25. Narendranathan M, Chriyan A. Lack of association between cassava consumption and tropical pancreatitis syndrome. J Gastroenterol Hepatol 1994; 9:282–5.

26. Bernard JP, Sahel J, Giovannini M et al. Pancreas divisium is a probable cause of acute pancreatitis: a report of 137 cases. Pancreas 1990; 5:248–54.

27. Cotton PB. Congenital anomaly of pancreas divisum can cause obstructive pain and pancreatitis. Gut 1980; 21:105–14.

28. Delhaye M, Engelholm L, Cremer M. Pancreas divisum: congenital anatomic variant or anomaly? Contribution of endoscopic retrograde dorsal pancreatography. Gastroenterology 1985; 89:951–8.

29. Loftus EV Jr, Olivares-Pakzak BA, Adkins MC et al. Members of the Pancreas Clinic, Pancreatic Surgeons of Mayo Clinic. Intraductal papillary-mucinous tumours of the pancreas: clinicopathological features, outcome, and nomenclature. Gastroenterology 1996; 110:1909–18.

30. Bess MA, Edis AJ, van Heerden JA. Hyperparathyroidism and pancreatitis. Chance or a causal association? JAMA 1980; 243:246–7.

31. Madrazo-de la Garza GA, Hill ID, Lebenthal E. Hereditary pancreatitis. In: Go VLM, DiMagno EP, Gardner JD et al. (eds) The pancreas: biology, pathobiology and disease, 2nd edn. New York: Raven Press, 1993; pp. 1095–101.

32. Le Bodic L, Bignon JD, Raguenes O et al. The hereditary pancreatitis gene maps to long arm of chromosome 7. Hum Mol Genet 1996; 5:549–54.

33. Whitcomb DC, Preston RA, Aston CE et al. A gene for hereditary pancreatitis maps to chromosome 7q35. Gastroenterology 1996; 110:1975–80.

34. Whitcomb DC. Hereditary pancreatitis: new insights into acute and chronic pancreatitis. Gut 1999; 45:317–22.

35. Lowenfels AB, Maisonneuve P, DiMagno EP et al. Hereditary pancreatitis and the risk of pancreatic cancer. J Natl Cancer Inst 1997; 89:442–6.

Key paper highlighting the strong risk of cancer developing in patients with hereditary pancreatitis.

36. Hall P de la M, Wilentz RE, de Klerk W et al. Premalignant conditions of the pancreas. Pathology 2002; 34: 504–17.

37. Misra SP, Dwivedi M. Do gallstones cause chronic pancreatitis? Int J Pancreatol 1991; 10:97–102.

38. Cohn JA, Friedman KJ, Noone PG et al. Relation between mutations of the cystic fibrosis gene and idiopathic pancreatitis. N Engl J Med 1998; 339:653–8.

39. Sharer N, Schwarz M, Malone G et al. Mutations of the fibrosis gene in patients with chronic pancreatitis. N Engl J Med 1998; 339:645–52.

40. DiMagno EP. Toward understanding (and management) of painful chronic pancreatitis. Gastroenterology 1999; 116:1252–7.

41. Layer P, Hironori Y, Kalthoff L et al. The different courses of early- and late-onset idiopathic and alcoholic chronic pancreatitis. Gastroenterology 1994; 107:1481–7.

42. Levy P, Menzelxhiu A, Palliot B et al. Abdominal radiotherapy is a cause for chronic pancreatitis. Gastroenterology 1993; 105:905–9.

43. Breuer-Katschinski BD, Bracht J, Tietjen-Harms S et al. Physical activity at work and the risk of chronic pancreatitis. Eur J Gastroenterol Hepatol 1996; 8:399–402.

44. Reber HA, Roberts C, Way LW. The pancreatic duct mucosal barrier. Am J Surg 1979; 137:128–34.

45. Layer P, Hotz J, Schmitz-Moormann HP et al. Effects of experimental chronic hypercalcemia on feline exocrine pancreatic secretion. Gastroenterology 1982; 82:309–16.

46. Daghorn JC (1993) Lithostatine. In: Go VLW, DiMagno EP, Gardner JD et al. (eds) The pancreas: biology, pathobiology, and disease, 2nd edn. New York: Raven Press, pp. 253–63.

47. Freedman SD, Sakamoto K, Venu RP. GP2, the homologue to the renal cast protein uro-modulin, is

a major component of intraductal plugs in chronic pancreatitis. J Clin Invest 1993; 92:83–90.

48. Giorgi D, Bernard JP, De Caro A et al. Pancreatic stone protein. I. Evidence that it is encoded by a pancreatic messenger ribonucleic acid. Gastroenterology 1985; 89:381–6.

49. Giorgi D, Bernard JPO, Ranquir S et al. Secretory pancreatic stone protein messenger RNA. Nucleotide sequence and expression in chronic calcifying pancreatitis. J Clin Invest 1989; 84:100–6.

50. Schmiegel W, Buchert M, Kalthoft H et al. Immunochemical characterisation and quantitative distribution of pancreatic stone protein in sera and pancreatic secretion in pancreatic disorders. Gastroenterology 1990; 99:1421–30.

51. Lohse J, Schmid D, Sarles H. Pancreatic citrate and protein secretion of alcoholic dogs in response to graded doses of caerulein. Pflügers Arch 1983; 397:141–3.

52. Lohse J, Pfeiffer A. Duodenal total and ionised calcium secretion in normal subjects, chronic alcoholics, and patients with various stages of chronic alcoholic pancreatitis. Gut 1984; 25:874–80.

53. Noronha M, Bapista A, Bordalo O. Sequential aspects of pathology in chronic alcoholic disease of the pancreas. In: Gyr KE, Singer MV, Sarles H (eds) Pancreatitis – concepts and classification. Amsterdam: Elsevier, Excerpta Medica International Congress Series No. 642, 1984; pp. 61–5.

54. Noronha M, Bordalo O, Dreiling DA. Alcohol and the pancreas. II. Pancreatic morphology of advanced alcoholic pancreatitis. Am J Gastroenterol 1981; 76:120–4.

55. Bordalo O, Bapista A, Dreiling D et al. Early pathomorphological pancreatic changes in chronic alcoholism. In: Gyr KE, Singer MV, Sarles H (eds) Pancreatitis – concepts and classification. Amsterdam: Elsevier, Excerpta Medica International Congress Series No. 642, 1984; pp. 57–65.

56. Apte M, Wilson JS, Korsten MA et al. Effects of ethanol and protein deficiency on pancreatic digestive and lysosomal enzymes. Gut 1995; 36:287–93.

57. Klöppel G, Maillet B. Chronic pancreatitis: evolution of the disease. Hepatogastroenterology 1991; 38:408–12.

58. Klöppel G, Maillet B. The morphological basis for the evolution of acute pancreatitis into chronic pancreatitis. Virchow's Arch Pathol Anat 1992; 420:1–4.

59. Braganza JM. Pancreatic disease: a casualty of hepatic 'detoxification'. Lancet 1983; ii:1000–3.

60. Singer MW, Gyr K, Sarles H. Revised classification of pancreatitis. Report of the Second International Symposium on the Classification of Pancreatitis in Marseille, France, March 28–30, 1984. Gastroenterology 1985; 89:683–5.

61. Walsh TN, Rodes J, Theis BA et al. Minimal change chronic pancreatitis. Gut 1992; 33:1566–71.

62. Stolte M, Weib W, Vokholz H et al. A special form of segmental pancreatitis: 'groove pancreatitis'. Hepatogastroenterology 1982; 29:198–208.

63. Brokman D, Buchler M, Malfertheiner P et al. Analysis of nerves in chronic pancreatitis. Gastroenterology 1988; 94:1459–69.

64. Büchler M, Weihe E, Friess H et al. Changes in peptidergic innervation in chronic pancreatitis. Pancreas 1992; 7:183–92.

65. Di Sebastiano P, Fink T, Weihe E et al. Immune cell infiltration and growth-associated protein 43 expression correlate with pain in chronic pancreatitis. Gastroenterology 1997; 112:1648–55.

66. Lowenfels AB, Maisonneuve P, Cavallini G et al. Pancreatitis and the risk of pancreatic cancer. N Engl J Med 1993; 328:1433–7.

67. Karlson BM, Ekbom A, Josefsson S et al. The risk of pancreatic cancer following pancreatitis: an association due to confounding? Gastroenterology 1997; 587–92.

68. Bornman PC, Marks IN, Girdwood AH et al. Pathogenesis of pain in chronic pancreatitis – an ongoing enigma. World J Surg 2003; 27:1175–82.

69. Braganza JM. The pathogenesis of chronic pancreatitis. Q J Med 1996; 89:243–50.

70. Patel AG, Toyama MT, Alvarez C et al. Pancreatic interstitial pH in human and feline chronic pancreatitis. Gastroenterology 1995; 109:1639–45.

71. Bockman DE, Buchler M, Malfertheiner P et al. Analysis of nerves in chronic pancreatitis. Gastroenterology 1988; 94:1459–69.

72. Karanjia ND, Widdison AL, Leung F et al. Compartment syndrome in experimental chronic obstructive pancreatitis: effects of decompressing the main pancreatic duct. Br J Surg 1994; 81:259–64.

73. Ammann RW, Muellhaupt B and Zurich Pancreatitis Study Group. The natural history of pain in alcoholic chronic pancreatitis. Gastroenterology 1999; 116:1132–40.

74. Ammann RW, Akovbiantz A, Largadier F et al. Course and outcome of chronic pancreatitis. Longitudinal study of a mixed medical-surgical series of 245 patients. Gastroenterology 1984; 86:820–8.

75. Gallagher PJ, McLauchlin G, Bornman PC et al. Diagnostic pitfalls and therapeutic strategies in the treatment of pancreatic duct haemorrhage. HPB Surg 1997; 10:293–7.

76. Lankisch PG. Function tests in the diagnosis of chronic pancreatitis. Int J Pancreatol 1993; 14:9–20.

77. Niederau C, Grendell JH. Diagnosis of chronic pancreatitis. Gastroenterology 1985; 88:1973–5.

78. Gilinsky NH, Bornman PC, Girdwood AH et al. The diagnostic yield of ERCP in the diagnosis of pancreatic carcinoma. Br J Surg 1986; 73:539–43.

Two papers indicating that ultrasonography, CT imaging and ERCP combined result in a high sensitivity and specificity for the diagnosis of chronic pancreatitis.

79. Carter DC. Cancer of the head of pancreas or chronic pancreatitis? A diagnostic dilemma. Surgery 1992; 111:602–3.

80. Fritscher-Ravens A, Brand L. Comparison of endoscopic ultrasound-guided fine needle aspiration for focal pancreatic lesions in patients with normal parenchyma and chronic pancreatitis. Am J Gastroenterol 2002; 97(11): 2768–75.

81. Brand B, Pfaff T, Binmoeller KF et al. Endoscopic ultrasound of differential diagnosis of focal pancreatic lesions, confirmed by surgery. Scand J Gastroenterol 2000; 11:1221–8.

82. Axon ATR, Classen M, Cotton PB et al. Pancreatography in chronic pancreatitis: international definitions. Gut 1984; 25:1107–12.

83. Lankisch PG, Seidensticker F, Otto J et al. Secretin-pancreozymin test (SPT) and endoscopic retrograde cholangiopancreatography (ERCP): both are necessary for diagnosing or excluding chronic pancreatitis. Pancreas 1996; 12:149–52.

84. Girdwood AH, Hatfield ARW, Bornman PC et al. Structure and function in non-calcific pancreatitis. Dig Dis Sci 1984; 298:721–6.

85. Helander A. Biological markers in alcoholism. J Neural Transm Suppl 2003; 66:15–32.

86. Kondo T, Hayakawa T, Noda A et al. Follow-up study of chronic pancreatitis. Gastroenterol Jpn 1981; 16:46–56.

87. Bornman PC, Girdwood AH, Marks IN et al. The influence of continued alcohol intake, pancreatic duct hold-up and pancreatic insufficiency on the pain pattern in chronic non-calcific and calcific pancreatitis: a comparative study. Surg Gastroenterol 1982; 1:5–9.

88. Ink O, Labayle D, Buffet C et al. Painful alcoholic chronic pancreatitis: relations between pain, alcohol withdrawal and pancreatic surgery. Gastroenterol Clin Biol 1984; 8:419–25.

89. Banks PA. Medical strategy in chronic pancreatitis. In: Carter DC, Warshaw AL (eds) Pancreatitis. Edinburgh: Churchill Livingstone, 1989; pp. 133–47.

90. Bornman PC, Marks IN, Girdwood AH et al. Is pancreatic duct obstruction or stricture a major cause of pain in calcific pancreatitis? Br J Surg 1980; 67:425–8.

91. Gullo L, Barbara W, Labó G. Effect of cessation of alcohol use on the course of pancreatic dysfunction in alcoholic pancreatitis. Gastroenterology 1988; 95:1063–8.

92. Marks IN, Girdwood AH, Bank S et al. The prognosis of alcohol-induced calcific pancreatitis. S Afr Med J 1980; 57:640–3.

93. Lewis KS, Ham NH. Tramadol: a new centrally acting analgesic. Am J Health Syst Pharm 1997; 54:643–52.

94. Leung JWC, Bowen-Wright M, Aveling W et al. Coeliac plexus block for pain in pancreatic cancer and chronic pancreatitis. Br J Surg 1983; 70:730–2.

95. Madsen P, Hansen E. Coeliac plexus block versus pancreaticogastrostomy for pain in chronic pancreatitis. A controlled randomised trial. Scan J Gastroenterol 1985; 20:1217–20.

96. Myhre I, Hilstedt I, Troimier B et al. Monitoring of celiac plexus block in chronic pancreatitis. Pain 1989; 38: 269–74.

97. Gress F, Schmitt C, Sherman S et al. Endoscopic ultrasound-guided celiac plexus block for managing abdominal pain associated with chronic pancreatitis: A prospective single center experience. Am J Gastroenterol 2002; 96:409–16.

98. Maher JW, Johnlin FC, Pearson P. Thoracoscopic splanchnicectomy for chronic pancreatitis pain. Surgery 1996; 120(4):603–10.

99. Ihse I, Zoucas E, Gyllstedt E et al. Bilateral thoracoscopic splanchnicectomy: Effects on pancreatic pain and function. Ann Surg 1999; 230;785–91.

100. Moodley J, Singh B, Shaik AS et al. Thorascopic splanchnicectomy: Effects on pancreatic pain and function. Ann Surg 1999; 23;785–91.

101. Buscher HCJL, Jansen JBMJ, van Dongen R et al. Long-term results of bilateral thoracoscopic splanchnicectomy in patients with chronic pancreatitis. Br J Surg 2002; 89:158–62.

102. Cuschieri A, Shimi SM, Crosthwatie G et al. Bilateral endoscopic splanchnicectomy through a posterior thorascopic approach. J R Coll Surg Edin 1994; 39:44–7.

103. Makarewicz W, Stefaniak T, Kossakowska M et al. Quality of life improvement after videothorascopic splanchnicectomy in chronic pancreatitis patients: case control study. World J Surg 2003; 27:906–11.

104. Larvin MM, McMahon MJ, Puntis MCA et al. Marked placebo responses in chronic pancreatitis: final results of a controlled trial of Creon therapy. Br J Surg 1992; 79:457 (abstr.).

105. Isaksson G, Ihse I. Pain reduction by an oral pancreatic enzyme preparation in chronic pancreatitis. Dig Dis Sci 1983; 28:97–102.

106. Slaff J, Jacobson D, Tillman CR et al. Protease specific suppression of pancreatic exocrine secretion. Gastroenterology 1984; 87:44–52.

107. Halgreen H, Pedersen NT, Worning H. Symptomatic effect of pancreatic enzyme therapy in patients with chronic pancreatitis. Scand J Gastroenterol 1986; 21:104–8.

108. Mossner J, Secknus R, Meyer J et al. Treatment of pain with pancreatic extracts in chronic pancreatitis: results of a prospective placebo-controlled multicentre trial. Digestion 1992; 53:54–66.

109. Malesci A, Gaia E, Fioretta A et al. No effect of long-term treatment with pancreatic extract on recurrent abdominal pain in patients with chronic pancreatitis. Scand J Gastroenterol 1995; 30:392–8.

   Initial enthusiastic response for the use of pancreatic replacement therapy for pain has not been supported by the disappointing results of these two randomised controlled trials.

110. Malfertheiner P, Mayer D, Büchler M et al. Treatment of pain in chronic pancreatitis by inhibition of pancreatic secretion with octreotide. Gut 1995; 36:450–4.

111. Toskes PP, Forsmark CE, DeMeo MT et al. Octreotide for the pain of chronic pancreatitis: results of a multicentre placebo-controlled dose-ranging pilot study. Pancreas (in press).

   Randomised trial showing benefit in using octreotide for pancreatic pain.

112. Kalvaria I, Bornman PC, Marks IN et al. The spectrum and natural history of common bile duct stenosis in chronic alcohol induced pancreatitis. Ann Surg 1989; 210:608–13.

113. Bornman PC, Kalvaria I, Girdwood AH et al. Clinical relevance of cholestasis syndrome in chronic pancreatitis: the Cape Town experience. In: Beger HG, Buchler M, Ditschuneit H et al. (eds) Chronic pancreatitis. Berlin: Springer-Verlag, 1990; pp. 256–9.

114. Huizinga W, Spitalls J, Thomson S et al. Chronic pancreatitis with biliary obstruction. Ann R Coll Surg Engl 1992; 74: 119–23.

115. Carter DC. Pancreatitis and the biliary tree: The continuing problem. Am J Surg 1988; 155:10–17.

116. Wilson D, Auld CD, Schlinkert R et al. Hepatobiliary complications in chronic pancreatitis. Gut 1989; 30:520–7.

117. Deviere J, Devaere S, Baize M et al. Endoscopic biliary drainage in chronic pancreatitis. Gastrointest Endosc 1990; 36:96–100.

118. Kiehne K, Folsch UR, Nitsche R. High complication rate of bile duct stents in patients with chronic alcoholic pancreatitis due to non-compliance. Endoscopy 2000; 32; 377–80.

119. Draganove P, Hoffman B, Marsch W et al. Long-term outcome in patients with benign biliary strictures treated endoscopically with multiple stents. Gastrointest Endosc 2002; 55:680–6.

120. Farnbacher MJ, Rabenstein R, Ell C et al. Is endoscopic drainage of common bile duct stenoses in chronic pancreatitis up-to-date? Am J Gastroenterol 2000; 95:1466–71.

121. Deviere J, Cremer M, Baize M et al. Management of common bile duct strictures caused by chronic pancreatitis with metal mesh self-expandable stents. Gut 1994; 35:122–6.

122. Nealon WH, Walser E. Main pancreatic ductal anatomy can direct choice of modality for treating pancreatic pseudocyst (surgery versus percutaneous drainage). Ann Surg 2002; 235:751–8.

123. Beckingham IJ, Krige JEJ, Bornman PC et al. Endoscopic management of pancreatic pseudocysts. Br J Surg 1997; 84:1638–45.

124. Beckingham IJ, Krige JEJ, Bornman PC et al. Long-term outcome of endoscopic drainage of pancreatic pseudocysts. Am J Gastroenterol 1999; 94:71–4.

   Early prospective studies demonstrating encouraging results for endoscopic drainage of pseudocysts.

125. Wiersma MJ. Endosonography-guided cyst-duodenostomy with therapeutic ultrasound endoscope. Gastrointest Endosc 1996; 44:611–17.

126. Gomes-Cerezo J, Barbado Cano A, Suarez I et al. Pancreatic ascites: study of therapeutic options by analysis of case reports and case series between the years 1975 and 2000. Am J Gastroenterol 2003; 93(3):568–77.

127. Kozarek RA. Endoscopic therapy of complete and partial pancreatic duct disruption. Gastrointest Endosc Clin North Am 1998; 8:39–53.

128. Sarforafas GH, Sarr MG, Farley DR et al. The significance of sinistral portal hypertension complicating chronic pancreatitis. Am J Surg 2000; 179:129–33.

129. DuVal MK. Caudal pancreaticojejunostomy for chronic relapsing pancreatitis. Ann Surg 1954; 140:775–85.

130. Delcore R, Rodriguez FJ, Thomas JH et al. The role of pancreaticojejunostomy in patients without dilated pancreatic ducts. Am J Surg 1994; 168:598–601.

131. Izbicki JR, Bloechle C, Broering DC et al. Longitudinal V-shaped excision of the ventral pancreas for small duct disease in severe chronic pancreatitis. Prospective evaluation of a new surgical procedure. Ann Surg 1998; 227(2):213–19.

132. Puestow CB, Gillesby WJ. Retrograde surgical drainage of the pancreas for chronic relapsing pancreatitis. Arch Surg 1958; 76:898–907.

133. Partington PF, Rochelle REC. Modified Puestow procedure for retrograde drainage of the pancreatic duct. Ann Surg 1960; 152:1037–43.

134. Prinz RA, Greenlee HB. Pancreatic duct drainage in 100 patients with chronic pancreatitis. *Ann Surg* 1981; 194:313–18.

135. Holmberg TJ, Isaacsson T, Ihse I. Long-term results in pancreaticojejunostomy in chronic pancreatitis. Surg Gynecol Obstet 1985; 160:339–46.

136. Noguiera CED, Dani R. Evaluation of the surgical treatment of chronic calcifying pancreatitis. Surg Gynecol Obst 1985;161:117.

137. Bradley EL. Long-term results of pancreatico-jejunostomy in patients with chronic pancreatitis. Am J Surg 1987; 153:207–13.

138. Adolff M, Schloegel M, Arnaud JP et al. Role of pancreatojejunostomy in the treatment of chronic pancreatitis: study of 105 operated patients. Chirurgie 1991; 117:251–7.

139. Wilson TG, Hollands MJ, Little JM. Pancreato-jejunostomy for chronic pancreatitis. Aust NZ J Surg 1992; 62:111–15.

Prospective studies demonstrating modest long-term benefit of pancreaticojejunostomy for pancreatic pain.

140. Markowitz JS, Rattner DW, Warshaw AL. Failure of symptomatic relief after pancreatojejunal decompression for chronic pancreatitis. Arch Surg 1994; 129:374–80.

141. Frey CF, Smith GJ. Description and rationale for a new operation for chronic pancreatitis. Pancreas 1987; 2:701–5.

Original description of the Frey operation.

142. Frey CF, Mikura K. Local resection of the head of the pancreas combined with longitudinal pancreatico-jejunostomy in the management of patients with chronic pancreatitis. Ann Surg 1994; 220:492–507.

143. Izibicki JR, Bloechle C, Knoefel WT et al. Duodenum-preserving resection of the head of the pancreas in chronic pancreatitis: a prospective, randomised trial. Ann Surg 1995; 221:350–8.

Randomised controlled trial in 61 patients showing no difference in pain relief between extended drainage or resection but an apparent improvement in quality of life with the former procedure.

144. Frey CF, Ho HS. Distal pancreatectomy in chronic pancreatitis. In: Trede M, Carter DC (eds) Surgery of the pancreas, 2nd edn. New York: Churchill Livingstone, 1997; pp. 347–55.

145. Howard TJ, Maiden CL, Smith HG et al. Surgical treatment of obstructive pancreatitis. Surgery 1995; 118:727–34.

146. Rattner DW, Fernandez-del Castillo C, Warshaw AL. Pitfalls of distal pancreatectomy for relief of pain in chronic pancreatitis. Am J Surg 1996; 171:142–6.

147. Sawyer R, Frey CF. Is there still a role for distal pancreatectomy in surgery for chronic pancreatitis? Am J Surg 1994; 168:6–9.

148. Saforafas GH, Sarr MG, Rowlands CM et al. Post-obstructive chronic pancreatitis. Results with distal resection. Arch Surg 2001; 136:643–7.

149. Beger HG, Imaizumi T. Duodenum-preserving head resection in chronic pancreatitis. J Hepatobil Pancreat Surg 1995; 2:13–18.

150. Morel P, Mathey P, Corboud H et al. Pylorus-preserving duodenopancreatectomy: long-term complications in comparison with a Whipple procedure. World J Surg 1990; 14:642–7.

151. Martin RF, Rossi RL, Leslie KA. Long-term results of pylorus preserving pancreatoduodenectomy for chronic pancreatitis. Arch Surg 1996; 131:247–52.

152. Keuse E, van Laarhoven CJHM, Eddes EH et al. Size of the pancreatic head as a prognostic factor for the outcome of Beger's procedure for painful chronic pancreatitis. Br J Surg 2003; 90:320–4.

153. Buchler M, Friess H, Muller MW et al. Randomised trial of duodenum-preserving pancreatic head resection versus pylorus preserving Whipple in chronic pancreatitis. Am J Surg 1995; 169:65–9.

Randomised trial showing no obvious benefit when a duodenum-preserving operation is performed.

154. Jimenez RE, Castillo CF, Rattner DW et al. Pylorus-preserving pancreatico-duodenectomy in the treatment of chronic pancreatitis. World J Surg 2003; 27:1211–16.

155. Gall FP, Gebhardt C, Meister R et al. Severe chronic cephalic pancreatitis: use of partial duodeno-pancreatectomy with occlusion of the pancreatic duct in 289 patients. World J Surg 1989; 13:809.

156. Rossi RL, Rothschild J, Braasch JW et al. Pancreato-duodenectomy in the management of chronic pancreatitis. Arch Surg 1987; 122:416.

157. Moreaux J. Long-term follow-up study of 50 patients with pancreaticoduodenectomy for chronic pancreatitis. World J Surg 1984; 8:346.

158. Traverso LW, Kozarek RA. The Whipple procedure for severe complications of chronic pancreatitis. Arch Surg 1993; 128:1047.

159. Beger HG, Buchler M. Duodenum-preserving resection of head of pancreas in chronic pancreatitis: results after duodenum-preserving resection of the head of pancreas. Pancreas 1995; 11:77–85.

Equivalent outcome with or without duodenum preservation in partial pancreatic resection for chronic pancreatitis.

160. Bloechle C, Izbicki JR, Knoefel WT et al. Quality of life in chronic pancreatitis: results after duodenum-preserving resection of the head of the pancreas. Pancreas 1995; 11:77–85.

161. Frey CF, Suzuki M, Isaji S et al. Pancreatic resection for chronic pancreatitis. Surg Clin North Am 1989; 69:499–528.

162. Trede M, Schwall G. The complications of pancreatectomy. Ann Surg 1988; 207:39–47.

163. Rossi RL, Soeldner JS, Braasch JW et al. Long-term results of pancreatic resection and segmental pancreatic autotransplantation for chronic pancreatitis. Am J Surg 1990; 159:51–8.

164. Dafoe DC, Naji A, Perloff LJ et al. Pancreatic and islet autotransplantation. Hepatogastroenterology 1990; 37:307–15.

165. White SA. Pancreas resection and islet auto-transplantation for end-stage chronic pancreatitis. Ann Surg 2001; 233:423–31.

166. Kozarek RA, Traverso LW. Endoscopic treatment of chronic pancreatitis: an alternative to surgery? Dig Surg 1996; 13:90–100.

     Systematic review of collective series suggesting that endoscopic treatment of pancreatic pain varied from 50 to 85% with moderate long-term follow-up.

167. Rosch T, Daniel S, Scholtz M et al. Endoscopic treatment of chronic pancreatitis: A multicenter study of 1000 patients with long-term follow-up. Endoscopy 2002; 34(10):765–71.

168. Adamek HE, Jakobs R, Buttmann A et al. Long-term follow-up of patients with chronic pancreatitis and pancreatic stones treated with extracorporeal shock wave lithotripsy. Gut 1999; 45:402–5.

169. Morgan DE, Smith JK, Hawkings K et al. Endoscopic stent therapy in advanced chronic pancreatitis: Relationships between ductal changes, clinical response, and stent patency. Am J Gastroenterol 2003; 98(4):821–6.

170. Smith MT, Sherman S, Ikenberry SO et al. Alterations in pancreatic duct morphology following polyethylene pancreatic stent therapy. Gastrointest Endosc 1996; 44:268–75.

171. Sherman S, Hawes RH, Savides TJ et al. Stent-induced pancreatic ductal and parenchymal changes: correlation of endoscopic ultrasound with ERCP. Gastrointest Endosc 1996; 44:276–82.

172. Di Magno EP. Towards understanding and management of painful chronic pancreatitis. Gastroenterology 1991; 116:1252–7.

173. Sherman I, Lehman GA, Hawes RH et al. Pancreatic ductal stones: frequency of successful endoscopic removal and improvement in symptoms. Gastrointest Endosc 1991; 37:511–17.

174. Lankish PG, Banks PA. Chronic pancreatitis: treatment of pancreatic insufficiency. Berlin: Springer-Verlag, 1998; pp. 316–25.

175. Steer ML, Waxman I, Freedman S. Chronic pancreatitis. N Engl J Med 1995; 332:1482–90.

     Excellent review of the natural history and management of chronic pancreatitis.

176. Eckhauser FE, Strodel WE, Krol JA et al. Near-total pancreatectomy for chronic pancreatitis. Surgery 1984; 96:599–607.

177. Braganza JM. Pathogenesis of chronic pancreatitis. Q J Med 1996; 89:243–50.

178. Salim AS. Role of oxygen-derived free radical scavengers in the treatment of recurrent pain produced by chronic pancreatitis – a new approach. Arch Surg 1991; 126:1109–14.

179. Bilton D, Schofield D, Mei G et al. Placebo-controlled trials of antioxidant therapy with S-adensylmethionine in patients with recurrent non-gallstone pancreatitis. Drug Invest 1994; 8:10–20.

180. Uden S, Schofield D, Miller PF et al. Antioxidant therapy for recurrent pancreatitis: biochemical profiles in a placebo controlled trial. Aliment Pharmacol Ther 1992; 6:229–40.

181. Warshaw AL, Banks PA, Del Castillo CF. AGA Technical Review: Treatment of pain in chronic pancreatitis. Gastroenterology 1998; 115:765–76.

Thirteen

Pancreatic cancer

Paul F. Ridgway and
Kevin C. Conlon

INTRODUCTION

Cancer of the pancreas remains a lethal disease associated with insidious onset in most sufferers. Despite resection with curative intent, overall survival approximates to 5% at 5 years. This figure is unchanged over the last quarter of a century.

However, recent improvements in preoperative imaging and staging strategies, coupled with improvements in perioperative care, have led to a resurgence of interest in this deadly cancer. A degree of optimism is also seen in the role and efficacy of adjuvant therapies combined with better understanding of the molecular basis of the disease.

Pancreatic neoplasia covers a broad spectrum of disease, encompassing benign and malignant pathology of both exocrine and endocrine function. As exocrine ductal adenocarcinomas and periampullary lesions account for 95% of malignant pancreatic lesions, they will form the focus of this chapter.

EPIDEMIOLOGY

An estimated 30 700 new cases of adenocarcinoma of the pancreas will occur in the USA each year, with 30 000 ensuing disease-related deaths.[1] The UK figures mirror this, with 3673 women and 3086 men diagnosed with the disease in 1999.[2] This confers a 1 in 96 lifetime risk in men (11th commonest) and a 1 in 95 risk in women (7th commonest). Male and female rates are thought to be equivalent, although there may be some bias related to the relative longevity of females.[3] Peak incidence for the disease occurs between the seventh and eighth decades of life, this form of cancer being very rare under the age of 30. In American populations, ethnicities such as African and Hawaiian confer a higher incidence than Caucasian, whereas Hispanic and Asian appear to be at slightly lower risks of developing the disease.[4] Overall it is felt that the incidence of pancreatic cancer is rising, particularly in Europe, although this observation is subject to reporting basis related to improved diagnostics. In the USA the incidence increased three-fold over the first three-quarters of the 20th century but has stabilised since.[5]

RISK FACTORS

Several risk factors to the development of cancer have been proposed based on cohort and case-control studies.

Smoking

Cigarette smoking is associated with a trebling of risk. In 1986, the International Agency for Research on Cancer (IARC) classified smoking as a proven carcinogen with respect to cancer of the pancreas.

Observational studies suggest that a dose-dependent relationship exists, necessitating long-term exposure.[6,7]

The precise carcinogen in cigarette smoke is unknown. The time in which cigarette smoking exerts its negative influence is also subject to debate; however, certain observational studies seem to point towards the latter stages of carcinogenesis, particularly in the 15 years preceding development.[8]

Alcohol

The role of heavy alcohol consumption in the development of pancreatic cancer is controversial. An association has been reported in at least two case–control studies,[9,10] although others question this relationship.[11] The IARC working group analysis dismissing alcohol as a factor predates these studies.[12]

Diet

Detailed case–control and cohort dietary analysis forms the mainstay of data regarding the association of diet and cancer development. Diets high in saturated fat have a suggested contributing role[13] although the data are not robust. Total energy intake has been also suggested,[14] although there are confounding issues such as increased body mass index (BMI) and over-reporting. Obesity itself has a positive association, with a relative risk of 1.72.[15] Height also has a proposed increased risk, although this may simply represent a surrogate for diet as a child.[15] Other positive and negative associations include vitamin C (protective),[13,14,16] fibre (protective),[13,16] and caffeine (negative),[17] but these are hotly disputed and probably play minimal roles at best.

Occupation

Workers exposed to ionising radiation, aluminium, acrylamide,[18] and halogenated hydrocarbons[19] have been reported to have a somewhat increased risk of developing adenocarcinoma of the pancreas.[3] In particular, the dry-cleaning industry is subject to a relative risk in the region of 1.5.[19,20] But, these data are considered weak overall and particular associations are controversial.

Past medical history

Interest has been paid to patients with chronic pancreatitis and diabetes. It has been suggested that increased risk is at its maximal shortly after diagnosis.[21] Whether these conditions have similar causal factors, represent precursors or are directly implicated in the carcinogenesis pathway is uncertain. In the case of pancreatitis, the risk of cancer approximates to normality after 10 years; with diabetes a positive association lasts beyond the 5-year mark. Other conditions linked with pancreatic cancer include Gardner's syndrome, and multiple endocrine neoplasia type 1 (neuroendocrine cancers).

Hereditary pancreatic cancer

The true extent of inherited patterns of pancreatic cancers have only recently become known. Previously, despite various reports of pancreatic cancer families,[22,23] the disease was not thought to have a significant familial preponderance. Silverman et al.[24] demonstrated a significantly increased risk of developing pancreatic cancer where a first-degree relative suffered the disease, in particular if the index case smoked. This was confirmed in a large US cohort study suggesting an odds ratio of 1.5 among first-degree relatives.[25] Seven percent of pancreatic cancers (over and above controls) are now thought to have some genetic relationship.[26] There exist known familial conditions such as Peutz–Jeghers syndrome[27] and the STK11/LLLLKB1 gene, BRCA2 expression[28] and atypical multiple mole syndrome (p16 inactivated in 95% of sporadic cancers) may predispose to pancreatic cancer.[29] Links with familial adenomatous polyposis, BRCA1 and von Hippel–Lindau have been suggested but not confirmed as conferring increased risk.

 Over recent decades there has been a steady rise in the incidence of pancreatic cancer, which is strongly associated with cigarette smoking.

PRECURSOR LESIONS

Defining precursor lesions and identifying factors with respect to pancreatic cancer development has proven difficult, due in part to the lack of a robust animal model for the disease. Despite this short-coming, molecular pathways characterising the change to the neoplastic phenotype have been better elucidated in recent times. The advent of micro-array chip analysis of normal and pathological pancreatic tissue represents a significant step forward not only in the efficiency of investigation but in identifying novel patterns for study. Tumour suppressor gene p16 has received much interest as over 95% of pancreatic cancers demonstrate a loss of function. This is usually due to homozygous deletions, loss of heterozygosity or promoter methylation.[30] Occasionally this can be an inherited defect. The K-*ras* gene product mediates signal transduction in the growth factor receptors, and mutations to this pathway are present in over 90% of ductal lesions.[31] Alteration in cell-cycle regulation, in particular inhibition of entry in S phase, accomplished by p53 protein, is lost in over 50% of cases.[32] Other targets include transforming growth factor β (TGFβ) receptor genes, BRCA2, HER-2/NEU, DPC4, MKK4 and EBER-1.

Workers for Johns Hopkins University have recently proposed pancreatic intraepithelial neo-plasms (PanIN; 1A→1B→2→3)[33] as the precursor lesions to invasive carcinoma in the pancreas. The model is similar to that of ductal carcinoma in situ (DCIS) of the breast or adenomatous polyps in

colorectal cancer. The lesions display atypical mucinous epithelium replacing the physiological cuboidal epithelium. The evidence for PanIN being true premalignant states is largely circumstantial although pressing. These lesions were first described adjacent to resected adenocarcinoma[34] more commonly than in non-neoplastic pancreas. The more atypical PanIN-2 and 3 were seen exclusively in neoplastic pancreas. These lesions also display similar genetic aberrations to the frankly invasive samples. In particular, the percentage of p16 and K-*ras* mutations increases the more atypical the PanIN. These data have heralded development of a tumorigenesis model[35] involving sequential progression from PanIN 1a→invasive adeno-carcinoma (**Fig. 13.1**). Similarly to breast DCIS, the natural progression and history of these lesions remain to be elucidated.

PRESENTATION

The majority of patients present with symptoms that are vague and non-specific (**Box 13.1**). Frequently, symptoms are assigned retrospectively when alarm signs such as jaundice finally occasion presentation. As a result disease is commonly widespread at diagnosis, and reports suggest in the region of 80% continue to present with irresectable disease.[36]

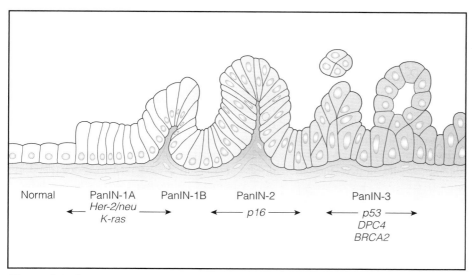

Figure 13.1 • Diagrammatic repesentation of PanIN progression to invasive carcinoma. Reproduced from Wilentz RE et al. Cancer Res 2000; 60(7):2002–6, with permission.

Box 13.1 · Symptoms/signs suggestive of pancreatic neoplasm

- Obstructive jaundice (+/− pain)
- Unexplained weight loss
- Endoscopy-negative epigastric/back symptoms
- Late-onset diabetes without antecedent risks
- Signs of malabsorption without defined cause
- None

The classical Courvoisier syndrome (palpable gall-bladder in the presence of painless jaundice) occurs in less than 25%. Jaundice may represent either primary disease causing biliary obstruction or advanced disease in the porta hepatis nodes. Pain is a more common symptom than physicians usually appreciate.[37] This may occur due to involvement of the visceral afferent nerves (and may be a portent of irresectability) or be related to an induced local pancreatitis. Weight loss is not necessarily a metastatic feature as in other epithelial tumours and, with pain, form the most tangible symptom and sign. Body and tail lesions tend to present insidiously and are therefore frequently advanced by the time symptoms appear.

Virchow's node (left supraclavicular node associated with upper gastrointestinal (GI) malignancy), thrombophlebitis migrans (non-specific paraneoplastic sign named after Trousseau) and Sister Mary Joseph nodule (umbilical metastatic lesion via the falciform ligament) are well described features of advanced disease. Blumer's shelf (rectally palpable rectovesical or rectovaginal mass) occurs exceptionally and is not usually sought as part of routine examination.

The most useful aide in disease diagnosis is an index of suspicion. Vague epigastric symptoms and weight loss in the presence of normal endoscopy and preliminary radiology should initiate further detailed investigation.

INVESTIGATION

Serology

Haematological and hepatic biochemical measurements are largely unhelpful in diagnosis although they may be deranged secondary to the tumour. Haemoglobin may be somewhat diminished secondary to occult loss although significant reductions can be seen with invading ampullary lesions. The picture of obstructive jaundice may be detected by investigating liver biochemistry, and alterations in bilirubin and alkaline phosphatase are the usual abnormalities. Hyperamylasaemia is not the rule and suggests a significant degree of obstruction or local pancreatitis. A raised pro-thrombin time suggests hepatic dysfunction secondary to metastases. Hyperglycaemia is non-specific and occurs in at least 20% of patients. The exact aetiology of this is unclear as glucose homeostasis is usually preserved until less than 10% of islet function remains. However, peripheral glucose resistance is present in >50% and may account for the abnormal glucose tolerance tests in the majority of patients.

Markers

There are a myriad of tumour markers available. The most valuable is a glycoprotein, carbohydrate antigen 19-9 (CA19-9; 0–37 U/mL). Initially it was based on a monoclonal antibody to colorectal cancer cell lines. As with all markers it has sensitivity and specificity issues. Falsely elevated CA19-9 is documented in non-malignant conditions such as pancreatitis, hepatic dysfunction and jaundice (failure to excrete). Levels higher than 200 U/mL confer a 90% sensitivity, and levels in the thousands are associated with high specificity (but also irresectability). Patients expressing Lewis blood group antigens (a and b) may have elevated levels.[38] CA19-9 is related to prognosis, and in particular if it is elevated preresection it can be used to predict recurrence postoperatively.[39] Levels exceeding a median of 243 U/mL for those undergoing primary chemoradiotherapy for locoregionally advanced disease also signify poorer median survival (7.1 vs. 12.3 months).[40] Although CA19-9 is primarily a marker of ductal adenocarcinoma, certain endocrine pancreatic tumours with ductal differentiation may also express the marker.[41] CA19-9 is probably not useful as a screening test in asymptomatic populations.[42]

Other markers, namely carcinoembryonic antigen (CEA), CA242, CA50, SPAN-1, DU-PAN2 and

(a)

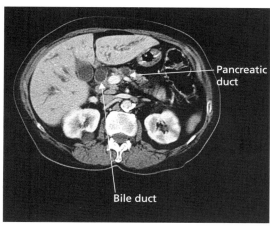

Pancreatic duct

Bile duct

(b)

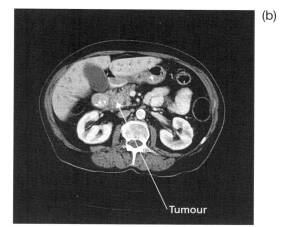

Tumour

Figure 13.2 • CT scan demonstrating **(a)** biliary and pancreatic duct obstruction caused by a carcinoma of the head of the pancreas **(b)**.

CAM-17.1, are proposed as having application in pancreatic neoplasms although relative insensitivity or unavailability limits their usefulness in practice.[43]

Diagnosis

Multiple diagnostic modalities are available for investigation. Transabdominal (TA) ultrasound (US) is obtained commonly in the jaundiced patient. It is often the first investigation in the jaundiced patient as its sensitivity for determining cholelithiasis is superior to that of computed tomography (CT). Common bile duct dilatation (>7 mm; >10 mm in cholecystectomised patients) is an indirect sign together with pancreatic duct dilatation (>2 mm). The primary pancreatic lesion is often visible together with liver metastases and ascites if present. TAUS is operator dependent and is not as sensitive as CT at detecting smaller lesions.[44,45]

Thin-cut contrast-enhanced multislice (1.25-mm sliced) pancreas protocol helical CT is the radiological investigation of choice (**Figs 13.2** and **13.3**). Intravenous and oral contrast is utilised, and scans are performed in three phases (non-contrast, venous and arterial). It is approximately 90% sensitive for lesions greater than 2 cm, although this drops to approximately 60% for smaller lesions. Apart from diagnosing the neoplasm, good-quality CT has advanced imaging to the point where it is useful in determining resectability. Metastatic lesions can be demonstrated, and more subtle parameters such as

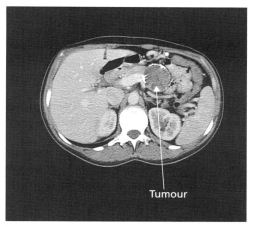

Tumour

Figure 13.3 • CT scan of a 42-year-old woman with a solid pseudopapillary tumour in the body of her pancreas. Diagnosis was made after an incidental calcification was noted on routine abdominal radiograph.

portal vein or superior mesenteric artery involvement can be determined. It is noteworthy, however, that small volume liver and peritoneal disease is missed frequently.

Magnetic resonance imaging (MRI) has evolved significantly in recent years. Its predilection for defining soft tissue has seen it overtake CT in many areas. Although this has not happened yet for the pancreas, the combination of T1/T2-weighted imaging with magnetic resonance cholangio-pancreatography (MRCP) is useful as the primary tumour can be visualised together with its relationship to biliary and pancreatic ducts as well as peripancreatic vasculature. T1-weighted images demonstrate the lesion with decreased signal, and on T2 the signal can be variable. The main use of T2 images is in MRCP after the intravenous injection of gadolinium-based contrast.

Endoscopic retrograde cholangiopancreatography (ERCP) is reserved mainly to characterise obstructive intraductal lesions and to relieve biliary obstruction in selected cases. Non-invasive MRCP is replacing ERCP as a diagnostic modality in this area. Endoscopic ultrasound (EUS) is useful in determining lesions that are equivocal on CT, allowing fine-needle aspiration if diagnosis is required.

Positron emission tomography (PET) has not been fully evaluated in diagnosis of pancreatic cancer; having variable sensitivities (c. 71%) and specificities (c. 64%) for demonstrating the pancreatic primary,[45] it does not define anatomical detail. It is not useful in determining local resectability since its main use is in demonstrating metastases although it is important to remember that hyperglycaemia (present in 15% of cases) may induce false negatives.

Cytology/histology

High-quality thin-slice pancreas CT forms the mainstay of diagnosis. Many tertiary referral centres forego histological or cytological confirmation prior to embarking on resection. The need for preoperative pathological confirmation depends in part on the radiological experience as well as the therapeutic philosophy and experience of the treating institution's surgeons. However, in such cases patients should be specifically counselled of a 10% rate of resection for benign disease. Conversely, due to the sclerotic nature of the adenocarcinomas a negative fine-needle aspirate should not deter the attending surgeon when there is robust CT evidence of neoplasia.

If neoadjuvant therapy is considered, histological confirmation is mandatory. This can be accomplished by transabdominal biopsy (US/CT) or endoscopy [ERCP/endoscopic ultrasound (EUS) + fine needle aspiration cytology (FNAC)].

It is accepted that helical CT scanning undertaken to a strict pancreas protocol is the radiological investigation of choice in the diagnosis and staging of pancreatic cancer.

ADVANCED STAGING TECHNIQUES

Laparoscopy

Laparoscopic strategies for staging of cancers have become increasing relevant in recent times. Both laparoscopy and laparoscopic ultrasound (**Fig. 13.4**) have proven roles in assessing those suffering from selected pancreatic neoplasms.[46,47] Laparoscopy may be performed immediately before conversion[48–50] to laparotomy or as an interval staging measure.[51,52] The added value of laparoscopy over state-of-the-art dynamic multislice CT remains up to 38% (**Table 13.1**).[51,53]

The main aim of staging laparoscopy is to mimic the open procedure with the minimum of access-related trauma. There exists some considerable controversy regarding its employment. Although in specialist hands it appears to correctly stage in the region of 11–35% more cases, critics extrapolate from open data suggesting that laparoscopy should only influence 10% of cases. These data include ampullary lesions, where laparoscopy classically only affects management where small-volume liver or rarely peritoneal disease is discovered (**Fig. 13.5**) (also in colour, Plate 12, facing p. 20).

Those who oppose minimal access staging suggest that a significant proportion of patients require surgical bypass and therefore laparoscopic staging should only be used if this would not be contemplated at laparotomy.[54,55] This is countered

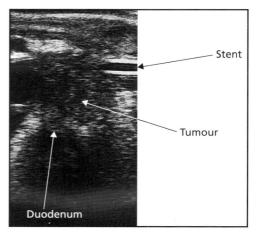

Figure 13.4 • Laparoscopic ultrasound characterising an ampullary carcinoma.

Table 13.1 • Percentage upstaged based on advanced minimal access staging strategies

Author	Year	N	Resectable on CT	CT resectable, laparoscopy irresectable	Percentage upstaged
Bemelman	1995	70	70	16	23
Conlon	1996	115	115	41	37
Andren-Sanberg	1998	60	60	11	18
Catheline	1999	26	26	8	31
Pierabissa	1999	50	42	10	24
Reddy	1999	109	99	70	71
Jimenez	2000	125	70	39	56
Conlon	2000	577	577	211	37
Total		**1132**	**1059**	**406**	**38**

Modified from Conlon et al.[127]

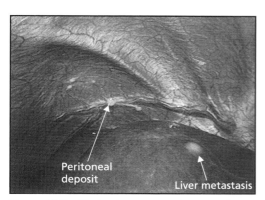

Figure 13.5 • Staging laparoscopy demonstrating small-volume hepatic and peritoneal deposits not seen on pancreas protocol CT. See also Plate 12, facing p. 20.

by the Memorial Sloan Kettering Cancer Center's experience from New York,[56] where only 3% of those defined as irresectable required subsequent palliative open bypass. Indeed, the authors went on to suggest that these data argue against the use of routine gastric or biliary bypass. This opinion is challenged by a randomised trial from Baltimore[57] investigating 43 patients who were randomised to no prophylactic gastroenterostomy when 19% (8) required subsequent gastric bypass. These data indicate that the matter remains open for interpretation and requires further investigation.

Concern has been expressed regarding the biological effect of insufflant gas (CO_2) on viable intraperitoneal tumour.[58–60] In particular, its hypoxic and acidic nature had been suggested as a possible facilitator for tumour seeding at port sites. This concern does not appear to be a clinically significant issue demonstrable on retrospective clinical analysis,[61] although the potential biological effects remain to be fully elucidated.[62]

The staging strategy mirrors open surgery via minimal access. It is helpful to mark the definitive incision thus allowing ports to be placed along the planned bilateral subcostal wound. A 10-mm port is placed in the right upper quadrant after induction of the pneumoperitoneum via the infraumbilical port site. A further 5-mm port is placed left of the midline. General laparoscopy is performed with an angled (usually 30-degree) lens looking for small-volume peritoneal and liver metastases not normally seen on CT. The liver is examined systematically and usually all but segment 7 can be viewed. If hepatic or peritoneal deposits are demonstrated then biopsy for frozen section histology is taken and the procedure is terminated if positive. Should there be no evidence of metastases, the hepatico-duodenal ligament is inspected for nodal disease. The lesser sac is opened by incising the gastrocolic omentum. This is achievable in approximately 80%. Once the sac is open it is inspected for tumour, and biopsies of the primary may be performed. In certain centres, mobilisation of the duodenum is performed to more faithfully mimic the open procedure although the authors believe that in the majority of cases this is unnecessary. When neoadjuvant therapies become more efficacious, there is no doubt that laparoscopic strategies will become increasingly important to define a group that may be suitable for downstaging similar to advanced rectal lesions. Inadequacy in chemotherapy and radiotherapy preclude consideration of this strategy at present.

Other staging techniques

Where the radiology (CT or MRI) suggests involvement of portal vein, endoscopic ultrasound may be useful to characterise further the presence and degree of invasion. Indeed, endoscopic ultrasound may also help define benign conditions mimicking cancer such as sclerosing pancreatitis or atypical choledocholithiasis. Using the stomach or duodenal wall as a sonic window, it can give fine anatomical detail including pancreas, gallbladder, common bile duct, coeliac axis and liver. While it is operator dependent, it has been reported to pick up lesions as small as 5 mm, where CT and MRI are less sensitive below 2 cm. EUS is extremely useful in defining small periampullary lesions[63] and has similar efficacy to ERCP. Vertical arrays can facilitate placement of fine needles for biopsy. Angiography to stage pancreatic cancer is no longer used routinely. ERCP for staging is reserved primarily for lesions involving the common bile duct where knowledge of extent of involvement is desirable. Even this function is largely being replaced by MRCP. ERCP's primary role is in the relief of lower biliary obstruction; similarly, percutaneous transhepatic cholangiography (PTC) is now used exclusively in relief of more proximal lesions.

There is strong evidence that laparoscopy provides additional information in the staging of pancreatic cancer over conventional radiological investigation but there remains debate on its impact on quality of survival in centres favouring open operative palliative techniques.

PATHOLOGY

Ductal adenocarcinomas account for 90–95% of all tumours (**Table 13.2**). It is probably best to regard tumours of the pancreas according to cellular differentiation:

- exocrine (ductal/acinar)
- endocrine: B cells (insulin), A cells (glucagon), δ cells (somatostatin)
- mesenchymal cells.

Table 13.2 • Common histotypes of pancreatic cancer

Differentiation	Histotype	Comment
Ductal (95%)	Adenocarcinoma Medullary Adenosquamous Serous cystadenocarcinoma Mucinous cystadenocarcinoma Intraductal papillary mucinous	Head (75%), body (20%), tail (5%), ampulla ?Better prognosis Poorer prognosis Very rare Similar prognosis to ductal Prognosis dependent on classification as benign or malignant
Mixed (<0.1%)	Pancreatoblastoma Solid-pseudopapillary	Young onset (15 years), good (c.75%) survival Women in their 30s. Rarely metastasise
Glandular (4%)	Acinar cell	Head (60%), body (20%), tail (20%)
Undifferentiated (<5%)	Giant-cell/sarcomatoid/osteoclast	Median survival 2 months
Neuroendocrine (1%)	Gastrinomas, insulinomas, VIPomas	Survival related to histotype and mitoses
Mesenchymal	Schwannoma, liposarcoma, malignant fibrous histiocytoma	Rare
Metastases	Lymphoma Breast, lung, colorectal, melanoma, gastric, renal cell	Involves the pancreas in 25%

Ductal adenocarcinoma can occur anywhere in the gland; however, in clinical practice the head of the gland appears to be the predominant site. Microscopically there is intense stromal fibrosis. The PanINs (1–3) are thought to represent precursor lesions (see above). The presence of perineural invasion is an independent poor prognostic factor.[64] Metastatic spread is usually to liver, peritoneum and lungs. Case reports of cutaneous metastases are also documented. Variants of ductal carcinoma exist and are summarised in **Table 13.2**. Medullary cancer is a poorly differentiated ductal cancer with a relatively better outcome than common pancreatic ductal cancer. There may also be an inherited component to this cancer.[65] Adenosquamous cancer is a rare cancer that contains glandular and squamous elements. It is associated with a dismal prognosis and with a preceding history of chemotherapy and radiotherapy.[66]

Cystic neoplasms of the pancreas are rare, accounting for 1% of pancreatic neoplasms and 10% of pancreatic cysts.[67] They are more common in women and usually occur in the sixth decade but have a wide range.[68] Serous cystadenomas are large, well-circumscribed tumours containing central calcification. The mucinous cystadenomas tend to be more heterogeneous. Although they tend to be as large as serous tumours their cellular architecture varies widely within the individual specimen. The reports of mucinous cystadenomas that metastasise probably represent sampling error of a primary cystadenocarcinoma. Intraductal papillary mucinous neoplasm (IPMN) was first described in the 1980s by Morohoshi and colleagues.[69] It is not cystic although it produces copious mucin, and this can be seen classically at ERCP where mucin can be observed discharging through the ampulla.[70] IPMNs generally are given an excellent prognosis although papillary mucinous carcinomas occur and are potentially fatal.[71]

Acinar cell carcinoma is derived from glandular epithelium and accounts for about 4% of pancreatic cancers. Twenty percent of these patients can develop subcutaneous fat necrosis, especially in the lower limbs, thought to be due to lipase production by the tumour.[72] They also tend to be larger, with a higher proportion occurring in the body and tail when compared with the distribution of typical ductal adenocarcinoma. Prognosis, however, is roughly equivalent.[73]

Undifferentiated carcinoma can be either sarcomatoid (giant-cell) or osteoclast-like giant-cell tumours. These rare tumours have minimal differentiation and are associated with a bleak median prognosis of 2 months. Osteoclast representation confers a slightly better prognosis, but is also associated with a poor survival. Other tumours such as solid pseudopapillary, lymphoma and pancreaticoblastoma occur occasionally.

The pancreatic endocrine tumours represent a spectrum of disease, and their clinical course is dependent on histotype. There is sometimes considerable difficulty in classifying malignant phenotypes on histology when the normal surrogates are less useful. Indirect markers such as size, mitotic rate (>10 per high-power field), and presence of necrosis are therefore relied upon. As a guide, tumours less than 2 cm are usually benign whereas those above 3 cm frequently metastasise.[74] Overall, approximately 10% of incidental pancreatic neuroendocrine tumours found are malignant although this varies considerably depending on histotype. Gastrinomas are associated with hypersecretion of gastrin and Zollinger–Ellison syndrome. Most are malignant but progress slowly.[75] Metastases to liver and bone usually herald end stages of disease progression. Insulinomas are nearly always benign. They present classically with postprandial syncope, although median time to diagnosis tends to be protracted in the absence of clinical suspicion. Neurological diagnoses are assigned frequently prior to the tumour discovery.[76] Other neuroendocrine tumours include A cell, δ cell, VIPomas, ACTH (adrenocorticotropic hormone) and PTH (parathyroid hormone) cell tumours.

Mesenchymal tumours such as liposarcomas, malignant fibrous histiocytoma and schwannomas are all associated rarely with primary growth in the pancreas. Behaviour and survival from these tumours are similar to when they occur elsewhere in the body. Metastatic tumours do occur in the pancreas, with breast, colorectal, renal and melanoma being the most common.[77]

TREATMENT

Treatment strategy in pancreatic cancer is defined by stage (**Table 13.3**) (**Fig. 13.6**). The major decision point is whether the patient is suitable

Table 13.3 • American Joint Committee on Cancer TNM staging, 2002[128]

Tumour (T)	Node (N)	Metastasis (M)
T1: <2 cm within pancreas	N0: no nodes	M0: no metastases
T2: >2 cm within pancreas	N1: positive nodes	M1: spread to distant organs or non-regional nodes (e.g. aorto-caval)
T3: Adjacent extrapancreatic spread (duodenum, bile duct)		
T4: Non-adjacent spread (stomach, colon, large vasculature)		
Stage I: T1,2 N0 M0		
Stage II: T3 N0 M0		
Stage III: T1,2,3 N1 M0		
Stage IVA: T4 any N M0		
Stage IVB: any T any N M1		

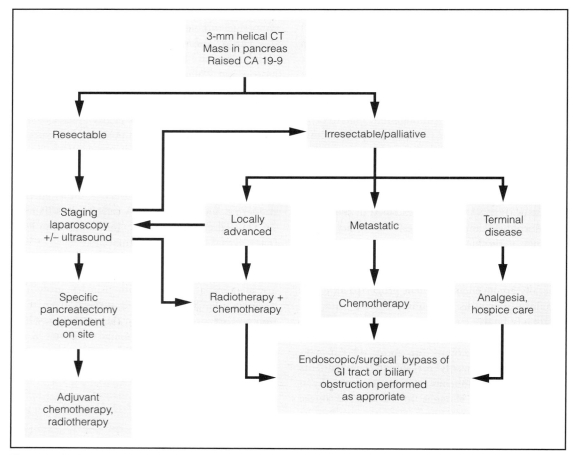

Figure 13.6 • Treatment algorithm for patients with pancreatic cancer.

for resectional therapy requiring some form of pancreatectomy. Unfortunately, less than 20% are in this group at presentation.

Resection

Surgical resection offers the only chance of long-term survival, yet prognosis is poor even with resection.

If jaundice is an intercurrent presenting symptom it is controversial whether biliary decompression should be undertaken. Available evidence suggests an increased risk of perioperative sepsis and pancreatic fistula as well as wound infections.[78–83] The authors' practice is not to decompress the bile duct preoperatively, unless symptoms and signs of cholangitis or secondary signs of hyperbilirubinaemia are present. Coagulopathy, if present, is treated three days prior to resection with vitamin K.

It is important to remember that despite surgery with curative intent, median survival ranges between 11 and 18 months, with less than 10% alive at 5 years. Patient selection despite apparent resectability is therefore paramount. Cardiovascular and respiratory performance must be fully evaluated, and age in itself is not a contraindication.[84,85] Leaving aside the oncological aspects, which are difficult to use as quality measures when ultimate prognosis is relatively poor, pancreatic resections previously were associated with significant mortality. It is only recently that they have been shown to be safe with acceptable mortality risks. It appears that high-volume (over seven resections per year) institutions appear to have lowest mortality (c. 1%) and morbidity figures.[84,86,87] This seems to be independent of hospital size[88] and probably represents the development of medical, nursing and radiological skill based on repetition and familiarity in dealing with these patients.

PANCREATICO-DUODENECTOMY

In 1935, Whipple described, to the American Surgical Association, three cases where ampullary cancers were treated by two-stage pancreatico-duodenectomy.[89] Later, in the 1940s, it was described as a one-stage procedure and although technical variations have since been described, it remains the mainstay of surgical therapy for tumours of the pancreatic head and neck.[90]

The patient is positioned supine under general anaesthesia, and prophylactic antibiotics to cover biliary pathogens are administered. A bilateral subcostal 'roof-top' is our incision of choice. Standard laparotomy is performed to confirm laparoscopic staging findings. The right colon is mobilised exposing the third and fourth parts of the duodenum. Extended Kocherisation of the duodenum is performed. This allows a tumour in the head of pancreas to be palpated and views of the left renal vein. The aortocaval and portal vein (PV) nodal packages are dissected and the respective vessels are skeletonised. At this point resectability is finally assessed as extensive involvement of the confluence of the portal vein/superior mesenteric vein (SMV) may herald termination of the procedure. Trial dissection allows this assessment to be made by passing one finger along the PV from above, the other along the SMV to establish the plane. It is important to remember that short segments of the PV can be resected if necessary and therefore an involved PV does not necessarily denote irresectability.

The remaining porta hepatis is dissected and nodes are cleared. Cholecystectomy is performed to allow higher ligation of the bile duct by maximising common hepatic duct length. The common hepatic duct is transected just proximal to the insertion of the cystic duct. It is our practice to send a biliary aspirate for routine culture and sensitivity as postoperative infective complications tend to involve biliary organisms.[81] The common bile duct is mobilised distally and the hepaticoduodenal ligament is dissected along its length, taking care to identify and preserve the common hepatic artery and PV. The gastroduodenal artery is ligated while care is taken not to damage an aberrant right hepatic artery.

In a conventional Whipple's operation the distal stomach is resected. This is the authors' favoured approach as resection includes the nodes along the greater and lesser curves, reduces stomach emptying dysfunction postoperatively, diminishes the density of parietal cells and theoretically reduces the risk of gastritis. The stomach is transected at the antrum along with the attached omentum. The proximal jejunum along with its mesentery is transected and the mobilised duodenum and jejunum is delivered back under the ligament of Treitz.

The pancreas is transected between four stay sutures (to facilitate haemostasis in the marginal arteries) after the uncinate process is dissected from the superior mesenteric vessels. Retroperitoneal dissection allows the tumour and nodal package to be delivered en bloc. If any doubt exists regarding the adequacy of tumour clearance, the pancreatic resection margin should be sent for frozen section histology.

Reconstruction is undertaken involving three anastomoses. The usual order is the biliary anastomosis followed by the pancreatic and finally the gastric. The pancreatic anastomosis has been the subject of research interest fuelled by desire to decrease pancreatic leaks and fistulas. In particular, pancreatico-gastrostomy versus the usual pancreatico-jejunostomy has been compared in a number of trials both randomised[91] and non-randomised.[92] These data suggest a marginal decrease in fistula rates with pancreatico-gastric reconstruction although these differences are not clinically significant and have not induced a widespread change in operative strategy, with jejunal reconstruction still favoured.

The nature of the pancreatic reconstruction is subject to individual variation. The authors' favour a two-layered pancreatico-jejunal anastomosis with mucosa-to-mucosa reconstruction. Choledocho-jejunostomy is performed in a similar manner (end to side) leaving gastro-jejunostomy until the end. We perform washout with warmed water for the theoretical hypotonic tumoricidal action.

We do not place abdominal drains routinely after Whipple's operation, based on the evidence supplied by the randomised New York experience[93] in which drains failed to decrease the rate of intra-abdominal collections and fistulas. We therefore reserve drains for selected cases only.

Complications following pancreatic resection include wound infection (10%), delayed gastric emptying (20%) and intra-abdominal collections/fistulas (12.5–15%). Mostly these complications can be dealt with either conservatively or using interventional radiologically placed drains.[93] Less than 5% require re-operation.

PYLORUS-PRESERVING PANCREATICO-DUODENECTOMY (PPPDR)

Although described over 50 years, the data supporting PPPDR have not been clear-cut. It is attractive to preserve the distal stomach and duodenum to diminish nutritive, dumping and bile reflux sequelae.[94] Watson described the first PPPDR in 1944.[95] However, this procedure did not become popular until the last two decades. PPPDR has similar morbidity and mortality rates to Whipple's operation.[96,97] Potentially, median blood losses and operative time in the PPPDR group are marginally less. Survival is unchanged and quality of life assessments are limited by their retrospective methodology.[98] Detractors of PPPDR point to delayed gastric emptying as potential cause for concern with this procedure.[99]

The procedure dictates conventional mobilisation up to where the stomach requires transection. In PPPDR the right gastric artery is preserved and the duodenum is transected at least 2 cm distal to the pylorus. Reconstruction is usually accomplished by duodeno-jejunostomy or gastro-jejunostomy, both probably equivalent in terms of postoperative function.[100]

EXTENDED LYMPH NODE DISSECTION

It is the authors' practice to perform extended lymphadenectomy in the majority of cases. At the time of presentation most tumours have involved lymph nodes beyond the gland.[101] Even 50% of the sub-2-cm tumours have lymph-node involvement.[102] Ishikawa and colleagues were the first to demonstrate increased median (but not long-term) survival following extended lymph node dissection.[103] Others suggest that due to the propensity for pancreatic cancer to demonstrate perineural spread that resection should also include the neural tissue.[104] Outside Japan, findings of increased survival have not been proven statistically. These studies fail to demonstrate the increased morbidity that one would expect with the radical operation, although in our experience there is invariably increased ascites in those who undergo extended lymphadenectomy. A subsequent trial from Johns Hopkins Hospital[105] demonstrated extended lymphadenectomy to be comparable with standard resection in terms of morbidity and early mortality, and a suggested 5% survival advantage at 1 year in those who survived although this was not proven statistically. The follow-up trial[106] with expanded numbers (294) suggested slightly increased morbidity in the radical group coupled with protracted hospital stay. There is no sustainable survival advantage seen at the

3-year point, although supporters of radical resection suggest that the available data are still underpowered to answer this point. We believe that clearance of the left gastric and aortocaval nodes increases the specificity of staging and therefore predicted prognosis and increases the likelihood of a negative surgical margin.

DISTAL PANCREATECTOMY

Distal pancreatectomy is performed for resectable tumours of the body and tail of the pancreas. This operation is used rarely for carcinoma as almost always the tumour is irresectable due to direct involvement of the middle colic vessels or metastases. Hence, the procedure is reserved usually for more benign lesions.

Once again a bilateral subcostal incision is favoured for access. The neck of the pancreas is dissected free from the portal vein and the splenic flexure of the colon is taken down. It is standard to resect with the spleen although in certain circumstances (and hence all patients are vaccinated prophylactically against encapsulated organisms, *Haemophilus influenzae* B, meningococcus C and pneumococcus) it is possible to resect while leaving the spleen.[107] If the spleen is to be taken, then early posterior mobilisation and sequential artery and vein ligation are performed to minimise blood loss. The residual gland is oversewn once resection has been performed between stay sutures.

TOTAL PANCREATECTOMY

Some suggest that pancreatic cancer is a multicentric disease and therefore advocate total pancreatec tomy. The first total pancreatectomy was performed by Rockey and colleagues in 1943.[108] Support in the 1970s for the procedure was probably related to the inadequacies of standard pancreatico-duodenectomy as opposed to benefits of total resection.[109] Although total pancreatectomy can be performed safely, the outcome is so dismal in cases of adenocarcinoma[110] as to call into question the indication for the operation.

Resectional surgery is possible in less than 20% of all cases but there is increasing evidence that operative mortality is reduced when patients are managed in high-volume institutions.

Pylorus-preserving pancreatico-duodenectomy has similar morbidity and mortality rates to Whipple's

operation and there is insufficient evidence to favour one procedure over the other.

The role of extended lymph node dissection remains controversial but there is no evidence that extended lymphadenectomy prolongs duration of survival.

Surgical palliation

With efficacious laparoscopic staging the role of surgical bypass is giving away to endoscopic bilary and GI tract stenting. Nevertheless surgical bypass techniques are still used occasionally.

OBSTRUCTIVE JAUNDICE

Obstructive jaundice and its secondary symptoms of nausea, anorexia, pruritus and progressive malnutrition may require surgical palliation. Hyperilirubinaemia causes hepatic, coagulation and myocardial dysfunction and can lead to early death in sufferers. In particular the pruritus may be debilitating and resistant to medical therapies such as antihistamines and bile salt binders such as cholestyramine. Endoscopic stenting during ERCP is now favoured for low lesions whereas percutaneous radiologically placed stents are reserved for higher common hepatic obstructions.

Surgical options include:

- choledocho-duodenostomy
- choledocho-jejunostomy
- cholecysto-jejunostomy
- hepatico-jejunostomy.

Choledocho-jejunostomy is the procedure of choice in patients with a median life expectancy of 6 months or more since cystic duct obstruction may arise from tumour progression over time.

The short-term mortality, morbidity and efficacy of operative versus non-operative interventions for biliary obstruction are equivalent.[111] In-hospital stay is longer in the surgery group. Introduction of clinical pathways in high-volume centres may serve to diminish both morbidity and in-hospital stay.[112]

UPPER GI TRACT OUTFLOW OBSTRUCTION

Gastric and more commonly duodenal outlet obstruction is said to occur in 20% of patients. Once hyperbilirubinaemic states have been addressed persistent nausea and vomiting should alert the attending physician that upper GI obstruction is present. Obviously if biliary obstruction is being dealt with at the time of open operation, prophylactic duodenal bypass should be considered. It is estimated by meta-analysis that 13% would require subsequent bypass if not performed at that time with a further 20% dying with duodenal outlet symptoms.[113] Randomised data suggest comparable figures (19%)[57] requiring bypass. These data have been criticised by some centres where laparoscopic staging is routine, suggesting that only 2–3% require surgical bypass, which may be accomplished laparoscopically.[56]

Contrast radiology is the investigation of choice in the non-operative setting. Minimal access laparoscopic gastro-jejunostomy is probably the management of choice where the local expertise exists. Luminal endoscopically placed stents may have a role in future although these techniques are in their infancy.

PAIN

Back pain is a feature seen in up to 90% of pancreatic cancers and despite improved palliative care, analgesic regimens may not meet the patient's requirements. Lillemoe et al.[114] examined the efficacy of chemical splanchnicectomy in a randomised placebo-controlled trial. They reported significantly improved long-term pain scores as well as a survival advantage in those who received splanchnicectomy.

Adjuvant therapies

Surgery with curative intent still has a disappointing 5-year survival rate of 10–15%. Indeed, median survival ranges between 11 and 18 months. Therapy failure must represent progression of micrometastases present at the time of surgery.[101] Even in lymph node-negative tumours, survival is rare beyond 40 months.[115] Thus chemoradiotherapy treatment was considered an attractive proposition. The Gastrointestinal Tumor Study Group (GITSG) reported on the first prospective randomised trial,[116,117] and reported a 20- versus 11-month median survival after adjuvant chemoradiotherapy based on 5-fluorouracil (5-FU), Adriamycin (doxorubicin) and mitomycin C (FAM). This study was criticised based on the delay in entering the treatment arm of up to 10 weeks post surgery, suggesting that only the fit patients were entered into the study. It is difficult to equivocate regarding the longer-term survival, where 19% were still living at 10 years versus none in the surgery-alone group.

The European Study Group for Pancreatic Cancer 1 trial demonstrated a median 5.7-month increased survival when the entire chemotherapy groups were compared to the observational postoperative group.[118] This translated to only a 1.5-month trend when analysed separately and suggested a detrimental effect on survival with radiotherapy. Gemcitabine-based therapies are currently undergoing phased trials.[119–121] Like 5-FU, gemcitabine is a synergistic radiosensitiser. The Radiation Therapy Oncology Group initiated a prospective randomised trial in 1998 comparing 5-FU and gemcitabine. Peer-reviewed results are awaited.

There has been disappointment[122] with antiangiogenic metalloprotease inhibitors[123] and hormonal-based therapies,[124,125] as well as immunotherapy, which has largely stalled in early phased trials.

Chemoradiation in locally advanced and metastatic disease

It is hard to argue on best evidence that chemoradiation in these settings has a place outside controlled trials as the case is far from clear cut. There is some evidence that quality of life is improved with gemcitabine and may confer minimal survival benefit.[123,124] Research is ongoing into finding a more efficacious additive agent to gemcitabine.

Neoadjuvant therapy

Intuitively, neoadjuvant multimodal strategies for pancreatic cancer should represent a significant area of interest, as 80% are irresectable at presentation. Neoadjuvant therapy theoretically should be efficacious as chemoradiation therapy works best on well-oxygenated tissue, and pretreatment may diminish the chance of tumour seeding at laparotomy. Patients inappropriate for resection may also be selected on the evidence of disease progression at the time of restaging (affecting 15–25%). Some prospective evidence exists suggesting a small response rate in terms of downstaging $(10-25\%)^{125}$ without any increase in postoperative complication rates.[126] However, there is not enough evidence to recommend neoadjuvant strategies as a routine.

There is now strong evidence that adjuvant chemotherapy improves duration of survival in pancreatic cancer.

FUTURE AREAS OF INTEREST

The last decade has seen considerable improvements in diagnostic modalities as well as advances in minimally invasive and endoscopic management of complications of pancreatic cancer. The surgical questions regarding pylorus preservation and extended lymph node dissection are well advanced, and elective resection can be performed safely. It is therefore disappointing that neoadjuvant strategies appear to confer little or no survival advantages, thus identifying the area where most investigation is needed. Immunotherapies held great promise although delivery systems and potency have underined the failure of standard therapies to materialise. Today complete surgical therapy with adjuvant chemoradiation represents the best available therapy for this disease, and lifetime survival rates of 5% remain a challenge for the future.

Key points

- Pancreatic cancer is associated with poor prognosis despite surgery with curative intent.
- Pancreatic cancer is strongly associated with cigarette smoking.
- Pancreatic protocol CT forms the mainstay of imaging.
- Preoperative staging is enhanced by focused laparoscopy although this is controversial.
- Resectional surgery is only possible in 20% of cases.
- There is increasing evidence to justify postoperative adjuvant therapy.

REFERENCES

1. Jemal A, Murray T, Samuels A et al. Cancer statistics, 2003. CA Cancer J Clin 2003; 53:5–26.
2. Cancer Research UK. Cancer Statistics. London: CRUK Press, 2003.
3. Weiderpass E, Partanen T, Kaaks R et al. Occurrence, trends and environment etiology of pancreatic cancer. Scand J Work Environ Health 1998; 24:165–74.
4. Miller BA, Kolonel LN, Bernstein I et al. Racial/ethnic patterns of cancer in the United States 1988–92. Bethesda, MD: NIH, 1996.
5. Lillemoe KD, Yeo CJ, Cameron JL. Pancreatic cancer: state-of-the-art care. CA Cancer J Clin 2000; 50:241–68.
6. Howe GR, Jain M, Burch JD et al. Cigarette smoking and cancer of the pancreas: evidence from a population-based case-control study in Toronto, Canada. Int J Cancer 1991; 47:323–8.
7. Boyle P, Maisonneuve P, Bueno de Mesquita B et al. Cigarette smoking and pancreas cancer: a case control study of the search programme of the IARC. Int J Cancer 1996; 67:63–71.
8. Cameron JL. Pancreatic Cancer. London: BC Decker, 2001.
9. Olsen GW, Mandel JS, Gibson RW et al. A case-control study of pancreatic cancer and cigarettes, alcohol, coffee and diet. Am J Public Health 1989; 79:1016–19.
10. Zheng W, McLaughlin JK, Gridley G et al. A cohort study of smoking, alcohol consumption, and dietary factors for pancreatic cancer (United States). Cancer Causes Control 1993; 4:477–82.
11. Ahlgren JD. Epidemiology and risk factors in pancreatic cancer. Semin Oncol 1996; 23:241–50.
12. International Agency for Research on Cancer. Alcohol drinking. IARC monograph evaluating carcinogen risks in humans. Lyon: IARC, 1988.
13. Howe GR, Burch JD. Nutrition and pancreatic cancer. Cancer Causes Control 1996; 7:69–82.
14. Silverman DT, Swanson CA, Gridley G et al. Dietary and nutritional factors and pancreatic cancer: a case-control study based on direct interviews. J Natl Cancer Inst 1998; 90:1710–9.
15. Michaud DS, Giovannucci E, Willett WC et al. Physical activity, obesity, height, and the risk of pancreatic cancer. JAMA 2001; 286:921–9.
16. Kalapothaki V, Tzonou A, Hsieh CC et al. Nutrient intake and cancer of the pancreas: a case-control study in Athens, Greece. Cancer Causes Control 1993; 4:383–9.
17. MacMahon B, Yen S, Trichopoulos D et al. Coffee and cancer of the pancreas. N Engl J Med 1981; 304:630–3.

18. Marsh GM, Lucas LJ, Youk AO et al. Mortality patterns among workers exposed to acrylamide: 1994 follow up. Occup Environ Med 1999; 56:181–90.

19. Anttila A, Pukkala E, Sallmen M et al. Cancer incidence among Finnish workers exposed to halogenated hydrocarbons. J Occup Environ Med 1995; 37:797–806.

20. Blair A, Stewart PA, Tolbert PE et al. Cancer and other causes of death among a cohort of dry cleaners. Br J Ind Med 1990; 47:162–8.

21. Everhart J, Wright D. Diabetes mellitus as a risk factor for pancreatic cancer. A meta-analysis. JAMA 1995; 273:1605–9.

22. MacDermott RP, Kramer P. Adenocarcinoma of the pancreas in four siblings. Gastroenterology 1973; 65:137–9.

23. Ehrenthal D, Haeger L, Griffin T et al. Familial pancreatic adenocarcinoma in three generations. A case report and a review of the literature. Cancer 1987; 59:1661–4.

24. Silverman DT, Schiffman M, Everhart J et al. Diabetes mellitus, other medical conditions and familial history of cancer as risk factors for pancreatic cancer. Br J Cancer 1999; 80:1830–7.

25. Coughlin SS, Calle EE, Patel AV et al. Predictors of pancreatic cancer mortality among a large cohort of United States adults. Cancer Causes Control 2000; 11:915–23.

26. Ghadirian P, Boyle P, Simard A et al. Reported family aggregation of pancreatic cancer within a population-based case-control study in the Francophone community in Montreal, Canada. Int J Pancreatol 1991; 10:183–96.

27. Giardiello FM, Welsh SB, Hamilton SR et al. Increased risk of cancer in the Peutz–Jeghers syndrome. N Engl J Med 1987; 316:1511–14.

28. Ozcelik H, Schmocker B, Di Nicola N et al. Germline BRCA2 6174delT mutations in Ashkenazi Jewish pancreatic cancer patients. Nat Genet 1997; 16:17–18.

29. Goldstein AM, Fraser MC, Struewing JP et al. Increased risk of pancreatic cancer in melanoma-prone kindreds with p16INK4 mutations. N Engl J Med 1995; 333:970–4.

30. Schutte M, Hruban RH, Geradts J et al. Abrogation of the Rb/p16 tumor-suppressive pathway in virtually all pancreatic carcinomas. Cancer Res 1997; 57:3126–30.

31. Almoguera C, Shibata D, Forrester K et al. Most human carcinomas of the exocrine pancreas contain mutant c-K-*ras* genes. Cell 1988; 53:549–54.

32. Pellegata NS, Sessa F, Renault B et al. K-*ras* and p53 gene mutations in pancreatic cancer: ductal and nonductal tumors progress through different genetic lesions. Cancer Res 1994; 54:1556–60.

33. Hruban RH, Adsay NV, Albores-Saavedra J et al. Pancreatic intraepithelial neoplasia: a new nomenclature and classification system for pancreatic duct lesions. Am J Surg Pathol 2001; 25:579–86.

    Description of the new classification system for pancreatic cancer.

34. Cubilla AL, Fitzgerald PJ. Morphological lesions associated with human primary invasive non-endocrine pancreas cancer. Cancer Res 1976; 36:2690–8.

35. Wilentz RE, Iacobuzio-Donahue CA, Argani P et al. Loss of expression of Dpc4 in pancreatic intra-epithelial neoplasia: evidence that DPC4 inactivation occurs late in neoplastic progression. Cancer Res 2000; 60:2002–6.

36. Singh SM, Longmire WP Jr, Reber HA. Surgical palliation for pancreatic cancer. The UCLA experience. Ann Surg 1990; 212:132–9.

37. Kelsen D. Neoadjuvant therapy for upper gastrointestinal tract cancers. Curr Opin Oncol 1996; 8:321–8.

38. Safi F, Schlosser W, Kolb G et al. Diagnostic value of CA 19–9 in patients with pancreatic cancer and nonspecific gastrointestinal symptoms. J Gastrointest Surg 1997; 1:106–112.

39. Safi F, Roscher R, Beger HG. Tumor markers in pancreatic cancer. Sensitivity and specificity of CA 19-9. Hepatogastroenterology 1989; 36:419–23.

    Important paper that summarises well the role of CA19-9 in pancreatic cancer.

40. Micke O, Bruns F, Kurowski R et al. Predictive value of carbohydrate antigen 19-9 in pancreatic cancer treated with radiochemotherapy. Int J Radiat Oncol Biol Phys 2003; 57:90–7.

41. Kamisawa T, Tu Y, Egawa N et al. Ductal and acinar differentiation in pancreatic endocrine tumors. Dig Dis Sci 2002; 47:2254–61.

42. Kim JE, Lee KT, Lee JK et al. Clinical usefulness of carbohydrate antigen 19-9 as a screening test for pancreatic cancer in an asymptomatic population. J Gastroenterol Hepatol 2004; 19:182–6.

43. Moossa AR, Gamagami RA. Diagnosis and staging of pancreatic neoplasms. Surg Clin North Am 1995; 75:871–90.

44. Ishiguchi T, Maruyama K, Fukatsu H et al. Radiologic diagnosis of pancreatic carcinoma. Semin Surg Oncol 1998; 15:23–32.

45. Sendler A, Avril N, Helmberger H et al. Preoperative evaluation of pancreatic masses with positron emission tomography using 18F-fluorodeoxyglucose: diagnostic limitations. World J Surg 2000; 24:1121–9.

46. van Dijkum EJ, de Wit LT, van Delden OM et al. Staging laparoscopy and laparoscopic ultrasonography in more than 400 patients with upper

gastrointestinal carcinoma. J Am Coll Surg 1999; 189:459–65.

47. Pisters PW, Lee JE, Vauthey JN et al. Laparoscopy in the staging of pancreatic cancer. Br J Surg 2001; 88:325–37.

48. Reed WP, Mustafa IA. Laparoscopic screening of surgical candidates with pancreatic cancer or liver tumors. Surg Endosc 1997; 11:12–4.

49. Conlon KC, Dougherty E, Klimstra DS et al. The value of minimal access surgery in the staging of patients with potentially resectable peripancreatic malignancy. Ann Surg 1996; 223:134–40.

  Author's seminal paper describing the role and value of minimal access surgery in staging of peripancreatic cancer.

50. Holzman MD, Reintgen KL, Tyler DS et al. The role of laparoscopy in the management of suspected pancreatic and periampullary malignancies. J Gastrointest Surg 1997; 1:236–44.

51. Jimenez RE, Warshaw AL, Rattner DW et al. Impact of laparoscopic staging in the treatment of pancreatic cancer. Arch Surg 2000; 135:409–14; discussion 414–15.

52. Conlon KC, Brennan MF. Laparoscopy for staging abdominal malignancies. Adv Surg 2000; 34:331–50.

53. Catheline JM, Turner R, Rizk N et al. The use of diagnostic laparoscopy supported by laparoscopic ultrasonography in the assessment of pancreatic cancer. Surg Endosc 1999; 13:239–45.

54. Luque-de Leon E, Tsiotos GG, Balsiger B et al. Staging laparoscopy for pancreatic cancer should be used to select the best means of palliation and not only to maximize the resectability rate. J Gastrointest Surg 1999; 3:111–17; discussion 117–18.

55. Pietrabissa A, Caramella D, Di Candio G et al. Laparoscopy and laparoscopic ultrasonography for staging pancreatic cancer: critical appraisal. World J Surg 1999; 23:998–1002; discussion 1003.

56. Espat NJ, Brennan MF, Conlon KC. Patients with laparoscopically staged unresectable pancreatic adenocarcinoma do not require subsequent surgical biliary or gastric bypass. J Am Coll Surg 1999; 188:649–55; discussion 655–7.

57. Lillemoe KD, Cameron JL, Hardacre JM et al. Is prophylactic gastrojejunostomy indicated for unresectable periampullary cancer? A prospective randomized trial. Ann Surg 1999; 230:322–8; discussion 328–30.

  Two key papers arguing the role for and against prophylactic gastroenterostomy in palliation of pancreatic cancer.

58. Ridgway PF, Ziprin P, Jones TL et al. Laparoscopic staging of pancreatic tumors induces increased invasive capacity in vitro. Surg Endosc 2003; 17:306–10.

59. Ridgway P, Smith A, Ziprin P et al. Pneumoperitoneum augmented tumour invasiveness is abolished by matrix metalloprotease blockade. Surg Endosc 2002; 16:533–6.

60. Ziprin P, Ridgway PF, Peck DH et al. Laparoscopic enhancement of tumour cell binding to the peritoneum is inhibited by anti-intercellular adhesion molecule-1 monoclonal antibody. Surg Endosc 2003; 17:1812–17.

61. Shoup M, Brennan MF, Karpeh MS et al. Port site metastasis after diagnostic laparoscopy for upper gastrointestinal malignancies: an uncommon entity. Ann Surg Oncol 2002; 9:632–6.

62. Ziprin P, Ridgway PF, Peck DH et al. The theories and realities of port-site metastases: a critical appraisal. J Am Coll Surg 2002; 195:395–408.

63. Legmann P, Vignaux O, Dousset B et al. Pancreatic tumors: comparison of dual-phase helical CT and endoscopic sonography. Am J Roentgenol 1998; 170:1315–22.

64. Nagakawa T, Mori K, Nakano T et al. Perineural invasion of carcinoma of the pancreas and biliary tract. Br J Surg 1993; 80:619–21.

65. Wilentz RE, Goggins M, Redston M et al. Genetic, immunohistochemical, and clinical features of medullary carcinoma of the pancreas: A newly described and characterized entity. Am J Pathol 2000; 156:1641–51.

66. O'Connor TP, Wade TP, Sunwoo YC et al. Small cell undifferentiated carcinoma of the pancreas. Report of a patient with tumor marker studies. Cancer 1992; 70:1514–19.

67. Warshaw AL, Compton CC, Lewandrowski K et al. Cystic tumors of the pancreas. New clinical, radiologic, and pathologic observations in 67 patients. Ann Surg 1990; 212:432–43; discussion 444–5.

68. Su CH, Tsay SH, Wu CC et al. Factors influencing postoperative morbidity, mortality, and survival after resection for hilar cholangiocarcinoma. Ann Surg 1996; 223:384–94.

69. Morohoshi T, Kanda M, Asanuma K et al. Intraductal papillary neoplasms of the pancreas. A clinicopathologic study of six patients. Cancer 1989; 64:1329–35.

70. Yamaguchi K, Tanaka M. Mucin-hypersecreting tumor of the pancreas with mucin extrusion through an enlarged papilla. Am J Gastroenterol 1991; 86:835–9.

71. Adsay NV, Conlon KC, Zee SY et al. Intraductal papillary-mucinous neoplasms of the pancreas: an analysis of in situ and invasive carcinomas in 28 patients. Cancer 2002; 94:62–77.

72. MacMahon HE, Brown PA, Shen EM. Acinar cell carcinoma of the pancreas with subcutaneous fat necrosis. Gastroenterology 1965; 49:555–9.

73. Holen KD, Klimstra DS, Hummer A et al. Clinical characteristics and outcomes from an institutional series of acinar cell carcinoma of the pancreas and related tumors. J Clin Oncol 2002; 20:4673–8.

74. Capella C, Heitz PU, Hofler H et al. Revised classification of neuroendocrine tumours of the lung, pancreas and gut. Virchows Arch 1995; 425:547–60.

75. Yu F, Venzon DJ, Serrano J et al. Prospective study of the clinical course, prognostic factors, causes of death, and survival in patients with long-standing Zollinger–Ellison syndrome. J Clin Oncol 1999; 17:615–30.

76. Dizon AM, Kowalyk S, Hoogwerf BJ. Neuro-glycopenic and other symptoms in patients with insulinomas. Am J Med 1999; 106:307–10.

77. Sperti C, Pasquali C, Liessi G et al. Pancreatic resection for metastatic tumors to the pancreas. J Surg Oncol 2003; 83:161–6; discussion 166.

78. Hatfield AR, Tobias R, Terblanche J et al. Pre-operative external biliary drainage in obstructive jaundice. A prospective controlled clinical trial. Lancet 1982; 2:896–9.

79. McPherson GA, Benjamin IS, Hodgson HJ et al. Pre-operative percutaneous transhepatic biliary drainage: the results of a controlled trial. Br J Surg 1984; 71:371–5.

80. Pisters PW, Hudec WA, Hess KR et al. Effect of preoperative biliary decompression on pancreatico-duodenectomy-associated morbidity in 300 con-secutive patients. Ann Surg 2001; 234:47–55.

81. Povoski SP, Karpeh MS Jr, Conlon KC et al. Pre-operative biliary drainage: impact on intraoperative bile cultures and infectious morbidity and mortality after pancreaticoduodenectomy. J Gastrointest Surg 1999; 3:496–505.

82. Povoski SP, Karpeh MS Jr, Conlon KC et al. Association of preoperative biliary drainage with postoperative outcome following pancreatico-duodenectomy. Ann Surg 1999; 230:131–42.

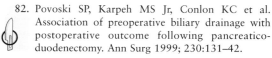

Paper highlighting the contribution of biliary stenting to operative morbidity.

83. Cooperman AM. Pancreatic cancer: the bigger picture. Surg Clin North Am 2001; 81:557–74.

84. Yeo CJ, Cameron JL, Sohn TA et al. Six hundred fifty consecutive pancreaticoduodenectomies in the 1990s: pathology, complications, and outcomes. Ann Surg 1997; 226:248–57; discussion 257–60.

85. Fong Y, Blumgart LH, Fortner JG et al. Pancreatic or liver resection for malignancy is safe and effec-tive for the elderly. Ann Surg 1995; 222:426–34; discussion 434–7.

86. Luft HS, Bunker JP, Enthoven AC. Should operations be regionalized? The empirical relation between surgical volume and mortality. N Engl J Med 1979; 301:1364–9.

87. Sosa JA, Bowman HM, Gordon TA et al. Importance of hospital volume in the overall management of pancreatic cancer. Ann Surg 1998; 228:429–38.

88. Cooperman AM, Schwartz ET, Fader A et al. Safety, efficacy, and cost of pancreaticoduodenal resection in a specialized center based at a community hospital. Arch Surg 1997; 132:744–7; discussion 748.

89. Whipple AO, Parson WB, Mullins CR. Treatment of carcinoma of the ampulla of Vater. Ann Surg 1935; 102:763–79.

90. Whipple AO. The rationale of radical surgery for cancer of the pancreas and ampullary region. Ann Surg 1941; 114:612–15.

91. Yeo CJ, Cameron JL, Maher MM et al. A prospec-tive randomized trial of pancreaticogastrostomy versus pancreaticojejunostomy after pancreatico-duodenectomy. Ann Surg 1995; 222:580–8; discussion 588–92.

Trial showing no difference in outcome for pancreatic anastomotic techniques employed at pancreatico-duodenectomy.

92. Takano S, Ito Y, Watanabe Y et al. Pancreatico-jejunostomy versus pancreaticogastrostomy in reconstruction following pancreaticoduodenectomy. Br J Surg 2000; 87:423–7.

93. Conlon KC, Labow D, Leung D et al. Prospective randomized clinical trial of the value of intra-peritoneal drainage after pancreatic resection. Ann Surg 2001; 234:487–93; discussion 493–4.

Author's own report showing no benefit for continuing drainage following pancreatic resection.

94. Klinkenbijl JH, van der Schelling GP, Hop WC et al. The advantages of pylorus-preserving pancreatoduodenectomy in malignant disease of the pancreas and periampullary region. Ann Surg 1992; 216:142–5.

95. Watson K. Carcinoma of the ampulla of Vater. Successful radical resection. Br J Surg 1944; 31:368–73.

96. Seiler CA, Wagner M, Sadowski C et al. Randomized prospective trial of pylorus-preserving vs. classic duodenopancreatectomy (Whipple procedure): initial clinical results. J Gastrointest Surg 2000; 4:443–52.

Randomised trial showing no benefit for pylorus-preserving pancreaticoduodenectomy.

97. Zerbi A, Balzano G, Leone BE et al. Clinical presen-tation, diagnosis and survival of resected distal bile duct cancer. Dig Surg 1998; 15:410–16.

98. Kozuschek W, Reith HB, Waleczek H et al. A comparison of long term results of the standard Whipple procedure and the pylorus preserving pancreatoduodenectomy. J Am Coll Surg 1994; 178:443–53.

99. Cooperman AM, Kini S, Snady H et al. Current surgical therapy for carcinoma of the pancreas. J Clin Gastroenterol 2000; 31:107–13.

100. Konishi M, Ryu M, Kinoshita T et al. Pathophysiology after pylorus-preserving pancreatoduodenectomy: a comparative study of pancreatogastrostomy and pancreatojejunostomy. Hepatogastroenterology 1999; 46:1181–6.

101. Fortner JG, Klimstra DS, Senie RT et al. Tumor size is the primary prognosticator for pancreatic cancer after regional pancreatectomy. Ann Surg 1996; 223:147–53.

102. Birk D, Fortnagel G, Formentini A et al. Small carcinoma of the pancreas. Factors of prognostic relevance. J Hepatobiliary Pancreat Surg 1998; 5:450–4.

103. Ishikawa O, Ohigashi H, Sasaki Y et al. Adjuvant therapies in extended pancreatectomy for ductal adenocarcinoma of the pancreas. Hepatogastroenterology 1998; 45:644–50.

104. Hiraoka T, Uchino R, Kanemitsu K et al. Combination of intraoperative radiation with resection of cancer of the pancreas. Int J Pancreatol 1990; 7:201–7.

105. Yeo CJ, Cameron JL, Sohn TA et al. Pancreaticoduodenectomy with or without extended lymphadenectomy for periampullary adenocarcinoma: comparison of morbidity and mortality and short-term outcome. Ann Surg 1999; 229:613–22.

106. Yeo CJ, Cameron JL, Lillemoe KD et al. Pancreaticoduodenectomy with or without distal gastrectomy and extended retroperitoneal lymphadenectomy for periampullary adenocarcinoma, part 2: randomized controlled trial evaluating survival, morbidity, and mortality. Ann Surg 2002; 236:355–66; discussion 366–8.

   Reports of trial showing no benefit for extended lymphadenectomy at time of pancreaticoduodenectomy for pancreatic cancer.

107. Shoup M, Brennan MF, McWhite K et al. The value of splenic preservation with distal pancreatectomy. Arch Surg 2002; 137:164–8.

108. Rockey EW. Total pancreatectomy for carcinoma: case report. Ann Surg 1943; 118:603–11.

109. Ihse I, Anderson H, Andren S. Total pancreatectomy for cancer of the pancreas: is it appropriate? World J Surg 1996; 20:288–93; discussion 294.

110. Karpoff HM, Klimstra DS, Brennan MF et al. Results of total pancreatectomy for adenocarcinoma of the pancreas. Arch Surg 2001; 136:44–7; discussion 48.

111. Watanapa P, Williamson RC. Surgical palliation for pancreatic cancer: developments during the past two decades. Br J Surg 1992; 79:8–20.

112. Pitt HA, Murray KP, Bowman HM et al. Clinical pathway implementation improves outcomes for complex biliary surgery. Surgery 1999; 126(4):751–6; discussion 756–8.

113. Sarr MG, Cameron JL. Surgical management of unresectable carcinoma of the pancreas. Surgery 1982; 91:123–33.

114. Lillemoe KD, Cameron JL, Kaufman HS et al. Chemical splanchnicectomy in patients with unresectable pancreatic cancer. A prospective randomized trial. Ann Surg 1993; 217:447–55; discussion 456–7.

115. Warshaw AL, Fernandez-del Castillo C. Pancreatic carcinoma. N Engl J Med 1992; 326:455–65.

116. Kalser MH, Ellenberg SS. Pancreatic cancer. Adjuvant combined radiation and chemotherapy following curative resection. Arch Surg 1985; 120:899–903.

117. Gastrointestinal Tumor Study Group. Further evidence of effective adjuvant combined radiation and chemotherapy following curative resection of pancreatic cancer. Cancer 1987; 59:2006–10.

118. Neoptolemos JP, Dunn JA, Stocken DD et al. Adjuvant chemoradiotherapy and chemotherapy in resectable pancreatic cancer: a randomised controlled trial. Lancet 2001; 358:1576–85.

119. Pipas JM, Mitchell SE, Barth RJ Jr et al. Phase I study of twice-weekly gemcitabine and concomitant external-beam radiotherapy in patients with adenocarcinoma of the pancreas. Int J Radiat Oncol Biol Phys 2001; 50:1317–22.

120. Crane C, Janjan N, Evans D et al. Toxicity and efficacy of concurrent gemcitabine and radiotherapy for locally advanced pancreatic cancer. Int J Gastrointest Cancer 2001; 29:9–18.

121. Crane CH, Janjan NA, Evans DB et al. Toxicity and efficacy of concurrent gemcitabine and radiotherapy for locally advanced pancreatic cancer. Int J Pancreatol 2001; 29:9–18.

122. Bramhall SR, Rosemurgy A, Brown PD et al. Marimastat as first-line therapy for patients with unresectable pancreatic cancer: a randomized trial. J Clin Oncol 2001; 19:3447–55.

123. Burris HA 3rd, Moore MJ, Andersen J et al. Improvements in survival and clinical benefit with gemcitabine as first-line therapy for patients with advanced pancreas cancer: a randomized trial. J Clin Oncol 1997; 15:2403–13.

   Randomised trial showing significant benefit for gemcitabine in advanced pancreatic cancer.

124. Sherman WH, Fine RL. Combination gemcitabine and docetaxel therapy in advanced adenocarcinoma of the pancreas. Oncology 2001; 60:316–21.

125. Farrell TJ, Barbot DJ, Rosato FE. Pancreatic resection combined with intraoperative radiation therapy for pancreatic cancer. Ann Surg 1997; 226:66–9.

126. Snady H, Bruckner H, Cooperman A et al. Survival advantage of combined chemoradiotherapy compared with resection as the initial treatment of patients with regional pancreatic carcinoma. An outcomes trial. Cancer 2000; 89:314–27.

127. Conlon KC, McMahon RL. Minimally invasive surgery in the diagnosis and treatment of upper gastrointestinal tract malignancy. Ann Surg Oncol 2002; 9:725–37.

128. American Joint Committee on Cancer. AJCC Cancer Staging Manual, 6th edn., Greene FL (ed.). Springer-Verlag, 2002.

Fourteen

Hepatobiliary and pancreatic trauma

Rowan W. Parks and
O. James Garden

INTRODUCTION

Despite its relatively protected location, the liver is the most frequently injured intra-abdominal organ,[1] although splenic injuries are more common following blunt abdominal trauma.[2] Associated injuries to other organs, uncontrolled haemorrhage from the liver and subsequent development of septic complications contribute significantly to morbidity and death.[3]

This chapter will address the presentation, initial assessment and management of patients with liver injury. The selection criteria for conservative management will be discussed together with the indications for operative intervention. The factors guiding operative decision-making and the available therapeutic options at operation will be examined. The spectrum of complications and likely outcomes after liver trauma will be reviewed. This chapter will also address the management of patients with traumatic (non-iatrogenic) injury to the extrahepatic bile duct system and also the management of pancreatic injury. It is not always possible in clinical practice to separate these injuries into clearly distinct categories. Therefore, this chapter reviews current evidence and provides practical guidance based on the evidence available.

LIVER TRAUMA

Mechanisms of liver injury

Blunt and penetrating trauma are the two principal mechanisms for trauma to the liver and pancreas. Road traffic accidents account for the majority of blunt injuries, whereas knife and gunshot wounds constitute the major cause of penetrating injuries. In the UK, blunt trauma predominates, and in our institution the ratio of blunt to penetrating liver trauma in a series of 75 patients over a 10-year period was 3:2.[4] Whilst this is typical for other European centres,[5,6] it differs from the experience in South Africa, where penetrating injuries account for 66% of liver trauma,[7] and in North America, where up to 86% of liver injuries are penetrating wounds.[8,9]

Two types of blunt liver trauma have been described – deceleration (shearing) trauma and crush injury. Deceleration injuries occur in road traffic accidents and in falls from a height where there is movement of the liver relative to its diaphragmatic attachments.[10] Crush injuries follow direct trauma to the abdomen over the liver area. The two types of injury may coexist but tend to produce somewhat different types of liver injury.

Deceleration or shearing injuries create lacerations in the hepatic parenchyma, typically between the right posterior section (segments 6 and 7) and the right anterior section (segments 5 and 8), which can extend to involve major vessels. In contrast, a direct blow to the abdomen, by a fist or any blunt object, may lead to a crush injury, with damage to the central portion of the liver (segments 4, 5 and 8). Compression between the right lower ribs and the spine may also cause bleeding from the caudate lobe (segment 1).[11] Blunt trauma can rupture Glisson's capsule and can also lead to subcapsular or intra-parenchymal haematoma formation. Penetrating injuries are usually associated with gunshot or stab wounds, with the former usually resulting in more tissue damage due to the cavitation effect as the bullet traverses the liver substance.

Injury to the hepatic veins and juxtahepatic vena cava can occur as a result of shearing stress in blunt trauma. It is worth noting that there may not be initial exsanguinating haemorrhage as the weight of the liver may provide some compression.[12]

Classification of liver injury

The severity of liver trauma ranges from a minor capsular tear, with or without parenchymal injury, to extensive disruption involving both lobes of the liver with associated hepatic vein or vena caval injury. The American Association for the Surgery of Trauma has adopted for general use the classifi-cation of liver injury described initially in 1989 by Moore and colleagues[13] and revised subsequently in 1994[14] (**Table 14.1**). The hepatic injury grade is calculated from assessment of the liver injury using information derived from radiological study, oper-ative findings or autopsy report. Where there are multiple injuries to the liver the grade is advanced by one stage. Grade I or II injuries are considered minor; they represent 80–90% of all cases and usually require minimal or no operative treatment. Grade III–V injuries are generally considered severe and often require surgical intervention, while grade VI lesions are regarded as incompatible with survival. Schweizer and colleagues have described a protocol-based liver trauma management system employing this classification system that permits lesser injuries to be treated non-operatively and allows more appropriate selection of patients for operative treatment.[15]

The initial assessment and management of an injured patient should proceed according to the Advanced Trauma Life Support (ATLS) guidelines of the American College of Surgeons Committee on Trauma.[16] The initial focus of attention is on the patient's airway, breathing and circulation. The

Table 14.1 • Hepatic injury scale used by the American Association for the Surgery of Trauma

Grade		Description
I	Haematoma	Subcapsular, <10% surface area
	Laceration	Capsular tear, <1 cm parenchymal depth
II	Haematoma	Subcapsular, 10–50% of surface area Intraparenchymal <10 cm in diameter
	Laceration	1–3 cm parenchymal depth, <10 cm in length
III	Haematoma	Subcapsular, >50% surface area or expanding; ruptured subcapsular or parenchymal haematoma; intraparenchymal haematoma >10 cm or expanding
	Laceration	>3 cm parenchymal depth
IV	Laceration	Parenchymal disruption involving 25–75% of hepatic lobe or 1–3 Couinaud segments within a single lobe
V	Laceration	Parenchymal disruption involving >75% of hepatic lobe or >3 Couinaud segments within a single lobe
	Vascular	Juxtahepatic venous injuries – retrohepatic cava, major hepatic veins
VI	Vascular	Hepatic avulsion

Note: advance one grade for multiple injuries up to grade III.

airway is secured, intravenous access established and fluid resuscitation commenced.

The role of 'aggressive' high-volume fluid replacement in trauma victims has been questioned, with evidence suggesting that excessive fluid replacement is associated with adverse outcome.[17] As this evidence came from an American series that included a large proportion of relatively young, previously fit adults suffering from penetrating trauma to the torso, with ready access to trauma centres, the results may not necessarily be applicable to practice in other countries.

Diagnosis of liver injury

In penetrating abdominal trauma, hepatic injury should be considered in any patient with a wound to the abdomen. Hepatic injury should also be considered in patients with penetrating low thoracic wounds and also in posterior penetrating wounds below a coronal plane at the tips of the scapulae.[12]

Patients with major hepatic injury may present with profound clinical shock and abdominal distension. Hypotension resistant to fluid resuscitation combined with gross abdominal distension constitutes an indication for immediate laparotomy. The operative management options for patients in this situation will be discussed in detail subsequently. Emergency room thoracotomy with cross clamping of the descending thoracic aorta is a dramatic intervention but even in centres where this technique is advocated the outcome is poor.

In Feliciano's series of 1000 patients with liver trauma treated during a 5-year period, 45 patients underwent emergency room thoracotomy for control of haemorrhage related to their liver injury and all died.[8] Similarly, in an 11-year review of 783 patients who sustained liver trauma in Scotland, 11 patients underwent an unsuccessful laparotomy or thoraco-laparotomy in the emergency room.[18]

Emergency room surgery remains a potentially life-saving manoeuvre in patients with significant intrathoracic injury who may have a coexistent liver injury. However, there is little place for this intervention in patients with a predominant abdominal injury. These patients are better served by rapid assessment and transport to the operating theatre.

In less dramatic situations, with a patient who is haemodynamically stable or responds to fluid resuscitation, appropriate investigations can be employed to obtain more information regarding the liver injury and to ascertain whether there is coexisting intra-abdominal visceral injury. During the initial survey a detailed clinical history is taken. Particular attention is paid to the mechanism of a road traffic accident, with supplemental information from ambulance crew, witnesses or police being used to piece together a picture of the accident. Speed of vehicle, position of occupant in vehicle, use of seatbelts, employment of airbag restraint systems and a history of ejection of the patient from the vehicle are important items of information. Conscious patients may complain of abdominal pain. Shoulder tip pain may arise from blood in the subdiaphragmatic space causing phrenic nerve irritation.

As resuscitation proceeds, a detailed physical examination is carried out. On inspection, attention is paid to the presence of anterior abdominal wall bruising, which may indicate compression from a seatbelt, and flank bruising, which may indicate retroperitoneal extravasation of blood. Signs of localised or generalised peritonitis are recorded in the conscious patient. In this context it should be noted that although there is evidence that the use of opiate analgesia will not significantly obscure physical signs in patients with acute abdominal pain,[19] these findings have not been confirmed in abdominal trauma patients where the situation may be complicated by head injury, alcohol intoxication or the requirement for assisted ventilation.

Baseline investigations consist of blood count (for haemoglobin and haematocrit), blood for cross-matching, serum urea and electrolytes, serum amylase and coagulation screen. An erect chest radiograph and a plain abdominal film can be taken if the patient is sufficiently stable. In the context of diagnosing liver injury, features that may be of relevance include fractures of the lower ribs, elevation of the right hemidiaphragm and loss of the psoas shadow suggesting retroperitoneal bleeding. Retroperitoneal perforation of the duodenum may give rise to soft tissue shadowing in the right upper quadrant, and loss of the psoas shadow and extra-luminal gas may occasionally be noted.

Following initial assessment, patients who are conscious but have haemodynamic instability resistant to fluid resuscitation and with clinical signs of peritonitis should undergo laparotomy. In patients who are haemodynamically stable and have suspected liver injury further diagnostic tests may be undertaken at this stage to define the nature of the injuries. An ideal test will establish the presence and extent of any liver injury together with providing information on concomitant visceral injury.

Diagnostic peritoneal lavage (DPL) has been advocated in patients with impaired conscious levels and equivocal physical signs.[20] DPL may help in the diagnosis of hollow visceral injury. However, a DPL that yields a positive result for blood will provide no information regarding either the site or the nature of the injury, and in the context of liver injury may lead to patients undergoing surgery where they may be better treated non-operatively.

An alternative test that may be used in the trauma room is abdominal ultrasonography. Several recent prospective studies have reported that ultrasonography can be performed with a sensitivity of 82–88% and a specificity of 99% in detecting intra-abdominal injuries, but it remains critically dependent on the skill of the operator. Recognising this, the multicentre North American FAST study (Focused Assessment for the Sonographic examination of the

Trauma patient) attempted to increase the reliability of ultrasound scanning in abdominal trauma by adhering to an agreed protocol for scanning that sequentially surveyed for haemopericardium and then the right upper quadrant, left upper quadrant and pelvis for haemoperitoneum in patients with potential truncal injuries.[21]

The FAST study demonstrated a significant correlation between haemoperitoneum in the right upper quadrant and injury to the liver, and suggested that adherence to a pre-agreed protocol increased the reliability of ultrasound assessment of abdominal trauma.[21] Other centres have also reported that ultrasound is a reliable 'first' test for the assessment of a patient with suspected liver trauma.[22]

However, an important cautionary note comes from the study carried out by Richards and colleagues.[23] In a series of 1686 abdominal ultrasound scans for trauma, 71 patients had bowel or mesenteric injury, and 30 patients had a negative ultrasound scan (43% false-negative rate).

Computed tomography (CT) is the 'gold standard' investigation for the evaluation of a patient with suspected liver trauma[24–27] (Fig. 14.1). The use of

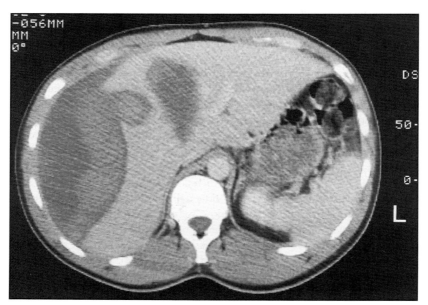

Figure 14.1 • CT scan of a 25-year-old male who sustained a blunt injury to the right chest wall but was admitted to hospital haemodynamically stable. The scan shows a substantial subcapsular haematoma associated with an intraparenchymal laceration. This patient was managed successfully without operation.

intravenous contrast may help in the detection of non-viable parenchyma. CT has high sensitivity and specificity for detecting liver injuries; these attributes increase as the time between injury and scanning increases, as haematomas and lacerations become better defined.[28] The more widespread use of CT has resulted in greater sophistication in the interpretation of the CT features of liver trauma. Fang and colleagues reported six patients (of a series of 194 undergoing CT for liver injury) who demonstrated intraparenchymal 'pooling' of intravenous contrast that correlated strongly to the presence of ongoing haemorrhage.[29] Yokota and Sugimoto[30] described 'periportal tracking', which consists of a circumferential area of low attenuation around the portal triad on contrast-enhanced CT. Periportal tracking is thought to represent blood or fluid within the condensation of the Glissonian sheath around the portal structures and indicates the presence of injury to structures in the portal triad. If the sign is present in the periphery of the liver it may alert the clinician to the presence of a peripheral bile duct injury that in turn may present as a bile leak. Addition of oral contrast medium does not appear to add to the diagnostic yield of CT in the assessment of liver injury.[31]

In order to maintain a balanced perspective it is worthwhile considering some of the limitations of CT in the assessment of liver trauma. The CT-defined grade of injury may differ from the grade of liver injury found at operation, with the predominant tendency being to overdiagnose the grade of injury on CT as compared with subsequent operative findings.[32] Croce et al. concluded that CT should not be used in isolation to estimate blood loss and that CT may not provide an accurate assessment of the extent of a liver laceration in some areas of the liver – specifically in the vicinity of the falciform ligament.

Bearing the above limitations in mind, CT will help define the extent of the liver injury and will be of value in the detection of injury to other intra-abdominal viscera, in particular pancreatic injury. CT will allow the liver injury to be graded and thus will provide objective information that is mandatory if non-operative treatment is to be contemplated. Further refinements now permit accurate three-dimensional image reconstruction,[33] and technical modifications such as helical CT combined with

intravenous contrast allow demonstration of the biliary tree (CT cholangiography).[34]

OTHER DIAGNOSTIC MODALITIES FOR THE ASSESSMENT OF LIVER INJURY

Newer non-invasive imaging techniques such as magnetic resonance imaging (MRI) have the advantage of being free of ionising radiation, but increased cost aside, the time taken to produce a scan means that this technique is not yet widely used in the trauma setting.[35] Angiography may be used as a complementary investigation to CT.[36] In this context it is of value in patients with high-grade liver injury and may be combined with therapeutic angiographic embolisation for ongoing blood loss or haemobilia.

Other diagnostic modalities may be used in specific situations. Endoscopic retrograde cholangio-pancreatography (ERCP) may help in delineation of the biliary tree in patients with liver trauma,[37] and endoscopic transpapillary stents may be used as a therapeutic modality to treat biliary leaks.[38]

Diagnostic laparoscopy has been used successfully in patients with abdominal trauma,[39–41] and therapeutic laparoscopic techniques for managing liver injuries using fibrin glue have also been described.[42] However, in the specific context of liver trauma, the authors have concerns about the use of laparoscopy because general anaesthesia, muscle relaxation and the creation of a pneumoperitoneum may decompress a stable perihepatic haematoma. Furthermore, laparoscopic assessment of the injured liver may not provide sufficient detail concerning parenchymal injury. For these reasons, the role of laparoscopy has yet to be established in the assessment of liver injuries.

In the initial management of suspected liver trauma, there is little evidence to support the use of emergency room thoracotomy. Ultrasound is reliable for the initial assessment of a patient with suspected liver trauma.

Management of liver injury: selection of patients for non-operative management

The feasibility of non-operative management of patients with intra-abdominal solid organ injury was first established in paediatric surgery and has extended gradually to adult practice. Richie and Fonkalsrud described successful conservative management of four patients with liver injury in an era before the availability of CT scans.[43] Further indirect evidence for the feasibility of a non-operative approach came from a report published by White and Cleveland[44] in the same year. They reported a consecutive series of 126 patients with liver trauma, all of whom underwent laparotomy. Interestingly, 67 patients in this series (53%) had placement of a drain to the subhepatic space as their only liver-related surgical intervention at laparotomy. Subsequent studies have recognised that 50–80% of liver injuries stop bleeding spontaneously and this has led to a non-operative approach for blunt liver trauma in selected patients.[45–48]

Non-operative management of liver trauma is now a well-established treatment option. Trunkey's group in Portland, Oregon, first defined in 1985 the following criteria for the selection of patients for non-operative management:

- haemodynamic stability
- absence of peritoneal signs
- availability of good-quality CT
- an experienced radiologist
- ability to monitor patients in an intensive care setting
- facility for immediate surgery (and by implication, availability of an experienced liver surgeon)
- simple liver injury with <125 mL of free intraperitoneal blood
- absence of other significant intra-abdominal injuries.[49]

Farnell and colleagues extended the threshold of haemoperitoneum to 250 mL and described specific liver injuries suitable for non-operative management.[50] Feliciano subsequently suggested that any blunt hepatic injury, regardless of its magnitude, should be managed without operation if the patient was haemodynamically stable and had a haemoperitoneum of less than 500 mL.[51] The degree of liver injury amenable to successful non-operative management has gradually extended over recent years, and most authors now believe that the ultimate decisive factor in favour of non-operative management is haemodynamic stability of the patient at presentation or after initial resuscitation, irrespective of the grade of liver injury on CT or the amount of haemoperitoneum.[52–55]

A 22-month prospective study from Memphis of the initial non-operative treatment of haemodynamically stable blunt hepatic trauma patients compared outcome to a matched cohort of blunt hepatic trauma patients treated operatively.[56] The study reported that of 136 patients with blunt trauma, 24 (18%) underwent emergency surgery. Of the remaining 112 patients, 12 (11%) failed conservative management (for causes not related to the liver injury in 7) and the remaining 100 patients were successfully treated without operation. Of these, 30% had minor injuries (grades I–II) but 70% had major injuries (grades III–V). This study concluded that non-operative management is safe for haemodynamically stable patients and that this was independent of the CT-delineated grade of the liver injury. The blood transfusion requirement and the incidence of abdominal complications were lower in the non-operatively treated group.

Reporting a single institutional experience, Boone and colleagues stated that 46 (36%) of 128 consecutive patients with blunt liver trauma were treated non-operatively with success, including 23 patients with grade III and IV injuries.[52] A review of 495 patients from the recent literature noted a success rate for non-operative treatment of 94%.[57] This was accomplished with a mean transfusion rate of 1.9 units, a complication rate of 6% and a mean hospital stay of 13 days. There were no liver-related deaths, nor were there any missed enteric injuries.

The current consensus view is that successful selection of patients for conservative treatment after blunt abdominal trauma cannot be carried out by CT scanning alone but that an overall assessment of suitability for conservative management must take into account the findings of careful repeated clinical examination and the results of close monitoring of haemodynamic and haematological parameters.[58–64] If non-operative management is selected, haemodynamic instability is the predominant indication for intervention early in the clinical course whilst intervention (often radiological or endoscopic) may be required later for management of bile leak or intrahepatic collections.

If a non-operative strategy is selected it should be borne in mind that the risk of hollow organ injury increases in proportion to the number of solid organs injured[65] and that there is a small but significant risk of delayed haemorrhage.[66] However, it appears that the natural course of liver injuries is more analogous to that of lung or kidney injuries, rather than splenic injuries, in that any deterioration is usually gradual, with a fall in haemoglobin level or an increase in fluid requirement, rather than acute haemodynamic decompensation.[67] Therefore with close supervision, patients who fail with an initial non-operative approach can be detected early and treated appropriately.

After the initial selection of a non-operative management strategy, routine follow-up CT is used widely to monitor the injury. Although some authors suggest there is little evidence that follow-up CT provides additional information and rarely changes management,[68] a recent study reported that follow-up CT scan at a mean of 10 days after surgical intervention showed a 49% incidence of liver-related complications, most of which required subsequent intervention.[69]

There is a broad consensus of opinion that a gunshot wound to the abdomen is an indication for laparotomy.[70,71] The increasing use of non-operative management has led to this strategy being challenged in selected patients with isolated gunshot wounds of the liver;[72] however, this approach is associated with the risk of failure to detect concomitant intra-abdominal visceral injury and at present there is insufficient evidence to justify a non-operative strategy in gunshot wounds of the liver.

 Non-operative management is safe for haemodynamically stable patients with CT scan evidence of liver injury.

Operative management of liver injury

GENERAL STRATEGY

Primary operative intervention is indicated for liver injury if the patient is haemodynamically unstable despite adequate initial resuscitation. Important prerequisites for a successful outcome are: adequate blood, platelets, fresh frozen plasma and cryo-precipitate; an intensive care unit; the necessary diagnostic facilities to monitor and detect potential complications; and an experienced liver surgeon. Although this is the ideal, patients with liver trauma often present initially to surgeons without specialist hepatobiliary experience and without the facilities available in liver surgery units. The surgeon operating on a patient in this situation should therefore attempt to control bleeding without causing further complications. It is in this context that there is a role for packing of the liver. This was popularised in the UK by Calne, who advocated liver packing followed by transfer of the patient to the care of a specialist hepatobiliary surgeon.[73]

CHOICE OF INCISION

A long midline incision is widely employed for an emergency laparotomy. It has the advantages that it can be made rapidly, extended proximally (to enter the chest after median sternotomy) or distally as required, and access to the liver can be improved by converting the incision into a 'T' by adding a right transverse component, or to a 'Y' by adding a right lateral thoracotomy. In our experience, extension of the incision into the chest is exceptional. In situations where operation is being carried out after initial conservative management, for example for treatment of bile leakage or resectional debridement, primary subcostal incision with fixed costal margin retraction affords excellent access to the liver.

INTRA-OPERATIVE ASSESSMENT

Once the abdomen has been entered, blood and clots should be removed and packs inserted into each quadrant of the abdomen. A thorough laparotomy is performed in a systematic manner to identify all intra-abdominal injuries. Any perforations in the bowel should be sutured immediately to minimise contamination. Significant liver haemorrhage can usually be controlled initially by direct pressure using packs, although additional techniques that may be employed include: temporary digital compression of the free edge of the lesser omentum (Pringle manoeuvre) (**Fig. 14.2**); bimanual compression of the liver; or manual compression of the aorta above the coeliac trunk. At this point, further evaluation of the extent of liver injury should be delayed until the anaesthetist has replenished

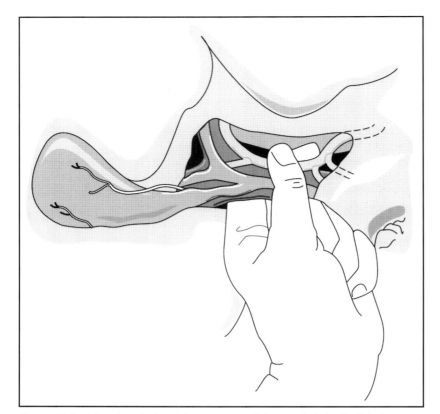

Figure 14.2 • Manual occlusion of the structures of the portal triad – the Pringle manoeuvre. From Rob and Smith's Operative Surgery – Hepatobiliary Surgery. London: Chapman & Hall, 1996. Reprinted by permission of Hodder Arnold.

adequately the intravascular volume and stabilised the blood pressure. Attempts to evaluate the liver injury before adequate resuscitation may result in further blood loss and worsening hypotension and acidosis.

The packs can be gently removed to allow a detailed evaluation of the type and extent of the liver injury. It should be borne in mind that a subcapsular haematoma may cover an area of ischaemic tissue and that parenchymal lacerations may be associated with damage to segmental bile ducts.[74] Many liver injuries will have stopped bleeding spontaneously by the time of surgery. If there is active bleeding, a Pringle manoeuvre can be used diagnostically and compression can be maintained with an atraumatic vascular clamp if haemorrhage decreases (**Fig. 14.3**). The clamp should be occluded only to the degree necessary to compress the blood vessels and not to injure the common bile duct. A normal liver can tolerate

inflow occlusion for up to 1 hour;[75] however, the ability of a damaged liver to tolerate ischaemia may be impaired. If haemorrhage is unaffected by portal triad occlusion, major vena cava injury or atypical vascular anatomy should be suspected. Hepatic outflow control may also be required. Access to the suprahepatic cava can be gained by an experienced liver surgeon, and slings may be placed around the hepatic veins following mobilisation of the liver from its peritoneal attachments. Total vascular occlusion of the liver requires control of the inferior vena cava below the liver in addition to the supra-hepatic cava but is likely to be poorly tolerated by an injured liver.[76,77]

PERIHEPATIC PACKING

In situations where it is thought that definitive control of haemorrhage cannot be obtained, the liver injury can be packed, the incision closed and

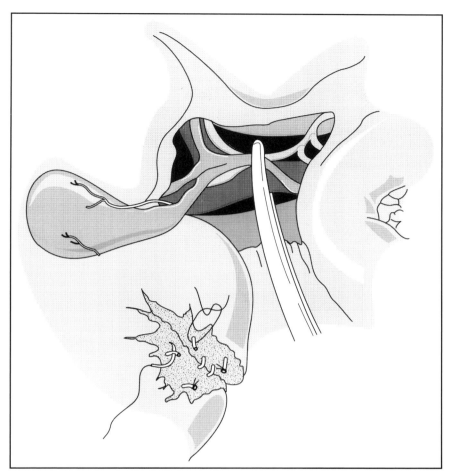

Figure 14.3 • Occlusion of the structures in the portal triad using a soft non-crushing clamp. From Rob and Smith's Operative Surgery – Hepatobiliary Surgery. London: Chapman & Hall, 1996. Reprinted by permission of Hodder Arnold.

the patient transferred for definitive treatment. Packing can also be employed as a holding manoeuvre in patients who are critically unstable, coagulopathic or acidotic and therefore would not tolerate a prolonged operative procedure. As packing is thus a widely applicable procedure, some attention should be devoted to technical considerations. The packs should not be inserted into the liver substance itself, as this will tend to distract the edges of the parenchymal tear and encourage continued bleeding. Rather, the technique of packing involves manual closure or approximation of the parenchyma, followed by sequential placing of dry abdominal packs or a single rolled gauze around the liver and directly over the injury in an attempt to provide tamponade to a bleeding wound

(**Fig. 14.4**). Most surgeons employ skin closure only, leaving the fascia for primary closure at the subsequent procedure for pack removal. The presence of packs, combined with massive oedema of the bowel, may lead to difficulties in wound closure. If this is encountered, a mesh can be inserted to prevent further compromise of ventilation and bowel viability, and to avoid pressure necrosis of the liver.[78]

A study from Cape Town reported that packing controlled haemorrhage in 18 of 22 patients with major haemorrhage from liver injuries.[79] The four patients in whom packing did not control bleeding were found to have a major vascular injury.

The principal complications and limitations of perihepatic packing can be considered in the 'early'

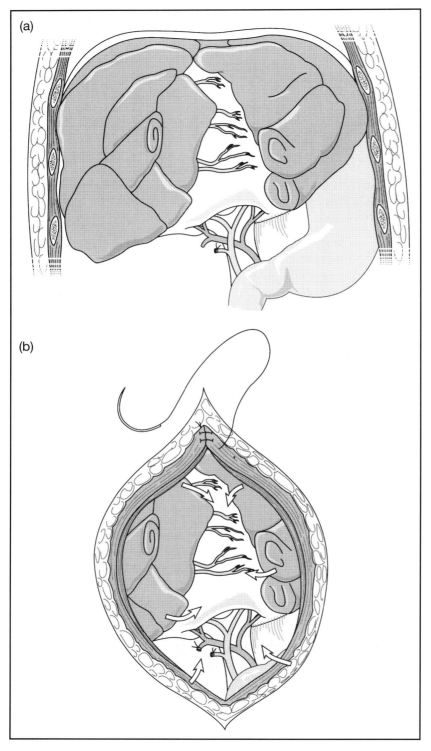

Figure 14.4 • (a) Placement of gauze packs around the liver to compress the fracture. (b) Closure of the incision provides additional compression. Reproduced with permission from Blumgart LH (ed.) Surgery of the liver and biliary tract, 2nd edn. Edinburgh: Churchill Livingstone, 1994.

and 'late' categories. Early complications include failure to control haemorrhage. However, this is relatively uncommon as even in patients with caval or hepatic venous injuries, packing may control haemorrhage.[80] Concerns may also be raised about the potential for compromise of caval blood flow by packing, although this may be avoided by monitoring caval pressure if this technique is available.[81] The principal late complication of packing is infection, and Krige and colleagues reported that leaving the packs in situ for more than 3 days was associated with a high incidence of infective complications.[79] Perihepatic packing is an indication for intravenous antibiotic administration.[82]

TECHNIQUES FOR SURGICAL HAEMOSTASIS

Exposed bleeding vessels can be suture-ligated, clipped or repaired to achieve haemostasis. The ultrasonic dissector is useful in removing damaged and non-viable hepatic parenchyma whilst exposing blood vessels. Diathermy coagulation can also be used and in this context the argon beam coagulator, which 'sprays' the diathermy current on an argon beam, is invaluable as it produces surface eschar without the diathermy probe becoming adherent to the liver surface.[83] The argon beam coagulator also has the advantage of producing less hepatic tissue necrosis than conventional diathermy, which is an advantage in a potentially contaminated operative field. Another substance that has been used to secure haemostasis is fibrin glue, which consists of concentrated human fibrinogen and clotting factors to which aprotinin, a fibrinolysis inhibitor, is added.[84,85] In an experimental porcine major liver trauma model, dry fibrin dressings provided better haemostasis than conventional gauze dressings.[86] There are, however, concerns about the use of fibrin glue in humans. Fatal hypotension following application of fibrin glue into a deep hepatic laceration has been reported.[87]

Liver sutures are absorbable sutures on a curved blunt-tipped needle often used in conjunction with a bolster of haemostatic material.[88] These can be used to approximate a fissured parenchymal injury and thus control haemorrhage as an alternative to exploration of the depths of the injury. The disadvantages of this technique are that vessels may continue to bleed resulting in a cavitating haematoma, bile duct injuries may not be detected, and the suture itself may cause further bleeding, ischaemia or intrahepatic bile duct injury.[89]

Stone and Lamb reported that the greater omentum could be employed as a pedicled flap to fill a defect in the liver parenchyma and may help stop oozing from the low-pressure venous system of the liver parenchyma.[90] The use of an absorbable polyglactin perihepatic mesh particularly for major parenchymal disruptions has also been reported.[91–93] This technique is not indicated where juxtacaval or hepatic vein injury is suspected. Advocates of mesh wrapping claim that it can provide the benefits of packing without the disadvantages normally associated with packing. In particular, a second laparotomy is not required routinely and, as mesh wrapping does not increase intra-abdominal volume or pressure, abdominal closure is much easier and respiratory or renal function are less compromised.[94] However, there is some concern about the amount of time needed to apply the mesh wrap in a haemodynamically unstable patient who might be best treated with rapid insertion of perihepatic packs, and as yet there is insufficient general experience with this technique.

RESECTIONAL DEBRIDEMENT

This technique involves removal of devitalised liver tissue down to normal parenchyma using the lines of the injury, rather than anatomical planes, as the boundaries of the resection.[95]

Bismuth categorised this as a 'secondary' surgical technique to be carried out using the techniques of liver surgery.[11] The optimum timing may be to combine debridement with pack removal, as necrotic tissue will be well demarcated at 48 h post-injury. Resectional debridement is by definition 'non-anatomical' and may expose segmental bile ducts. Bile ducts exposed in the periphery of the liver should be ligated in order to prevent post-operative bile leaks into a central hepatic cavity, as this troublesome complication will not necessarily be treatable by endoscopic transampullary biliary stenting. It is better to anticipate and avoid this complication.

ANATOMICAL LIVER RESECTION

The practical difficulties of undertaking formal anatomical liver resection in a patient with a significant liver injury, who will frequently have associated shock, coagulopathy and concomitant injury, are such that this type of treatment is not widely used. It is generally accepted that anatomical resections should be reserved for situations in which no other procedure adequately achieves haemostasis, such as with deep liver lacerations involving major vessels and/or bile ducts, where there is extensive devascularisation or if there is major hepatic venous bleeding.

Strong reported a single-centre series of 37 patients undergoing anatomical resection for liver trauma from an institutional experience of 287 patients with liver injury treated over a 13-year period.[96] Twenty-seven of these patients underwent right hemihepatectomy and overall there were three postoperative deaths (8% mortality rate). However, these excellent results achieved by a technically skilled liver surgeon and his unit may not be reproduced if the technique were more widely used.

SELECTIVE LIGATION OF THE HEPATIC ARTERY

Selective ligation of the hepatic artery is no longer a commonly used technique and is not mentioned frequently in contemporary reports. It may be used when intrahepatic manoeuvres have failed and when persistent re-bleeding occurs on unclamping the hepatic pedicle. Mays reported the use of this technique in 60 patients.[97] In this series the right hepatic artery was ligated selectively in 36 patients, the left hepatic artery in 15 patients, and the main hepatic artery in 9 patients. No cases of liver failure or necrosis were observed but it seems likely that modern liver surgical approaches have rendered ligation an uncommon manoeuvre in liver injury. Hepatic arterial ligation to control haemorrhage should only be performed when other manoeuvres have failed, when selective ligation has failed and when pedicle clamping has been demonstrated to arrest haemorrhage. Acute gangrenous cholecystitis is a well-recognised complication of hepatic artery ligation, and cholecystectomy should be performed if the main hepatic artery or right hepatic artery is ligated.[98]

MANAGEMENT OF HEPATIC VENOUS AND RETROHEPATIC CAVAL INJURY

Suspicion that one of these serious injuries is present should be raised if the Pringle manoeuvre fails to arrest haemorrhage. In this situation it is vital that a systematic approach be adopted. Injudicious mobilisation of the liver can cause exsanguination or embolisation of air or detached fragments of liver parenchyma.[12] Therefore it is important to exclude anatomical vascular variants. For example, there may be bleeding from the left liver due to the presence of a left hepatic artery arising from the left gastric artery or there may be bleeding from the right liver due to an aberrant right hepatic artery. The commonest anatomical variation in the origin of the right hepatic artery is the persistence of the right primordial hepatic artery where the right hepatic artery arises from the superior mesenteric artery.[99] This is present in approximately 15% of cases and the aberrant right hepatic artery can usually be found running just to the right and slightly posterior to the structures in the porta hepatis. These anatomical variants should be considered and excluded. During this process, active bleeding can be reduced or arrested by perihepatic packing. Persistent bleeding despite exclusion of anatomical variants may then indicate the presence of hepatic venous or retrohepatic caval injury. These injuries account for about 10% of liver trauma cases,[100] and there is no clear consensus on an optimal management strategy. Total vascular exclusion (clamping of the inferior vena cava and suprahepatic cava in addition to the Pringle manoeuvre) may be used. However, clamping the vena cava will seriously compromise venous return in a situation of major trauma and seems unwise. Veno-venous bypass (shunt from common femoral vein to left internal jugular or axillary vein) has the advantage of preserving venous return. Atriocaval shunting has also been described and, combined with a Pringle manoeuvre, allows total vascular isolation of the liver. Chen and colleagues reported on a series of 19 patients with blunt juxtahepatic venous injury from a group of 92 patients with blunt liver trauma over a 2-year period.[101] Five patients with isolated left hepatic vein injuries were treated with the use of veno-venous bypass with no mortality. Ten of the 20 patients with isolated right hepatic vein injury were treated using an atriocaval shunt but the mortality in these 20 patients was 18 (80%) with one survivor in both the shunted and non-shunted groups. Of four patients with combined right and left hepatic vein injury, one was treated by liver transplantation but all four patients in this group died. The overall mortality rate in patients with juxtahepatic vein injury was 63%. The opportunity to optimise the outcome in patients with these serious injuries probably lies in packing followed by transfer to a specialist liver surgery unit.

EX VIVO SURGERY AND LIVER TRANSPLANTATION

Ringe and Pichlmayr[102] reported a consecutive series of eight patients with severe liver trauma treated by total hepatectomy followed by liver transplantation. These patients had all undergone prior surgery for trauma, which had been followed by severe complications – uncontrollable bleeding in four and massive necrosis in four. Where a donor liver was not immediately available a temporary portacaval shunt was used as a bridging procedure. There was a high mortality in this group, with six out of eight patients dying from multiple organ failure or sepsis. The authors conclude that total hepatectomy can be a potentially life-saving procedure in exceptional emergencies in patients with major liver injuries. Heparinised coated tubes such as the Gott shunt can be used to bridge caval defects if total hepatectomy and excision of a caval segment is required in order to obtain haemostasis.[103] The shunt acts as a temporary bridge during the anhepatic phase and has been reported to remain patent over an 18-h period. Whilst experience of this sort of surgery is extremely infrequent, awareness of the therapeutic potential is useful and small series continue to report encouraging results.[104]

Complications of liver trauma

COMPLICATIONS OF NON-OPERATIVE MANAGEMENT

Complications of non-operative management of liver trauma can be considered in three main categories. First, it should be borne in mind that complications can arise as a result of inappropriate selection of a patient for conservative management. If a patient has continued bleeding this may present as episodes of hypotension requiring fluid and blood replacement, impaired renal function, impaired respiratory function (due to diaphragmatic splinting by intra-abdominal haematoma) and there may be evidence of coagulopathy. These features represent not so much a 'complication' as the natural progression of

a patient with continued active intra-abdominal bleeding, and in such a case the policy of non-operative intervention will require reappraisal.

The second group of complications are those relating to coexisting injuries that have not been recognised at the time of initial presentation or become apparent after initial delay. Bile leaks may manifest as biliary peritonitis or as a localised bile collection. ERCP is useful in diagnosing the source of a bile leak in patients with liver trauma treated non-operatively and also in postoperative patients.[37] Perforations of the intestine are also at risk of being missed as the signs of abdominal tenderness may be attributed to intra-abdominal blood from the liver injury. The risk of missing this type of injury can be minimised by regular careful clinical observation. Intestinal perforation may become apparent on serial ultrasound or CT scanning by detection of the presence of free intraperitoneal fluid or gas. In Sherman's series of patients with liver trauma treated non-operatively, 4 out of 30 (13%) patients initially treated without operation subsequently required laparotomy.[54] These were due to splenic injury in three patients and renal injury in one patient. Although the grade of injury to these organs is not specified, in all cases the injuries became apparent after a period of clinical observation. However, the authors concluded that this risk of missed solid organ injury does not obviate the benefits of initial non-operative management.

The third category of complication relates to the late complications of liver injury. Liver injury may give rise to a transient increase in liver transaminase enzymes, which may commence as soon as 15 min after injury.[105] Persistent elevation of these enzymes suggests significant liver injury. Septic complications such as intra-abdominal abscess and bile leak are recognised late complications and may require radiological, endoscopic or surgical intervention.

POSTOPERATIVE COMPLICATIONS AFTER SURGERY FOR LIVER TRAUMA

The complications after liver surgery for trauma are similar to those encountered after any form of liver surgery. Haemorrhage in the immediate postoperative period may be due to coagulopathy related to large-volume transfusion and may require correction with fresh frozen plasma and platelet concentrates. If there is no evidence of a significant coagulopathy and bleeding continues, selective

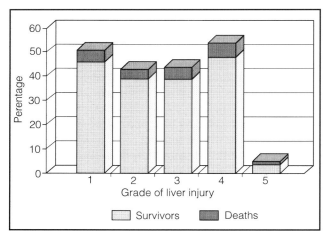

Figure 14.5 • Outcome after liver injury. Note that the overall outcome will be influenced by the severity of coexisting injuries. Reproduced with permission from Schweizer W et al. Br J Surg 1993; 80:86–8, Blackwell Publishing Ltd.

mesenteric angiography may provide diagnostic information and may permit therapeutic embolisation, although re-laparotomy is generally indicated to assess the source of bleeding and to remove retained blood and clot.[106] Bleeding in the later postoperative period may be due to haemobilia or bleeding from the biliary tree into the gut. It has been reported to occur in 1.2% of patients with liver trauma.[107] Postoperative sepsis may be due to infected collections of bile or blood or related to devitalised segments of liver parenchyma. Ultrasound and CT scanning are of value in diagnosis and these modalities may be used to guide placement of drains. Bile leakage from a drain site is not uncommon and usually ceases spontaneously; however, if it persists, ERCP may be all that is required to define the site of the leak and allow temporary stent placement. Arteriovenous fistula is not an uncommon complication after injury in many sites of the body and can manifest after liver injury as an arterioportal fistula.[108] Large fistulas can result in portal hypertension.

Outcome after liver injury

The outcome after liver trauma is related not only to the severity of the injury but also to the severity of any associated injury.[8] Most series report mortality rates of approximately 10–15%; however, the large variation in case mix between different centres makes comparison difficult. In a large series of 1000 cases of liver trauma from Houston, an overall mortality of 10.5% was reported.[8] White

and Cleveland reported a similar mortality rate in 1972, with eight deaths occurring in a consecutive series of 126 patients (6.3%).[44] The results of liver trauma in the series reported by Schweizer et al.,[15] which compared outcome to grade of injury, are shown in graphic form in Fig. 14.5. The mortality rate was 11% for grade I injuries, 10% for grade II injuries, 13% for grade III and IV injuries, and 33% in the small number of grade V injuries. The overall mortality was 12% (21 deaths in 175 patients). The mechanism of injury has an important bearing on the mortality rate, with blunt trauma carrying a higher mortality rate (10–30%) than penetrating liver trauma (0–10%). While most early deaths seem to be due to uncontrolled haemorrhage and associated injuries, most late deaths result from head injuries and sepsis with multiple organ failure.[9,109,110]

EXTRAHEPATIC BILIARY TRACT TRAUMA

Non-iatrogenic injury to the extrahepatic biliary tract is uncommon and encountered only rarely by surgeons outside specialist hepatobiliary centres. Most injuries are due to penetrating rather than blunt abdominal trauma. Biliary tract injury is diagnosed rarely before operation and is often only recognised incidentally at laparotomy. Extrahepatic bile duct injury due to blunt trauma is only rarely associated with injury to the portal vein or hepatic artery. This may be explained by the increased length, tortuosity and elasticity of the vascular structures. Furthermore, a vascular injury, especially portal vein rupture, is likely to be associated with a high immediate mortality.

Incidence of biliary injury

The reported incidence of injury to the extrahepatic biliary system varies between 1 and 5% of patients who sustain abdominal trauma.[111] In a review of 5070 patients who sustained blunt and penetrating abdominal trauma, Penn reported a 1.9% incidence of gallbladder injury.[112] Soderstrom and colleagues identified 31 patients (2.1%) with gallbladder injury in a group of 1449 patients who sustained blunt abdominal trauma and underwent exploratory laparotomy.[113] In a further review of 949 patients undergoing laparotomy for acute trauma, there were 32 injuries to the gallbladder (3.4%) and 5 to the common bile duct (0.5%).[114] Burgess and Fulton reported that over a 5-year period, 24 out of 184 patients with abdominal trauma had extrahepatic bile duct or gallbladder injury as well as liver injury.[115] They reported that this injury was often seen with severe hepatic trauma and in association with multiple organ injury. Dawson and colleagues reviewed the results of treatment of all patients with porta hepatis injuries presenting to a level 1 trauma centre in Seattle over an 11-year period.[116] A total of 21 patients (0.21% of 10 500 admissions) had injuries to the portal triad, of whom 11 (52%) died. Isolated extrahepatic bile duct injury occurred in four of these patients. Injuries to the portal vein or hepatic artery, either in isolation or in association with extrahepatic bile duct injury, were associated with the worst prognosis. Of note is the fact that in none of the 21 cases was the diagnosis of the injury made preoperatively. The male to female ratio is usually reported as approximately 5:1.[117,118] However, Bade and colleagues reported a male to female ratio of 25:1, which may reflect the higher number of injuries from stab wounds seen in a South African population.[119] Most series report a median age of approximately 30 years,[114,117,119] and there are many reports in children.

Classification of biliary injury

The gallbladder is the most frequently injured part of the extrahepatic biliary tract. The largest reported series of extrahepatic biliary tract injuries consists of 53 patients, of whom 45 (85%) sustained injury to the gallbladder and 8 (15%) had an injury to the bile duct.[119] Kitahama and colleagues reported the gallbladder to be involved in 32 (80%) of 40 patients, while ductal injury occurred in 12 (30%), some patients having multiple injuries.[117]

Injury to the gallbladder resulting from blunt trauma can be classified as either contusion, avulsion or perforation. In addition to these three main types of injury, Penn added traumatic cholecystitis as a pathological entity.[112] The most common type of gallbladder injury is perforation. Avulsion of the gallbladder may refer to the organ being partially or completely torn from the liver bed, while still attached to the bile duct, or it may signify complete separation from all attachments with the organ lying free in the abdomen. Contusion is probably under-reported, as it will be recognised only if laparotomy is performed. The natural course of an untreated gallbladder contusion is not known, although it is likely that the majority resolve without further complication. It has been speculated that an intramural haematoma might result in necrosis of the gallbladder wall and result in a subsequent perforation. There have been a number of reports of delayed rupture of the gallbladder,[120–122] and it is plausible that unrecognised contusion of the gallbladder might lead to such a delayed presentation.

Bile duct injury is classified according to the site of injury and according to whether the transection is partial or complete. Partial duct injuries are often referred to as 'tangential' wounds. Penetrating injuries can affect any part of the extrahepatic biliary system; however, the commonest sites of injury due to blunt trauma are at the point where the common bile duct enters the pancreas and where the biliary confluence exits from the liver. These sites are at points of maximum fixation, which accounts for their propensity to injury.

Isolated injury to the extrahepatic biliary tract is very uncommon. The liver is the organ most commonly injured in association with biliary tract trauma. Liver damage occurs in approximately 80% of cases, with the duodenum, stomach, colon and pancreas being the next most frequently reported. Associated vascular injuries are relatively rare; however, inferior vena cava and portal vein injuries are more commonly reported than those to the hepatic artery, renal vessels or aorta.

Presentation and diagnosis of biliary injury

Clinical presentation of the vast majority of bile duct injuries can be divided into two broad categories. The first contains patients in whom clinical signs or associated injury lead to laparotomy with early diagnosis and surgical management (early presentation); these patients generally present with hypovolaemic shock or signs of an acute abdomen. The second category of patient has a delay (greater than 24 h) in diagnosis and definitive therapy (delayed presentation). These patients comprise over half the cases (53.2%) in a review of combined series.[123] In addition, a third category of patient, representing a very small proportion of those who sustain a bile duct injury, may present with obstructive jaundice months or even years after the initial trauma (late presentation).[118,124] In these patients, the bile duct injury is always isolated. Compromise of the blood supply to the duct may occur either at the time of the primary injury or at operation during the Pringle manoeuvre, and this may contribute to the development of a late biliary stricture.[125,126] Bourque and colleagues reported that the delay between clinical presentation and surgical intervention for isolated bile duct injury averaged 18 days, with a range from several hours to 60 days.[127] Michelassi and Ranson reported that biliary injury was not recognised at initial operation in 11 (12%) of 91 patients with extrahepatic biliary tract trauma,[123] whereas Dawson and Jurkovich reported that 41% of bile duct injuries were missed at initial laparotomy.[128]

If a non-operative course of management for abdominal trauma is adopted, suspicion of an extrahepatic bile duct injury may be raised by CT scan evidence of a central liver injury involving the porta hepatis or the head of the pancreas, the presence of fluid collections in the subhepatic space, or evidence of periportal tracking of haematoma.[30] The diagnostic procedure of choice is ERCP, and if a duct injury is identified, this may be treated by endoscopic stenting.[129]

Intraoperative recognition of biliary tract injury requires a high index of suspicion. The presence of free bile in the peritoneal cavity, or the presence of bile staining in the hepatoduodenal ligament or retroperitoneum, is a sign of injury to the extra-hepatic biliary tract. Biliary tract injury must also be suspected if there is profuse bleeding from the hepatic artery or portal vein, particularly following blunt trauma, as the bile duct is also likely to be injured.[130] Penetrating wounds near the porta hepatis require careful examination. If routine dissection does not reveal the location of the injury, fine-needle intraoperative cholangiography via the gallbladder or common bile duct may identify the site. Cystic duct cholangiography should be considered after cholecystectomy for traumatic gallbladder injury to avoid missing an associated bile duct injury.[131]

It is possible for a patient who has sustained blunt abdominal trauma to be discharged from hospital only to return days or weeks later with a combination of symptoms and signs, including jaundice, abdominal distension, nausea, vomiting, anorexia, abdominal pain, low-grade fever or weight loss – a clinical picture similar to that seen in patients with intraperitoneal bile leakage following cholecystectomy. When jaundice develops after abdominal trauma, missed extrahepatic biliary injury must be considered.

Operative management of biliary injury

Many patients with extrahepatic biliary tract injury present in shock due to associated haemorrhage, and the priority at laparotomy is to identify and control haemorrhage. The report of Dawson and colleagues demonstrates that these patients are at risk of exsanguinating on the operating table.[116] Injuries to the gallbladder are best treated by cholecystectomy. Primary repair of a clean and simple partial or complete transection of the common duct using absorbable sutures such as 4/0 polydioxanone over a T-tube inserted through a separate choledochotomy has been described. However, this type of repair is not appropriate if there is any evidence of duct contusion, loss of ductal tissue or possible injury to the hepatic artery as this may increase the risk of late development of an ischaemic stricture. In general, it is therefore safer to recommend that most injuries should be managed by fashioning a biliary-enteric anastomosis with a Roux-en-Y segment of jejunum. This is in keeping with the advice of specialists in the field of iatrogenic bile duct injury for repair by primary Roux-en-Y choledocho-jejunostomy or hepatico-jejunostomy.[132]

Outcome after biliary injury

Injuries of this nature are associated with a mortality rate of 10% from concomitant injuries.[117] Septic complications and bile leakage account for most of the early morbidity and may require operative intervention. Late morbidity after repair of a traumatic biliary tract injury is unusual; however, jaundice or episodes of ascending cholangitis suggest a stricture of the ductal system.

PANCREATIC TRAUMA

Injuries to the pancreas are uncommon, accounting for 1–4% of severe abdominal injuries and usually occurring in young men.

Mechanisms of pancreatic injury

Deceleration injury is a major mechanism of blunt pancreatic injury with the region of the junction between the head and body being at risk of transection across the vertebral column. The deep location of the pancreas means that considerable force is needed to cause an injury and this level of force may often be sufficient to damage other organs.[133]

Diagnosis of pancreatic injury

Pancreatic injury should be suspected in any patient with penetrating trauma to the trunk, particularly if the entry site is between the nipples and the iliac crest, and in any patient with blunt compression trauma of the upper abdomen.[133] In an early study, Moretz and colleagues found that there was no reliable correlation between serum amylase and pancreatic injury.[134]

In a later report, Takashima and colleagues retrospectively studied admission serum amylase values in a series of 73 patients with blunt pancreatic trauma treated in a single institution over a 16-year period.[135] Sixty-one (84%) of these patients had a raised serum amylase level. Of interest, the serum amylase level was found to be abnormal in all patients admitted more than 3 hours after trauma.

Bearing in mind the practicality that patients with pancreatic injury will simultaneously be undergoing evaluation to exclude concomitant intra-abdominal visceral injury, contrast-enhanced CT has been the investigation of choice.[136–138] Reported CT features of pancreatic injury include free intraperitoneal fluid, localised fluid in the lesser sac, retroperitoneal fluid, pancreatic oedema or swelling and changes in the peripancreatic fat.[139] The presence of fluid in the lesser sac between the pancreas and the splenic vein is reported by Lane and colleagues to be a reliable sign in blunt pancreatic injury.[139] However, Sivit and Eichelberger reported that fluid separating the pancreas and the splenic vein is rarely the only abnormal CT finding in pancreatic injury.[140] It should be borne in mind that many of these CT features are also seen in acute pancreatitis[141] (and furthermore that acute pancreatitis may occur as a result of blunt abdominal trauma).[142] There is also evidence that CT tends to underdiagnose pancreatic injury. Akhrass and colleagues evaluated the clinical course of 72 patients with pancreatic injury admitted over a 10-year period.[143] Seventeen of these patients underwent CT as part of their initial assessment and this was reported as normal in nine. Eight of these patients underwent laparotomy (principally for suspected associated splenic injury) and three were found to have pancreatic injury requiring distal pancreatectomy. Newer, non-invasive imaging modalities such as magnetic resonance pancreatography have been reported in the assessment of patients with suspected pancreatic trauma.[144] Increased sophistication with the use of this technique may allow for accurate assessment of pancreatic ductal integrity.[145]

Classification of pancreatic injury

Of the various proposed classification schemes Lucas suggested in an early report that appropriate treatment be formulated according to the type of injury.[146] This classification system divides pancreatic injuries into three groups:

- grade I – superficial contusion with minimal damage
- grade II – deep laceration or transection of the left portion of the pancreas
- grade III – injury of the pancreatic head.

A more complex system of classification taking into account the frequent coexistence of duodenal and pancreatic injuries was proposed by Frey and Wardell[147] (**Table 14.2**). The most common site of injury is the junction of the neck and body of the pancreas. The relative frequency of pancreatic injuries reported in collected reviews is represented in **Fig. 14.6**.

Initial management of pancreatic injury

In a major retrospective clinical casenote review of pancreatic trauma from six hospitals, Bradley and colleagues demonstrated a significant association between pancreas-related morbidity and injury to the main pancreatic duct.[148] Delayed intervention (due to delay in recognition of main pancreatic duct injury) was associated with high morbidity. CT was unreliable for the assessment of main pancreatic ductal integrity and an accurate assessment required ERCP.[148]

Assessment of the integrity of the main pancreatic duct is critical to the treatment of pancreatic injury. In patients with a suspected pancreatic injury (who are haemodynamically stable), ERCP is indicated to assess major duct integrity.[149] Demonstration of an intact main pancreatic duct at ERCP in a patient with suspected isolated pancreatic injury may allow for a trial of non-operative management.[150,151]

Operative management of pancreatic injury

The mainstay of treatment remains operative as pancreatic injuries are usually diagnosed at laparotomy.[152,153] The important principles at operation are to gain good access to allow thorough inspection of the gland.[154] Access to the lesser sac is best done by creating a window in the gastrocolic omentum outside the gastroepiploic arcade to allow examination of the body of the pancreas. A Kocher manoeuvre is necessary to permit palpation of the

Table 14.2 • Classification of pancreatic injury proposed by Frey and Wardell

Pancreatic injury	
Class I	Capsular damage, minor gland damage (P_1)
Class II	Body or tail pancreatic duct transection, partial or complete (P_2)
Class III	Major duct injury involving the head of the pancreas or the intrapancreatic common bile duct (P_3)
Duodenal injury	
Class I	Contusion, haematoma or partial-thickness injury (D_1)
Class II	Full-thickness duodenal injury (D_2)
Class III	Full-thickness injury with >75% circumference injury or full-thickness duodenal injury with injury to the extrahepatic common bile duct (D_3)
Combined pancreatico-duodenal injuries	
Type I	P_1D_1, P_2D_1, or D_2P_1
Type II	D_2P_2
Type III	D_3P_{1-2} or P_3D_{1-2}
Type IV	D_3P_3

Reproduced with permission from Frey CF, Wardell JW. Injuries to the pancreas. In Trede M, Carter DC (eds) Surgery of the pancreas. Edinburgh: Churchill Livingstone, 1993.

head of the pancreas between thumb and fingers. A thorough inspection of the base of the transverse mesocolon is also undertaken. Injury to the pancreas is suspected if retroperitoneal haemorrhage can be seen through the base of the mesocolon or the lesser omentum. Absence of any sign of haemorrhage over the pancreas and duodenum makes injury unlikely.

Experience of patients with pancreatic injury from Durban led to the recommendation for operative treatment of patients with penetrating or gunshot injury and signs of peritoneal irritation.[155] In this large series of 152 patients with pancreatic trauma presenting during a 5-year period, 63 patients had been shot, 66 stabbed and 23 had blunt trauma. The mainstay of treatment was exploratory laparotomy followed by drainage of the pancreatic injury site. Large-bore soft silastic drains were used

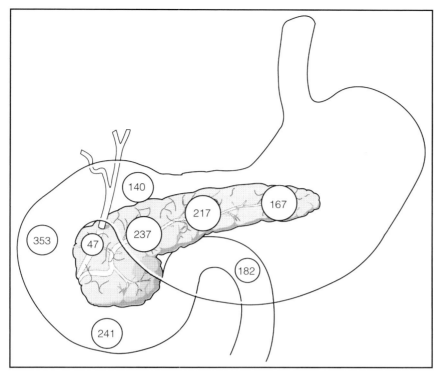

Figure 14.6 • Distribution of pancreatic injuries in the world literature. Note the preponderance of injuries in the junctional area of the neck of the gland. Reproduced with permission from Trede M, Carter DC (eds) Surgery of the pancreas. Edinburgh: Churchill Livingstone, 1993.

to minimise the risk of drain erosion into a major vessel. The mortality rates in these groups were 8% after gunshot injury, 2% after stab wounds and 10% after blunt trauma. The majority of these deaths were attributed to damage of other organs. The proportions of patients developing pancreatic fistulas in the three groups were 14%, 9% and 13%, respectively. The authors concluded that 'conservative' surgical drainage (avoiding pancreatic resection) was justified after pancreatic injury. This large contemporary report lends weight to the treatment plan proposed by Lucas for grade I injuries, which consists of passive closed drainage using a wide-bore drain.

Simplified management guidelines based on the treatment protocols developed during the treatment of 124 pancreatic injuries at the University of Tennessee[152] also advocate simple drainage alone for proximal pancreatic injuries. There were 37 (30%) patients with proximal injuries. The 'pancreas-related' morbidity was 11% – principally

the sequelae of pancreatic fistulas. Of 87 distal pancreatic injuries, the integrity of the main pancreatic duct was not established in 54 (62%). Patients thought to have a high probability of duct transection were treated by distal pancreatectomy. A concern with simple drainage for injuries in the head of the pancreas is persistent pancreatic fistula, and thus a surgical alternative is to drain the head of the pancreas into a Roux-en-Y limb of jejunum using the type of modified Peustow procedure described by Partington and Rochelle.[156]

Moncure and Goins described their experience over a 6-year period with a consecutive series of 44 patients with pancreatic injury,[157] of which penetrating abdominal trauma accounted for the majority of cases. Class I pancreatic injuries occurred in 55% of patients and the majority were managed by simple drainage. Grade II injuries occurred in 18% and grade III injuries in 21%. Coexistent duodenal injuries were treated by primary closure in 21%, and more complex duodenal exclusion techniques were used in 20%. Their most frequent complications were intra-abdominal abscess (31%) and pancreatic fistulas (16%). Craig and colleagues report similar results in a series of 13 patients with blunt pancreatic trauma treated over a 10-year period.[158]

Severe Lucas grade III injuries involving the head of the pancreas, duodenum and distal bile duct represent a major challenge, but fortunately are relatively rare, occurring in approximately 5% of all duodenal injuries.[159] The principles of treatment are to ensure that haemorrhage from concomitant injuries is dealt with first, as this is likely to be the major source of mortality.[160] Similarly a prolonged operative procedure should be avoided in a potentially unstable patient and the involvement of an experienced pancreatic surgeon is desirable. Duodenal injuries can be closed primarily or drained into a Roux loop. Bile duct injuries may be repaired primarily over a T-tube or drained into a Roux limb of jejunum. A gastric serosal patch may be used to protect a pancreatic stump closure line.[161] The large variety of operative procedures described for these complex injuries suggests that treatment has to be tailored to the individual injury complex and that no single procedure is likely to be uniformly applicable or successful. Very rarely, pancreatico-duodenectomy may be required for complex, severe pancreatic injuries with concomitant duodenal and distal bile duct injuries.[162,163] Clearly, this sort of resection should not be undertaken lightly in an individual suffering from shock and its sequelae, but rather like liver transplantation for trauma it is useful to have an index of awareness of the available therapeutic options.

Complications of pancreatic injury

Pancreas-specific complications include pancreatic abscess, pancreatic fistula[164] and pseudocyst. The principles underlying treatment are similar to those for treating these complications when they arise as a result of pancreatitis or pancreatic surgery. The Cape Town group reported that of a series of 64 patients with pancreatic trauma, pseudocysts developed in 15 patients (23%).[165] Endoscopic pancreatography demonstrated duct injury in eight. Patients with pseudocysts related to distal duct

injury were treated successfully by percutaneous aspiration. Three patients with duct injuries in the neck/body region underwent distal pancreatectomy. Pseudocysts related to ductal injury in the head of the pancreas were drained internally by Roux-en-Y cyst-jejunostomy. They concluded that traumatic pancreatic pseudocysts associated with a peripheral duct injury may resolve spontaneously whereas those associated with injuries to the proximal duct require surgical intervention. Treatment of a post-traumatic pseudocyst is based on the principles for treatment of this complication after inflammation. Whilst there is increasing evidence that endoscopic internal drainage is successful in the management of pseudocysts complicating chronic pancreatitis[166] this approach is less likely to be successful in managing acute postinflammatory pseudocysts. The management of the post-traumatic pseudocyst will depend on delay to presentation, presence of ongoing ductal leak, site of leak and presence of debris within the pseudocyst cavity.

The incidence of pancreatic fistula after surgery for trauma is dependent on the type of procedure, with some evidence that the fistula rate is higher after drainage procedures than after resection.[167] Inflammation of the pancreas after trauma behaves in much the same way as acute biliary or acute alcohol-induced pancreatitis with the possible exception that there is a higher incidence of development of local complications such as pseudocyst – possibly relating to the nature of duct disruption in trauma.[168] In Holland's series, 8 of 14 (57%) children with acute post-traumatic pancreatitis developed pseudocysts.

CONCLUSION

The contemporary management of patients with suspected liver, biliary or pancreatic injury involves detailed clinical assessment and resuscitation followed, in haemodynamically stable patients, by imaging investigations. If surgical intervention is required, the mainstay of treatment is to control haemorrhage. In European healthcare systems, the optimum care of the patient may consist of packing followed by transfer to a regional hepato-pancreatico-biliary unit. A paper by Hoyt and colleagues examining preventable causes of death in 72 151 admissions with abdominal trauma to

North American level I trauma centres identified abdominal injury as the cause of death in 287, with liver injury being responsible for 92.[169] Delays in packing were highlighted as a preventable cause of death, as was a need for better understanding of the endpoints to be achieved by packing. The conclusion of this large survey was that the management of liver injury remains a major technical challenge.

Key points

- Management of patients with suspected liver, biliary or pancreatic injury involves detailed clinical assessment and resuscitation.
- Haemodynamic instability resistant to fluid resuscitation associated with clinical signs of peritonism is an indication for immediate laparotomy.
- Patients who are haemodynamically stable or who respond to initial fluid resuscitation should undergo further imaging investigations.
- Laparotomy is required for patients with an abdominal gunshot wound.

Liver trauma
- Non-operative management of liver trauma is now a well-established treatment option.
- Significant liver haemorrhage can initially be controlled at operation by manual compression of the liver parenchyma, a Pringle manoeuvre or by compression of the aorta above the coeliac trunk.
- Perihepatic packing is a highly effective technique to control bleeding from the liver or juxtahepatic veins.
- Resectional debridement of non-viable hepatic parenchyma may be undertaken, but anatomical resection is rarely indicated.
- Other techniques to control haemorrhage include suture ligation of vessels, mesh wrapping of a liver lobe and selective hepatic arterial ligation.
- Postoperative complications include bile leakage or sepsis, and may require radiological, endoscopic or surgical intervention.

Extrahepatic biliary tract trauma
- This uncommon injury is more likely to be due to penetrating rather than blunt abdominal trauma.
- It is rarely diagnosed before operation and is usually recognised incidentally at laparotomy.
- Concomitant vascular injury of the portal vein or hepatic artery is rare.
- ERCP may demonstrate bile leakage and allow therapeutic insertion of a biliary stent.
- Definitive operative intervention for gallbladder trauma is cholecystectomy.
- Roux-en-Y hepatico-jejunostomy is the operation of choice for most injuries to the bile duct.

Pancreatic trauma
- Is most commonly diagnosed by CT; however, ERCP may be undertaken to assess pancreatic duct integrity and may allow therapeutic stenting if leakage of contrast is identified.
- Exploratory laparotomy and drainage of the pancreatic region remains the mainstay of surgical treatment.
- Selected injuries may be managed by either distal pancreatectomy, pancreatico-duodenectomy, or pancreatico-jejunostomy Roux-en-Y.

REFERENCES

1. Feliciano DV. Surgery for liver trauma. Surg Clin North Am 1989; 69:273–84.

2. Cox EF. Blunt abdominal trauma. A five year analysis of 870 patients requiring celiotomy. Ann Surg 1984; 199:467–74.

3. Beal SL. Fatal hepatic haemorrhage: an unresolved problem in the management of complex liver injuries. J Trauma 1990; 30:163–9.

4. John TG, Greig JD, Johnstone AJ et al. Liver trauma: a 10-year experience. Br J Surg 1992; 79:1352–6.

5. Watson CJ, Calne RY, Padhani AR et al. Surgical restraint in the management of liver trauma. Br J Surg 1991; 78:1071–5.

6. Talving P, Beckman M, Haggmark T et al. Epidemiology of liver injuries. Scand J Surg 2003; 92:192–4.

7. Krige JE, Bornman PC, Terblanche J. Liver trauma in 446 patients. S Afr J Surg 1997; 35:10–15.

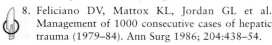

8. Feliciano DV, Mattox KL, Jordan GL et al. Management of 1000 consecutive cases of hepatic trauma (1979–84). Ann Surg 1986; 204:438–54.

    Large US series highlighting the injury pattern and management of liver trauma.

9. Fabian TC, Croce MA, Stanford GG et al. Factors affecting morbidity following hepatic trauma. A prospective analysis of 482 injuries. Ann Surg 1991; 213:540–7.

10. Parks RW, Chrysos E, Diamond T. Management of liver trauma. Br J Surg 1999; 86:1121–35.

11. Sherlock DJ, Bismuth H. Secondary surgery for liver trauma. Br J Surg 1991; 78:1313–17.

12. Donovan AJ, Berne TV. Liver and bile duct injury. In: Blumgart LH (ed.) Surgery of the liver and biliary tract, 2nd edn. Edinburgh: Churchill Livingstone, 1994; pp. 1221–42.

13. Moore EE, Shackford SR, Pachter HL et al. Organ injury scaling: spleen, liver and kidney. J Trauma 1989; 29:1664–6.

14. Moore EE, Cogbill TH, Jurkovich GJ et al. Organ injury scaling: spleen and liver (1994 revision). J Trauma 1995; 38:323–4.

15. Schweizer W, Tanner S, Baer HU et al. Management of traumatic liver injuries. Br J Surg 1993; 80:86–8.

16. American College of Surgeons Committee on Trauma. Advanced trauma life support student manual, 5th edn. Chicago: American College of Surgeons, 1995.

17. Bickell WH, Wall MJ Jr, Pepe PE et al. Immediate versus delayed fluid resuscitation for hypotensive patients with penetrating torso injuries. N Engl J Med 1994; 331:1105–9.

Aggressive fluid replacement may be associated with an adverse outcome in abdominal trauma.

18. Scollay JM, Beard D, Smith R et al. Eleven years of liver trauma: the Scottish experience. Br J Surg 2004; 91(Suppl. 1):24.

    Large population-based study describing liver injury management in Scotland.

19. Attard AR, Corlett MJ, Kidner NJ et al. Safety of early pain relief for acute abdominal pain. Br Med J 1992; 305:554–6.

20. Reed RL II, Merrell RC, Meyers WC et al. Continuing evolution in the approach to severe liver trauma. Ann Surg 1992; 216:524–38.

21. Rozycki GS, Ochsner MG, Feliciano DV et al. Early detection of hemoperitoneum by ultrasound examination of the right upper quadrant: a multi-center study. J Trauma 1998; 45:878–83.

22. McKenney MG, Martin L, Lentz K et al. 1000 consecutive ultrasounds for blunt abdominal trauma. J Trauma 1996; 40:607–12.

    Two studies supporting the use of abdominal ultra-sonography in the initial assessment of suspected liver injury.

23. Richards JR, McGahan JP, Simpson JL et al. Bowel and mesenteric injury: evaluation with abdominal US. Radiology 1999; 211:399–403.

24. Adam A, Roddie ME. Computed tomography of the liver and biliary tract. In: Blumgart LH (ed.) Surgery of the liver and biliary tract, 2nd edn. Edinburgh: Churchill Livingstone, 1994; pp. 243–70.

25. Safi F, Weiner S, Poch B et al. Surgical management of liver rupture. Chirurgie 1999; 70:253–8.

26. Cachecho R, Clas D, Gersin K et al. Evolution in the management of the complex liver injury at a Level I trauma center. J Trauma 1998; 45:79–82.

27. Strong RW. The management of blunt liver injuries. Aust NZ J Surg 1999; 69:609–16.

28. Toombs BD, Sandler CM, Rauschkolb EN et al. Assessment of hepatic injuries with computed tomography. J Comput Assist Tomogr 1982; 6:72–5.

29. Fang JF, Chen RJ, Wong YC et al. Pooling of contrast material on computed tomography mandates aggressive management of blunt hepatic injury. Am J Surg 1998; 176:315–19.

30. Yokota J, Sugimoto T. Clinical significance of periportal tracking on computed tomographic scan in patients with blunt liver trauma. Am J Surg 1994; 168:247–50.

31. Shankar KR, Lloyd DA, Kitteringham L et al. Oral contrast with computed tomography in the evaluation of blunt abdominal trauma in children. Br J Surg 1999; 86:1073–7.

32. Croce MA, Fabian TC, Kudsk KA et al. AAST organ injury scale: correlation of CT graded liver injuries and operative findings. J Trauma 1991; 31:806–12.

    Study highlighting the tendency of CT scanning to overdiagnose the severity of liver injury.

33. Goodman DA, Tiruchelvam V, Tabb DR et al. 3D CT reconstruction in the surgical management of hepatic injuries. Ann R Coll Surg Engl 1995; 77:7–11.

34. Dinkel HP, Moll R, Gassel HJ et al. Helical CT cholangiography for the detection and localisation of bile duct leakage. Am J Roentgenol 1999; 173:613–17.

35. Vock P. Magnetic resonance imaging. In: Blumgart LH (ed.) Surgery of the liver and biliary tract, 2nd edn. Edinburgh: Churchill Livingstone, 1994; pp. 271–82.

36. Hagiwara A, Yukioka T, Ohta S et al. Non-surgical management of patients with blunt hepatic injury: efficacy of transcatheter arterial embolization. Am J Roentgenol 1997; 169:1151–6.

37. Sugimoto K, Asari Y, Sakaguchi T et al. Endoscopic retrograde cholangiography in the non-surgical management of blunt liver injury. J Trauma 1993; 35:192–9.

38. Carrillo EH, Spain DA, Wohltmann CD et al. Interventional techniques are useful adjuncts in the non-operative management of hepatic injuries. J Trauma 1999; 46:619–22.

39. Sosa JL, Markley M, Sleeman D et al. Laparoscopy in abdominal gunshot wounds. Surg Laparosc Endosc 1993; 3:417–19.

40. Sosa JL, Arrillaga A, Puente I et al. Laparoscopy in 121 consecutive patients with abdominal gunshot wounds. J Trauma 1995; 208:62–6.

41. Hallfeldt KK, Trupka AW, Erhard J et al. Emergency laparoscopy for abdominal stab wounds. Surg Endosc 1998; 12:907–10.

42. Chen RJ, Fang JF, Lin BC et al. Selective application of laparoscopy and fibrin glue in the failure of non-operative management of blunt hepatic trauma. J Trauma 1998; 44:691–5.

43. Richie JP, Fonkalsrud EW. Subcapsular haematoma of the liver: non-operative management. Arch Surg 1972; 104:780–4.

44. White P, Cleveland RJ. The surgical management of liver trauma. Arch Surg 1972; 104:785–6.

45. Hammond JC, Canal DF, Broadie TA. Non-operative management of adult blunt hepatic trauma in a municipal trauma centre. Am Surg 1992; 58:551–5.

46. Pachter HL, Feliciano DV. Complex hepatic injuries. Surg Clin North Am 1996; 76:763–82.

47. Brammer RD, Bramhall SR, Mirza DF et al. A 10-year experience of complex liver trauma. Br J Surg 2002; 89:1532–7.

48. Coughlin PA, Stringer MD, Lodge JP et al. Management of blunt liver trauma in a tertiary referral centre. Br J Surg 2004; 91:317–21.

49. Meyer AA, Crass RA, Lim RC et al. Selective non-operative management of blunt liver injury using computed tomography. Arch Surg 1985; 120:781–4.

50. Farnell MB, Spencer MP, Thompson E et al. Non-operative management of blunt hepatic trauma in adults. Surgery 1988; 104:748–56.

51. Feliciano DV. Continuing evolution in the approach to severe liver trauma. Ann Surg 1992; 216:521–3.

52. Boone DC, Federle M, Billiar TR et al. Evolution of management of major hepatic trauma: identification of patterns of injury. J Trauma 1995; 39:344–50.

53. Durham RM, Buckley J, Keegan M et al. Management of blunt hepatic injuries. Am J Surg 1992; 164:477–81.

54. Sherman HF, Savage BA, Jones LM et al. Non-operative management of blunt hepatic injuries: safe at any grade? J Trauma 1994; 37:616–21.

55. Carrillo EH, Platz A, Miller FB et al. Non-operative management of blunt hepatic trauma. Br J Surg 1998; 85:461–8.

56. Croce MA, Fabian TC, Menke PG et al. Non-operative management of blunt hepatic trauma is the treatment of choice for hemodynamically stable patients. Results of a prospective trial. Ann Surg 1995; 221:744–53.

    This trial provides clear evidence to support a non-operative approach to management of liver injuries in haemodynamically stable patients.

57. Pachter HL, Hofstetter SR. The current status of nonoperative management of adult blunt hepatic injuries. Am J Surg 1995; 169:442–54.

58. Kudson MM, Lim RC Jr, Oakes DD et al. Non-operative management of blunt liver injuries in adults: the need for continued surveillance. J Trauma 1990; 30:1494–500.

59. Menegaux F, Langlois P, Chigot JP. Severe blunt trauma of the liver: study of mortality factors. J Trauma 1993; 35:865–9.

60. Clark DE, Cobean RA, Radke FR et al. Management of major hepatic trauma involving inter-hospital transfer. Am Surg 1994; 60:881–5.

61. Coburn MC, Pfeifer J, DeLuca FG. Non-operative management of splenic and hepatic trauma in the multiply injured pediatric and adolescent patient. Arch Surg 1995; 130:332–8.

62. Goff CD, Gilbert CM. Non-operative management of blunt hepatic trauma. Am Surg 1995; 61:66–8.

63. Dominguez Fernandez E, Aufmkolk M, Schmidt U et al. Outcome and management of blunt liver injuries in blunt trauma patients. Langenbecks Arch Surg 1999; 384:453–60.

64. Gross M, Lynch F, Canty T Sr et al. Management of pediatric liver injuries: a 13-year experience at a pediatric trauma centre. J Pediatr Surg 1999; 34:811–16.

65. Nance ML, Peden GW, Shapiro MB et al. Solid viscus injury predicts major hollow viscus injury in blunt abdominal trauma. J Trauma 1999; 43:618–22.

66. Shilyansky J, Navarro O, Superina RA et al. Delayed hemorrhage after non-operative management of blunt hepatic trauma in children: a rare but significant event. J Pediatr Surg 1999; 34:60–4.

67. Meredith JW, Young JS, Bowling J et al. Non-operative management of blunt liver trauma: the exception or the rule? J Trauma 1994; 36:529–34.

68. Ciraulo DL, Nikkanen HE, Palter M et al. Clinical analysis of the utility of repeat computed tomographic scan before discharge in blunt hepatic injury. J Trauma 1996; 41:821–4.

69. Demetriades D, Karaiskakis M, Alo K et al. Role of postoperative computed tomography in patients with severe liver injury. Br J Surg 2003; 90:1398–1400.

70. Cogbill TH, Moore EE, Jurkovich GJ et al. Severe hepatic trauma: a multicenter experience with 1335 liver injuries. J Trauma 1988; 28:1433–8.

71. Marr JDF, Krige JEJ, Terblanche J. Analysis of 153 gunshot wounds of the liver. Br J Surg 2000; 87:1030–4.

72. Demetriades D, Gomez H, Chahwan S et al. Gunshot injuries to the liver: the role of selective non-operative management. J Am Coll Surg 1999; 188:343–8.

73. Calne RY, McMaster P, Pentlon BD. The treatment of major liver trauma by primary packing with transfer of the patient for definitive treatment. Br J Surg 1978; 66:338–9.

74. Howdieshell TR, Purvis J, Bates WB et al. Biloma and biliary fistula following hepatorraphy for liver trauma: incidence, natural history and management. Am Surg 1995; 61:165–8.

75. Elias D, Desruennes E, Lasser P. Prolonged intermittent clamping of the portal triad during hepatectomy. Br J Surg 1991; 78:42–4.

76. Launois B, Jamieson GG. General principles of liver surgery. In: Launois B, Jamieson GG (eds) Modern operative techniques in liver surgery. Edinburgh: Churchill Livingstone, 1993; pp. 23–37.

77. Bismuth H, Castaing D, Garden OJ. Major hepatic resection under total vascular exclusion. Ann Surg 1989; 210:13–19.

78. Cue JI, Cryer HG, Miller FB et al. Packing and planned reexploration for hepatic and retroperitoneal hemorrhage: critical refinements of a useful technique. J Trauma 1990; 30:1007–13.

79. Krige JEJ, Bornman PC, Terblanche J. Therapeutic perihepatic packing in complex liver trauma. Br J Surg 1992; 79:43–6.
    Study reporting the use of perihepatic packing in 22 patients with hepatic trauma.

80. Ochsner MG, Jaffin JH, Golocovsky M et al. Major hepatic trauma. Surg Clin North Am 1993; 73:323–4.

81. Gadzijev EM, Stanisavljevic D, Mimica Z et al. Can we evaluate the pressure of perihepatic packing? Results of a study on dogs. Injury 1999; 30:35–41.

82. Watson CJE, Calne RY, Padhani AR et al. Surgical restraint in the management of liver trauma. Br J Surg 1991; 78:1071–5.

83. Postema RR, Kate JW, Terpstra OT. Less hepatic tissue necrosis after argon beam coagulator than after conventional electrocoagulation. Surg Gynecol Obstet 1993; 176:177–80.

84. Kram HB, Reuben BI, Fleming AW. Use of fibrin glue in hepatic trauma. J Trauma 1988; 28:1195–201.

85. Feliciano DV, Pachter HL. Trauma to the liver vasculature, aneurysm and arteriovenous fistula. In: Blumgart LH (ed.) Surgery of the liver and biliary tract, 2nd edn. Edinburgh: Churchill Livingstone, 1994; pp. 1243–57.

86. Holcomb JB, Pusateri AE, Harris RA et al. Effect of dry fibrin sealant dressings versus gauze packing on blood loss in grade V liver injuries in resuscitated swine. J Trauma 1999; 46:49–57.

87. Berguer R, Staerkel RL, Moore EE et al. Warning: fatal reaction to the use of fibrin glue in deep hepatic wounds. Case reports. J Trauma 1991; 31:408–11.

88. Wood CB, Capperauld I, Blumgart LH. Bioplast fibrin buttons for liver biopsy and partial hepatic resection. Ann R Coll Surg Engl 1976; 58:401–4.

89. Mays ET. The hazards of suturing certain wounds of the liver. Surg Gynecol Obstet 1976; 143:201–4.

90. Stone HH, Lamb JM. Use of pedicled omentum as an autogenous pack for control of haemorrhage in major injuries of the liver. Surg Gynecol Obstet 1975; 141:92–4.

91. Stevens SL, Maull KI, Enderson BL et al. Total mesh wrapping for parenchymal liver injuries: a combined experimental and clinical study. J Trauma 1991; 31:1103–9.

92. Jacobson LE, Kirton OC, Gomez GA. The use of an absorbable mesh wrap in the management of major liver injuries. Surgery 1992; 111:455–61.

93. Brunet C, Sielezneff I, Thomas P et al. Treatment of hepatic trauma with perihepatic mesh: 35 cases. J Trauma 1994; 37:200–4.

94. Reed RL, Merrell RC, Meyers WC et al. Continuing evolution in the approach to severe liver trauma. Ann Surg 1992; 216:524–38.

95. Cox EF, Flancbaum L, Dauterieve AH et al. Blunt trauma to the liver. Analysis of management and mortality in 323 consecutive patients. Ann Surg 1988; 207:126–34.

Large study advocating the use of simple suture techniques and resectional debridement to control haemorrhage after liver injury.

96. Strong RW, Lynch SV, Wall DR et al. Anatomic resection for severe liver trauma. Surgery 1998; 123:251–7.

Large single-centre experience supporting the limited use of hepatic resection for hepatic trauma.

97. Mays ET. Hepatic trauma. Curr Probl Surg 1976; 13:6–73.

98. Flint LM, Polk HC Jr. Selective hepatic artery ligation: limitations and failures. J Trauma 1979; 19:319–23.

99. Couinaud C. Surgical anatomy of the liver revisited. Tulle: L'Imprimerie Maugein et Cie., Paris, 1989.

100. Ricker DL, Morton JR, Okies JE et al. Surgical management of injuries to the vena cava: changing patterns of injury and newer techniques of repair. J Trauma 1971; 11:725–35.

101. Chen RJ, Fang JF, Lin BC et al. Surgical management of juxtahepatic venous injuries in blunt hepatic trauma. J Trauma 1995; 38:886–90.

102. Ringe B, Pichlmayr R. Total hepatectomy and liver transplantation: a life-saving procedure in patients with severe hepatic trauma. Br J Surg 1995; 82:837–9.

103. Lin PJ, Jeng LB, Chen RJ et al. Femoro-arterial bypass using Gott shunt in liver transplantation following severe hepatic trauma. Int Surg 1993; 78:295–7.

104. Ginzburg E, Shatz D, Lynn M et al. The role of liver transplantation in the subacute trauma patient. Am Surg 1998; 64:363–4.

105. Hellstrom G. The activity of glutamic-oxaloacetic and glutamic-pyruvic transaminases (GOT and GPT), ornithine-carbamoyl transferase (OCT) and alkaline phosphatase (AP) in serum in closed liver injury. An experimental study. Acta Chir Scand 1966; 131:476–84.

106. Wagner WW, Lundell CJ, Donovan AJ. Percutaneous angiographic embolisation for hepatic arterial hemorrhage. Arch Surg 1985; 120:1241–9.

107. Maurel J, Aouad K, Martel B et al. Post-traumatic hemobilia. How to treat? Ann Chir 1994; 48:572–5.

108. Oishi AJ, Nagorney DM, Cherry KJ. Portal hypertension, variceal bleeding and high output cardiac failure secondary to an intrahepatic arterioportal fistula. HPB Surg 1993; 7:53–9.

109. McInnis WD, Richardson JD, Aust JB. Hepatic trauma: pitfalls in management. Arch Surg 1977; 112:157–61.

110. Bender JS, Geller ER, Wilson RF. Intra-abdominal sepsis following liver trauma. J Trauma 1989; 29:1140–5.

111. Parks RW, Diamond T. Non-surgical trauma to the extrahepatic biliary tract. Br J Surg 1995; 82:1303–10.

112. Penn I. Injuries of the gallbladder. Br J Surg 1962; 49:636–41.

113. Soderstrom CA, Maekawa K, DuPriest RW Jr et al. Gallbladder injuries resulting from blunt abdominal trauma: an experience and review. Ann Surg 1981; 193:60–6.

114. Posner MC, Moore EE. Extrahepatic biliary tract injury: operative management plan. J Trauma 1985; 25:833–7.

115. Burgess P, Fulton RL. Gall bladder and extrahepatic biliary duct injury following abdominal trauma. Injury 1992; 23:413–14.

116. Dawson DL, Johansen KH, Jurkovich GJ. Injuries to the portal triad. Am J Surg 1991; 161:545–51.

117. Kitahama A, Elliott LF, Overby JL et al. The extrahepatic biliary tract injury: perspective in diagnosis and treatment. Ann Surg 1982; 196:536–40.

118. Busuttil RW, Kitahama A, Cerise E et al. Management of blunt and penetrating injuries to the porta hepatis. Ann Surg 1980; 191:641–8.

119. Bade PG, Thomson SR, Hirshberg A et al. Surgical options in traumatic injury to the extrahepatic biliary tract. Br J Surg 1989; 76:256–8.

120. Coulter DF. Traumatic delayed rupture of the gallbladder in a child aged 9. BMJ 1948; I:198.

121. Brickley HD, Kaplan A, Freeark RJ et al. Immediate and delayed rupture of the extrahepatic biliary tract following blunt abdominal trauma. Am J Surg 1960; 100:107–9.

122. Fielding JWL, Strachan CJL. Jaundice as a sign of delayed gallbladder perforation following blunt abdominal trauma. Injury 1975; 7:66–7.

123. Michelassi F, Ranson JHC. Bile duct disruption by blunt trauma. J Trauma 1985; 25:454–7.

124. Shorthouse AJ, Singh MP, Treasure T et al. Isolated complete transection of the common bile duct by blunt abdominal trauma. Br J Surg 1978; 65:543–5.

125. Pachter HL, Spencer FC, Hofstetter SR et al. Significant trends in the management of hepatic trauma: experience with 411 injuries. Ann Surg 1992; 215:492–502.

126. Gupta N, Solomon H, Fairchild R et al. Management and outcome of patients with combined bile duct and hepatic artery injuries. Arch Surg 1998; 133:176–81.

127. Bourque MD, Spigland N, Bensoussan AL et al. Isolated complete transection of the common bile duct due to blunt trauma in a child, and review of the literature. J Paediatr Surg 1989; 24:1068–70.

128. Dawson DL, Jurkovich GJ. Hepatic duct disruption from blunt abdominal trauma: case report and literature review. J Trauma 1991; 31:1698–702.

129. Jenkins MA, Ponsky JL. Endoscopic retrograde cholangiopancreatography and endobiliary stenting in the treatment of biliary injury resulting from liver trauma. Surg Laparosc Endosc 1995; 5:118–20.

130. Dawson DL, Johansen KH, Jurkovich GJ. Injuries to the portal triad. Am J Surg 1991; 161:545–51.

131. McFadden PM, Tanner G, Kitahama A. Traumatic hepatic duct injury: a new approach to surgical management. Am J Surg 1980; 139:268–71.

132. Bismuth H, Franco D, Corlette MB. Long-term results of Roux-en-Y hepaticojejunostomy. Surg Gynecol Obstet 1978; 146:161–7.

133. Johnson CD. Pancreatic trauma. Br J Surg 1995; 82:1153–4.

134. Moretz JA III, Campbell DP, Parker DE et al. Significance of serum amylase in evaluating pancreatic trauma. Am J Surg 1975; 130:739–41.

135. Takashima T, Sugimoto K, Hirata M et al. Serum amylase level on admission in the diagnosis of blunt injury to the pancreas: its significance and limitations. Ann Surg 1997; 226:70–6.

Report of 73 patients with blunt pancreatic trauma indicating that an early elevated serum amylase is indicative of pancreatic injury.

136. Procacci C, Graziani R, Bicego E et al. Blunt pancreatic trauma. Role of CT. Acta Radiol 1997; 38:543–9.

137. Asensio JA, Demetriades D, Hanpeter DE et al. Management of pancreatic injuries. Curr Probl Surg 1999; 36:325–419.

138. Patel SV, Spencer JA, el-Hasani S et al. Imaging of pancreatic trauma. Br J Radiol 1998; 71:985–90.

Studies providing evidence for the value of CT imaging in pancreatic trauma.

139. Lane MJ, Mindelzun RE, Sandhu JS. CT diagnosis of blunt pancreatic trauma: importance of detecting fluid between the pancreas and the splenic vein. Am J Roentgenol 1994; 163:833–5.

140. Sivit CJ, Eichelberger MR. CT diagnosis of pancreatic injury in children: significance of fluid separating the splenic vein and the pancreas. Am J Roentgenol 1995; 165:921–4.

141. Powell JJ, Singh KK, Storey S et al. Prognostic value of early contrast-enhanced computed tomography in acute pancreatitis. Proceedings of the 3rd world congress of the IHPBA 1999; pp. 336–7.

142. McKay CJ, Evans S, Sinclair M et al. High early mortality rate from acute pancreatitis in Scotland, 1984–95. Br J Surg 1999; 86:1302–5.

143. Akhrass R, Kim K, Brandt C. Computed tomography: an unreliable indicator of pancreatic trauma. Am Surg 1996; 62:647–51.

144. Nirula R, Velmahos GC, Demetriades D. Magnetic resonance cholangiopancreatography in pancreatic trauma: a new diagnostic modality? J Trauma 1999; 47:585–7.

145. Takehara Y. MR pancreatography: technique and applications. Top Magn Reson Imaging 1996; 8:290–301.

146. Lucas CE. Diagnosis and treatment of pancreatic and duodenal injury. Surg Clin North Am 1977; 57:49–65.

147. Frey CF, Wardell JW. Injuries to the pancreas. In: Trede M, Carter DC (eds) Surgery of the pancreas. Edinburgh: Churchill Livingstone, 1993; pp. 565–89.

148. Bradley E, Young PR Jr, Chang MC et al. Diagnosis and initial management of pancreatic trauma: guidelines from a multi-institutional review. Ann Surg 1998; 227:861–9.

149. Hayward SR, Lucas CE, Sugawa C et al. Emergent endoscopic retrograde cholangiopancreatography: a highly specific test for acute pancreatic trauma. Arch Surg 1989; 124:745–6.

150. Firstenberg MS, Volsko TA, Sivit C et al. Selective management of paediatric pancreatic injuries. J Pediatr Surg 1999; 34:1142–7.

151. Keller MS, Stafford PW, Vane DW. Conservative management of pancreatic trauma in children. J Trauma 1997; 42:1097–110.

Studies reporting the utility of ERCP in the diagnosis and mangement of pancreatic injuries.

152. Patton JH Jr, Lyden SP, Croce MA et al. Pancreatic trauma: a simplified management guideline. J Trauma 1997; 43:234–9.

Large single-centre study describing useful management guidelines for pancreatic injury.

153. Akhrass R, Jaffe MB, Brandt CP et al. Pancreatic trauma: a ten-year multi-institutional experience. Am Surg 1997; 63:598–604.

154. Asensio JA, Demetriades D, Berne JD et al. A unified approach to the surgical exposure of pancreatic and duodenal injuries. Am J Surg 1997; 174:54–60.

155. Madiba TE, Mokoena TR. Favourable prognosis after surgical drainage of gunshot, stab or blunt trauma of the pancreas. Br J Surg 1995; 82:1236–9.

156. Partington PF, Rochelle REL. Modified Puestow procedure for retrograde drainage of the pancreatic duct. Ann Surg 1960; 152:1037–43.

157. Moncure M, Goins WA. Challenges in the management of pancreatic and duodenal injuries. JAMA 1993; 85:767–72.

158. Craig MH, Talton DS, Hauser CJ et al. Pancreatic injuries from blunt trauma. Am Surg 1995; 61:125–8.

159. Feliciano DV, Martin TD, Cruse PA et al. Management of combined pancreatoduodenal injuries. Ann Surg 1987; 205:673–80.

160. Martin TD, Feliciano DV, Mattox KL et al. Severe duodenal injuries. Treatment with pyloric exclusion and gastrojejunostomy. Arch Surg 1983; 118:631–5.

161. Kluger Y, Alfici R, Abbley B et al. Gastric serosal patch in distal pancreatectomy for injury: a neglected technique. Injury 1997; 28:127–9.

162. Verma GR, Wig JD. Pancreatoduodenectomy in abdominal trauma: a viable alternative. Indian J Gastroenterol 1997; 16:26–7.

163. Feliciano DV, Bitondo CG, Burch JM et al. Management of traumatic injuries to the extrahepatic biliary ducts. Am J Surg 1985; 150:705–9.

164. Ridgeway MG, Stabile BE. Surgical management and treatment of pancreatic fistulas. Surg Clin North Am 1996; 76:1159–73.

165. Lewis G, Krige JEJ, Bornman PC et al. Traumatic pancreatic pseudocysts. Br J Surg 1993; 80:89–93.

166. Beckingham IJ, Krige JE, Bornman PC et al. Endoscopic management of pancreatic pseudocysts. Br J Surg 1997; 84:1638–45.

167. Young PR Jr, Meredith JW, Baker CC. Pancreatic injuries resulting from pancreatic trauma: a multi-institution review. Am Surg 1998; 64:838–43.

168. Holland AJ, Davey RB, Sparnon AL et al. Traumatic pancreatitis: long-term review of initial non-operative management in children. J Pediatr Child Health 1999; 35:78–81.

169. Hoyt DB, Bulger EM, Knudson MM et al. Death in the operating room: an analysis of a multicenter experience. J Trauma 1994; 37:426–38.

Index

Note
Page numbers followed by 'f' indicate figures, those followed by 't' indicate tables or boxes.
The following abbreviations have been used:
CBD, common bile duct
HCC, hepatocellular carcinoma
TIPS, transjugular intrahepatic porto-systemic shunts

NHS Staff Library at St James's

To renew this book, please phone **0113 2065638**, or e-mail **leedsth-tr.stafflibraries@nhs.net**. You can also renew this book online using the NHS library catalogue. Please ask library staff for details.

24 /5/19